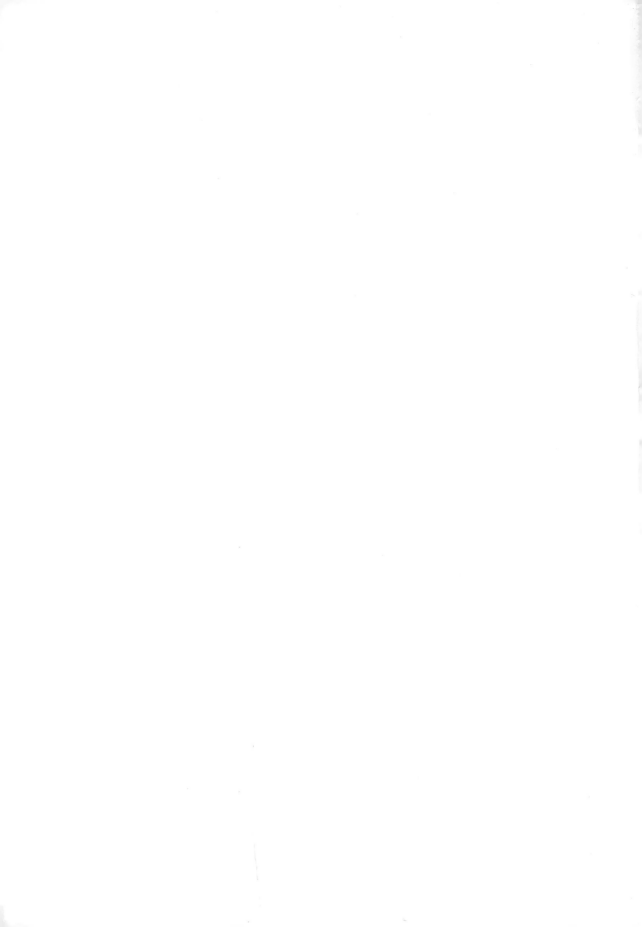

Netter's Cardiology

Netter's Cardiology

Edited by

Marschall S. Runge, MD, PhD
**The University of North Carolina
School of Medicine, Chapel Hill**

E. Magnus Ohman, MB, FRCPI
**The University of North Carolina
School of Medicine, Chapel Hill**

Illustrations by Frank H. Netter, MD

Contributing Illustrators

John A. Craig, MD
Carlos A. G. Machado, MD
David Mascaro
Enid Hatton
Steven Moon
Kip Carter

Icon Learning Systems · Teterboro, New Jersey

Published by Icon Learning Systems LLC, a subsidiary of MediMedia USA, Inc.
Copyright © 2004 MediMedia, Inc.

FIRST EDITION

ISBN 1-92900705-1

Library of Congress Catalog No 2003114073

Printed in the U.S.A.

NOTICE

Every effort has been taken to confirm the accuracy of the information presented and to describe generally accepted practices. Neither the publisher nor the authors can be held responsible for errors or for any consequences arising from the use of the information contained herein, and make no warranty, expressed or implied, with respect to the contents of the publication.

Before prescribing pharmaceutical products, readers are advised to check the product information currently provided by the manufacturer of each drug to be administered to verify the recommended dose, the method and duration of administration, and the contraindications. It is the responsibility of the treating physician, relying on experience and knowledge of the patient, to determine dosages and the best treatment for the patient. Neither the publisher nor the editors assumes any responsibility for any injury and/or damage to persons or property.

Executive Editor: Paul Kelly
Editorial Director: Greg Otis
Managing Editor: Jennifer Surich
Editorial Assistant: Nicole Zimmerman
Production Editing: Stephanie Klein
Digital Asset Manager: Karen Oswald
Graphic Artist: Colleen Quinn
Director of Manufacturing: Mary Ellen Curry

Binding and Printing by Banta Book Group
Digital Separations by R.R. Donnelly and Page Imaging

10   9   8   7   6   5   4   3   2   1

ACKNOWLEDGMENTS

Developing a new textbook on cardiovascular diseases was a major undertaking not only for us, but also for many other dedicated individuals.

First, we thank the contributing authors. All are current or former faculty members at the University of North Carolina School of Medicine, Chapel Hill, or have close ties to the institution. Without their intellect, dedication, and drive for excellence, *Netter's Cardiology* could not have been published.

Special recognition goes to John A. Craig, MD, and Carlos A.G. Machado, MD. They are uniquely talented physicians–artists who, through their work, brought to life important concepts in medicine in the new and updated figures included in this text.

We also thank Paul Kelly, Jennifer Surich, Stephanie Klein, Greg Otis, and their colleagues in the editorial and production offices of Icon Learning Systems for their care and commitment in developing this new text. Special thanks goes to Carolyn Kruse for her excellent editing.

We are also indebted to Ms. Angela Clotfelter-Rego, whose superb organizational skills enabled this text to become a reality.

We would especially like to acknowledge our families: our wives—Susan Runge and Elspeth Ohman—whose constant support, encouragement and understanding made completion of this text possible; our children—Thomas, Elizabeth, William, John, and Mason Runge and Edward, Elsa-Maria, and Henry Ohman—who inspire us and remind us that there is life beyond the word processor; and finally our parents—whose persistence, commitment, and work ethic got us started on this road many, many years ago.

Marschall S. Runge, MD, PhD, was born in Austin, Texas and was graduated from Vanderbilt University with a BA in General Biology and a PhD in Molecular Biology. He received his medical degree from the Johns Hopkins School of Medicine and trained in internal medicine at the Johns Hopkins Hospital. He was a cardiology fellow and junior faculty member at the Massachusetts General Hospital. Dr. Runge's next position was at Emory University, where he directed the Cardiology Fellowship Training Program. He then moved to the University of Texas Medical Branch in Galveston where he was Chief of Cardiology and Director of the Sealy Center for Molecular Cardiology. He came to UNC in 2000 as Chairman of the Department of Medicine. Dr. Runge is board certified in internal medicine and cardiovascular diseases and has spoken and published widely on topics in clinical cardiology and vascular medicine. He maintains an active clinical practice in cardiovascular diseases and medicine, in addition to his teaching and administrative activities in the Department of Medicine.

E. Magnus Ohman, MB, FRCPI, was born in Stockholm, Sweden and was graduated from the Royal College of Surgeons of Ireland in Dublin. He completed his residency at St. Laurence's Hospital and St. Vincent's Hospital in Dublin. He was a cardiology fellow at Duke University, where he remained for the next decade, attaining the rank of Associate Professor of Medicine. He was also Assistant Director of the Duke Critical Care Transport Program and Codirector of the Duke Clinical Research Institute. Dr. Ohman was recruited to UNC in 2001 as the Ernest and Hazel Craige Professor of Cardiovascular Medicine, Chief of the Division of Cardiology, and Director of the UNC Heart Center. He is also an Adjunct Professor of Clinical Epidemiology at the School of Public Health. Dr. Ohman maintains a busy clinical schedule as an interventional cardiologist and consultant. He is also active in research and currently serves as Executive Codirector of the CRUSADE National Quality Improvement Initiative. Dr. Ohman lectures internationally and has published extensively in the field of cardiovascular medicine, making contributions in many fields.

In the past half-century, amazing advances in the prevention, diagnosis and treatment of cardiovascular diseases have occurred. The randomized clinical trials completed in this field dwarf those in other disciplines, both in size and in number. For this reason, the use of evidenced-based medicine is more widespread in this field than in any other. This explosion of information will likely continue with the completion of the human genome project and the implementation of new gene-based strategies.

Although such advances are welcome, they present a challenge for practicing physicians. Up-to-date information is the currency of those who strive to provide the very best care for their patients. Sorting through the enormous repositories of information can be problematic, and clinicians often do not know where to turn. Several outstanding comprehensive textbooks are available, as are electronic texts and countless journals and synopses of the latest research. Most practitioners have come to realize that there is no single best way to "keep up" and that the efficient utilization of time is key.

The year 2003 saw the publication of *Netter's Internal Medicine*, a new approach to the need for complete yet concise information on the diagnosis and treatment of common diseases. In that book, the artwork of one of medicine's greatest teachers, the late Frank H. Netter, MD, was combined with text by authors associated with the University of North Carolina School of Medicine, Chapel Hill, in a format that provides readers with up-to-date, easily accessible information about patient care.

Following the success of *Netter's Internal Medicine*, we decided to create an analogous textbook of cardiovascular diseases. Once again, the use of Dr. Netter's artwork, along with the contributions of his protégés, gave us the opportunity to offer a useful, practical resource for busy, time-pressured clinicians. Our goal has been to provide the essentials of clinical practice in cardiovascular disease in a readable and understandable format. Thus, in chapters that can be read and understood in a short period of time, this text covers the most common clinical problems in cardiovascular diseases that are encountered by practicing clinicians. It assumes that the reader has a basic understanding of the pathobiology of cardiovascular diseases, and therefore focuses on the clinical concepts that guide diagnosis and treatment.

There are two primary reasons that make us believe that this text will be useful for clinicians. The first is the knowledgeable and experienced authors whom we called upon to contribute to it. In our institution we are privileged to work with many highly qualified physicians known for both their research and their clinical expertise. To write on each topic, we invited the person generally recognized by our UNC colleagues as the most expert in the field, the one that they themselves call upon when faced with a clinical dilemma. In some areas we extended our author pool to include internationally recognized experts at other institutions, all of whom trained at UNC, were previously on the faculty here, or have close ties to the institution. We then asked those experts to examine the great quantity of data available, extract that which is essential to a practical understanding of the topic and present it in a standardized, logical format with an emphasis on clinical decision-making. Thus, this text is written by authors who specialize in many different areas of cardiovascular medicine but who share a common approach to patients with cardiovascular diseases. By inviting authors principally from within our own institution we have been able to maintain the focus and format of this book and thus serve our readers' interests.

Second, as with *Netter's Internal Medicine*, we relied on the work of Dr. Netter to inform us and inspire us during the creation of this text. The longer we study Dr. Netter's illustrations, the more our admiration grows for this unique physician–artist. Time and again he captures the essentials of a medical subject in a way that is both immediate and memorable. Because so many changes have occurred in the field of cardiovascular diseases since Dr. Netter's death, this text required the development of many new art plates. John A. Craig, MD, and Carlos A.G. Machado, MD, both worthy successors to Dr. Netter, once again spent countless hours creating artwork that carries on the Netter tradition in an outstanding manner.

We believe we have created in *Netter's Cardiology* a highly useful resource for all clinicians who treat patients with cardiovascular diseases—from the young to the old, from trainees to experienced practitioners. We hope that after reading this text you will agree.

Marschall S. Runge, MD, PhD
Marion Covington Distinguished Professor
Chairman, Department of Medicine
The University of North Carolina
  School of Medicine, Chapel Hill

E. Magnus Ohman, MB, FRCPI
Ernest and Hazel Craige Professor
Chief, Division of Cardiology
Director, UNC Heart Center
The University of North Carolina
  School of Medicine, Chapel Hill

Frank H. Netter, MD

Frank H. Netter was born in 1906 in New York City. He studied art at the Art Student's League and the National Academy of Design before entering medical school at New York University, where he received his M.D. degree in 1931. During his student years, Dr. Netter's notebook sketches attracted the attention of the medical faculty and other physicians, allowing him to augment his income by illustrating articles and textbooks. He continued illustrating as a sideline after establishing a surgical practice in 1933, but he ultimately opted to give up his practice in favor of a full-time commitment to art. After service in the United States Army during World War II, Dr. Netter began his long collaboration with the CIBA Pharmaceutical Company (now Novartis Pharmaceuticals). This 45-year partnership resulted in the production of the extraordinary collection of medical art so familiar to physicians and other medical professionals worldwide.

Icon Learning Systems acquired the Netter Collection in July 2000 and continues to update Dr. Netter's original paintings and to add newly commissioned paintings by artists trained in the style of Dr. Netter.

Dr. Netter's works are among the finest examples of the use of illustration in the teaching of medical concepts. The 13-book Netter Collection of Medical Illustrations, *which includes the greater part of the more than 20,000 paintings created by Dr. Netter, became and remains one of the most famous medical works ever published. The Atlas of Human Anatomy, first published in 1989, presents the anatomical paintings from the Netter Collection. Now translated into 11 languages, it is the anatomy atlas of choice among medical and health professions students the world over.*

The Netter illustrations are appreciated not only for their aesthetic qualities but, more importantly, for their intellectual content. As Dr. Netter wrote in 1949, ". . . clarification of a subject is the aim and goal of illustration. No matter how beautifully painted, how delicately and subtly rendered a subject may be, it is of little value as a medical illustration if it does not serve to make clear some medical point." Dr. Netter's planning, conception, point of view, and approach are what inform his paintings and what makes them so intellectually valuable.

Frank H. Netter, MD, physician and artist, died in 1991.

CONTRIBUTORS

All the contributors are associated with the University of North Carolina School of Medicine at Chapel Hill, unless otherwise noted

Marschall S. Runge, MD, PhD
Marion Covington Distinguished Professor of Medicine
Professor and Chairman, Department of Medicine

E. Magnus Ohman, MB, FRCPI
Ernest and Hazel Craige Professor of Cardiovascular Medicine
Professor and Chief, Division of Cardiology
Director, UNC Heart Center

Kirkwood F. Adams, Jr, MD
Associate Professor of Medicine and
Radiology
Director, Heart Failure Program
Division of Cardiology

Ali Akbary, MD
Cardiac Electrophysiologist
Carolina Cardiology Associates
Highpoint, North Carolina

Nitish Badhwar, MD
Assistant Professor of Medicine
Division of Cardiology, Electrophysiology
Service
University of California, San Francisco
San Francisco, California

Thomas M. Bashore, MD
Professor of Medicine
Division of Cardiology
Duke University Medical Center
Durham, North Carolina

Mark S. Bleiweis, MD
Cardiothoracic Surgeon
Medical Director, Children's Heart Institute
Children's Hospital of Orange County
Orange, California

Christoph Bode, MD, PhD
Chairman of Medicine
Department of Cardiology and Angiology
University of Freiburg
Freiburg, Germany

Edith E. Bragdon, PhD
Adjunct Post Doctoral Associate of Medicine
Division of Cardiovascular Medicine
University of Florida
Gainesville, Florida

Bruce R. Brodie, MD
Clinical Professor of Medicine
University of North Carolina Teaching Service
Director, LeBauer Cardiovascular Research
Foundation
Moses Cone Heart and Vascular Center
Greensboro, North Carolina

Philip A. Bromberg, MD
Bonner Distinguished Professor of Medicine
Division of Pulmonary and Critical Care
Medicine
Scientific Director, Center for Environmental
Medicine, Asthma, and Lung Biology

Scott H. Buck, MD
Associate Professor of Pediatrics
Division of Pediatric Cardiology

Wayne E. Cascio, MD
Professor of Medicine
Division of Cardiology
Center for Environmental Medicine, Asthma
and Lung Biology

Christopher D. Chiles, MD
Instructor of Medicine
Division of Cardiology

CONTRIBUTORS

David R. Clemmons, MD
Sarah Graham Kenan Professor of Medicine
Chief, Division of Endocrinology and
Metabolism
Associate Chair for Research

Romulo E. Colindres, MD, MSPH
Professor of Medicine
Director, Hypertension Clinic
Division of Nephrology and Hypertension

John L. Cotton, MD
Associate Professor of Pediatrics
Director, Pediatric Echocardiography
Laboratory
Division of Pediatric Cardiology

Gregory J. Dehmer, MD
Professor of Medicine
Texas A&M College of Medicine
Director, Division of Cardiology
Scott & White Clinic
Temple, Texas

Robert B. Devlin, PhD
Chief, Clinical Research Branch
Division of Human Studies
National Health and Environmental Effects
Research
Environmental Protection Agency
Research Triangle Park, North Carolina

Mary Anne Dooley, MD, MPH
Associate Professor of Medicine
Division of Rheumatology and Immunology

Stephanie H. Dunlap, DO
Assistant Professor of Medicine
Section of Cardiology
Rush University
Chicago, Illinois

Joseph J. Eron, MD
Associate Professor of Medicine
Director, Clinical Core, UNC Center for AIDS
Research

Associate Director, General Clinical Research
Unit
Division of Infectious Diseases

Steven W. Falen, MD, PhD
Director of Nuclear Medicine and PET
Services
Department of Radiology
Riverside Regional Medical Center
Newport News, Virginia

Mark A. Farber, MD
Assistant Professor of Surgery and
Interventional Radiology
Director, UNC Endovascular Institute
Division of Vascular Surgery

Elman G. Frantz, MD
Associate Professor of Pediatrics
Director, Pediatric Cardiac Catheterization
Laboratory
Division of Pediatric Cardiology

Markus Frey, MD
Assistant Professor of Medicine
Department of Cardiology and Angiology
University of Freiburg
Freiburg, Germany

Leonard S. Gettes, MD
Distinguished Professor of Medicine
Division of Cardiology

Ajmal Masood Gilani, MD
Assistant Professor of Neurology
Section of Adult Neurology

Lee R. Goldberg, MD
Interventional Cardiologist
Tucson, Arizona

Thomas R. Griggs, MD
Professor of Medicine and Pathology
Division of Cardiology

Colin D. Hall, MBChB
Professor of Neurology
Vice Chairman, Department of Neurology

Eileen M. Handberg, PhD, ARNP
Assistant Professor of Medicine
Director, Clinical Programs
Division of Cardiovascular Medicine
University of Florida
Gainesville, Florida

Milan J. Hazucha, PhD
Associate Professor of Medicine
Division of Pulmonary and Critical Care
Medicine
Center for Environmental Medicine, Asthma
and Lung Biology

G. William Henry, MD
Professor of Pediatrics
Chief, Division of Pediatric Cardiology

Margaret C. Herbst, RN, MSN
Clinical Instructor of Medicine
Division of Cardiology

Lisa B. Hightow, MD, MPH
Instructor of Medicine
Division of Infectious Diseases

Alan L. Hinderliter, MD
Associate Professor of Medicine
Division of Cardiology

S. Adil Husain, MD
Cardiothoracic Surgeon
Orange County Thoracic and Cardiovascular
Surgeons
Orange, California

Parag Kale, MD
Assistant Professor of Medicine/Cardiology
Division of Cardiology
Case Western Reserve University & University
Hospitals
Cleveland, Ohio

Blair A. Keagy, MD
Professor of Surgery
Chief, Division of Vascular Surgery

Meera Kelley, MD
Clinical Associate Professor of Medicine
Division of Infectious Diseases

Eileen A. Kelly, MD
Director, Women's Heart Program
Division of Cardiology
Evanston Northwestern Healthcare
Evanston, Illinois

Hanna Kelly, MD
Instructor of Medicine
Division of Hematology and Oncology

Chin K. Kim, MD
Instructor of Medicine
Division of Cardiovascular Medicine
University of Florida
Gainesville, Florida

Christopher R. Kroll, MD
Interventional Cardiologist
Heart Group of the Carolinas
Concord, North Carolina

Daniel J. Lenihan, MD
Associate Professor of Medicine
Associate Director, Cardiomyopathy Service
Department of Cardiology
MD Anderson Cancer Center
Houston, Texas

James P. Loehr, MD
Associate Professor of Pediatrics
Division of Pediatric Cardiology

Tift Mann, MD
Interventional Cardiologist
Director, Wake Heart Research
Wake Heart Center
Raleigh, North Carolina

CONTRIBUTORS

Anthony Mathur, MB, BChir, MRCP, PhD
Consultant Cardiologist
Department of Cardiology
The London Chest Hospital
London, England

Matthew A. Mauro, MD
Professor of Radiology and Surgery
Vice Chairman, Department of Radiology

Robert Mendes, MD
Instructor of Surgery
Division of Vascular Surgery

Venu Menon, MBBS
Assistant Professor of Medicine and
Emergency Medicine
Director, Coronary Care Unit
Director, Chest Pain Unit
Division of Cardiology

Michael R. Mill, MD
Professor of Surgery
Chief, Division of Cardiothoracic Surgery
Director, Heart and Heart-Lung Transplant
Programs
Director, UNC Comprehensive Transplant
Center

Peter Mills, BM, Bch, BSc, FRCP
Consultant Cardiologist
Department of Cardiology
The London Chest Hospital
London, England

Timothy A. Mixon, MD
Assistant Professor of Medicine
Texas A&M College of Medicine
Division of Cardiology
Scott & White Hospital
Temple, Texas

Timothy C. Nichols, MD
Professor of Medicine and Pathology
Director, Francis Owen Blood Research
Laboratory
Division of Cardiology

José Ortiz, MD
Assistant Professor of Medicine/Cardiology
Division of Cardiology
Case Western Reserve University & University
Hospitals
Cleveland, Ohio

Alden M. Parsons, MD
Resident, Division of General Surgery

Paresh K. Patel, MD
Interventional Cardiologist
Houston, Texas

Cam Patterson, MD
Henry A. Foscue Distinguished Professor of
Medicine and Cardiology
Director, Carolina Cardiovascular Biology
Center

Kristine B. Patterson, MD
Clinical Assistant Professor of Medicine
Division of Infectious Diseases

Srikanth Ramachandruni, MD
Clinical Assistant Professor of Medicine
Division of Cardiovascular Medicine
University of Florida
Gainesville, Florida

Blair V. Robinson, MD
Assistant Professor of Pediatrics
Division of Pediatric Cardiology

Bryon E. Rubery, MD
Instructor of Medicine
Division of Cardiology

William E. Sanders, Jr, MD, MBA
Associate Professor of Medicine and
Pathology
Director, Clinical Cardiac Electrophysiology
Division of Cardiology

Melvin M. Scheinman, MD
Professor of Medicine and Walter H.
Shorenstein Endowed Chair in Cardiology
Division of Cardiology, Electrophysiology
Service
University of California, San Francisco

Richard S. Schofield, MD
Associate Professor of Medicine
Division of Cardiovascular Medicine
University of Florida
Chief, Cardiology Section
North Florida/South Georgia Veterans Health
System
Gainesville, Florida

Sanjeev Shah, MD
Resident, Department of Medicine

Richard G. Sheahan, MD
Associate Professor of Medicine
Division of Cardiology

David S. Sheps, MD, MSPH
Professor of Medicine
Associate Director, Division of Cardiovascular
Medicine
University of Florida
Gainesville, Florida

Brett C. Sheridan, MD
Assistant Professor of Surgery
Division of Cardiothoracic Surgery

Yevgeniy Sheyn, MD
Instructor of Medicine
Division of Rheumatology and Immunology

Ross J. Simpson, Jr, MD, PhD
Professor of Medicine
Director, Lipid and Prevention Clinics
Division of Cardiology

Sidney C. Smith, Jr, MD
Professor of Medicine
Director, Center for Cardiovascular Science

and Medicine
Division of Cardiology

Mark A. Socinski, MD
Associate Professor of Medicine
Division of Hematology and Oncology
Director, Multidisciplinary Thoracic Oncology
Program
Lineberger Comprehensive Cancer Center

Peter J.K. Starek, MD
Professor of Surgery
Division of Cardiothoracic Surgery

Jeff P. Steinhoff, MD
Instructor of Medicine
Division of Cardiology

Steven R. Steinhubl, MD
Associate Professor of Medicine
Associate Director, Cardiac Catheterization
Laboratory
Division of Cardiology

George A. Stouffer, MD
Associate Professor of Medicine
Director, Cardiac Catheterization Laboratory
Director, Interventional Cardiology
Division of Cardiology

Carla A. Sueta, MD, PhD
Associate Professor of Medicine
Division of Cardiology

Walter A. Tan, MD, MS
Assistant Professor of Medicine and
Radiology
Director, Vascular Medicine Program
Division of Cardiology

David A. Tate, MD
Associate Professor of Medicine
Division of Cardiology

Gregory H. Tatum, MD
Clinical Fellow

CONTRIBUTORS

Division of Cardiology
Children's Hospital of Pittsburgh
Pittsburgh, Pennsylvania

Georgeta D. Vaidean, MD, MPH
Cardiovascular Epidemiology Program
Department of Epidemiology

Richard A. Walsh, MD
John H. Hord Professor of Medicine
Chairman, Department of Medicine
Physician-in-Chief, University Hospitals of
Cleveland
Case Western Reserve University & University
Hospitals
Cleveland, Ohio

Park W. Willis IV, MD
Professor of Medicine and Pediatrics
Associate Chief, Division of Cardiology
Director, Adolescent and Adult Congenital
Cardiac Clinic
Medical Director, Cardiac Graphics
Laboratory
Director, Adult Training Program in
Cardiovascular Medicine
Division of Cardiology

TABLE OF CONTENTS

TABLE OF CONTENTS

TABLE OF CONTENTS

X. AFFECTING HEART DISEASE–FUTURE DIRECTIONS
Section Editor: Marschall S. Runge

Section I
INTRODUCTION

Chapter 1

The History and Physical Examination

Marschall S. Runge and E. Magnus Ohman

The ability to determine whether disease is present or absent—and how that patient should be treated—is the ultimate goal for clinicians evaluating patients with suspected heart disease. Despite the number of diagnostic tests available, never has the importance of a careful history and physical examination been greater. Selection of the most appropriate test and therapeutic approach for each patient can only result from establishing the prior probability of disease, an assessment based on a skillfully performed history and physical examination. Opportunities for error in this judgment are abundant. Screening patients for coronary risk using a broad and unfocused panel of laboratory and noninvasive tests instead of a history and physical examination is inappropriate. While entire texts have been written on cardiac history and physical examination, this chapter specifically focuses on features of the cardiac history and the cardiovascular physical examination that help discern the presence or absence of heart disease.

THE CONCEPT OF PRIOR PROBABILITY

The history and physical examination should enable the clinician to establish the prior probability of heart disease: that is, the likelihood that the symptoms reported by the patient result from heart disease. A reasonable goal is to establish a patient's risk of heart disease as "low," "intermediate," or "high." One demonstration of this principle in clinical medicine is the assessment of patients with chest pain, in which the power of exercise stress testing to accurately diagnose coronary heart disease (CHD) depends on the prior probability of disease. In patients with very low risk of CHD based on clinical findings, exercise stress testing resulted in a large number of false-positive test results. Because 15% or less of exercise stress tests produce positive results in individuals without CHD, use of this test in a low-risk population can result in an adverse ratio of false-positive:true-positive test results and unnecessary cardiac catheterizations. Conversely, in patients with a very high risk of CHD based on clinical findings, exercise stress testing can result in false-negative test results—an equally undesirable outcome because patients with significant coronary artery disease (CAD) and their physicians may be falsely reassured that no further evaluation or treatment is necessary.

Emphasis is increasing on quantifying prior probability to an even greater degree using various mathematical models. This is a useful approach in teaching and may be clinically feasible in some diseases. However, for the majority of patients with suspected heart disease, categorizing risk as low, intermediate, and high is appropriate, reproducible, and feasible in a busy clinical practice. Therefore, obtaining the history and physical examination represents a key step before any testing, to minimize use of inappropriate diagnostic procedures.

THE HISTORY

A wealth of information is available to clinicians who perform a careful assessment of the patient's history. Key components are assessment of the chief complaint; careful questioning for related, often subtle, symptoms that may further define the chief complaint; and determination of other factors that help categorize the likelihood of disease. Major symptoms of heart patients include chest discomfort, dyspnea, palpitations, and syncope or presyncope.

Chest Discomfort

Determining whether chest discomfort results from a cardiac cause is often a challenge. The most common cause of chest discomfort is myocardial ischemia, which produces **angina pectoris**. Many causes of angina exist, and the differential diagnosis for chest discomfort is extensive (Table 1-1). Angina that is reproducible and constant in frequency and severity is often referred to as *stable angina*. For the purposes of this chapter, stable angina is a condition that occurs when CAD is present and coronary blood flow cannot be increased to accommodate for increased myocardial demand. However, as discussed in chapters 7 through 9, there are many causes of myocardial ischemia, including fixed coronary artery stenoses and endothelial dysfunction, which leads to reduced vasodilatory capacity.

A description of chest discomfort can help establish whether the pain is angina or of another origin. First, a description of the quality and location of the discomfort is essential (Fig. 1-1). Chest discomfort because of myocardial ischemia may be described as pain, a tightness, a heaviness, or simply an uncomfortable and difficult-to-describe feeling. The discomfort can be localized to the mid chest or epigastric area or may be characterized as pain in related areas, including the left arm, both arms, the left jaw, or the back. The radiation of chest discomfort to any of these areas increases the likelihood of the discomfort being angina. Second, the duration of the discomfort is important because chest discomfort due to cardiac causes generally lasts minutes. Therefore, pain of very short duration ("seconds" or "moments"), regardless of how typical it may be of angina, is less likely to be of cardiac origin. Likewise, pain that lasts for hours, on many occasions, in the absence of objective evidence of myocardial infarction (MI), is not likely to be of coronary origin. Third, the presence of accompanying symptoms should be considered. Chest discomfort may be accompanied by other symptoms (including dyspnea, diaphoresis, or nausea), any of which increase the likelihood that the pain is cardiac in origin. However, the presence of accompanying symptoms is not needed to define the discomfort as angina. In addition, factors that precipitate or relieve the discomfort should be evaluated. Angina typically occurs during physical exertion, during emotional stress, or in other circumstances of increased myocardial oxygen demand. When

Table 1-1
Differential Diagnosis of Chest Discomfort

Cardiovascular

Ischemic
- Coronary atherosclerosis (angina pectoris)
    Stable coronary disease
- Unstable coronary syndrome
- Aortic stenosis
- Hypertrophic cardiomyopathy
- Aortic regurgitation
- Mitral regurgitation
- Severe systemic hypertension
- Severe RV/pulmonary hypertension
- Severe anemia/hypoxia

Nonischemic
- Aortic dissection
- Pericarditis
- Mitral valve prolapse syndrome: autonomic dysfunction

Gastrointestinal

- Gastroesophageal reflux disease (GERD)
- Esophageal spasm
- Esophageal rupture
- Hiatal hernia
- Cholecystitis

Pulmonary

- Pulmonary embolus
- Pneumothorax
- Pneumonia
- COPD
- Pleurisy

Neuromusculoskeletal

- Thoracic outlet syndrome
- Degenerative joint disease of the cervical or · thoracic spine
- Costochondritis
- Herpes zoster

Psychogenic

- Anxiety
- Depression
- Cardiac psychosis
- Self-gain

RV indicates right ventricular.

Figure 1-1

Pain of Myocardial Ischemia

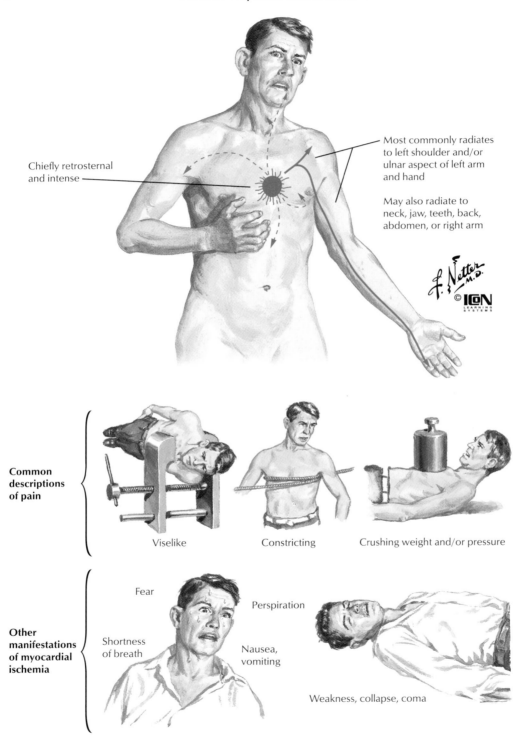

Chiefly retrosternal and intense

Most commonly radiates to left shoulder and/or ulnar aspect of left arm and hand

May also radiate to neck, jaw, teeth, back, abdomen, or right arm

Common descriptions of pain

Viselike   Constricting   Crushing weight and/or pressure

Other manifestations of myocardial ischemia

Fear

Perspiration

Shortness of breath

Nausea, vomiting

Weakness, collapse, coma

exercise precipitates chest discomfort, relief after cessation of exercise substantiates the diagnosis of angina. Sublingual nitroglycerin also relieves angina, generally over a period of minutes. Instant relief or relief after longer periods lessens the likelihood that the chest discomfort was angina.

Although an exercise history is important in assessing CHD risk, individuals, especially sedentary ones, may have anginalike symptoms that are not related to exertion. These include postprandial and nocturnal angina or angina that occurs while the individual is at rest. As described herein, **"rest-induced angina,"** or the new onset of angina, connotes a different pathophysiology than effort-induced angina. Angina can also occur in persons with fixed CAD and increased myocardial oxygen demand due to anemia, hyperthyroidism, or similar conditions (Table 1-2). Angina occurring at rest, or with minimal exertion, may denote a different pathophysiology, one involving platelet aggregation and clinically termed **"unstable angina"** or an **"acute coronary syndrome"** (see chapter 8).

Patients with heart disease need not present with chest pain at all. **Anginal equivalents** include dyspnea during exertion, abdominal discomfort, fatigue, or decreased exercise tolerance. Clinicians must be alert to and specifically ask about these symptoms. Often, a patient's family member or spouse notices subtle changes in endurance in the patient or that the individual no longer performs functions that require substantial physical effort. Sometimes patients may be unable to exert themselves due to comorbidities. For instance, the symptoms of myocardial ischemia may be absent in patients with severe peripheral vascular disease who have limiting claudication. One should also be attuned to subtle or absent symptoms in individuals with diabetes mellitus (including type I and type II diabetes), a "coronary risk equivalent" as defined by the Framingham Risk Calculator.

When considering the likelihood that CHD accounts for a patient presenting with chest discomfort or any of the aforementioned variants, assessment of the cardiac risk factor profile is important. The Framingham Study first codified the concept of cardiac risk factors. Although clinicians had long thought these were important

Table 1-2
Conditions That Cause Increased Myocardial Oxygen Demand

- Hyperthyroidism
- Tachycardia of various etiologies
- Hypertension
- Pulmonary embolism
- Pregnancy
- Psychogenic
- Central nervous system stimulants
- Exercise
- Psychological stress
- Fever

factors, their quantification has become increasingly important. Cardiac risk factors determined by the Framingham Study include a history of cigarette smoking, diabetes mellitus, hypertension, or hypercholesterolemia; a family history of CHD (including MI, sudden cardiac death, and first-degree relatives having undergone coronary revascularization); age; and sex (male). Although an attempt has been made to rank these risk factors, all are important, with a history of diabetes mellitus being perhaps the single most important factor. Subsequently, a much longer list of potential predictors of cardiac risk has been made (Table 1-3). An excellent, easy to use model for predicting risk is the Framingham Risk Calculator, as described in the Adult Treatment Panel III (ATP III) guidelines.

Symptoms suggestive of vascular disease require special attention. Peripheral vascular disease may mask CHD because the individual may not be able to exercise sufficiently to provoke angina. A history of stroke, transient ischemic attack, or atheroembolism in any vascular distribution is usually evidence of significant vascular disease. Sexual dysfunction in men is not an uncommon presentation of peripheral vascular disease. Raynaud's-type symptoms should also be elicited, since the presence of such symptoms is suggestive of abnormal vascular tone and function, and increases the risk that coronary heart disease is present.

Determining whether the patient has stable or unstable angina is as important as making the diagnosis of angina. Stable angina is important

Table 1-3
Cardiac Risk Factors

- Diabetes
- Smoking
- High BP
- High cholesterol
- Hyperlipidemia
- Sedentary lifestyle
- High-fat diet
- Stress
- "Metabolic syndrome"
- Family history of CHD (including history of MI, sudden cardiac death, and first-degree relatives who underwent coronary revascularization)
- Age
- Male sex

CHD indicates coronary heart disease; MI, myocardial infarction.

Table 1-4
Canadian Cardiovascular Society Classification of Angina Pectoris

I Ordinary physical activity, for example, walking or climbing stairs, does not cause angina; angina occurs with strenuous, rapid, or prolonged exertion at work or recreation.

II Slight limitation of ordinary activity; for example, angina occurs when walking or stair climbing after meals, in cold, in wind, under emotional stress or only during the few hours after awakening, when walking more than two blocks on the level, or when climbing more than one flight of ordinary stairs at a normal pace and during normal conditions.

III Marked limitation of ordinary activity; for example, angina occurs when walking one or two blocks on the level or when climbing one flight of stairs during normal conditions and at a normal pace.

IV Inability to carry on any physical activity without discomfort; angina syndrome may be present at rest. comfort; angina syndrome may be present at rest.

From Campeau L. Grading. F angina pectoris. *Circulation* 1976;54:522.

to evaluate and treat, but does not necessitate emergent intervention. The diagnosis of unstable angina, or acute coronary syndrome, carries a significant risk of MI or death in the immediate future. The type of symptoms reported by patients with stable and unstable angina differ little, and the risk factors for both are identical. Indeed, the severity of symptoms is not necessarily greater in patients with unstable angina, just as a lack of chest discomfort does not rule out significant CHD. The important distinction between stable and unstable coronary syndromes rests in whether the onset is new or recent and/or progressive. The initial presentation of angina is, by definition, unstable angina. Although for a high percentage of individuals this may merely represent the first recognizable episode of angina. For those with unstable angina, the risk of MI in the near future is markedly increased. Likewise, when the patient experiences angina in response to decreased levels of exertion or when exertional angina has begun to occur at rest, these urgent circumstances require immediate therapy. The treatment of stable angina and acute coronary syndromes is discussed in chapters 7 and 8. The Canadian Cardiovascular Society Functional Classification of Angina Pectoris is a useful guide for everyday patient assessment (Table 1-4). Categorizing patients according to their class of symptoms is rapid and precise and can be used in follow-up. Class IV describes the typical patient with

acute coronary syndrome.

Finally, it is important to distinguish those patients who have noncoronary causes of chest discomfort from those with CHD. Patients with gastroesophageal reflux disease (GERD) often present with symptoms that are impossible to distinguish from angina. In numerous studies, GERD is the most common diagnosis in patients who undergo diagnostic testing for angina and are found not to have CHD. The characteristics of the pain can be identical. Because exercise can increase intraabdominal pressure, GERD may be exacerbated with exercise, especially after meals. Symptoms from GERD can also be relieved with use of sublingual nitroglycerin. GERD can also result in early morning awakening (as can unstable angina) but tends to awaken individuals 2 to 4 hours after going to sleep, rather than 1 to 2 hours before arising, as is the case with unstable angina. Other causes (Table 1-1) of anginalike pain can be benign, or suggestive of other high-risk syndromes, such as aortic dissection. Many of these "coronary mimics" can be ruled out by patient history, but others, such as valvular aortic stenosis, can be confirmed or excluded by physical examination. The goal of taking the history is to alert the clinician to entities that can be confirmed or excluded by physical examination, or that necessitate further diagnostic testing.

Dyspnea, Edema, and Ascites

Dyspnea can accompany angina pectoris or it can be an anginal equivalent. Dyspnea can also reflect congestive heart failure (CHF) or occur because of noncardiac causes. The key to understanding the etiology of dyspnea is a clear patient history, which is then confirmed by a targeted physical examination.

Dyspnea during exertion that quickly resolves at rest or with use of nitroglycerin may be a result of myocardial ischemia. It is important to establish the amount of activity necessary to provoke dyspnea, the reproducibility of these symptoms, and the duration of recovery. As with angina, dyspnea as an anginal equivalent or an accompanying symptom tends to occur at a given workload or stress level—dyspnea occurring one day at low levels of exertion, but not prompted by vigorous exertion on another day is less likely to be an anginal equivalent.

In patients with CHF, dyspnea reflects left ventricular (LV) dysfunction (Fig. 1-2). Although most commonly LV systolic dysfunction is the cause of the dyspnea, dyspnea also occurs in individuals with preserved LV systolic function and severe diastolic dysfunction. These two entities present differently, however, and physical examination can distinguish them. With LV systolic dysfunction, dyspnea tends to gradually worsen, and its exacerbation is more variable than that of exertional dyspnea resulting from myocardial ischemia, although both are due to fluctuations in pulmonary arterial volume and left atrial filling pressures. Typically, patients with LV systolic dysfunction do not recover immediately after exercise cessation or use of sublingual nitroglycerin, and the dyspnea may linger for longer periods. *Orthopnea*, the occurrence of dyspnea when recumbent, or paroxysmal nocturnal edema provides further support for a presumptive diagnosis of LV systolic dysfunction. Patients with LV diastolic dysfunction tend to present abruptly with severe dyspnea that resolves more rapidly in response to diuretic therapy than does dyspnea caused by LV sys-

tolic dysfunction. The New York Heart Association (NYHA) Classification for CHF (Table 1-5) is extremely useful in following patients with CHF and provides a simple and rapid means for longitudinal assessment. The NYHA Classification also correlates well with prognosis. Patients who are NYHA Class I have a low risk of death or hospital admission within the following year. In contrast, the annual mortality rate of those with NYHA Class IV symptoms exceeds 30%.

As with chest discomfort, the differential diagnosis of dyspnea is broad, encompassing many cardiac and noncardiac causes (Table 1-6). Congenital heart disease, with or without pulmonary hypertension, can cause exertional dyspnea. Patients with significant intra- or extracardiac shunts and irreversible pulmonary hypertension (Eisenmenger's syndrome) are dyspneic during minimal exertion and often at rest. It is also possible to have dyspnea because of acquired valvular heart disease, usually from aortic or mitral valve stenosis or regurgitation. All of these causes should be easily distinguished from CHD or CHF by physical examination. Primary pulmonary causes of dyspnea must be considered, with COPD and reactive airways disease (asthma) being most common. Again, a careful history for the risk factors (e.g., cigarette smoking, industrial

Table 1-5
New York Heart Association Classification of CHF

Class I	Patients with no limitation of activities; they have no symptoms after ordinary activities.
Class II	Patients with slight, mild limitation of activity; they are comfortable at rest or during mild exertion.
Class III	Patients with marked limitation of activity; they are comfortable only at rest.
Class IV	Patients who should be at complete rest, confined to a bed or a chair; any physical activity brings on discomfort and symptoms occur at rest.

From the Criteria Committee of the New York Heart Association. *Diseases of the Heart and Blood Vessels: Nomenclature and Criteria for Diagnosis*. Boston. Brown; 1964.

Figure 1-2

Physical Examination
Left-Sided Cardiac Heart Failure

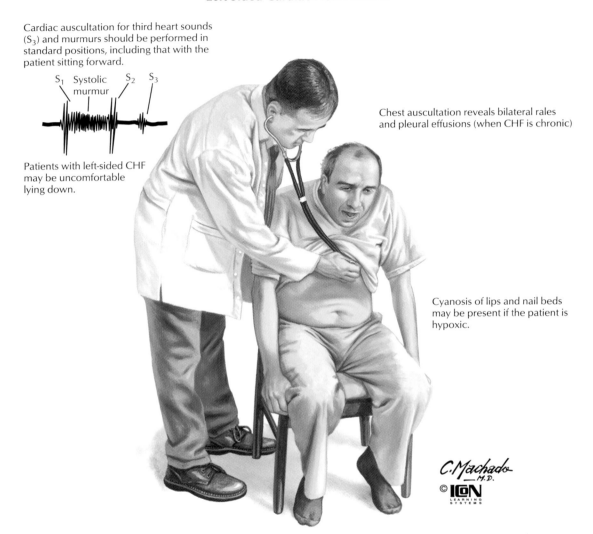

Cardiac auscultation for third heart sounds (S_3) and murmurs should be performed in standard positions, including that with the patient sitting forward.

S_1 Systolic S_2 S_3
murmur

Patients with left-sided CHF may be uncomfortable lying down.

Chest auscultation reveals bilateral rales and pleural effusions (when CHF is chronic)

Cyanosis of lips and nail beds may be present if the patient is hypoxic.

C. Machado
— M.D.
© ICON
LEARNING SYSTEMS

exposure, allergens) associated with these entities and an accurate physical examination should distinguish primary pulmonary causes from dyspnea due to CHD or CHF.

Peripheral edema and ascites are physical examination findings consistent with right ventricular (RV) failure. These findings are included in the history because they may be part of the presentation. Although patients often comment on peripheral edema, with careful questioning, they may also identify increasing abdominal girth consistent with ascites. Important questions on lower extremity edema include determination of whether the edema is symmetric (unilateral edema suggests alternate diagnoses) and whether the edema improves or resolves with elevation of the lower extremities. The finding of "no resolution overnight" argues against RV failure as an etiology. In addition, for peripheral edema and ascites, it is important to ask questions directed toward determining the presence of anemia, hypoproteinemia, or other causes. The differential diagnosis of edema is broad and beyond the scope of this chapter.

Table 1-6
Differential Diagnosis of Dyspnea

Pulmonary

- Reactive airways disease (asthma)
- COPD
- Emphysema
- Pulmonary edema
- Pulmonary hypertension
- Lung transplant rejection
- Infection
- Interstitial lung disease
- Pleural disease
- Pulmonary embolism
- Respiratory muscle failure
- Exercise intolerance

Cardiac

- Ischemic heart disease/angina pectoris
- Right-sided heart failure
- Aortic stenosis or regurgitation
- Arrhythmias
- Dilated cardiomyopathy
- Hypertrophic cardiomyopathy
- CHF
- Mitral regurgitation or stenosis
- Mediastinal abnormalities
- Pericardial tuberculosis
- Transposition of the great arteries

Other

- Blood transfusion reaction
- Measles

CHF indicates congestive heart failure.

Palpitations and Syncope

It is normal to be aware of the sensation of the heart beating, particularly during or immediately after exertion or emotional stress. *Palpitations* refer to an increased awareness of the heart beating. Patients use many different descriptions, including a "pounding or racing of the heart," the feeling that their heart is "jumping" or "thumping" in their chest, the feeling that the heart "skips beats" or "races," or countless other descriptions. A history showing that palpitations have begun to occur during or immediately after exertion, and not at other times, raises the concern that

these sensations reflect ventricular ectopy associated with myocardial ischemia. It is more difficult to assess the significance of palpitations occurring at other times. Supraventricular and ventricular ectopy may occur at any time and may be benign or morbid. As discussed in chapters 20, 22, and 23, ventricular ectopy is worrisome in patients with a history of MI or cardiomyopathy. Lacking this information, clinicians should be most concerned if lightheadedness or presyncope accompanies palpitations.

Syncope generally indicates an increased risk for sudden cardiac death and is usually a result of cardiovascular disease and arrhythmias. If a syncopal episode is a presenting complaint, the patient should be admitted for further assessment. In approximately 85% of patients, the cause of syncope is cardiovascular. In patients with syncope, one must assess for CHD, cardiomyopathy, and congenital or valvular heart disease. In addition, neurocardiogenic causes represent a relatively common and important possible etiology for syncope. Table 1-7 shows the differential diagnosis for syncope. It is critical to determine whether syncope really occurred. A witness to the episode and documentation of an intervening period are very helpful. In addition, with true syncope, injuries related to the sudden loss of consciousness are common. However, an individual who reports recurrent syncope (witnessed or unwitnessed) but has never injured him- or herself may not be experiencing syncope. This is not to lessen the concern that a serious underlying medical condition exists, but rather to reaffirm that the symptoms fall short of syncope, with its need for immediate evaluation.

THE PHYSICAL EXAMINATION

There are several advantages to obtaining patient history before the physical examination. First, the information gained in the history directs the clinician to pay special attention to aspects of the physical examination. For instance, a history consistent with CHD necessitates careful inspection for signs of vascular disease; a history suggestive of CHF should make the clinician pay particular attention to the presence of a third heart sound. Second, the history allows the clinician to establish a rapport with patients, to assure patients that he or she is interested in their well-

Table 1-7
Causes of Syncope

Cardiogenic

- · Mechanical
  - Outflow tract obstruction
  - Pulmonary hypertension
  - Congenital heart disease
  - Myocardial disease—low output states

- · Electrical
  - Bradyarrhythmias
  - Tachyarrhythmias

- · Neurocardiogenic
  - Vasovagal (vasodepression)
  - Orthostatic hypotension

Other

- · Peripheral neuropathy
- · Medications
- · Primary autonomic insufficiency
- · Intravascular volume depletion
- · Reflex
- · Cough
- · Micturition
- · Acute pain states
- · Carotid sinus hypersensitivity

being, and that the physical examination is an important part of a complete evaluation. In this light, the therapeutic value of the physical examination to the patient should not be underestimated. In spite of the emphasis on technology today, even the most sophisticated patients expect to be examined, to have their hearts listened to, and to be told whether worrisome findings exist or the examination results were normal.

General Inspection and Vital Signs

Much useful information can be gained by an initial "head-to-toe" inspection and assessment of vital signs. For instance, truncal obesity may signal the presence of type II diabetes or the metabolic syndrome. Cyanosis of the lips and nail beds may indicate underlying cyanotic heart disease. Hairless, dry-skinned lower extremities or distal ulceration may indicate peripheral vascular disease. Other findings are more specific

(Fig. 1-3). Abnormalities of the digits are found in atrial septal defect; typical findings of Down's syndrome indicate an increased incidence of ventricular septal defect or more complex congenital heart disease; hyperextensible skin and lax joints are suggestive of Ehlers-Danlos syndrome; and tall individuals with arachnodactyly, lax joints, pectus excavatum, and an increased arm–height ratio may have Marfan's syndrome. These represent some of the more common morphologic phenotypes in individuals with heart disease. Vital signs can also be helpful. Although normal vital signs do not rule out CHD, marked hypertension may signal cardiac risk, whereas tachycardia, tachypnea, and/or hypotension at rest suggest CHF.

Important Components
of the Cardiovascular Examination

The clinician should focus efforts on those sites that offer a window into the heart and vasculature. Palpation and careful inspection of the skin for secondary changes because of vascular disease or diabetes is important. Lips, nail beds, and fingertips should be examined for cyanosis (including clubbing of the fingernails) and, when indicated, for signs of embolism. Examination of the retina using an ophthalmoscope can reveal evidence of longstanding hypertension, diabetes, or atheroembolism, denoting underlying vascular disease. Careful examination of the chest, including auscultation, can help to differentiate causes of dyspnea. The presence of dependent rales is consistent with left-sided heart failure. Pleural effusions can result from longstanding LV dysfunction or noncardiac causes, and can be present with predominantly right-sided heart failure, representing transudation of ascites into the pleural space. Hyperexpansion with or without wheezing suggests a primary pulmonary cause of dyspnea, such as COPD or reactive airways disease. The presence of wheezing rather than rales does not rule out left-sided heart failure. It is not uncommon to hear wheezing with left-sided CHF. Most commonly, wheezing from left-sided CHF is primarily expiratory. Inspiratory and expiratory wheezing, particularly with a prolonged inspiratory:expiratory ratio is more likely to be caused by intrinsic lung disease.

Figure 1-3

Physical Examination: General Inspection

Ehlers-Danlos syndrome

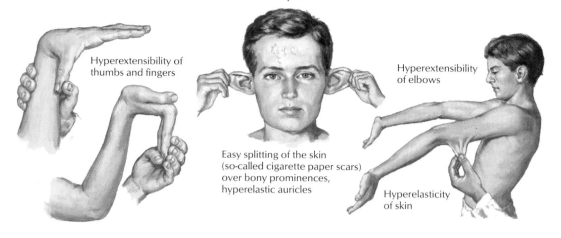

Hyperextensibility of thumbs and fingers

Easy splitting of the skin (so-called cigarette paper scars) over bony prominences, hyperelastic auricles

Hyperextensibility of elbows

Hyperelasticity of skin

Marfan's syndrome

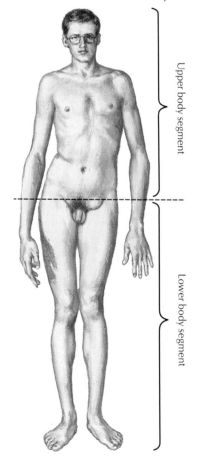

Upper body segment

Lower body segment

Walker-Murdoch wrist sign. Because of long fingers and thin forearm, thumb and little finger overlap when patient grasps wrist.

Down's syndrome

Typical facies seen in Down's syndrome

Upward slanting eyes contrasting with ethnic group

Small mouth with protruding tongue

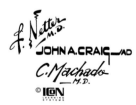

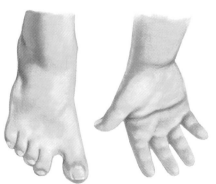

Wide gap between the first and second toes

"Simian" crease on the palm

Figure 1-4 ## Important Components of Cardiac Examination

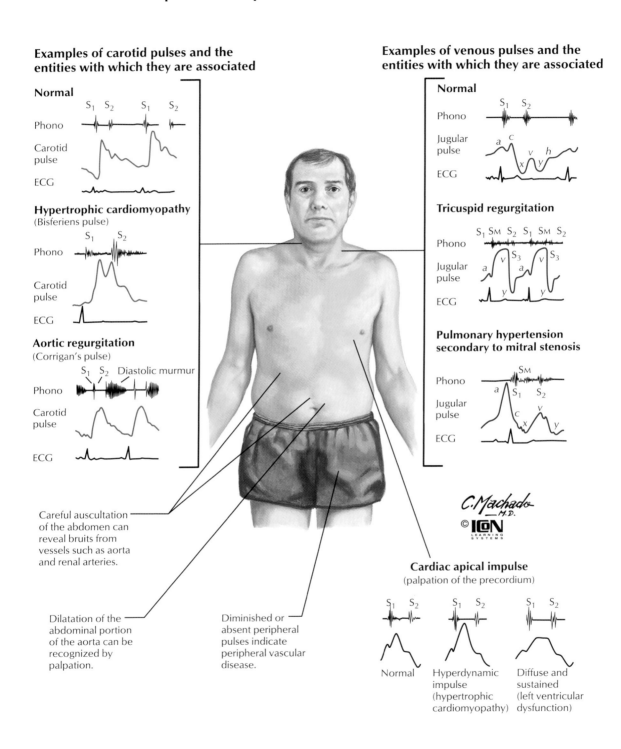

Examples of carotid pulses and the entities with which they are associated

Normal

Phono

Carotid pulse

ECG

Hypertrophic cardiomyopathy
(Bisferiens pulse)

Phono

Carotid pulse

ECG

Aortic regurgitation
(Corrigan's pulse)

Phono

Carotid pulse

ECG

Examples of venous pulses and the entities with which they are associated

Normal

Phono

Jugular pulse

ECG

Tricuspid regurgitation

Phono

Jugular pulse

ECG

Pulmonary hypertension secondary to mitral stenosis

Phono

Jugular pulse

ECG

Careful auscultation of the abdomen can reveal bruits from vessels such as aorta and renal arteries.

Dilatation of the abdominal portion of the aorta can be recognized by palpation.

Diminished or absent peripheral pulses indicate peripheral vascular disease.

C. Machado
—M.D.
© ICON
LEARNING
SYSTEMS

Cardiac apical impulse
(palpation of the precordium)

Normal

Hyperdynamic impulse (hypertrophic cardiomyopathy)

Diffuse and sustained (left ventricular dysfunction)

The vascular examination is an important component of a complete evaluation. The quality of the pulses, in particular the carotid and the femoral pulses, can identify underlying disease (Fig. 1-4). Diminished or absent distal pulses indicate peripheral vascular disease. The examiner should also auscultate for bruits over both carotids, over the femoral arteries, and in the abdomen. Abdominal auscultation should be performed, carefully listening for aortic or renal bruits, in the mid abdominal area before abdominal palpation, which can stimulate increased bowel sounds. Distinguishing bruits from transmitted murmurs in the carotid and abdominal areas can be challenging. When this is a concern, carefully marching out from the heart using the stethoscope can be helpful. If the intensity of the murmur or bruit continually diminishes farther from the heart, it becomes more likely that this sound originates from the heart, rather than from a stenosis in the peripheral vasculature. Much information is available about the peripheral vascular examination, but by following the simple steps outlined herein, the examiner can gather the majority of the accessible clinical information.

Examination of the jugular venous pulsations is a commonly forgotten step. Jugular venous pressure, which correlates with right atrial pressure and RV diastolic pressure, should be estimated initially with the patient lying with the upper trunk elevated 30°. In this position, at normal jugular venous pressure, no pulsations are visible. This correlates roughly to a jugular venous pressure less than 6 to 10 cm. The absence of jugular vein pulsations with the patient in this position can be confirmed by occluding venous return by placing a fingertip parallel to the clavicle in the area of the sternocleidomastoid muscle. The internal and external jugular veins should partially fill. Although with normal jugular venous pressure examination of the waveforms is less important, the head of the examination table can be lowered until the jugular venous pulsations are evident. When the jugular venous pulsations are visible at 30°, the examiner should note the waveforms. It is possible to observe and time the a and v waves by simultaneously timing the cardiac apical impulse or the carotid impulse on the contralateral side. An exaggerated a wave is consistent with increased atrial filling pressures because of tricuspid valve stenosis or increased RV diastolic pressure. A large v wave generally indicates tricuspid valve regurgitation, a finding easily confirmed by auscultation.

Finally, before cardiac auscultation, it is important to palpate the precordium. This is the easiest way to identify dextrocardia. Characteristics of the cardiac impulse can also yield important clues about underlying disease. Palpation of the precordium is best performed from the patient's right side with the patient lying flat. The cardiac apical impulse is normally located in the fifth intercostal space along the midclavicular line. Most examiners use the fingertips to palpate the apical impulse. It is often possible to palpate motion corresponding to a third or fourth heart sound. Use of the fingertips offers fine detail on the size and character of the apical impulse. A diffuse and sustained apical impulse is consistent with LV systolic dysfunction. Patients with hypertrophic cardiomyopathy, in contrast, often have a hyperdynamic apical impulse. *Thrills*, palpable vibrations from loud murmurs or bruits, can also be palpated.

The RV impulse, if identifiable, is located along the left sternal border. Many clinicians prefer to palpate the RV impulse with the base of the hand, lifting the fingertips off the chest wall. In RV hypertrophy a sustained impulse can be palpated and the fingertips then can be placed at the LV impulse to confirm that the two are distinct. In patients with a sustained RV impulse, the examiner should again look for prominent a and v waves in the jugular venous pulsations.

Cardiac Auscultation

Hearing and accurately describing heart sounds is arguably the most difficult part of the physical examination. For this reason and because of the commonplace use of echocardiography, many clinicians perform a cursory examination. The strongest arguments for performing cardiac auscultation carefully are to determine whether further diagnostic testing is necessary; to correlate findings of echocardiography with the clinical examination so that, in longitudinal follow-up, the clinician can determine progression of disease without repeating echocardiography at each visit; and because the more a clinician makes these correlations, the better his or her skills in auscultation will become and the better his or her patients will be served. It should also be noted that, with normal general cardiac physical examination results, the absence of abnormal heart sounds, and a normal electrocardiogram, the use of echocardiography for evaluation of valvular or congenital heart disease is not indicated. Furthermore, if there are no symptoms of CHF or evidence of hemodynamic compromise, echocardiography is not indicated for assessment of LV function. Practice guidelines from cardiologists and generalists agree on this point, as do third-party insurers. It is neither appropriate nor feasible to replace a careful cardiovascular examination using auscultation with more expensive testing.

However, echocardiography has revolutionized the quantitative assessment of cardiovascular hemodynamics: that is, the severity of valvular and congenital heart disease. No longer is it necessary for the clinician to make an absolute judgment on whether invasive assessment (cardiac catheterization) is needed to further define hemodynamic status or whether the condition is too advanced to allow surgical intervention. Therefore, cardiac auscultation is an extremely important screening technique for significant hemodynamic abnormalities and an important means by which the physician can longitudinally follow patients with known disease.

There are several keys to excellence in auscultation. Foremost is the ability to perform a complete general cardiac physical examination, as described previously. The findings help the examiner focus on certain auscultatory features. Second, it is important to use a high-quality stethoscope. Largely dictated by individual preference, clinicians should select a stethoscope that has bell and diaphragm capacity both (for optimal appreciation of low- and high-frequency sounds, respectively) and that fits the ears comfortably and is well insulated so that external sounds are minimized. Third, it is important to perform auscultation in a quiet environment. Particularly as skills in auscultation are developing, trying to hone these in the hall of a busy emergency room or on rounds while others are speaking is time spent poorly. Additionally, taking the time to

return to see a patient with interesting findings detected during auscultation, and repetition, are keys to becoming competent in auscultation.

The patient should be examined while he or she is in several positions: while recumbent, while in the left lateral decubitus position, and while sitting forward. Every patient is different and, using all three positions, the examiner can optimize the chance that soft heart sounds can be heard. Likewise, it is important to listen carefully at the standard four positions on the chest wall (Fig. 1-5), as well as over the apical impulse and RV impulse (if present). It is also best to isolate different parts of the examination in time. Regardless of the intensity of various sounds, it is best to always perform the examination in the same order so that the presence of a loud murmur, for instance, does not result in failure to listen to the other heart sounds.

Listen for S_1 (the first heart sound) first. As with jugular venous pulsations, the heart sounds can be timed by simultaneously palpating the cardiac apical impulse or the carotid upstroke. Even the most experienced clinician occasionally needs to time the heart sounds. Is a single sound present, or is the first heart sound split? Is a sound heard before S_1, indicating an S_4? Next, listen to the second heart sound. Normally the first component (A_2, the aortic valve closing sound) is louder than the second component (P_2, the pulmonic valve closing sound). A louder second component may indicate increased pulmonary pressure. A more subtle finding is a reversal of A_2 and P_2 timing that occurs with left bundle branch block and in some other circumstances. Additionally, it is important to assess whether A_2 and P_2 are normally split or whether they are widely split with no respiratory variation—a finding suggestive of an atrial septal defect. The examiner should then listen carefully for a third heart sound. An S_3 is often best heard over the tricuspid or mitral areas and is a low-frequency sound. It is heard best with the bell and is often not heard with the diaphragm.

After characterizing these heart sounds, it is time to listen carefully for murmurs. Murmurs are classified according to their intensity, their duration, their location, and their auscultatory characteristics: crescendo, decrescendo, blowing, among others. It is also important to note

Figure 1-5

Cardiac Auscultation
Precordial areas of auscultation

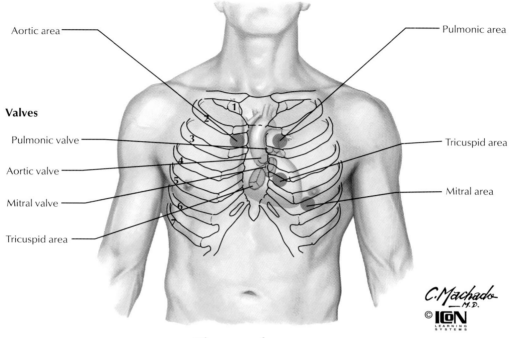

Aortic area

Pulmonic area

Valves

Pulmonic valve

Aortic valve

Mitral valve

Tricuspid area

Tricuspid area

Mitral area

C. Machado
— M.D.
© ICON
LEARNING SYSTEMS

Diagrams of murmurs

Innocent murmur

S_1 | S_2

Innocent murmur with widely split S_2

S_1 A_2 P_2

Systolic murmur from increased pulmonic flow followed by fixed, widely split S_2 (Atrial septal defect)

S_1 ES A_2 P_2

Systolic murmur followed by widely split S_2

S_1 A_2 P_2

Murmur and ejection click (pulmonary hypertension)

S_1 EC S_2

Holosystolic murmur (acute mitral regurgitation)

S_1 S_2

Systolic murmur (chronic mitral regurgitation) with S_3 and S_4 (dilated cardiomyopathy)

S_4 S_1 S_2 S_3

Holosystolic murmur (IVSD or mitral or tricuspid regurgitation)

S_1 S_2

Late systolic murmur following midsystolic click (mitral prolapse)

S_1 A_2 P_2

Click

Ejection sound followed by a murmur that extends through A_2 with widely split S_2 and the presence of S_4 (moderate pulmonary stenosis)

S_4 S_1 A_2 P_2

EC

Continuous murmur (patent ductus arteriosus)

S_1 S_2

Diastolic murmur (aortic or pulmonary regurgitation)

S_1 S_2

Long diastolic murmur following opening snap (mitral stenosis)

S_1 S_2 OS

Figure 1-6

Maneuvers

Vascular resistance and venous return are altered by maneuvers used to modify auscultatory findings of many different etiologies. Mitral valve prolapse is used here to exemplify the use of some of these maneuvers.

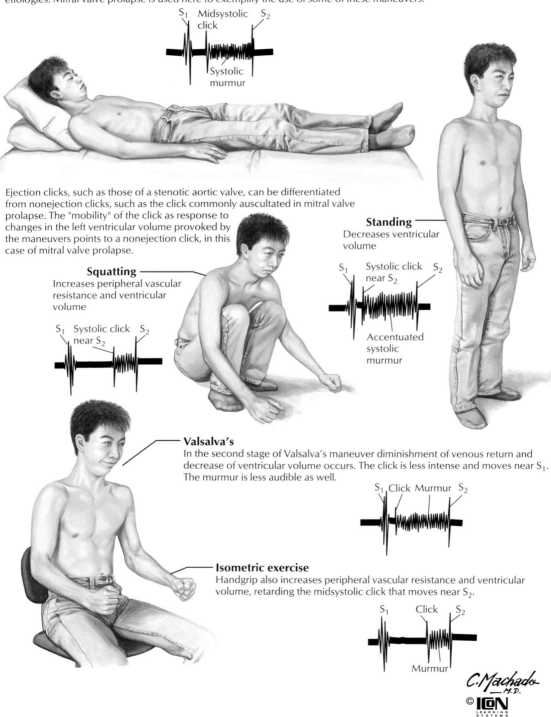

Ejection clicks, such as those of a stenotic aortic valve, can be differentiated from nonejection clicks, such as the click commonly auscultated in mitral valve prolapse. The "mobility" of the click as response to changes in the left ventricular volume provoked by the maneuvers points to a nonejection click, in this case of mitral valve prolapse.

Standing
Decreases ventricular volume

S_1 Systolic click S_2
near S_2

Accentuated systolic murmur

Squatting
Increases peripheral vascular resistance and ventricular volume

S_1 Systolic click S_2
near S_2

Valsalva's
In the second stage of Valsalva's maneuver diminishment of venous return and decrease of ventricular volume occurs. The click is less intense and moves near S_1. The murmur is less audible as well.

S_1 Click Murmur S_2

Isometric exercise
Handgrip also increases peripheral vascular resistance and ventricular volume, retarding the midsystolic click that moves near S_2.

S_1 Click S_2

Murmur

C.Machado
M.D.

© ICON
LEARNING SYSTEMS

the site where the murmur is loudest and whether the murmur radiates to another area of the precordium or to the carotids. All of these features contribute to determining the origin of the murmur, the likelihood that it represents an acute or chronic process, and how it affects the diagnostic and therapeutic approaches. Most importantly, it is necessary for clinicians to judge whether a murmur represents cardiac disease or is innocent. Innocent murmurs, also termed "flow murmurs," are common in children. More than 60% of children have innocent murmurs. Innocent murmurs become less common in adults; however, an innocent murmur can still be found into the fourth decade of life. Alterations in hemodynamics induced by pregnancy, anemia, fever, hyperthyroidism, or any state of increased cardiac output can produce an innocent murmur. These murmurs are generally midsystolic and heard over the tricuspid or pulmonic areas and do not radiate extensively. They are often loudest in thin individuals. Innocent murmurs do not cause alterations in the carotid pulse and do not coexist with abnormal cardiac impulses or with other abnormalities, such as extra heart sounds (S_3 and S_4), in adults. In elderly individuals, a common finding is a systolic murmur that shares auditory characteristics with the murmur of aortic stenosis; however, carotid upstrokes are normal. This finding, aortic sclerosis, may necessitate confirmation by echocardiography. It represents sclerosis of the aortic leaflets, but without significant hemodynamic consequence.

The characteristics of the most common and hemodynamically important murmurs are shown in Figure 1-5. As noted previously, the murmur is defined not only by its auditory characteristics, but also by the company it keeps. Often the key to excellence in auscultation is being thorough in all aspects of the cardiovascular examination.

Maneuvers

No discussion of cardiac auscultation would be complete without the use of maneuvers to accentuate auscultatory findings. As shown in Figure 1-6, patient positioning can alter peripheral vascular resistance or venous return, accentuating murmurs that are modulated by these changes. Murmurs associated with fixed valvular lesions change little with changes in position

or the maneuvers illustrated in Figure 1-6. Thus, these maneuvers are most useful for diagnosing entities in which hemodynamic status affects murmurs. The two classic examples are the click and murmur of mitral valve prolapse, as shown here, and the aortic outflow murmur of hypertrophic cardiomyopathy (not shown).

FUTURE DIRECTIONS

Handheld echocardiography machines can be carried on the shoulder and have a small transducer that can obtain echocardiographic images of sufficient quality to quantify murmurs and assess LV dysfunction. Although these portable echocardiographic machines have advantages and have been incorporated in medical school curricula at many institutions, they have not yet replaced the stethoscope, nor are they likely to do so.

The roles of cardiac history and physical examination have changed. Before the noninvasive testing of today, astute clinicians were the arbiters of whether invasive diagnostic testing was needed, based largely on examination findings alone. Today, it is believed that the role of the clinician is to use physical examination findings to establish the prior probability of cardiovascular disease, whether CHD, valvular heart disease, or congenital heart disease, thereby determining the need for further testing. In the continual quest for improved noninvasive testing, it is likely that a clinician's skill will continue to evolve as the interplay between history taking, physical examination, and diagnostic testing further develops.

REFERENCES

American College of Cardiology Foundation. Clinical Statements/Guidelines. Available at: http://www.acc.org/clinical/statements.htm.

American Heart Association. Heart Profilers. Available at: http://www.americanheart.org/presenter.jhtml?identifier=3000416.

Diamond GA, Forrester JS. Analysis of probability as an aid in the clinical diagnosis of coronary–artery disease. N Engl J Med 1979;300:1350–1358.

European Society of Cardiology. Available at: http://www.escardio.org.

Harvey WP. Cardiac Pearls [videorecording]. Atlanta: Emory Medical Television Network; 1981.

Hurst JW, Morris DC. Chest Pain. Futura Publishing; 2001.

National Heart, Lung and Blood Institute. Third Report of the Expert Panel on Detection, Evaluation, and Treatment of High Blood Cholesterol in Adults (Adult Treatment Panel III). Available at: http://www.nhlbi.nih.gov/guidelines/cholesterol/index.htm.

Chapter 2
Coronary Atherosclerosis

Cam Patterson and Marschall S. Runge

Cardiovascular diseases (CVD)—coronary artery disease, hypertension, congestive heart failure, and stroke—are the leading cause of death and disability in elderly individuals in the Western world (Fig. 2-1). In the United States, the CVD death toll is nearly 1 million each year, and the estimated cost of CVD treatment was $326.6 billion for the year 2000; the future holds increases in the incidence of CVD. This is particularly a problem as the population ages. The United States Census Bureau projects that nearly one in four individuals will be 65 years of age or older by the year 2035, and adults older than 65 years of age are two and a half times more likely to have hypertension and four times more likely to have coronary heart disease than are those in the 40- to 49-year age group.

Although the prevalence of atherosclerotic disease continues to increase in developed countries, death rates from cardiovascular diseases have decreased by more than a third in the past two decades. This effect is due to primary and secondary prevention strategies and to improvements in the care and rehabilitation of patients with atherosclerotic diseases.

In spite of this encouraging news, atherosclerotic diseases remain an enormous challenge for the clinician, for several reasons. Many preventive strategies involve lifestyle changes that test the compliance of even the most devoted patients. The disease itself progresses silently for decades before symptoms develop, and the initial clinical presentation of atherosclerotic disease is often a catastrophic event, such as MI, stroke, or sudden cardiac death (SCD). The diagnosis of atherosclerotic disease, particularly through noninvasive methods, is imperfect, and the clinical manifestations of atherosclerotic diseases are often subtle and easily mistaken for causes that are more benign. Therefore, although the diagnosis and treatment of atherosclerotic diseases remain of paramount importance, the promise of future advances rests in a more detailed understanding of atherosclerosis, leading to earlier diagnosis and prevention that is ultimately more effective.

ETIOLOGY AND PATHOGENESIS

Atherosclerotic plaques lead to clinical events (angina, myocardial infarction [MI]) by two mechanisms. First, with gradual enlargement, plaques may obstruct blood flow within epicardial vessels, resulting in ischemia to the myocardial tissue dependent on the blood supply of the affected vessel. Alternatively, plaques may become symptomatic because of acute rupture or thrombosis, resulting in catastrophic acute occlusion of a vessel, the hallmark of MI. Indeed, the two mechanisms are apt to be linked because less catastrophic (and subclinical) episodes of plaque rupture are probably one of the mechanisms by which nonocclusive plaques enlarge to become symptomatic.

The concept that endothelial injury is an inciting event in atherosclerosis is common to most theories of pathogenesis. Endothelial injury is a component of the earliest stages of *atherosclerosis*, the formation of lesions that can be detected only at autopsy, the fatty streak (Fig. 2-2). Most of the well-characterized risk factors for atherosclerosis (hypertension, diabetes mellitus, cigarette smoking, hyperlipidemia, advanced age, elevated plasma homocysteine concentrations) injure the endothelium, initiating a chain of events, all attributes of atherosclerosis: smooth muscle cell proliferation, inflammatory cell recruitment, and lipid deposition within the blood vessel (Fig. 2-3). Oxidative stress and inflammation have been proposed as common features of atherosclerotic risk factors that lead to endothelial cell injury, raising the possibility that antioxidant and/or anti-inflammatory strategies may be beneficial to prevent or treat atherosclerosis.

Endothelial injury and the subsequent events that occur in the vessel wall initiate the progression from stable to unstable atherosclerotic plaques,

Figure 2-1

Angina Pectoris

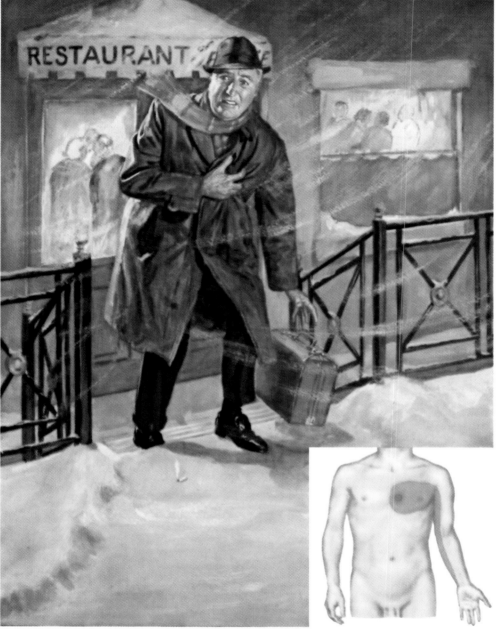

Common precipitating factors in angina pectoris:
Heavy meal, exertion, cold, smoking

Characteristic distribution of
pain in angina pectoris

Figure 2-2

Atherogenesis: Fatty Streak Formation

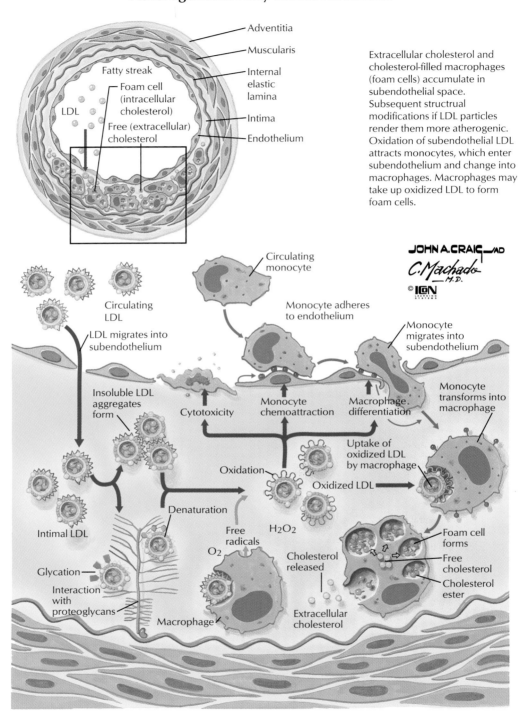

Adventitia
Muscularis
Internal elastic lamina
Fatty streak
Foam cell (intracellular cholesterol)
LDL
Intima
Free (extracellular) cholesterol
Endothelium

Extracellular cholesterol and cholesterol-filled macrophages (foam cells) accumulate in subendothelial space. Subsequent structrual modifications if LDL particles render them more atherogenic. Oxidation of subendothelial LDL attracts monocytes, which enter subendothelium and change into macrophages. Macrophages may take up oxidized LDL to form foam cells.

JOHN A. CRAIG _AD
C. Machado _M.D.
©ICON

Circulating monocyte
Monocyte adheres to endothelium
Monocyte migrates into subendothelium
Circulating LDL
LDL migrates into subendothelium
Insoluble LDL aggregates form
Cytotoxicity
Monocyte chemoattraction
Macrophage differentiation
Monocyte transforms into macrophage
Uptake of oxidized LDL by macrophage
Oxidation
Oxidized LDL
Denaturation
Intimal LDL
Free radicals
H_2O_2
Foam cell forms
Free cholesterol
Cholesterol ester
O_2
Glycation
Cholesterol released
Interaction with proteoglycans
Macrophage
Extracellular cholesterol

Figure 2-3

Atherogenesis: Fibrous Plaque Formation

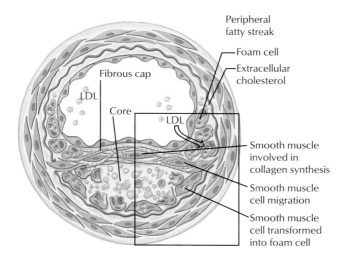

Peripheral
fatty streak

Foam cell

Extracellular
cholesterol

Fibrous cap

LDL

Core

LDL

Smooth muscle
involved in
collagen synthesis

Smooth muscle
cell migration

Smooth muscle
cell transformed
into foam cell

Fibrous plaque larger than fatty
streak and occupies more of arterial
lumen. Thickened cap synthesized
by modified smooth muscle cells.
Central core consists of extracellular
cholesterol. Foam cells surrounding
core derived primarily from smooth
muscle cells. Fatty streaks may
continue to form at periphery of
plaque.

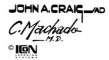

**Cholesterol accumulation
continues at plaque**

Fibrous cap forms over

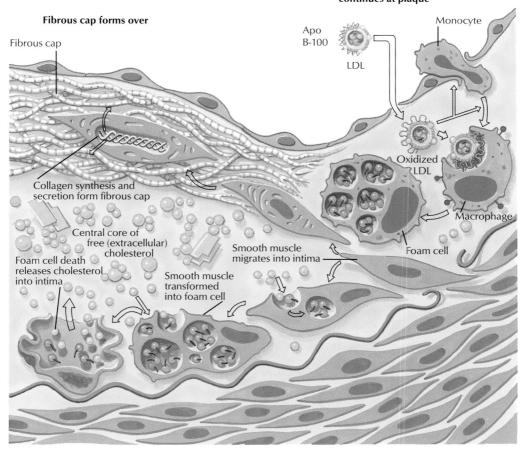

Fibrous cap

Apo
B-100

LDL

Monocyte

Oxidized
LDL

Macrophage

Collagen synthesis and
secretion form fibrous cap

Central core of
free (extracellular)
cholesterol

Foam cell

Foam cell death
releases cholesterol
into intima

Smooth muscle
migrates into intima

Smooth muscle
transformed
into foam cell

ultimately leading to the rupture of unstable plaques, thrombosis of the vessel, and, in many cases, MI (Fig. 2-4). Lesion development in the medium and small vessels of cerebral vessels leads to stroke and in renal and mesenteric vasculature contributes to diabetic complications.

An abundance of evidence suggests that atherosclerotic lesions, at least in part, result from an excessive inflammatory response. For example, although elevated low-density lipoprotein (LDL) is a risk factor for premature atherosclerosis, the LDL must undergo oxidative modification to cause damage to the arterial wall. Cytokines, growth factors, and oxidative stress may also contribute to atherosclerosis by mechanisms that are independent of LDL oxidation. Any of these mediators can rapidly react with and inactivate nitric oxide, enhancing proatherogenic mechanisms such as leukocyte adhesion to endothelium, impaired vasorelaxation, and platelet aggregation (Fig. 2-5).

Numerous adaptive changes in vascular structure occur with aging in healthy individuals. These changes include increases in arterial stiffening, aortic root size, and aortic wall thickness (which resembles the increased intimal medial thickness during early atherogenesis) and measurable abnormalities in vascular function, such as enhanced arterial systolic and pulse pressure. Collagen content is increased but elastin content is decreased.

Throughout the spectrum of atherogenesis, smooth muscle cells play a pivotal role. Smooth muscle cells are not terminally differentiated and can undergo phenotypic modulation, reverting to cells capable of proliferation, migration, and secretion of mediators involved in these processes. These modulated smooth muscle cell phenotypes have potentially opposing functions because they can repair vascular damage but can also contribute to vascular disease such as hypertension and atherosclerosis. In arteries prone to develop atherosclerosis, and in the sites of plaque destabilization and rupture, the terminal events in lesion progression—the number of smooth muscle cells—is often decreased. Because smooth muscle cells are important in maintaining plaque stability (most of the interstitial collagen fiber deposition important for the tensile strength of the fibrous cap is secreted by SMCs), the paucity of SMCs increases the likelihood of plaque rupture. Therefore, it is likely that SMC proliferation is deleterious in the early stages of atherosclerotic lesion formation, whereas loss of SMCs (and decreased capacity for proliferation) in later stages increases the likelihood of plaque destabilization and clinical outcomes such as MI and stroke.

Advances in molecular biologic and genetic approaches promise a more detailed understanding of atherosclerosis and improved diagnostic and therapeutic methods. In the past two decades, an explosion of information based on identification of genes and proteins involved in experimental atherosclerosis has resulted in a better understanding of the biology of atherosclerosis. Unfortunately, these advances have generally not translated into better diagnostic testing. In addition, because with rare exceptions atherosclerosis is a multigenic disease, gene therapy and other similar approaches are less likely to offer therapeutic effectiveness (see chapter 62).

For the immediate future, it is likely that investigators will focus on the interplay between genetic and environmental factors. Current approaches include (1) identifying families of genes (using **DNA gene chip** or **microarray** technologies) that may predispose individuals to atherosclerosis development; (2) defining genetic–environmental interactions that accelerate atherosclerosis; (3) elucidating key cellular events in atherogenesis using genetic approaches, from initiation of gene expression to how vascular and myocardial cells deal with degraded proteins and other cellular components (see also chapter 62).

CLINICAL PRESENTATION

Understanding the symptoms of myocardial ischemia is essential in the context of atherosclerosis, and the brief descriptions provided represent an overview. These topics are discussed in more detail in other chapters (chapters 1, 7, 8, and 9). There are three classic clinical presentations of coronary atherosclerosis. The first is *angina pectoris*, the characteristic ischemia-induced chest pain. The chest pain of angina is typically retrosternal, with radiation to the arms and neck, and is often accompanied by dyspnea. Angina may occur predictably with exertion (stable angina) or, more ominously, at rest or in an accelerating pattern (unstable angina). The symptoms of stable angina are often subtle and difficult to distinguish from other

Figure 2-4

Atherogenesis: Unstable Plaque Formation

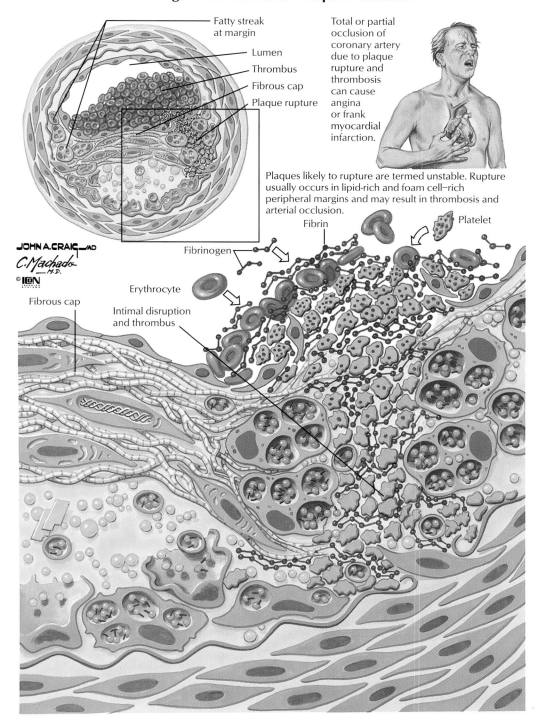

Fatty streak at margin

Lumen

Thrombus

Fibrous cap

Plaque rupture

Total or partial occlusion of coronary artery due to plaque rupture and thrombosis can cause angina or frank myocardial infarction.

Plaques likely to rupture are termed unstable. Rupture usually occurs in lipid-rich and foam cell–rich peripheral margins and may result in thrombosis and arterial occlusion.

Fibrin

Platelet

Fibrinogen

Erythrocyte

Fibrous cap

Intimal disruption and thrombus

JOHN A. CRAIG—MD
C. Machado—M.D.
©ICN

Figure 2-5

Risk Factors in Coronary Heart Disease

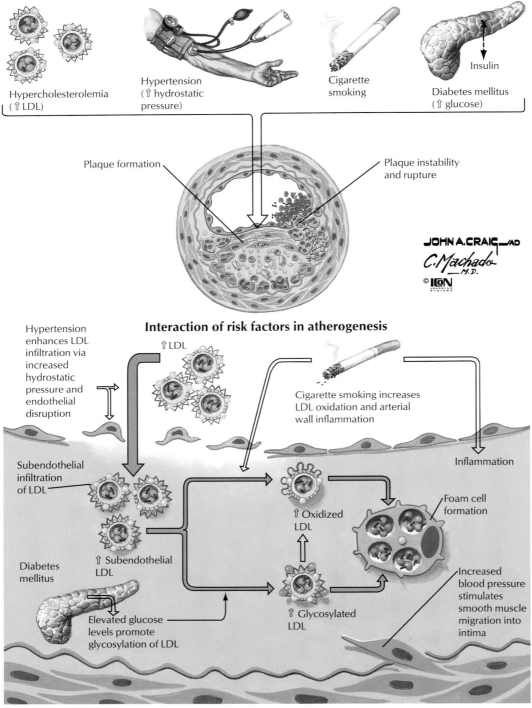

Hypercholesterolemia
(⇑ LDL)

Hypertension
(⇑ hydrostatic
pressure)

Cigarette
smoking

Insulin

Diabetes mellitus
(⇑ glucose)

Plaque formation

Plaque instability
and rupture

JOHN A.CRAIG—MD
C.Machado
—M.D.
©ICN

Interaction of risk factors in atherogenesis

Hypertension
enhances LDL
infiltration via
increased
hydrostatic
pressure and
endothelial
disruption

⇑ LDL

Cigarette smoking increases
LDL oxidation and arterial
wall inflammation

Inflammation

Subendothelial
infiltration
of LDL

⇑ Oxidized
LDL

Foam cell
formation

Diabetes
mellitus

⇑ Subendothelial
LDL

Elevated glucose
levels promote
glycosylation of LDL

⇑ Glycosylated
LDL

Increased
blood pressure
stimulates
smooth muscle
migration into
intima

causes of chest discomfort. This is particularly true in women, in whom the typical symptoms described herein are less commonly present.

If not treated promptly, unstable angina may be a harbinger of **MI**, the second classic presentation of atherosclerosis. Patients with MI frequently, but not exclusively, present with chest pain; however, unlike anginal pain, the pain of MI is typically unremitting and more severe and may be accompanied by autonomic symptoms, such as nausea and vomiting. Arrhythmias may ensue from ischemia-induced electrical instability of the myocardium. In severe cases, symptoms of heart failure because of acute left or right ventricular dysfunction may also be present. Ventricular dysfunction is an ominous sign in patients with MI and merits prompt attention.

The third presentation of atherosclerosis is **SCD** due to ventricular fibrillation, which is the first clinical manifestation of coronary atherosclerosis in about 25% of patients with the disease (see chapter 23). The only hope of survival for patients who present with SCD is prompt administration of cardiopulmonary resuscitation and ventricular defibrillation. A number of studies have demonstrated that community-based efforts to train the public in resuscitation techniques, to provide access to defibrillation devices, and to improve emergency medical access improve survival in out-of-hospital SCD (chapter 23). Resuscitation after SCD is more effective in patients admitted to the hospital, largely because of continuous electrocardiographic monitoring and the development of coronary care units that provide advanced care for patients who experienced MI.

It should be noted that more than 50% of patients with myocardial ischemia present with atypical symptoms ranging from "anginal equivalents" to nonspecific symptoms in the setting of acute MI. For this reason, a high index of clinical suspicion should endorse further diagnostic testing in individuals with atypical symptoms (chapter 1).

DIFFERENTIAL DIAGNOSIS

The identification of patients with coronary atherosclerosis is one of the classic dilemmas in clinical decision-making for three reasons. First, as much as 70% luminal obstruction by an atherosclerotic lesion is necessary to cause hemodynamically significant obstruction that results in myocardial ischemia and the symptoms of angina. Second, however, many lesions that rupture or undergo thrombosis and lead to MI are nonobstructive, and neither the identification of suspect lesions by angiography nor the early warning symptoms of angina necessarily forewarn of dramatic clinical presentations such as unstable angina or MI. Third, the symptoms of angina pectoris, and even MI, can be especially subtle and difficult to distinguish from other causes of chest discomfort, even for an experienced clinician. Moreover, oftentimes, cardiac symptoms are not recognized by the patient before an acute presentation (chapter 1). The failure to identify the symptoms of myocardial ischemia is one of the most common, and the most costly, clinical errors.

Typical anginal pain is frequently exertional and subsides predictably within a few minutes of rest. The pain may also be exacerbated by emotional stress and drug use, including tobacco and cocaine. The pain is often described as aching, pressure, heaviness, or squeezing. The diagnosis is further complicated by the number of other causes of chest discomfort, many of which are also medical emergencies. Other cardiovascular diseases, including **aortic dissection** and a**cute pericarditis**, may produce chest pain. More common cardiac, noncoronary causes of ischemic chest pain are **systemic hypertension** and endothelial dysfunction or **syndrome X**. Individuals with marked hypertension may experience exertional chest pain as a result of subendocardial ischemia, which often occurs in the absence of angiographically significant coronary stenosis. Similarly, patients with syndrome X experience effort-induced chest pain, probably due to subendocardial ischemia from the inability of the coronary arteries to undergo vasodilation normally. Based on the biology of atherosclerosis, as discussed previously herein, it is no surprise that considerable overlap exists between patients with hypertension and/or endothelial dysfunction and those with significant atherosclerotic lesions. Pulmonary causes of chest pain include **pulmonary embolism** and **pulmonary hypertension**, the latter of which may be exertional and difficult to distinguish from myocardial ischemia based on symptoms alone. Gastrointestinal diseases are very common, and frequently difficult to distinguish from angina pectoris based on medical history; **gastroesophageal reflux** and **esophageal spasm** frequently cause chest discomfort similar to angina, as can **gastritis** and **peptic ulcer disease**. Musculoskeletal conditions, such as **muscle strains** and **arthritis**, may produce angina-like symptoms. Finally, it is not uncommon for the distribution of **herpes zoster** pain to suggest angina pectoris to the clinician, particularly if the rash typical of herpes zoster has not yet appeared. Thus, the nonspecific nature of angina pectoris symptoms, plus the broad overlap with other common disorders, contributes to the difficulties in the diagnosis of coronary artery disease (CAD) based on signs and symptoms alone.

DIAGNOSTIC APPROACH

The suspicion of coronary atherosclerosis is raised by a careful history and physical examination—in particular, the solicitation of symptoms of angina pectoris and the consideration of potential risk factors for the development of atherosclerosis. A host of diagnostic methods are available for the clinician evaluating a patient for CHD (see chapters 3–6). The first step in the evaluation of patients suspected of having coronary atherosclerosis is 12-lead electrocardiography. In patients with MI, the characteristic abnormality detected is ST-segment elevation, whereas patients with angina may have evidence of prior myocardial injury (Q waves) or ST-segment depression, or a normal ECG. Other abnormalities may also occur and ST-segment changes may disappear when ischemic symptoms resolve. Electrocardiography is a relatively specific but not highly sensitive indicator of CAD, and a normal ECG never excludes coronary disease under any circumstances (chapter 3). When MI is suspected, cardiac markers (creatine kinase–MB and troponin T or I) should be monitored for evidence of myocardial injury.

Additional studies to test for atherosclerosis fall in two groups: functional studies and anatomical studies. Among the functional studies, the most straightforward is the exercise treadmill test, which detects ST depression during exercise as a marker for obstructive CAD. Although simple to perform and relatively specific, the sensitivity of exercise treadmill tests falls in the 70 to 80% range at best. The sensitivity of provocative studies such as the treadmill

test can be greatly enhanced by adding radionuclide scintigraphy, echocardiography, or PET (particularly when knowledge of myocardial viability is important). Functional studies have the advantage of being noninvasive and, although their sensitivities in detection of significant CAD are improving, they do not equal the gold standard sensitivity of coronary angiography. Typically, the predictive accuracy of any noninvasive test is best with severe multivessel CAD; the predictive accuracy of these tests in single-vessel CAD is in the range of 65 to 75%. Therefore, if the clinical suspicion is high and a definitive diagnosis is needed, anatomic evaluation (coronary angiography) should be considered even in individuals with negative noninvasive evaluation results.

The definitive anatomical test for CAD is coronary arteriography, which is the gold standard for diagnosis of coronary atherosclerosis (chapters 5 and 10). This is also the most invasive diagnostic procedure for atherosclerosis and, although the risks of angiography in otherwise healthy patients are very low, postprocedure complications occur in a small percentage of patients. Coronary arteriography provides detailed information about the size and extent of atherosclerotic lesions. Further definition of lesion characteristics can be performed using intravascular ultrasound (Fig. 2-6) or other imaging methods; however, these additional studies are more commonly used for research than for clinical purposes. In addition to its invasive nature, the other disadvantage of coronary arteriography is that functional information regarding the extent of ischemia from a given lesion is not provided; this may not matter in the case of severe stenoses, but in moderate stenoses (50–70%), it can be important.

MANAGEMENT AND THERAPY

The management of patients with coronary atherosclerosis depends on the initial presentation of the disease. For patients presenting with acute MI, thrombolysis or acute percutaneous revascularization need to be considered, if appropriate, combined with pharmacologic therapies, as described in detail in chapters 8 and 9. Patients with stable angina pectoris are generally treated with aspirin, β-blocker therapy, and nitrates as needed for symptoms (chapter 7). Percutaneous coronary intervention is an

Figure 2-6

Intravascular Ultrasonography

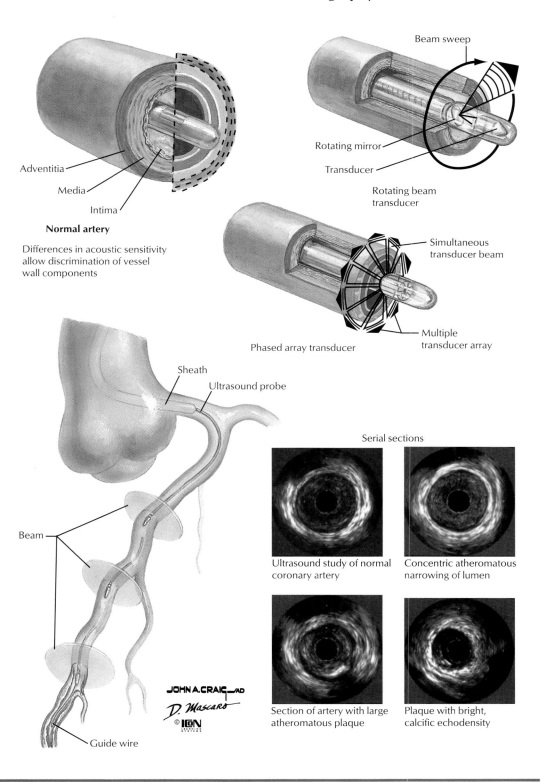

Adventitia

Media

Intima

Normal artery

Differences in acoustic sensitivity
allow discrimination of vessel
wall components

Beam sweep

Rotating mirror

Transducer

Rotating beam
transducer

Simultaneous
transducer beam

Multiple
transducer array

Phased array transducer

Sheath

Ultrasound probe

Beam

Serial sections

JOHN A. CRAIG_MD

D. Mascaro

© ICN

Guide wire

Ultrasound study of normal
coronary artery

Concentric atheromatous
narrowing of lumen

Section of artery with large
atheromatous plaque

Plaque with bright,
calcific echodensity

increasingly important therapy even in stable coronary syndromes (chapters 7 and 10). Coronary artery bypass surgery may be needed for patients with refractory angina or those with extensive coronary disease that is not amenable to percutaneous revascularization (chapter 11). In selected subsets—multivessel CAD in diabetic persons or in individuals with impaired left ventricular systolic function—coronary artery bypass surgery has proven to be effective.

Although well-validated therapies for the consequences of coronary atherosclerotic disease exist, specific therapies aimed at treating or preventing atherosclerosis itself are lacking. Risk factor modification largely prevents progression of atherosclerotic lesions that have formed (and lessens the formation of new lesions), but there is scant evidence that lesions can substantially regress, even with aggressive risk factor modification. Lipid-lowering agents—statins in particular—are thought to stabilize lesions through various mechanisms, ultimately decreasing the likelihood of plaque rupture, acute coronary syndrome, or cardiac death. Numerous studies have demonstrated risk reduction in individuals treated with use of statins. Similarly, aspirin therapy may prevent complications related to atherosclerosis by inhibiting platelet function, but aspirin probably has little effect on atherosclerotic lesions.

FUTURE DIRECTIONS

Several new approaches are under consideration as therapeutic methods for patients with atherosclerosis. Gene therapy approaches, particularly those designed to inhibit cell cycle events in smooth muscle cells within lesions, have been in development for several years, but little progress has been made in clinical application. Angiogenesis therapies are in phase 2 trials for patients with atherosclerotic disease, but this approach does not affect primary atherosclerotic lesions. Antioxidant strategies are under consideration to arrest or reverse atherosclerotic lesions, given the pleiotropic effects of oxidants on cellular events that accelerate the atherosclerotic process. Although the use of antioxidant vitamins has not been beneficial, more effective antioxidant strategies may be necessary to reverse or prevent the progression of lesion formation, and may optimally be targeted to patients with markers of high

levels of oxidative stress as detected noninvasively. Similarly, there is significant interest in therapies that diminish inflammation, but prospective randomized studies have yet to be completed.

Until the latter part of the 1950s, only palliative therapies were widely available to patients with atherosclerosis and its complications. Although huge strides have been taken in the approach to this disease, much progress remains to be made. First, specific serum markers of atherosclerosis would be hugely beneficial, not only for diagnosis, but as a screening tool for testing large populations at risk for atherosclerosis. Use of inflammatory markers, such as C-reactive protein levels, is an important step in this direction, but more sensitive and specific tests are needed. Second, improvements in the ability to analyze coronary artery anatomy noninvasively are needed; recent improvements in CT and MRI technologies are especially promising in this regard. Finally, development of specific therapies that can reverse or prevent atherosclerotic lesion development remains a hope for the future. Gene therapy remains promising if appropriate targets can be identified; safety issues, resolved. However, newer studies documenting the involvement of many redundant signaling pathways in atherogenesis, along with improvements in targeted pharmacologic therapies, probably indicate that pharmaceutical approaches will dominate future therapies.

REFERENCES

Haber E. Automatic detection and recording of cardiac arrhythmias. *JAMA* 1959;170:1782–1785.
Hollenberg M. Comparison of a quantitative treadmill exercise score with standard electrocardiographic criteria in screening asymptomatic young men for coronary artery disease. *N Engl J Med* 1985;313:600–606.
Lakatta EG. Age-associated cardiovascular changes in health: Impact on cardiovascular disease in older persons. *Heart Fail Rev* 2002;7:29–49.
Lefkowitz RJ, Willerson JT. Prospects for cardiovascular research. *JAMA* 2001;285:581–587.
National Institutes of Health. *National Heart, Lung, and Blood Institute Fact Book*. 2000.
Patterson C, Madamanchi N, Runge MS. The oxidative paradox: Another piece of the puzzle. *Circ Res* 2000;87:1074–1076.
Ridker PM, Cushman M, Stampfer MJ, Tracy RP, Hennekens CH. Inflammation, aspirin, and the risk of cardiovascular disease in apparently healthy men. *N Engl J Med* 1997;336:973–979.
Ross R. The pathogenesis of atherosclerosis: A perspective for the 1990s. *Nature* 1993;362:801–809.

Chapter 3
Electrocardiography

Leonard S. Gettes

In 1902, the Dutch physiologist Wilhelm Einthoven recorded the first ECG signals from humans. Since then, the number of recording leads has increased from 3 to 12, but the basic principles underlying electrocardiography are unchanged. Electrocardiography records from the body surface the voltage gradients created as myocardial cells sequentially depolarize and repolarize. It is the most commonly used technique to detect and diagnose cardiac disease and to monitor therapies that influence the electrical behavior of the heart. It is noninvasive, virtually risk free, and relatively inexpensive. Since its introduction, a large database has been assembled that correlates the ECG waveform recorded from the body surface to the clinical presentation of the patient, providing insight into the underlying electrical behavior of the heart and its modification by physiologic, pharmacologic, and pathologic events. This chapter discusses the relation of the ECG waveform to the underlying electrophysiologic properties of the heart and illustrates the changes in the ECG waveform induced by various events.

LEADS

Twelve leads are routinely used to record the body surface ECG: three bipolar limb leads: leads I, II, and III; three augmented limb leads: leads aVR, aVL, and aVF; and six unipolar chest leads: leads V_1 through V_6 (Fig. 3-1). In the bipolar limb leads, the negative pole for each of the leads is different, whereas in the unipolar chest leads, the negative pole is constant and created by the three limb leads. The positive chest lead is, in effect, an exploring lead that can be placed anywhere, provided the reader of the ECG knows its position. In children, for example, routine electrocardiography often includes placing leads on the right side of the chest wall in the positions referred to as V_3R and V_4R. Similar right-sided chest leads are often used in adults to diagnose right ventricular infarction, and one or more leads positioned on the back are sometimes used to diagnose posterior wall infarction.

The chest leads are much closer to the heart than are the limb leads and are influenced by the electrical activity directly under the recording lead. Changes in the relation of the individual chest lead to the heart may cause significant changes in the ECG waveform. For instance, if the lead is placed an interspace too high or too low, or if the patient is in a sitting rather than a supine position, the relation of the leads to the heart and the ECG waveform will change, potentially leading to misinterpretation unless the reader of the ECG is aware of the change from normal position.

ELECTROCARDIOGRAPHIC WAVEFORM

The ECG waveform consists of a P wave, a PR interval, a QRS complex, an ST segment, and T and U waves. Their relation to the underlying electrophysiologic events is shown in Figure 3-2. The P wave reflects depolarization of the atria, the QRS complex reflects depolarization of the ventricles, and the ST segment and T wave reflect repolarization of the ventricles. The cause of the U wave remains unclear. Sinus node depolarization occurs before the onset of the P wave, but the voltage gradients associated with sinus node depolarization are too small to be recorded on the body surface by the clinically used ECG machine. Therefore, this event is electrocardiographically silent. Similarly, the electrical activity of the atrioventricular (AV) junction, which occurs during the PR interval, is also electrocardiographically silent. Figure 3-3 is an example of a normal ECG.

P Wave

The P wave is caused by voltage gradients created by the sequential depolarization of atrial cells, indicated in Figure 3-2 by the upstroke of the atrial action potential. The sequence of atrial depolarization and time required to depolarize

Figure 3-1   ## Electrocardiographic Leads and Reference Lines

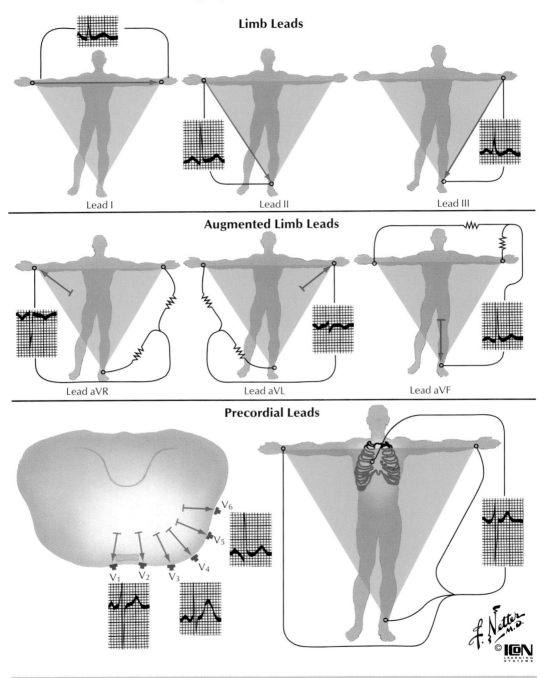

Limb Leads

Lead I   Lead II   Lead III

Augmented Limb Leads

Lead aVR   Lead aVL   Lead aVF

Precordial Leads

V₆
V₅
V₁ V₂ V₃ V₄

When current flows toward red arrowheads, upward deflection occurs in ECG
When current flows away from red arrowheads, downward deflection occurs in ECG
When current flows perpendicular to red arrows, no deflection or biphasic deflection occurs

Figure 3-2

Relation of Action Potential From the Various Cardiac Regions to the Body Surface ECG

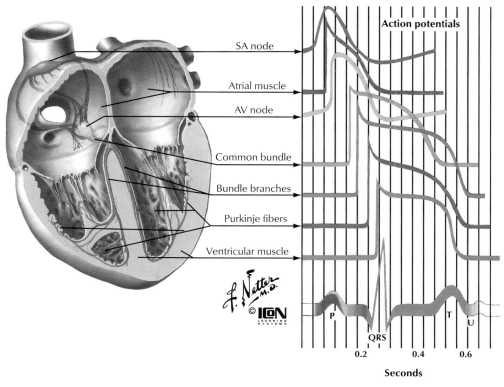

Figure 3-3

Normal ECG

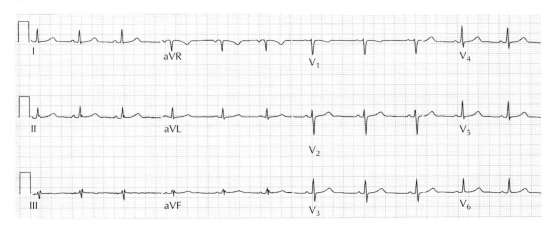

Example of a normal ECG recorded from a 24-year-old woman. Note that the P wave is upright in leads I and II and inverted in aVR. The QRS complex gradually changes from negative to V_1 to positive V_6. Note that the polarity of the T wave is similar to that of the QRS complex.

all cells of the two atria are reflected in the shape and duration of the P wave. Impulses arising in the sinus node depolarize the right atrium before the left atrium. For this reason, the vectorial direction of atrial depolarization is from right to left, from superior to inferior, and from anterior to posterior. This results in a P wave that is characteristically upright or positive in leads I, II, V_5, and V_6 and inverted in lead aVR (Fig. 3-3). In V_1, the P wave may be upright, biphasic, or inverted.

QRS Complex

The QRS complex reflects ventricular depolarization. Normally, depolarization of both ventricles occurs simultaneously, spreading from endocardium to epicardium and from apex to base. Because the left ventricle is three times the size of the right ventricle, its depolarization overshadows and largely obscures right ventricular (RV) depolarization. The spatial vector of the QRS complex reflects this left ventricular (LV) dominance and is directed to the left and posteriorly. The QRS complex is usually upright or positive in leads I, V_5, and V_6, the left-sided and more posterior leads, and negative or inverted in leads aVR and V_1, the most right-sided and more anterior leads (Fig. 3-3). It is only in situations such as right bundle branch block and profound RV hypertrophy that the electrical activity associated with RV depolarization can be identified.

ST Segment

During the ST segment, all ventricular action potentials are at their plateau voltage of approximately 0 mV, and no voltage gradients are generated. Therefore, the ST segment is at the same level on the ECG as the PR and TP segments, during which time the ventricular action potentials are at their resting phase of approximately −85 mV.

T Wave

The T wave occurs as the result of sequential repolarization of the ventricular cells. If the repolarizing sequence were the same as the depolarizing sequence, the T wave would be opposite in direction to the QRS complex. However, the normal T wave is generally upright (positive) in leads with an upright or positive QRS complex (leads I, V_5, and V_6) and inverted (negative) in leads with an inverted QRS complex (aVR and V_1) (Fig. 3-3). The QRS and T wave vectorial directions are similar because the sequence of repolarization is reversed, relative to the sequence of depolarization. This occurs because the duration of epicardial action potentials is shorter than that of the action potentials in the mid myocardium and subendocardium. Therefore, the cells on the epicardium are the first to repolarize, though they are the last to depolarize. The shorter duration of the epicardial action potential is attributed to two primary factors: The repolarizing ionic currents are slightly different in the epicardium, and cells of the specialized conducting systems have longer action potentials than the ventricular fibers and tend to prolong the action potentials of endocardial cells.

FACTORS THAT ALTER COMPONENTS OF THE BODY SURFACE ELECTROCARDIOGRAM

Factors that alter the sequence of depolarization and/or influence the upstroke of the action potential influence and alter the shape, duration, and vectorial direction of the P wave or the QRS complex, whereas factors that alter the sequence of repolarization and/or the phase of rapid repolarization influence the shape, duration, and vectorial direction of the T wave. The ST, TP, and PR segments are elevated or depressed by factors that introduce voltage gradients during these portions of the action potential. The interval from the onset of the QRS complex to the end of the T wave (the QT interval) is affected by factors that alter the time required for ventricular repolarization to occur, either by lengthening or shortening the plateau phase of the action potential, thereby influencing the duration of the ST segment, or by speeding or slowing the phase of rapid repolarization, thereby influencing the duration of the T wave. The route and the speed of conduction from the atria to the ventricles, which usually occurs via the AV node and specialized conducting system, influence the PR interval. Slowing of the impulse conduction anywhere in this pathway, but especially within the AV node, lengthens the PR interval. If bypass tracts that circumvent the AV nodal conduction pathway are present, conduction to the ventricles requires less time and the PR interval shortens.

P Wave

The duration of the P wave is lengthened by factors that prolong impulse propagation in the atria, such as fibrosis or hypertrophy. The shape of the P wave is modified by atrial hypertrophy, by the position of the heart within the chest, and by the site of origin of the impulses initiating atrial activation. For instance, in COPD, the diaphragm is depressed and the heart assumes a more vertical position. In this situation, the P wave will be altered. When the left atrium is hypertrophied, or when intra-atrial conduction is slowed, the terminal component of the P wave, which represents left atrial depolarization, will be affected and the P wave will change.

Impulses arising from an ectopic focus within the atria are associated with P waves in which the shape depends on the location of the focus and the sequence of atrial depolarization. If the ectopic focus is close to the sinus node, the P wave will resemble a normal sinus P wave. The further the ectopic focus is from the sinus node, the more abnormal will be the P-wave configuration. For instance, impulses arising in the inferior portion of the atria or in the AV node will depolarize the atria in a retrograde, superiorly oriented direction. The P wave will reflect this superior orientation and will be inverted in leads II, III, and aVF (Fig. 3-4).

PR Interval

The PR interval is prolonged by factors that slow AV nodal conduction, including an increase in vagal tone (because the AV node is richly supplied by vagal fibers) and by drugs that enhance vagal tone or diminish sympathetic tone, such as the digitalis glycosides and the β-adrenergic–blocking agents. Drugs that inhibit or block the calcium inward current, calcium channel blockers, also cause PR prolongation because calcium ions rather than sodium ions are responsible for the upstroke of the action potential in cells comprising the AV node upper portion. Diseases involving the AV node are another cause of PR prolongation. The PR interval is shortened when impulses reach the ventricles via a bypass tract to cause ventricular preexcitation.

QRS Complex

The QRS complex is altered both in shape and duration by abnormalities in the sequence of ventricular activation, such as right and left bundle branch block (Fig. 3-5A). Ventricular pre-excitation (as occurs in the Wolff-Parkinson-White Syndrome) also changes the sequence of ventricular activation and the shape and duration of the QRS complex, mimicking a bundle branch block (Fig. 3-5B). Loss of ventricular muscle also results in an abnormal QRS shape. ECG changes accompanying myocardial infarction are examples of this phenomenon (Fig. 3-6). Infarction results in abnormalities in the early portion of the QRS complex with creation of an abnormal Q wave in leads overlying the infarct region. In this way, the ECG abnormality localizes the infarction and suggests the vessel responsible for the infarct.

Drugs that block the sodium inward current, such as the type I antiarrhythmic drugs, slow the rate at which individual cells depolarize. This slows impulse propagation throughout the ventricle and causes diffuse lengthening of the QRS complex. However, the sequence of activation is not altered, so the QRS complex maintains its normal waveform. An increase in extracellular potassium, which makes the resting membrane potential of the individual action potential less negative, also slows interventricular conduction and the rate of cellular depolarization, causing uniform lengthening of the QRS complex and also characteristic peaking of T waves (Fig. 3-7). The QRS complex is also changed by ectopic beats and rhythms originating from an ectopic focus in the ventricle. The shape and duration of these ectopic beats reflect the site of origin.

The amplitude of the QRS complex is subject to a variety of factors: thickness of the LV and RV walls, presence of pericardial or pleural fluid, and amount of tissue between the heart and the chest wall. Age, sex, and race may also affect QRS amplitude. For instance, young adults have greater QRS voltages than older individuals, men have a greater QRS voltage than women, and black individuals tend to have greater QRS voltages than white individuals. In LV hypertrophy, the magnitude of left and posterior forces associated with LV depolarization increases, causing an increase in the positive QRS voltage, that is, the R wave, in the left-sided leads, V_5 and V_6, and an increase in the negative QRS voltage, that is, the S wave, in the right-sided chest leads.

Figure 3-4

Ectopic Atrial Rhythm

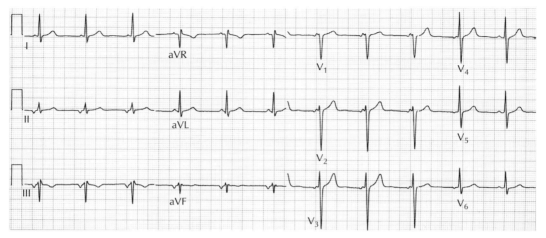

Electrocardiogram showing an ectopic atrial rhythm. It was recorded from a 59-year-old man. The polarity of the P wave is abnormal. It is inverted in leads II, III, and aVF and upright in lead aVR.

QRS duration may increase, reflecting the increased thickness of the left ventricle and there may be repolarization changes (Fig. 3-8). Pericardial and pleural effusion decreases QRS voltage in all leads. Infiltrative diseases, such as amyloidosis, may also decrease QRS voltage.

ST Segment and T Wave

The ST segment and T wave reflect the action potential plateau (ST segment), and the phase of rapid repolarization (T wave). These two components are often affected simultaneously by factors such as LV hypertrophy; cardioactive drugs, such as digitalis and the type I and type III antiarrhythmic agents; and a decreased concentration of serum potassium. In these situations, ST-segment and T-wave changes both occur. However, the ST segment and T wave may also be affected separately, resulting in ST-segment changes without T-wave changes or T-wave changes without ST-segment changes. The ST segment is altered by factors that induce voltage gradients during the plateau phase of the action potential. Acute myocardial ischemia causes the plateau voltage to become more negative in cells located within the ischemic zone, creating voltage gradients during the plateau phase between the ischemic and nonischemic regions. This phenomenon leads to generation of injury currents across the ischemic margin, which can cause either ST-segment elevation or depression, depending on whether acute ischemia is transmural or nontransmural (see Figs. 3-6 and 3-9). Acute pericarditis usually involves the entire precordial surface but does not affect deeper layers. Thus, the injury current generated is between the epicardium and deeper layers and, generally, leads to diffuse ST-segment elevation. There are also normally occurring differences in the early portion of the plateau of the action potential in cells from the epicardial and deeper layers. These differences may cause voltage gradients and result in ST-segment elevation. This form of ST-segment deviation, which occurs most frequently in younger males, is a normal variant and referred to as "early repolarization."

The duration of the ST segment and, thereby, the duration of the QT interval may be altered by changes in heart rate and by changes in extracellular calcium. Hypocalcemia and bradycardia lengthen the plateau of the action potential and cause lengthening of the ST segment and of the QT interval (Fig. 3-10). Hypercalcemia and tachycardia have the opposite effect. They shorten the plateau duration, the ST segment, and the QT interval.

The T wave can be influenced independent of the ST segment by factors that alter the sequence of repolarization. For example, sudden changes in heart rate may cause some

Figure 3-5

Bundle Branch Block

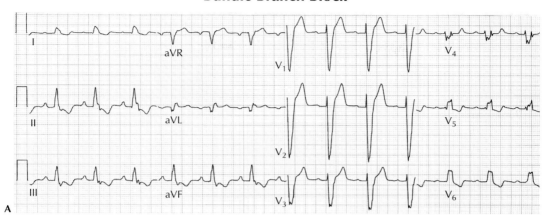

A

(**A**) Electrocardiogram showing left bundle branch block. It was recorded from a 73-year-old man. Note that the QRS complex is diffusely widened and is notched in leads V_3, V_4, V_5, and V_6. Note also that the T wave is directed opposite to the QRS complex. This is an example of a secondary T-wave change.

Ventricular Preexcitation

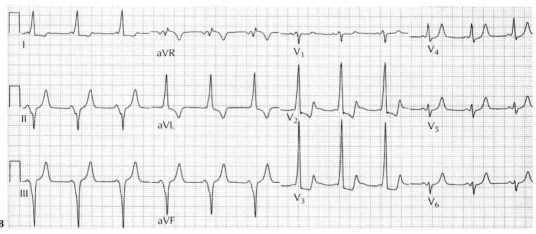

B

(**B**) ECG showing ventricular preexcitation. It is recorded from a 28-year-old woman. Note the short PR interval (0.9 seconds) and the widened QRS complex (0.134 seconds). The initial portion of the QRS complex appears slurred. This is referred to as a *delta wave*. This combination of short PR interval and widened QRS complex with a delta wave is characteristic of ventricular pre-excitation. Note also that the T wave is abnormal, another example of a secondary T-wave change.

action potentials to shorten or lengthen more rapidly and to a greater extent than other action potentials. This is an example of a functional rather than a pathologic T-wave change. Pathologic T-wave changes are those that occur with disease entities such as myocarditis and some cardiomyopathies. Inverted T waves may also persist after an ischemic event or myocardial infarction (Fig. 3-11). Changes in the sequence of repolarization also result from changes in the sequence of depolarization. These obligatory changes in repolarization result in "secondary" T-wave changes and are responsible for the ST-segment and T-wave changes accompanying bundle branch blocks and ventricular preexcitation (Figs. 3-5A and 3-5B).

Figure 3-6

Myocardial Ischemia, Injury, and Infarction

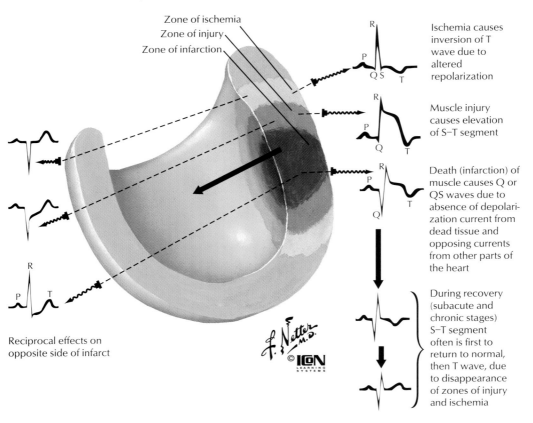

Zone of ischemia
Zone of injury
Zone of infarction

Ischemia causes inversion of T wave due to altered repolarization

Muscle injury causes elevation of S–T segment

Death (infarction) of muscle causes Q or QS waves due to absence of depolarization current from dead tissue and opposing currents from other parts of the heart

During recovery (subacute and chronic stages) S–T segment often is first to return to normal, then T wave, due to disappearance of zones of injury and ischemia

Reciprocal effects on opposite side of infarct

Figure 3-7

Changes Associated With Hyperpotassemia

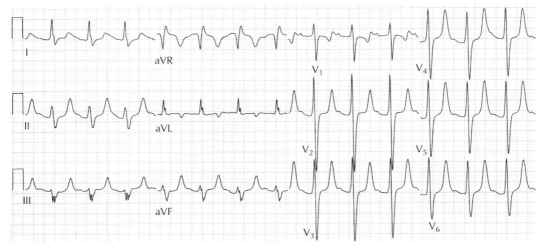

Example of the ECG changes associated with hyperpotassemia. It is recorded from a 29-year-old woman with chronic renal disease. The P wave is broad and difficult to identify in some leads. The QRS is diffusely widened (0.188 seconds) and the T wave is peaked and symmetrical. These changes are characteristic of severe hyperpotassemia and, in this patient, the serum potassium concentration was 8.2 mM.

Figure 3-8

ECG Changes of LV Hypertrophy

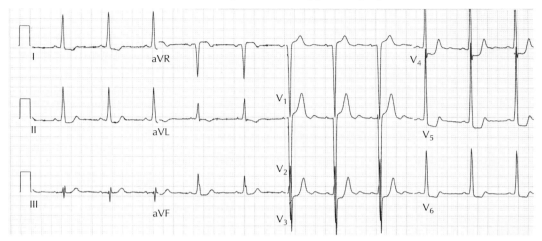

Example of the ECG changes of LV hypertrophy. It is recorded from an 83-year-old woman with aortic stenosis and insufficiency. Note the increase in QRS amplitude, the slight increase in QRS duration to 100 ms, and the ST-segment and T-wave changes.

Figure 3-9

ST-Segment Changes Associated
With an Acute Ischemic Event

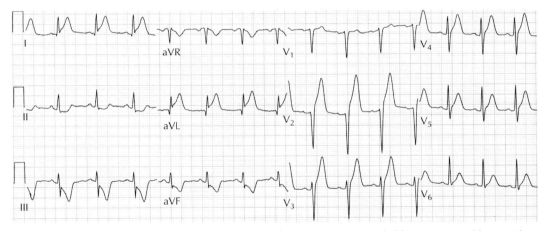

Example of ST-segment changes associated with an acute ischemic event. It is recorded from a 43-year-old man with chest pain. Note the ST-segment elevation in leads V1, aVL, and V2 through V6, and the ST-segment depression in leads III and aVF.

U Wave

The U wave follows the T wave. It may also arise within the terminal portion of the T wave and be difficult to distinguish from a notched T wave. Although the precise etiology of the U wave is not clear, an increase in its magnitude or a change in its polarity occurs with several clinical entities. An increase in U-wave amplitude is frequently associated with hypopotassemia and with some direct-acting cardiac drugs (Fig. 3-12A). Notching of the T wave, resembling an increase in U-wave amplitude and lengthening of the QT–U interval, also occurs in patients with congenital long QT syndrome (Fig. 3-12B), reflecting a genetic abnormality of one or more ionic channels responsible for repolarization.

Figure 3-10

ST-Segment and QT-Interval Changes Associated With Hypocalcemia

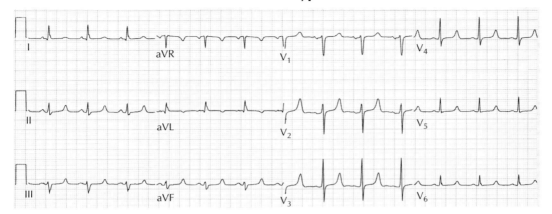

ST-segment and QT-interval changes associated with hypocalcemia. It is recorded from a 53-year-old man with chronic renal disease. The ST segment is prolonged, but the T wave is normal. The QT interval reflects ST-segment lengthening and is prolonged.

Figure 3-11

T-Wave Changes Induced by a Recent Ischemic Event

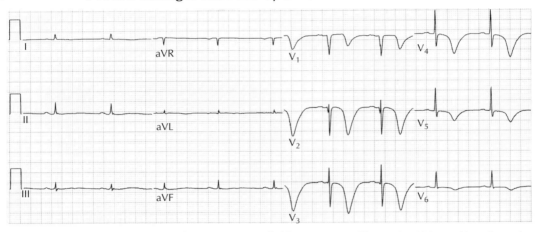

T-wave changes induced by a recent ischemic event, recorded from a 70-year-old man. The QT interval is prolonged and the T waves are markedly inverted in the precordial leads (V_1 through V_6). These changes gradually evolved over several days, and coronary angiography recorded the day this tracing was taken revealed a subtotal occlusion of the left anterior descending coronary artery.

Arrhythmias

Electrocardiography is indispensable in the diagnosis of brady- and tachyarrhythmias. For instance, a heart rate greater than 100 beats/min may have multiple causes, including sinus tachycardia, atrial and AV junctional tachycardia (Fig. 3-13A), atrial flutter, atrial fibrillation (Fig. 3-13B), and ventricular tachycardia (Fig. 3-13C). The rate and configuration of the P wave, its relation to the QRS complexes, and the shape and duration of the QRS complex establish the correct diagnosis. Abnormally slow heart rates may also be caused by several entities, including sinus bradycardia or sinoatrial or AV block (Fig. 3-13D). Again, the diagnosis can be established by noting the rate, regularity, and configuration of the P wave and

Figure 3-12

Changes Associated With Hypopotassemia

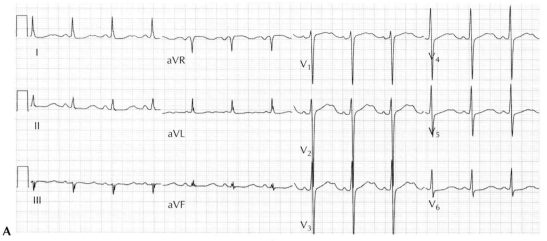

A

(**A**) Example of the changes associated with hypopotassemia. It is recorded from a 44-year-old man who was receiving long-term thiazide therapy. The QT interval is prolonged due to the presence of a U wave, which interrupts the descending limb of the T wave and is of equal amplitude to the T wave. In this patient, the serum potassium concentration was 2.7 mM.

Congenital Long QT Syndrome

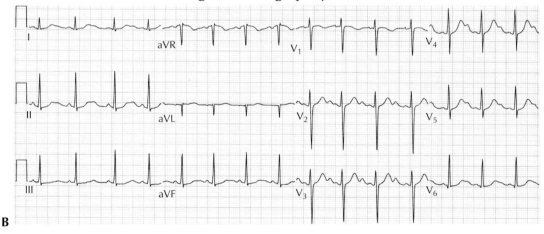

B

(**B**) Recorded from a 16-year-old girl with syncopal episodes that were documented to be due to rapid ventricular tachycardia. It is an example of long QT syndrome. The T wave is notched and prolonged in much the same way as was shown in the patient with hypopotassemia. However, in this patient, the serum potassium concentration was normal.

QRS complexes, the relation of the P wave to the QRS complexes, and the PR interval.

Irregular rhythms may be due to atrial and ventricular premature beats (Figs. 3-14A and 3-14B), atrial fibrillation (Fig. 3-13B), and incomplete (second degree) sinoatrial or AV block (Fig. 3-14C).

FUTURE DIRECTIONS

The ECG provides a window into the basic electrophysiologic properties of the heart and their modification by physiologic, pharmacologic, and pathologic causes. The ECG is relatively simple to obtain, reasonably inexpensive, and,

Figure 3-13

Abnormal Cardiac Rhythms

AV Nodal Reentrant Tachycardia

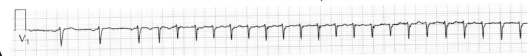

A

(**A**) Lead V$_1$ recorded from a patient with abnormal cardiac rhythms. This tracing shows the onset of AV nodal reentrant tachycardia in a 47-year-old man. There are three sinus beats followed by an atrial premature beat, which initiates a run of AV nodal reentrant tachycardia, with a rate of 170 beats/min.

Atrial Fibrillation

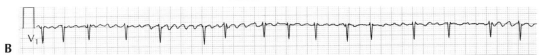

B

(**B**) Example of atrial fibrillation in a 50-year-old woman. Note the undulating baseline and the irregularly irregular QRS complexes, with a rate of 105 beats/min.

Ventricular Tachycardia

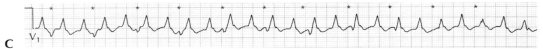

C

(**C**) Ventricular tachycardia with a rate of 150 beats/min from a 56-year-old man. The QRS complex is widened, and there is AV disassociation. The P waves, with an atrial rate of 73 beats/min, are marked with an asterisk.

Complete AV Block

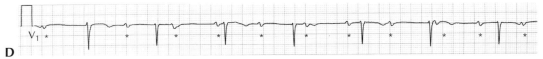

D

(**D**) Complete AV block from a 78-year-old woman. The atrial rate is 70 beats/min, and the ventricular rate is 46 beats/min. There is no relation between the P waves (marked with an asterisk) and the QRS complexes.

when correctly interpreted, of inestimable help in the diagnosis and treatment of a wide variety of cardiac diseases. Many proposed approaches have the goal of obtaining more precise, predictive information from the baseline ECG. Signal-averaged ECGs (SAECG) were developed as an attempt to more accurately predict the propensity of development of ventricular arrhythmias in an individual and to gauge the effectiveness of pharmacologic therapy. It has become evident that the SAECG offers only a limited amount of incremental information. There is much interest in computerized analysis of T-wave features as markers for the same events. It is likely that more powerful computerized analysis of ECG morphology will increase the usefulness of this test and its prognostic value, and that detailed analysis of the ECG will become increasingly important.

Figure 3-14

Irregular Cardiac Rhythms
Atrial Premature Beats

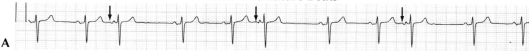

A

(**A**) Atrial premature beats (shown with an arrow) recorded from a 77-year-old man. In this example, there is an atrial premature beat after every two sinus beats. This is referred to as *atrial trigeminy*. Note that the shape of the premature P wave is different than that of the sinus P waves, reflecting its ectopic location.

Ventricular Premature Beats

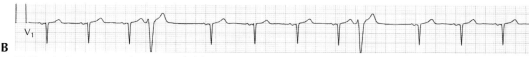

B

(**B**) Ventricular premature beats recorded from a 30-year-old man with no known heart disease.

Type I Second-Degree AV Block

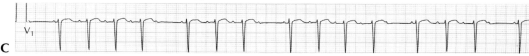

C

(**C**) Type I second-degree AV block with Wenckebach periodicity recorded from a 74-year-old man. There is progressive prolongation of the PR interval, followed by a blocked or nonconducted P wave. This leads to irregular groups of QRS complexes. In this example, there is 5:4 and 4:3 AV block. The atrial rate is 110 beats/min, and the ventricular rate is 90 beats/min.

REFERENCES

Chou TC. In: Surawicz B, Knilans TK, eds. *Chou's Electrocardiography in Clinical Practice: Adult and Pediatric.* 5th ed. Philadelphia: WB Saunders; 2001.

Gettes LS. *ECG Tutor* [CD-ROM]. Armonk, NY: Future Publishing; 2000.

Surawicz B. *Electrophysiologic Basis of ECG and Cardiac Arrhythmias.* Philadelphia: Williams & Wilkins; 1995.

Chapter 4

Noninvasive Cardiac Imaging

Christopher D. Chiles, Steven W. Falen, and Park W. Willis IV

Imaging techniques are central to the evaluation and management of patients with known or suspected heart disease. Technological advances in recent years have produced a broad spectrum of diagnostic imaging studies. Each study has advantages and appropriate clinical applications. The challenge for clinicians treating patients with cardiovascular diseases is to understand the applications and limitations of the available methodologies and use them effectively, but efficiently. This chapter focuses on technological aspects of cardiac imaging and the information that can be provided by each type of study. Chapter 6 discusses the selection of various diagnostic tests, including imaging studies, and paradigms for their use in the clinical setting.

PLAIN CHEST RADIOGRAPHY

The first cardiac imaging test developed, the chest x-ray (CXR), provides a means to assess the heart, the great vessels and the pulmonary veins, the lung fields and the mediastinum. On the basis of the differential density of myocardium, blood, vascular tissue, and the surrounding air-filled lung, the CXR portrays a radiographic silhouette.

In the standard posteroanterior projection (Fig. 4-1), the right mediastinal border of the heart is formed by the right atrium (the lower portion of the mediastinal border) and the superior vena cava, which appears above the right atrial border as a slight bulge or straightening. Superimposed on the superior vena cava is the ascending aortic arch, a short convexity along the upper right mediastinum. The right pulmonary artery courses under the ascending aorta and is visualized as a faint shadow with numerous fading branches. The azygos vein arches over the right main stem bronchus and connects to the superior vena cava. The upper left mediastinal border is composed of the prominent aortic arch (aortic knob), which tapers toward the mediastinum to a less prominent main pulmonary trunk. The left pulmonary artery projects laterally from the trunk and forms smaller branches. Below the pulmonary trunk, the superior left heart border is formed by the left atrial appendage and the lateral border of the left ventricle forms a convex or straight structure tapering to the left diaphragmatic border.

In the lateral projection, the lower third of the anterior border of the cardiac silhouette is formed by the apex and the outflow tract of the right ventricle, abutting in the lower quarter or third of the sternum and the anterior chest wall (Fig. 4-2). The upper two thirds is composed of the outflow portion of the right ventricle and the ascending aorta. The posterior wall of the left atrium forms most of the posterior border of the heart. Inferiorly, small portions of the right atrium and the inferior vena cava are profiled just above the diaphragm. Thus, with posteroanterior and lateral CXRs, the clinician can detect abnormalities directly and infer valvular or structural heart disease and abnormalities in the great vessels and the lungs.

Clinical Applications

Patients with heart disease may have any number of CXR abnormalities. The CXR is usually normal in uncomplicated coronary artery disease (CAD) but can help exclude aortic or lung disease in patients with chest pain. Coronary artery calcification on CXR correlates with significant obstructive disease, but the CXR is less sensitive than fluoroscopy or electron beam CT (see below) for detecting the presence of coronary artery calcification. The CXR can be abnormal when CAD is complicated by heart failure or a ventricular aneurysm. In patients with longstanding systemic arterial hypertension, secondary left ventricular hypertrophy can manifest as elongation of the cardiac silhouette along the left hemidiaphragm and a plump, or downwardly displaced, apex. There may be associated dilation of the aortic root and the left atrium.

Figure 4-1

Radiology and Angiocardiography

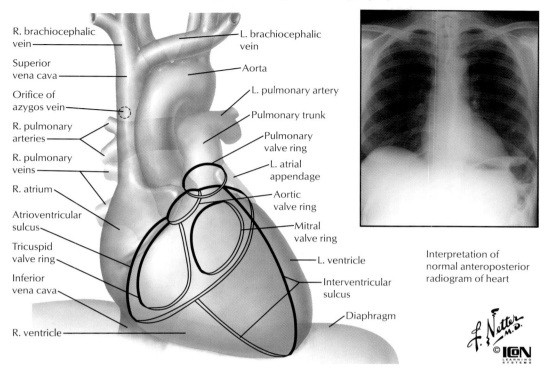

R. brachiocephalic vein

L. brachiocephalic vein

Superior vena cava

Aorta

Orifice of azygos vein

L. pulmonary artery

R. pulmonary arteries

Pulmonary trunk

R. pulmonary veins

Pulmonary valve ring

R. atrium

L. atrial appendage

Atrioventricular sulcus

Aortic valve ring

Tricuspid valve ring

Mitral valve ring

Inferior vena cava

L. ventricle

Interventricular sulcus

R. ventricle

Diaphragm

Interpretation of normal anteroposterior radiogram of heart

The CXR can also help confirm a diagnosis of valvular heart disease. For instance, in aortic stenosis, radiographic abnormalities include valvular calcification, poststenotic dilation of the aortic root and left ventricular hypertrophy. Chronic aortic regurgitation of significant degree causes left ventricular dilation. Mitral stenosis can result in radiographic evidence of valvular calcification, but surrounding soft-tissue densities make visualization difficult. A deliberately overpenetrated CXR can be useful in visualizing mitral valve calcification. However, because echocardiography is widely available and more sensitive in detecting valvular abnormalities, an overpenetrated CXR is rarely ordered today. Left atrial chamber dilation often can be detected as prominence of the left atrial appendage; marked left atrial enlargement can displace the border so that it becomes the most rightward cardiac structure, overlapping the right atrium and the superior vena cava. The two atrial structures, separated because of a small amount of interposed air-filled space in the pulmonary parenchyma, form a double density.

When associated pulmonary hypertension is present, mitral stenosis also causes pulmonary artery dilation. Chronic mitral regurgitation causes left atrial dilation and, when severe, left ventricular dilation.

The lateral CXR is the best view for distinguishing aortic and mitral valve calcification, and it is also useful for evaluating right ventricular and left atrial chamber dilation. Increased left ventricular size can be detected when the left ventricle extends posteriorly beyond the right atrium, forming the lower posterior heart border.

Coarctation of the aorta is commonly associated with radiographic signs of hypertension. The classic finding of "notching of ribs" 3 to 9 from dilated collateral internal mammary arteries is often also present. Tetralogy of Fallot commonly manifests as a "boot-shaped" heart, reflecting right ventricular hypertrophy; the aortic arch is right-sided in 25% of cases.

Because the pulmonary vessels are surrounded by lung, even minor changes in size and distribution (reflecting alterations in flow or pressure) are easily identified. The primary

Figure 4-2 **Radiology and Angiocardiography**

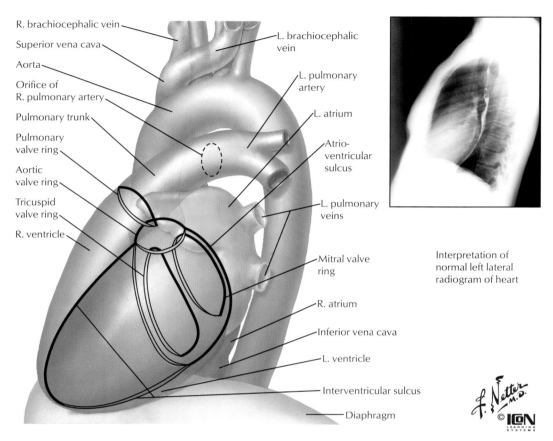

R. brachiocephalic vein
Superior vena cava
Aorta
Orifice of R. pulmonary artery
Pulmonary trunk
Pulmonary valve ring
Aortic valve ring
Tricuspid valve ring
R. ventricle

L. brachiocephalic vein
L. pulmonary artery
L. atrium
Atrio-ventricular sulcus
L. pulmonary veins
Mitral valve ring
R. atrium
Inferior vena cava
L. ventricle
Interventricular sulcus
Diaphragm

Interpretation of normal left lateral radiogram of heart

radiographic manifestation of left heart failure is pulmonary vasculature prominence, reflecting elevated left atrial filling pressure and pulmonary venous congestion. The lower-lobe peripheral vessels become less well defined and relatively small while the upper-lobe vessels remain well defined and increase in size. These changes become detectable when mean pulmonary venous pressure exceeds 15 mm Hg. As pressures rise to 20 mm Hg and above, fluid in the interlobular septa first appears at the lung bases, causing peripheral linear opacities perpendicular to the lateral pleural surface, the so-called Kerley's B lines. Pulmonary edema occurs when mean pulmonary venous pressure rises to 25 to 30 mm Hg and is typically a central, symmetric fluffy-appearing infiltrate with a butterfly appearance. Depending on etiology, generalized cardiomegaly or specific chamber enlargement can also occur.

Limitations

The CXR is limited because only the perimeter of the heart is visualized, because this technique does not differentiate between myocardium, valves, or blood pool, and because other methodologies are more accurate in assessing myocardial and valvular function.

COMPUTED TOMOGRAPHY

Since the development of CT, many applications and techniques have been pursued for patients with cardiovascular diseases, but applications in clinical practice have lagged behind investigative approaches. A major limitation of standard CT is that the scan acquisition time of 2 to 5 seconds results in limited resolution because of motion artifacts of the cardiac and respiratory cycles, even when corrected by "gating" the image to the cardiac cycle. This has led to the development of "spiral" or "helical" CT, where scan acquisition time is accelerated to 1 rotation per second. With this acceleration of acquisition time, spiral CT has become widely used for great vessel examination and evaluation of proximal pulmonary emboli. "Ultrafast" or electron beam CT (EBCT) has scan times of 50 msec. At this speed, the cardiac anatomy can be determined at high resolution in the beating heart. EBCT technology has been studied for evaluation of left ventricular wall mass, estimations of ejection fractions or stroke volumes, detection of wall thinning, and detection and quantitation of coronary calcification—as a surrogate marker for CAD.

Clinical Applications

Potential applications of standard CT include examination of the lungs for tumors or mass lesions, detection of pericardial disease, and examination of the great vessels and the pulmonary vasculature. In many of these areas, however, magnetic resonance imaging (MRI) has superseded CT (see below). CT with IV contrast is an excellent method for evaluating diseases of the aorta, such as aortic dissection or aneurysm. Because aortic dissection is life threatening and needs rapid diagnosis, many emergency departments prefer CT as an initial diagnostic approach. In addition, CT is a reliable, rapid, and widely used method for diagnosis of proximal pulmonary emboli. EBCT has emerged as a sensitive mode for evaluating the presence of coronary calcification. Because advanced coronary lesions generally contain calcium, detection (and quantitation) of coronary calcification by EBCT has been proposed as a noninvasive means of screening for CAD. The clinical application of EBCT screening for CAD has yet to be completely determined, as many coronary lesions that are lethal or clinically unstable are the softer, smaller plaques, lesions that are not calcium-rich. Cardiac tumors and pericardial disease may also be evaluated by CT. However echocardiography or cardiac MRI is superior for these pathologies.

Limitations

CT evaluation of the heart and the great vessels requires the use of IV contrast agents, which can be nephrotoxic. Patients with renal insufficiency or dye allergy require special precautions before they undergo imaging, but these problems are easily addressed. Although CT is an excellent method for imaging the aorta and the great vessels, standard CT, spiral CT, are EBCT not routinely used for evaluation of cardiac function. With rapid developments in MRI and echocardiography, the application of CT for cardiovascular imaging will likely be further limited in coming years.

ECHOCARDIOGRAPHY

Echocardiography is the most commonly used imaging technology for patients with cardiovascular disease. It utilizes high-frequency ultrasound to image cardiac and great vessel structure and blood flow. A complete transthoracic echocardiographic study includes the use of multiple ultrasound imaging methods, including M-mode, two-dimensional (2-D), and Doppler imaging.

Transthoracic 2-D echocardiography is the foundation of the clinical echocardiographic examination. Images from multiple planes (Fig. 4-3) provide reliable, portable, and reproducible evaluation of ventricular contractile performance, cardiac chamber sizes, valvular function, and pericardial disease. Doppler echocardiographic assessment of the direction and the velocity of blood flow within the heart is valuable in the detection and quantification of obstructive lesions and valvular regurgitation (Fig. 4-4). Transthoracic 2-D directed M-mode echocardiography is especially valuable in the evaluation of mitral and aortic valve motion in dynamic and fixed left ventricular outflow obstruction, in the timing of valve closure in aortic regurgitation, and in the assessment of pericardial disease. It also precisely measures cardiac chamber sizes and wall thickness and estimates left ventricular contractile performance.

Transesophageal echocardiography (TEE) can provide important complementary diagnostic information not available by transthoracic echocardiographic study and is used when better imaging of the heart or the great vessels is required. Exercise and pharmacologic stress echocardiography are very useful in the assessment of known or suspected CAD (see chapter 6).

Clinical Applications

Echocardiography is valuable in the assessment of coronary heart disease, even though the coronary arteries are not directly imaged. Echocardio-

Figure 4-3 **Transducer Positions in Echocardiographic Examination**

Parasternal position

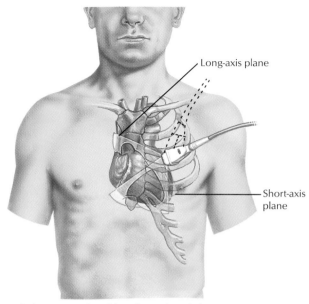

Long-axis plane

Short-axis plane

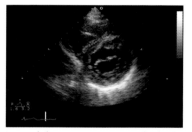

Normal long-axis view during systole

Normal short-axis view at mitral valve level

Left parasternal position allows views in long- and short-axis planes. Tilting transducer allows multiple sections.

Apical position

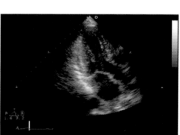

Normal apical long-axis view

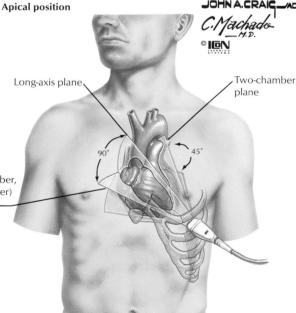

JOHN A. CRAIG, MD
C. Machado, M.D.
©ICON

Long-axis plane

Two-chamber plane

90°   45°

Transverse (four-chamber, five-chamber) plane

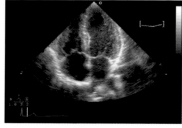

Normal apical four-chamber view

Apical studies imaged from point of maximal impulse toward base. Four-chamber plane passes through atrioventricular valves; upward tilt gives five-chamber plane. Counterclockwise rotation of 45° gives two-chamber plane. 90° rotation gives long-axis plane.

A

Figure 4-3 (cont.) **Transducer Positions in Echocardiographic Examination**

Subcostal position

Short-axis plane
(right ventricular
outflow)

90°

Four-chamber
plane

Subcostal position allows multiple short axis views;
90° rotation provides four-chamber view.

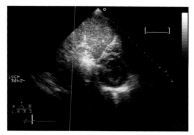

Subcostal short-axis view of the left
ventricle

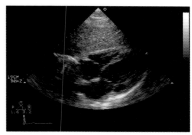

Subcostal four-chamber view

JOHN A. CRAIG—MD
C. Machado
—M.D.
©ICON
LEARNING
SYSTEMS

Suprasternal position

Plane gives sagittal section of aorta.

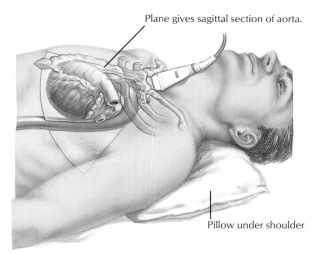

Pillow under shoulder

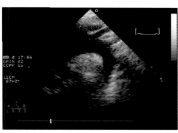

Suprasternal view of the aortic arch and
the origins of the left common carotid
and left subclavian

Suprasternal position uses plane of aortic arch to
provide views of aorta and mediastinum.

B

Figure 4-4

Principles of Doppler Echocardiography

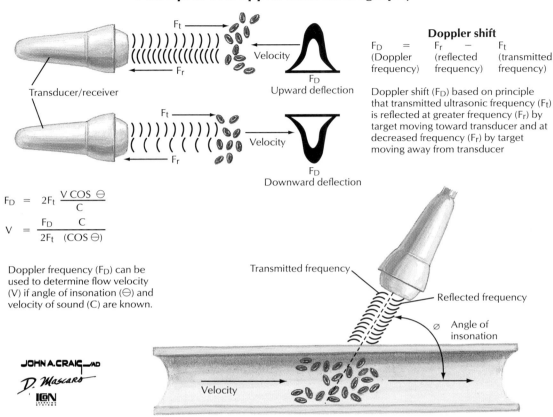

Transducer/receiver

F_t

Velocity

F_r

F_D

Upward deflection

F_t

Velocity

F_r

F_D

Downward deflection

Doppler shift

F_D	$=$	F_r	$-$	F_t
(Doppler frequency)		(reflected frequency)		(transmitted frequency)

Doppler shift (F_D) based on principle that transmitted ultrasonic frequency (F_t) is reflected at greater frequency (F_r) by target moving toward transducer and at decreased frequency (F_r) by target moving away from transducer

$$F_D = 2F_t \frac{V \cos \ominus}{C}$$

$$V = \frac{F_D}{2F_t} \frac{C}{(\cos \ominus)}$$

Doppler frequency (F_D) can be used to determine flow velocity (V) if angle of insonation ($\ominus$) and velocity of sound (C) are known.

Transmitted frequency

Reflected frequency

∅ Angle of insonation

Velocity

JOHN A. CRAIG—MD
D. Mascaro
IGN
LEARNING SYSTEMS

Dopper signal processing (waveform spectral analysis)

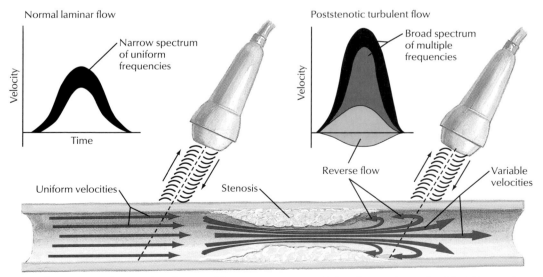

Normal laminar flow

Velocity

Narrow spectrum of uniform frequencies

Time

Uniform velocities

Stenosis

Poststenotic turbulent flow

Velocity

Broad spectrum of multiple frequencies

Reverse flow

Variable velocities

Laminar flow consists of zones of unidirectional flow of fairly uniform velocities, resulting in narrow Doppler spectral waveform of similar frequencies.

Turbulent flow made up of widely different velocities and reverse flow, creating waveform made up of broad spectrum of frequencies (spectral broadening)

graphic evidence of segmental ventricular contractile dysfunction is an excellent screen for
ischemic injury or infarction secondary to CAD.
However, the diagnosis of CAD is not absolute,
as segmental wall motion abnormalities can also
be caused by myocarditis and infiltrative myocardial diseases. In addition, multivessel CAD can
cause generally decreased ventricular contraction without segmental abnormalities, a circumstance generally necessitating further evaluation.

Echocardiography is the most reliable and
reproducible clinical laboratory method for the
initial diagnostic evaluation and follow-up of
patients with congenital and valvular heart disease, including the evaluation of right ventricular
and pulmonary arterial hypertension (see sections V and VIII). Anatomic information about the
nature of a congenital defect and its hemodynamic consequences, including the direction of
intracardiac shunts and pulmonary and systemic
flow, can be calculated by Doppler techniques.

In stenotic valvular lesions, M-mode techniques
are useful in assessing valvular thickness and
motion, ventricular chamber sizes and wall thickness measurements, and atrial chamber dimensions and in estimating the hemodynamic effects
of a valvular lesion. Transthoracic 2-D echocardiography shows a more complete picture of the
valvular, subvalvular, and annular structures, and
when 2-D echo is combined with Doppler ultrasound techniques, obstructive gradients can be
accurately measured and cross-sectional valve
area can be estimated. Regurgitant valvular
lesions can be accurately quantified by color flow
Doppler imaging (see also chapter 6). Clinical
decisions about medical therapy and operative
intervention for patients with valvular disease are
usually based on echocardiographic data, supplemented by information from cardiac catheterization. Echocardiography is the primary tool for
evaluating the presence and hemodynamic consequences of pericardial effusion. A thickened
pericardium and typical hemodynamic alterations can alert the clinician to the diagnosis of
pericardial constriction, but MRI and catheterization are usually needed for full evaluation. Analysis of Doppler-measured inflow into the ventricles
can be useful in differentiating between pericardial constriction and infiltrative cardiomyopathy
(see chapters 14 and 36).

In TEE, an ultrasound probe is passed into the
esophagus, posterior to the heart, to obtain
detailed images of the atria, the interatrial septum, the aorta, and the valvular structures. Proximity to the heart and absence of chest wall and
lung interference allow utilization of higher-fre-
quency ultrasound, yielding better resolution of
cardiac structures. TEE is most commonly
applied in the evaluation for atrial and ventricular septal defects, patent foramen ovale, valvular
vegetations, and atrial thrombus.

Echocardiographic stress testing, when combined with exercise stress testing or pharmacologic agents (usually dobutamine), is an accurate, noninvasive approach to determining the presence
and/or the severity of coronary heart disease. A
stress-induced segmental wall motion abnormality
usually indicates flow-limiting CAD. This technique
is more accurate than routine treadmill testing
across the spectrum of patients, including those
with single or multivessel CAD and those with normal or abnormal ECGs at rest. With advances in
echocardiographic imaging and because echocardiography is readily available and does not require
handling of radionuclides, the use of stress
echocardiography has expanded dramatically.

Limitations

Echocardiography is an operator-dependent
technique that requires considerable technical
skill, expertise, and patience on the part of the
physician or technician obtaining images. Image
acquisition is limited by obesity, chronic obstructive pulmonary disease, and patient discomfort
from chest wall injuries or recent surgery. Overall, however, echocardiography is relatively
inexpensive, portable, and well suited to many
settings. TEE is limited by its requirement of
sedation and esophageal intubation, and structural limitations prevent complete visualization
of the left ventricle. TEE is also more invasive and
carries with it the potential for complications,
including esophageal perforation and aspiration
of gastric contents.

NUCLEAR MYOCARDIAL PERFUSION IMAGING

Nuclear medicine imaging of the heart (also
called myocardial perfusion imaging [MPI]) utilizes
intravenously administered radiopharmaceuticals

to assess coronary blood flow to the myocardium. The radiopharmaceuticals used in MPI are taken up into the myocardium in proportion to blood flow. Images are usually taken after exercise or pharmacologic stress and compared with images taken at rest. In a normal study, there is homogeneous radiotracer uptake in the heart during stress and rest. Perfusion defects seen during stress that are either normal or better at rest are associated with myocardial ischemia (Fig. 4-5). Fixed perfusion defects in both the stress and the rest images that are associated with left ventricular focal wall motion defects are usually associated with scarring from a prior MI. Fixed perfusion defects with normal wall motion and thickening are usually attenuation artifacts caused by overlying breast or diaphragm. In addition to MPI studies, gated equilibrium radionuclide ventriculography studies can be performed to assess left ventricular performance. Analysis of the first-pass of a bolus of radiotracer can be used to evaluate right ventricular performance.

Clinical Applications

Myocardial perfusion imaging is well established as an effective clinical tool in the evaluation and management of CAD. It can be used to evaluate patients with either known or suspected CAD to assess for the presence, location, and severity of significant flow-limiting CAD. In patients who have had a prior myocardial infarction, MPI can be used to evaluate the size and severity of the infarct zone. Left ventricular ejection fractions can also be determined.

Like echocardiography, gated equilibrium radionuclide ventriculography is suited for determining left ventricular function and is particularly useful in patients who are difficult to image with echocardiography, as described above. In addition, gated equilibrium radionuclide ventriculography is often used to longitudinally assess left ventricular function in patients undergoing chemotherapy with cardiotoxic drugs and to evaluate the management of patients with congestive heart failure. Various parameters such as left ventricular ejection fraction, regional wall motion, heart volumes, and peak filling rate are measurable and quantifiable using this technique.

Limitations

Occasionally, obese patients or patients with breast implants are difficult to image using MPI or radionuclide ventriculography. More commonly, the converse is true; nuclear medicine approaches can be used in patients who are difficult to image by other techniques. Although image acquisition is easily standardized, image analysis software varies considerably and data interpretation from different centers may not be comparable, so careful interpretation is essential.

MAGNETIC RESONANCE IMAGING

Magnetic resonance imaging is an emerging technology in diagnostic cardiovascular imaging (Table 4-1). Magnetic resonance image acquisition relies on the interaction of hydrogen nuclei with an external magnetic field. An intrinsic property of hydrogen nuclei is their alignment with an applied static magnetic field. These magnetic moments precess about the applied magnetic field at a frequency called the Lamour frequency. When radiofrequency pulses tuned to the Lamour frequency are applied, the protons become "excited" and the net orientation of the magnetization of the nuclei deviates

Table 4-1
Common Cardiovascular Applications of MRI

· Measurement of right and left ventricular volume, mass, ejection fraction, and stroke volume.

· Pericardial thickness and visualization of pericardial cysts, and pericardial effusions.

· Cardiac tumors and masses.

· Specific for evaluation of right ventricular dysplasia.

· Evaluation and diagnosis of congenital heart disease.

· Excellent imaging method for the aorta and its major branches.

· Detection of coronary artery stenosis.
   Coronary MRA using IV contrast can detect proximal and middle vessel atherosclerotic stenosis in the coronary arteries.
   Left main and three-vessel disease can be reliably ruled out by MRA.

· Flow velocity measurement.

· Direct visualization of infarcts using delayed hyperenhancements.

MRA indicates magnetic resonance angiography.

Figure 4-5

Stress Nuclear Imaging

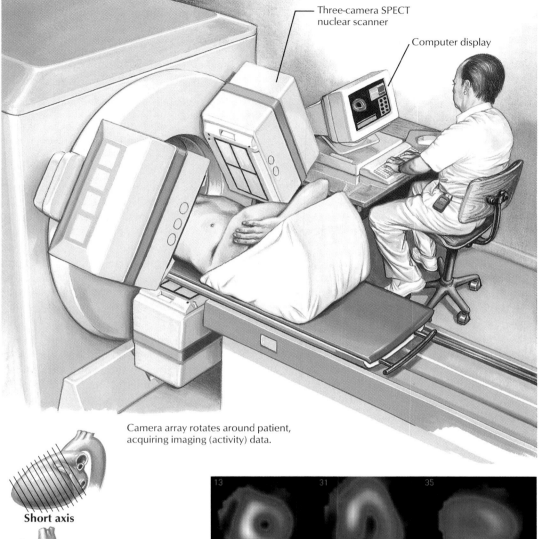

Three-camera SPECT nuclear scanner

Computer display

Camera array rotates around patient, acquiring imaging (activity) data.

Short axis

Horizontal long axis

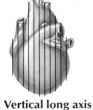

Vertical long axis

JOHN A. CRAIG—MD
C. Machado
—M.D.
© ICON
LEARNING SYSTEMS

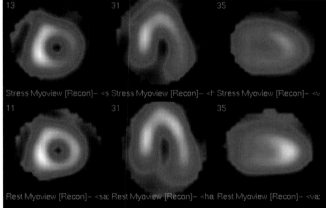

Computer reconstructs acquired image data into a series of tomographic slices displayed in three standard views: short axis, horizontal long axis, and vertical long axis.

Figure 4-6

Imaging Planes Used for MRI

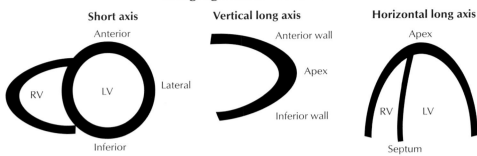

from alignment with the external magnetic field. In the presence of magnetic field gradients, the return of magnetization to equilibrium is measured. A magnetic resonance image is acquired by performing many repetitions of the above using different radiofrequency and gradient waveforms and is not a single snapshot of the imaged structure. In cardiac imaging, the signal must be gated to the electrocardiogram. Fast spin-echo and cine-gradient techniques are complementary methods for morphologic and functional heart evaluation. Standard imaging planes are the short axis, the horizontal axis, and vertical long axis (Fig. 4-6).

Clinical Applications

The use of MRI for cardiovascular imaging will likely increase, as it has for central nervous system, joint, and orthopedic imaging. The difference in contrast between flowing blood and the myocardium provides excellent visualization of the endocardium.

Limitations

Many patients with heart disease have pacemakers or internal defibrillators that preclude safe evaluation with MRI. Most valvular prostheses and intracoronary stents are not contraindications to MRI but may cause artifacts that obscure image quality. Coronary stents should be in place for 6 weeks before patients undergo MRI. Well-secured valves without dehiscence are safe, with the exception of older, Starr-Edwards valves. Because images are gated to the cardiac cycle, irregular heart rhythms (such as atrial fibrillation or frequent premature atrial or ventricular contractions) negatively affect image quality. The usual limitations of MRI, including claustrophobia and obesity, also apply to cardiac studies.

FUTURE DIRECTIONS

The role of cardiac imaging in the evaluation of cardiac disease will likely continue to expand. Imaging techniques are generally safe and increasingly provide valuable decision-making information. Novel approaches in echocardiography are becoming clinically useful. Three-dimensional echocardiography is available at many university centers. Myocardial contrast echocardiography has primarily been used in research, but it can evaluate the integrity of postinfarction microcirculation. PET scanning for myocardial viability is used with radiolabeled glucose to detect viable myocardium after infarction. Radiolabeled NH_4 has also been used for viability testing. New multidetector CT scanners can have temporal resolution as low as 65 msec, which results in fewer motion artifacts for evaluation of the heart and the vasculature, including coronary artery imaging. Finally, MRI is expected to make a significant impact in clinical use, with the potential to detect coronary stenosis, ischemia during stress, and myocardial viability in addition to providing valvular and functional information with a single imaging modality.

REFERENCES

Kim WY, Darias PG, Stuber M, et al. Coronary magnetic resonance angiography for the detection of coronary stenosis. *N Engl J Med* 2001;345:1863–1869.

Rumberger JA, Breen JF, Johnston DL. Magnetic resonance imaging and computed tomography of the heart and great vessels. In: Murphy JG, ed. *Mayo Clinic Cardiology Review.* New York: Lippincott, Williams & Wilkins; 2000:743–769.

Steiner RM. Radiology of the heart and great vessels. In: Braunwald E, Zipes DP, Libby P, eds. *Heart Disease: A Textbook of Cardiovascular Disease.* 6th ed. New York: Saunders; 2001:237–273.

Chapter 5

Diagnostic Coronary Angiography

George A. Stouffer

The ability to directly visualize coronary arteries was a seminal advance in the history of modern medicine and led directly to the development of the concept of transluminal angioplasty (first performed by Charles Dotter in 1964), CABG (first performed by Rene Favaloro in 1967), percutaneous transluminal peripheral angioplasty (first performed by Andreas Gruentzig in 1974), and percutaneous transluminal coronary angioplasty (first performed by Andreas Gruentzig in 1977). With the high prevalence of coronary heart disease (CHD) in industrialized countries and the advances made in its treatment, the use of diagnostic coronary angiography has continued to increase. In 2000, approximately 2,000,000 cardiac catheterizations were performed in the United States. This chapter focuses on the coronary anatomy and the technique of coronary angiography and its clinical use.

CORONARY ANATOMY AND ANOMALIES

The right coronary artery (RCA) arises from the right coronary sinus and runs in the right AV groove (Fig. 5-1). Generally, the conus artery and the sinoatrial artery arise from the RCA. In approximately 85% of individuals, the posterior descending coronary artery arises from the RCA (defined as a right dominant coronary circulation). The left main coronary artery arises from the left coronary sinus. Within a few centimeters of its origin, it divides into the left anterior descending (LAD) coronary artery (in the anterior interventricular groove), the left circumflex coronary artery (in the atrioventricular groove) and, in a minority of cases, a ramus intermedius artery.

Coronary artery anomalies are found in 1 to 1.5% of individuals (Fig. 5-2); most anomalies are benign. The most common anomaly is separate origins from the aorta of the LAD and left circumflex (i.e., absence of a left main coronary artery), which occurs in 0.4 to 1% of individuals and is occasionally associated with a bicuspid aortic valve. Clinically significant anomalies include origin of a coronary artery from the opposite coronary sinus (e.g., left main artery originating from the right coronary sinus), the presence of a single coronary ostium (and hence a single coronary artery), and origin of a coronary artery from the pulmonary artery.

TECHNIQUES

Coronary angiography delineates the course and size of the coronary arteries, identifies coronary anomalies, and provides information on the location and degree of any obstruction (Table 5-1). Coronary angiography is performed by injecting radiopaque contrast dye directly into the ostium of the left and right coronary arteries. Access to the aorta is usually gained via percutaneous puncture of the femoral artery; however brachial, radial, and axillary arteries can also be used for arterial access. Specific preformed catheters are passed over a guide wire into the aortic root; the selection of the catheter to be used depends on the access site and the coronary artery being investigated. The wire is removed and the coronary artery is cannulated with use of fluoroscopic guidance. Contrast dye is injected during cineradiography while blood pressure and ECG are continually monitored and sequential frames are recorded.

Complete evaluation of coronary arteries involves angiography in multiple projections (Figs. 5-3 and 5-4), necessitated by the difficulty of visualizing three-dimensional structures in two dimensions. These views are obtained by rotating the imaging system to different positions around the patient who lies supine on a radiolucent table. Views from the left or the right of the patient can be obtained by varying the degrees of angle. The imaging system can also be rotated from head (cranial) to toe (caudal)

INTRODUCTION

Figure 5-1   Coronary Arteries and Cardiac Veins

Sternocostal surface

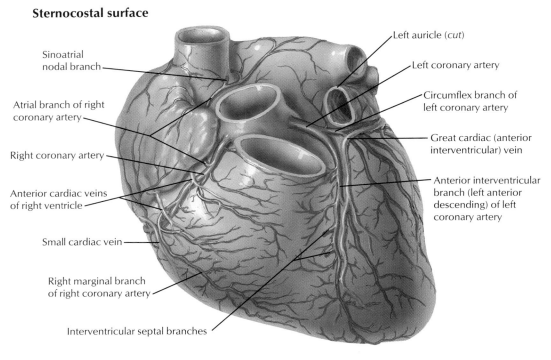

Sinoatrial nodal branch

Atrial branch of right coronary artery

Right coronary artery

Anterior cardiac veins of right ventricle

Small cardiac vein

Right marginal branch of right coronary artery

Interventricular septal branches

Left auricle (*cut*)

Left coronary artery

Circumflex branch of left coronary artery

Great cardiac (anterior interventricular) vein

Anterior interventricular branch (left anterior descending) of left coronary artery

Diaphragmatic surface

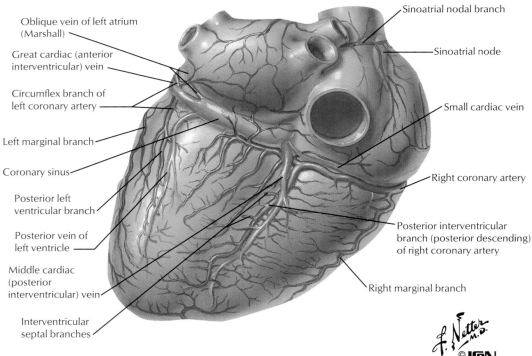

Oblique vein of left atrium (Marshall)

Great cardiac (anterior interventricular) vein

Circumflex branch of left coronary artery

Left marginal branch

Coronary sinus

Posterior left ventricular branch

Posterior vein of left ventricle

Middle cardiac (posterior interventricular) vein

Interventricular septal branches

Sinoatrial nodal branch

Sinoatrial node

Small cardiac vein

Right coronary artery

Posterior interventricular branch (posterior descending) of right coronary artery

Right marginal branch

Figure 5-2

Coronary Arteries and Cardiac Veins: Variations

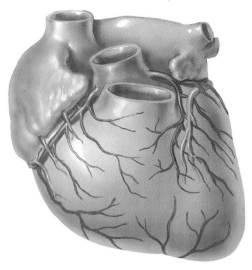

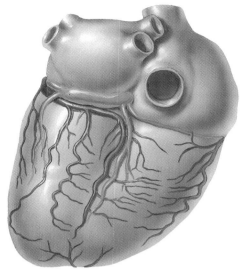

Anterior interventricular (left anterior descending) branch of left coronary artery very short. Apical part of anterior (sternocostal) surface supplied by branches from posterior interventricular (posterior descending) branch of right coronary artery curving around apex.

Posterior interventricular (posterior descending) branch derived from circumflex branch of left coronary artery instead of from right coronary artery

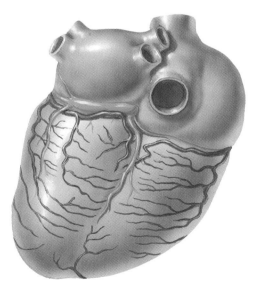

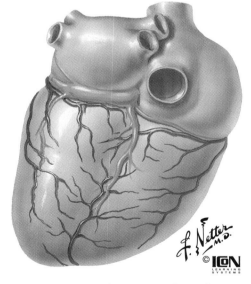

Posterior interventricular (posterior descending) branch absent. Area supplied chiefly by small branches from circumflex branch of left coronary artery and from right coronary artery.

Posterior interventricular (posterior descending) branch absent. Area supplied chiefly by elongated anterior interventricular (left anterior descending) branch curving around apex.

Figure 5-3

Coronary Arteries: Arteriographic Views

Left coronary artery: Left anterior oblique veiw

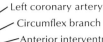

Left coronary artery

Circumflex branch

Anterior interventricular branch
(left anterior descending)

Diagonal branches of anterior
interventricular branch

Atrioventricular branch of circumflex branch

Left marginal branch

Posterolateral branches

(Perforating) interventricular septal branches

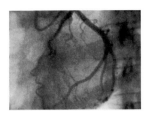

Arteriogram

Left coronary artery: Right anterior oblique view

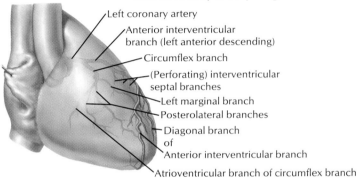

Left coronary artery

Anterior interventricular
branch (left anterior descending)

Circumflex branch

(Perforating) interventricular
septal branches

Left marginal branch

Posterolateral branches

Diagonal branch
of
Anterior interventricular branch

Atrioventricular branch of circumflex branch

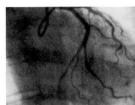

Arteriogram

Right coronary artery: Left anterior oblique view

Sinoatrial (SA) nodal branch

Right coronary artery

Atrioventricular (AV) nodal branch

Branches to back of left ventricle

Right marginal branch

Posterior interventricular branch
(posterior descending artery)

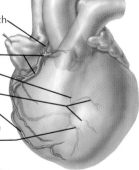

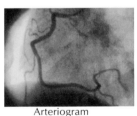

Arteriogram

Right coronary artery: Right anterior oblique view

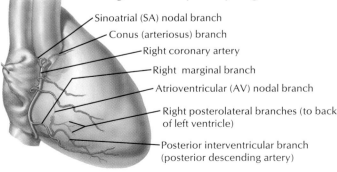

Sinoatrial (SA) nodal branch

Conus (arteriosus) branch

Right coronary artery

Right marginal branch

Atrioventricular (AV) nodal branch

Right posterolateral branches (to back
of left ventricle)

Posterior interventricular branch
(posterior descending artery)

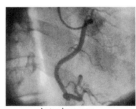

Arteriogram

Figure 5-4

Coronary Angiography

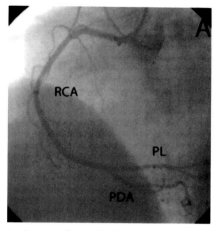

Angiogram of normal right coronary artery (RCA) and normal posterolateral (PL) and posterior descending (PDA) branches

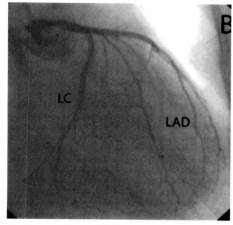

Angiogram of normal left anterior descending coronary artery (LAD) and left circumflex (LC) artery

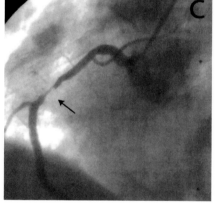

Angiographic demonstration of narrowing of RCA

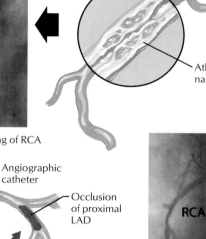

Angiographic catheter

RCA

Atherosclerotic narrowing of RCA

Angiographic catheter

Dye injection of RCA

Occlusion of proximal LAD

RCA

Collateral vessels

LAD

Angiogram demonstrating filling of LAD by dye injected into RCA via collateral vessels

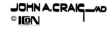

JOHN A. CRAIG—MD
© ICN

Table 5-1
Information Provided by Selective Coronary Angiography

- Origin of major coronary arteries
- Size of coronary arteries
- Course of coronary arteries
- Branches originating from large and medium coronary arteries
- Degree and location of lumen irregularities
- Presence of fistulas
- Presence of collaterals
- Presence of bridging
- Presence of large thrombus
- Aneurysms
- Spasm and response to nitroglycerin
- Coronary plaques—location, degree of narrowing, eccentricity, involvement of side branches, length

positions. Although there is an almost limitless combination of potential imaging positions, several standard approaches have been developed (as described herein) that allow full visualization of the coronary arteries in most patients.

In all cases, multiple views help to avoid foreshortening of specific areas and the potentially confounding feature of overlapping branches, and are obtained using caudal or cranial angulation in combination with left and right angulation. The most commonly used views for left coronary angiography include right anterior oblique (RAO) with cranial and caudal angulation, and left anterior oblique (LAO) with cranial and caudal angulation. The most commonly used views for RCA angiography include right anterior oblique and left anterior oblique projections with or without cranial angulation. Individual variation in coronary anatomy or location of stenoses often necessitates customization of projections. Standard nomenclature to define coronary segments has been developed by several groups, including the Coronary Artery Surgery Study investigators and the Bypass Angioplasty Revascularization Investigation investigators.

The usual method of analyzing angiograms in clinical practice identifies areas of relative narrowing, and then quantifies the degree of narrowing by comparing the minimal diameter of the narrowed coronary segment with that of an adjacent, normal-appearing reference segment. In many angiography suites, experienced observers estimate the degree of stenosis; however, stenosis can be quantified using calipers or quantitative computer angiography. Because atherosclerotic plaques are often eccentric, orthogonal views are needed to accurately determine the degree of obstruction.

Flow in coronary arteries can be estimated at the time of coronary angiography with a scale developed by the Thrombolysis in Myocardial Infarction (TIMI) investigators. Flow defined as TIMI 0 indicates a completely occluded artery. TIMI 1 flow describes a severe lesion in which dye passes the area of narrowing but does not extend to the distal portion of the vessel. With TIMI 2 flow, the distal vessel is opacified but not as rapidly as would be expected or as rapidly as nonobstructed vessels. TIMI 3 flow is "normal." The TIMI flow index has shown significant prognostic value. TIMI "frame counts," the number of frames necessary for dye to reach the distal portion of the vessel, are used as a quantitative index of flow.

Microvascular integrity can be assessed at the time of coronary angiography with use of angiographic myocardial blush scores. These scores, which measure contrast dye density and washout in the area of interest, correlate with LV functional recovery post-MI, and prognosis. In the setting of acute MI, myocardial blush scores add additional prognostic information to TIMI frame score and persistent ST elevation.

Coronary angiography can be performed separately or as part of cardiac catheterization or an interventional procedure. Most patients referred for diagnostic angiography also undergo left-sided heart catheterization and left ventriculography. Increasingly, these patients also undergo angiography of other vascular beds, as indicated. For example, patients with hypertension commonly undergo renal angiography; those with claudication undergo lower extremity artery angiography; and those with left internal mammary artery grafting to the LAD coronary artery undergo subclavian angiography (Fig. 5-5).

INDICATIONS

The most common indication for coronary angiography is to determine the presence, location, and severity of atherosclerotic lesions. Coronary angiography provides essential infor-

Figure 5-5

Angiographic Demonstration of Subclavian Steal

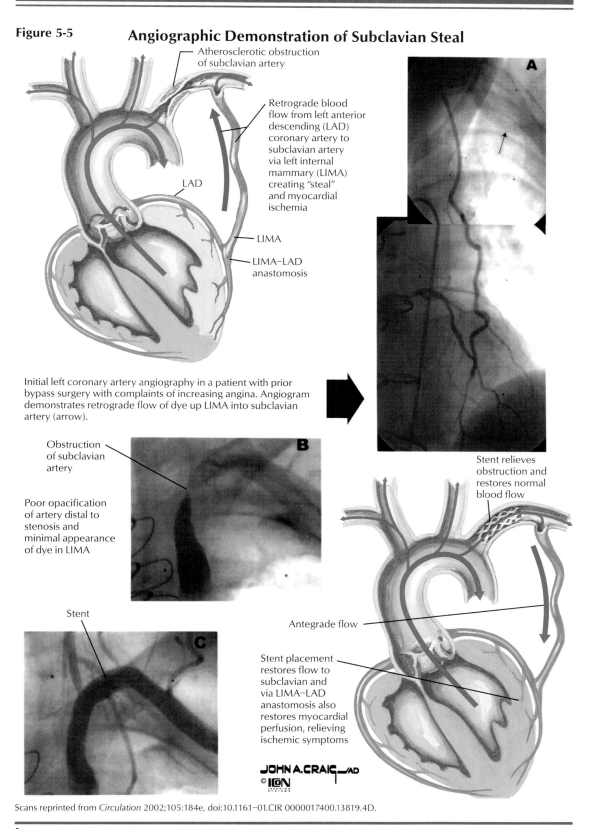

Atherosclerotic obstruction of subclavian artery

Retrograde blood flow from left anterior descending (LAD) coronary artery to subclavian artery via left internal mammary (LIMA) creating "steal" and myocardial ischemia

LAD

LIMA

LIMA–LAD anastomosis

Initial left coronary artery angiography in a patient with prior bypass surgery with complaints of increasing angina. Angiogram demonstrates retrograde flow of dye up LIMA into subclavian artery (arrow).

Obstruction of subclavian artery

Poor opacification of artery distal to stenosis and minimal appearance of dye in LIMA

Stent

Stent relieves obstruction and restores normal blood flow

Antegrade flow

Stent placement restores flow to subclavian and via LIMA–LAD anastomosis also restores myocardial perfusion, relieving ischemic symptoms

JOHN A. CRAIG ᴀᴅ
© ICN

Scans reprinted from *Circulation* 2002;105:184e, doi:10.1161–01.CIR 0000017400.13819.4D.

Table 5-2
Indications for Coronary Angiography

Percent of Patients	No. Patients (%)
Exertional Angina	51
Non–Q-wave MI	18
Congestive heart failure	9
Primary treatment of ST-elevation MI	7
Valvular heart disease	6
Cardiogenic shock	2
ST elevation post administration of thrombolytic agents (rescue angioplasty)	1
Miscellaneous	6
Annual evaluation after heart transplantation	
Hypertrophic cardiomyopathy with chest pain	
Constrictive pericarditis	
Congenital heart disease	
Preoperative evaluation for proximal aortic and/or aortic arch aneurysm repair	
Preoperative assessment for aortic dissection repair	
Evaluation prior to heart, lung, or liver transplantation	
Ventricular arrhythmias and/or survival of sudden cardiac death	
Abnormal stress tests in high-risk occupations (e.g., pilot)	
Postrevascularization ischemia	
Prospective heart transplant donor whose age and risk factor profile suggests the possibility of coronary artery disease	
Patient who is at high risk for coronary disease when other cardiac surgical procedures (e.g., pericardectomy) are planned	

The percentages reflect the relative volume at the University of North Carolina based on a random sample of 100 consecutive patients. MI indicates myocardial infarction.

mation in the diagnosis of CAD, in determining prognosis, and in decision-making regarding revascularization. Neither percutaneous coronary intervention nor CABG can occur without coronary angiography. More rarely, coronary angiography is used to diagnose anomalies, muscular bridging, fistula, spasm, emboli, aneurysms, and arteritis.

Indications for coronary angiography in a random sample of 100 consecutive patients at the University of North Carolina are listed in Table 5-2. The most common indication was for evaluation of symptomatic CAD—either stable angina or acute coronary syndrome. Less common indications include valvular heart disease; congestive heart failure; evaluation before heart, lung or liver transplant; periodic evaluation after heart transplant; and congenital heart disease. Indications for coronary angiography not included on this list are being a sudden cardiac death survivor, history of ventricular tachycardia, abnormal results of stress tests in high-risk occupations (e.g., pilot or bus driver), history of postrevascularization ischemia, and being a prospective heart transplant donor whose age and risk factor profile suggest possible CAD.

USE OF CORONARY ANGIOGRAPHY IN THE EVALUATION OF PATIENTS WITH CHEST PAIN—CLINICAL PRACTICE

The American Heart Association and American College of Cardiology publish guidelines on the indications for coronary angiography (http://circ.ahajournals.org/cgi/content/full/99/17/2345). Use of coronary angiography in specific conditions is assigned a rating (Table 5-3) of the weight of evidence that (1) supports the indication (class I and IIa), (2) argues against the indication (class III), or (3) is insufficient to support or refute the indication (class IIb). Because there are risks associated with coronary angiography, patients with class III indications should rarely, if ever, undergo the procedure. Referral for angiography with class II indications is a decision that involves the preferences of the referring physician and the patient; many patients with class IIa indications are referred for angiography, whereas it is less common for patients with class IIb indications to undergo coronary angiography. Despite the guidelines, marked differences exist in practice patterns among individual physicians, geographic regions within the United States, and different countries. In some areas, coronary angiography is considered to be the standard of care for particular conditions, whereas noninvasive approaches are favored elsewhere.

The two most important issues in the evaluation of patients with suspected ischemic chest pain are the identification of the extent of CAD and the delineation of LV function. This can be done either directly (e.g., cardiac catheterization) or indirectly (e.g., exercise treadmill testing). If patients have stable, exertional symptoms, an exercise treadmill test can provide diagnostic and prognostic information. In addition to ECG findings, the test provides information on symptoms during exercise, blood pressure response, and duration of exercise. Combining ECG monitoring with either nuclear imaging (to determine myocardial perfusion) or echocardiographic imaging (to determine LV function) during exercise enhances the sensitivity and specificity of treadmill testing (see chapters 4 and 6). Imaging is essential in patients in whom the ECG response cannot be interpreted (e.g., left bundle branch block or Wolfe-Parkin-

Table 5-3
Summary of AHA/ACC Classification Regarding Appropriateness of Procedures

Class	Definition
I	There is evidence and/or general agreement that coronary angiography is useful and effective.
IIa	There is conflicting evidence and/or a divergence of opinion about the usefulness/efficacy of performing coronary angiography, but the weight of evidence/opinion is in favor of usefulness/efficacy.
IIb	There is conflicting evidence and/or a divergence of opinion about the usefulness/efficacy of performing coronary angiography, with the usefulness/efficacy of coronary angiography being less well-established by evidence/opinion.
III	There is evidence and/or general agreement that the procedure is not useful/effective and in some cases may be harmful.

With permission from *J Am Coll Cardiol* 1999; 33:1756–1903. Table created using data in text ACC/AHA Guidelines for Coronary Angiography.

son-White syndrome). It is also extremely helpful in situations in which the sensitivity and/or specificity of exercise ECG is reduced, for example, in middle-aged females or concomitant with LV hypertrophy. Pharmacologic stress testing coupled with imaging is available for patients unable to exercise.

Evidence for flow-limiting CAD on stress testing is an indication to proceed to coronary angiography. Occasionally, further evaluation is not needed if patient symptoms are controlled by medical therapy and if information from the stress test (e.g., duration of exercise, extent of ischemia) suggests that patient prognosis is good. Rarely, patients with normal results of stress tests are referred for coronary angiography. These are patients with typical symptoms in whom results of the stress test are thought to be falsely negative.

In selected patients with stable symptoms and in all patients with unstable symptoms, cardiac catheterization is performed without prior stress testing. Included in this group are patients with symptoms highly typical of angina, congestive heart failure, prior MI, and prior revascularization and/or with symptoms at a low level of exertion (class III or IV). In addition, patients with unstable symptoms should be referred directly for catheterization. In particular, patients with unstable angina, recent non–Q-wave MI or acute ST-elevation MI should be referred for urgent or emergent angiography, with possible use of percutaneous intervention (see chapter 8).

CONTRAINDICATIONS

The only absolute contraindication to coronary angiography is lack of patient consent. However, relative contraindications reflect greatly increased associated risks in certain conditions. Acute renal failure or severe preexisting renal dysfunction, especially in diabetic individuals, identifies patients at high risk for contrast-induced nephropathy. Severe coagulopathy, active bleeding, or both limit the ability to anticoagulate the blood of patients for interventional procedures and increase the risk of vascular complications. Decompensated heart failure can lead to respiratory failure when the patient is required to remain supine during the procedure. Electrolyte abnormalities and/or digitalis toxicity can predispose the patient to malignant arrhythmias during contrast injection. Other relative contraindications include patient inability to cooperate, active infection, allergy to contrast agents, uncontrolled hypertension, severe peripheral vascular disease, and pregnancy.

LIMITATIONS

Coronary angiography outlines the lumen of the vessel but is unable to provide any information on wall thickness. Proper interpretation of stenosis severity involves identification of an appropriate reference segment with which to compare the abnormal section. Furthermore, even with the identification of a proper reference section, studies have shown that experienced observers are limited in their ability to consistently identify hemodynamically significant coronary stenoses.

These limitations have led to the development of technologies to supplement coronary angiography, including intravascular ultrasound and pressure wire analysis. Intravascular ultrasound provides two-dimensional cross-sectional images in which the three layers of the vessel (intima, media, and adventitia) can frequently be identified (see chapter 2). Luminal cross-sectional area, wall thickness, and plaque area can be identified and quantified. Additionally, calcium, thrombus, and dissection planes can be imaged. Intravascular ultrasound is clinically useful in the assessment of complex coronary lesions, left main coronary artery lesions, and results of interventional procedures.

Advances in technology have enabled pressure transducers to be attached to 0.014-in angioplasty wires, allowing determination of intracoronary pressure distal to coronary stenoses. By comparing distal coronary pressure with aortic pressure at rest and during conditions of maximal coronary hyperemia, fractional flow reserve can be calculated. Determination of fractional flow reserve is clinically useful in assessment of intermediate lesions (i.e., coronary lesions of unclear significance angiographically) and determination of adequate balloon angioplasty and/or stent placement.

COMPLICATIONS

The risk of major complications during coronary angiography, defined as death, MI, or stroke, is approximately 0.3%. If the definition is expanded to include vascular complications, arrhythmias, and contrast reactions, the rate is still less than 2%. Conditions that increase risk include shock, acute coronary syndrome, renal failure, left main CAD, severe valvular disease, increased age, peripheral vascular disease, prior anaphylactoid reaction to contrast media, and congestive heart failure. The risks of cardiac catheterization with coronary angiography are outlined in Table 5-4. Complication rates were remarkably consistent across registries from the 1980s. More recent registries have focused on complications associated with coronary interventions.

FUTURE DIRECTIONS

During the 40 years that diagnostic cardiac catheterization has been performed, continual

Table 5-4
Complications of Coronary Angiography

Year	1982	1989	1990
N	53,581	222,553	59,792
Death, %	0.14	0.10	0.11
MI, %	0.07	0.06	0.05
CVA, %	0.07	0.07	0.07
Arrhythmia, %	0.56	0.47	0.38
Vascular, %	0.57	0.46	0.43
Total, %	1.82	1.74	1.70

Rates of complications of coronary angiography and cardiac catherization as reported by registries of the Society for Cardiac Angiography and Intervention.

CVA indicates cerebrovascular accident or stroke; MI, myocardial infarction.

With permission from Kennedy JW. Complications associated with cardiac catheterization and angiography. *Cathet Cardiovasc Diagn* 1982;8:5–11; Johnson LW, Lozner EC, Johnson S, et al. Coronary arteriography 1984–1987: A report of the Registry of the Society for Cardiac Angiography and Interventions. I. Results and complications. *Cathet Cardiovasc Diagn* 1989;17:5–10; and Noto TJ Jr, Johnson LW, Krone R, et al. Cardiac catheterization 1990: A report of the Registry of the Society for Cardiac Angiography and Interventions (SCA&I). *Cathet Cardiovasc Diagn* 1991;24:75–83.

modifications of catheters, imaging approaches, and points of access have enabled the procedure to be performed more quickly and safely. Many investigators are now examining whether noninvasive approaches to coronary artery imaging (based on improvements in MRI or CT) will lessen the need for, or even replace, diagnostic coronary angiography. Regardless of whether it is the routine use of noninvasive imaging or further modifications of invasive imaging, one can be certain that further reduction in the morbidity and mortality rates associated with defining coronary anatomy will be achieved.

REFERENCES

Alderman EL, Stadius ML. The angiographic definitions of the Bypass Angioplasty Revascularization Investigation (BARI). *Coron Artery Dis* 1992;3:1189–1207.

Angelini P, Velasco JA, Flamm S. Coronary anomalies: Incidence, pathophysiology, and clinical relevance. *Circulation* 2002;105:2449–2454.

Gibson CM, Cannon CP, Murphy SA, et al. Relationship of TIMI myocardial perfusion grade to mortality after administration of thrombolytic drugs. *Circulation* 2000;101:124–130.

Pijls NH, de Bruyne B, Peels K, et al. Measurement of fractional flow reserve to assess the functional severity of coronary-artery stenoses. *N Engl J Med* 1996;334:1703–1708.

Poli A, Fetiveau R, Vandoni P, et al. Integrated analysis of myocardial blush and ST-segment elevation recovery after successful primary angioplasty: Real-time grading of microvascular reperfusion and prediction of early and late recovery of left ventricular function. *Circulation* 2002;106:313–318.

Ringqvist I, Fisher LD, Mock M, et al: Prognostic value of angiographic indices of coronary artery disease from the Coronary Artery Surgery Study (CASS). *J Clin Invest* 1983;71:1854–1866.

Scanlon PJ, Faxon DP, Audet AM, et al: ACC/AHA guidelines for coronary angiography. A report of the American College of Cardiology/American Heart Association Task Force on practice guidelines (Committee on Coronary Angiography). Developed in collaboration with the Society for Cardiac Angiography and Interventions. *J Am Coll Cardiol* 1999;33:1756–1824.

Sheehan FH, Braunwald E, Canner P, et al: The effect of intravenous thrombolytic therapy on left ventricular function: A report on tissue-type plasminogen activator and streptokinase from the Thrombolysis in Myocardial Infarction (TIMI Phase I) trial. *Circulation* 1987;75:817–829.

Chapter 6

Use of Diagnostic Testing

Anthony Mathur and Peter Mills

The physician confronted with a patient with suspected cardiovascular disease has a multitude of tests available to provide diagnostic and prognostic information. Chapters 3, 4, and 5 describe the various modalities for diagnosing cardiovascular diseases. This chapter focuses on the selection of the most appropriate test for individual patients.

Generally, the available cardiovascular diagnostic tests can be divided into two categories: tests that assess anatomy and tests that assess function. These categories are merging, as tests once used solely for anatomic purposes are modified to also assess function. The choice of test depends not only on the question being asked but also on the cost-effectiveness and predictive value of the test and the relative value of anatomic versus functional information. An anatomic assessment (using a test validated by comparison with coronary angiography) may be useful in some settings, but it does not eliminate the need for a functional assessment, which may be even more predictive of a patient's prognosis and need for further intervention. Thus, new imaging techniques must be carefully evaluated for accuracy, ability to provide the needed information, and cost-effectiveness compared to pre-existing methods of obtaining similar information. It should be noted that the initial description of the sensitivity and specificity of a diagnostic test may overestimate what can be achieved in practice. Initial publications usually describe the assessment of a diagnostic test under rigorous conditions by experienced operators in a highly selected population. The true measure of a test is its ability to produce reliable information in an everyday clinical environment.

This chapter reviews the available tests that most frequently provide diagnostic, prognostic, and cost-effective information in the evaluation of patients with suspected cardiovascular disease.

DIAGNOSTIC TESTS
Electrocardiography
The resting ECG is the most frequently performed investigation in evaluating patients with cardiovascular disease (see chapter 3). Electrocardiography is a highly versatile diagnostic test; it can provide information on a broad spectrum of clinical conditions, ranging from metabolic disturbances (e.g., hypo- and hyperkalemia) and pharmacologic toxicity to ischemic heart disease (e.g., acute myocardial infarction, unstable angina), arrhythmia, and pericardial disease (see chapter 3). With such versatility, this simple-to-perform test is cost-effective.

In the investigation of arrhythmias, Holter electrocardiographic monitoring augments the resting ECG by allowing the correlation of a patient's symptoms to the rhythm disturbance and the subsequent monitoring of the patient's response to treatment. Continuous ST-segment monitoring also collects prognostic data on patients who have had a coronary event.

Exercise electrocardiography is a relatively inexpensive investigation used in the diagnosis and management of coronary artery disease (CAD). However, with a sensitivity of approximately 67% and a specificity of 84% for the detection of significant CAD in an optimal setting (and much lower accuracy reported in other settings), the main value of exercise electrocardiography lies in excluding CAD in patients who have a low pretest likelihood of significant coronary stenoses. The choice of exercise electrocardiography to exclude CAD in a patient with a high prior probability (including multiple risk factors and a classic history of effort-induced angina; see chapter 1) would be neither useful to the patient nor cost-effective.

Echocardiography
Echocardiography provides a versatile and cost-effective method for assessing cardiac

anatomy and function (see chapter 4 for an overview of echocardiography). The greatest values of echocardiography are the capacity for simultaneous assessment of valvular, pericardial, myocardial, and extracardiac abnormalities. Because complex image processing is not needed, the results of the study are immediately available to the experienced echocardiographer. In addition, it is possible to perform echocardiography on critically ill patients who cannot be moved, or in other circumstances when a portable test is preferable. For these reasons, echocardiography is the preferred screening imaging test for further assessing suspected myocardial dysfunction. Moreover, the use of Doppler echocardiography (Doppler) to measure flow allows the measurement of peak velocity across valves, the mapping of regurgitant jets, the estimation of pulmonary artery pressures, and the detection of shunts (e.g., ventricular and atrial septal defects). The severity of valvular heart disease and its contribution to the clinical presentation can be determined immediately. Figures 6-1 and 6-2 illustrate the use of Doppler echocardiography in evaluation of mitral and aortic valve disease. For patients with chest pain, congestive heart failure, or arrhythmias, echocardiography provides a rapid means of determining underlying cardiovascular function.

Transesophageal echocardiography adds to the sensitivity of transthoracic echocardiography because views of the heart are not impeded by artifact related to the lungs or the chest wall. In addition, transesophageal echocardiography allows visualization of structures that are usually not well seen by transthoracic echocardiography (Figs. 6-1 and 6-2). The development of transesophageal echocardiography has also been an important advance in the management of patients who are undergoing cardiothoracic surgery, providing information on left ventricular (LV) function and the success of valvular repair. In addition, transesophageal echocardiography may allow a more accurate determination of valvular dysfunction and assessment for bacterial endocarditis, intracardiac thromboses, or both.

In addition to its usefulness in assessing valvular heart disease, echocardiography provides information on regional wall motion abnormali-ties suggestive of myocardial ischemia or necrosis in patients with CAD. The addition of pharmacologic or exercise-induced stress to detect inducible ischemia provides increased sensitivity and specificity compared with electrocardiographic exercise testing (Fig. 6-3; upper panel). In 21 studies, the sensitivity of exercise stress echocardiography averaged 84% (71–97%) and the specificity averaged 86% (64–100%). The use of echocardiography can be limited by technical considerations, including an inability to obtain diagnostic images in some patients (an estimated 15%). Stress echocardiography is indicated for individuals who have an intermediate prior probability of CAD and for individuals with abnormal ECGs or who are prescribed medications that can cause ECG abnormalities with stress (such as digoxin). In either of these cases the predictive value of exercise electrocardiography is substantially reduced, justifying the use of an imaging technique during stress.

Contrast Echocardiography

Injection into the circulation of contrast agents that reflect ultrasound helps demonstrate intracardiac shunts, improves resolution of cardiac structures, and enhances spectral Doppler signals of flow-through heart valves (Fig. 6-3; lower panel). Although contrast echocardiography is not indicated for all patients, it can enable quantification of the severity of an intracardiac shunt, thereby indicating whether invasive testing (cardiac catheterization) or surgery is needed.

Tissue Doppler

The processing of Doppler signals reflected by the myocardium gives two-dimensional directional information that allows better visualization of the endocardium and assessment of ventricular wall motion. Tissue Doppler is helpful for the assessment of regional wall abnormalities at rest or with stress. Although not needed in every study, tissue Doppler can be extremely useful in difficult-to-image individuals.

Radionuclide Testing

Radionuclide imaging assesses LV function and detects reversible ischemia secondary to CAD. As described in chapter 4, quantitative assessment of right and left ventricular ejection

Figure 6-1

Transesophageal Echocardiography

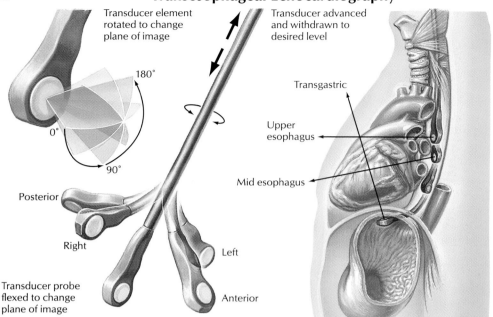

Transducer element rotated to change plane of image

Transducer advanced and withdrawn to desired level

180°

0°

90°

Posterior

Right

Left

Anterior

Transducer probe flexed to change plane of image

Transgastric

Upper esophagus

Mid esophagus

Positions and axes of image of esophageal probe

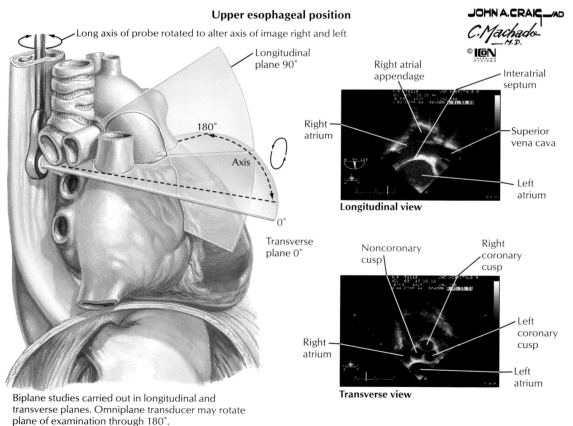

Upper esophageal position

Long axis of probe rotated to alter axis of image right and left

Longitudinal plane 90°

180°

Axis

0°

Transverse plane 0°

Biplane studies carried out in longitudinal and transverse planes. Omniplane transducer may rotate plane of examination through 180°.

JOHN A. CRAIG _MD_
C. Machado _M.D._
©ICON

Right atrial appendage

Interatrial septum

Right atrium

Superior vena cava

Left atrium

Longitudinal view

Noncoronary cusp

Right coronary cusp

Right atrium

Left coronary cusp

Left atrium

Transverse view

Figure 6-2

Transesophageal Echocardiography

Midesophagus position

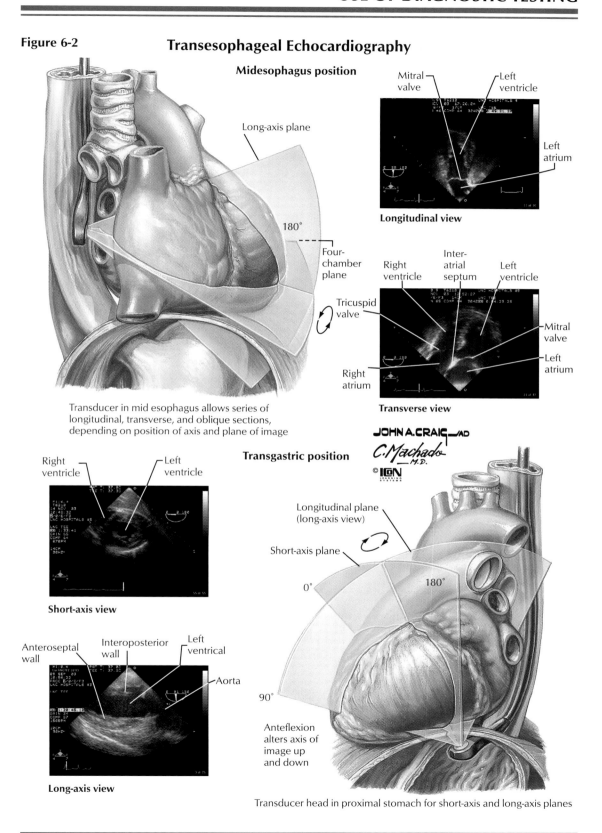

Long-axis plane

Mitral valve — Left ventricle

Left atrium

Longitudinal view

180°

Four-chamber plane

Inter-atrial septum

Right ventricle — Left ventricle

Tricuspid valve

Mitral valve

Right atrium

Left atrium

Transverse view

Transducer in mid esophagus allows series of longitudinal, transverse, and oblique sections, depending on position of axis and plane of image

JOHN A. CRAIG — MD
C. Machado — M.D.
© ICON

Right ventricle — Left ventricle

Short-axis view

Transgastric position

Longitudinal plane (long-axis view)

Short-axis plane

0°   180°

90°

Anteroseptal wall   Interoposterior wall   Left ventrical

Aorta

Anteflexion alters axis of image up and down

Long-axis view

Transducer head in proximal stomach for short-axis and long-axis planes

Figure 6-3

Exercise and Contrast Echocardiography

Left ventricle
Anteroseptal wall
Right ventricle
Aortic valve
Left atrium
Anterior leaflet mitral valve

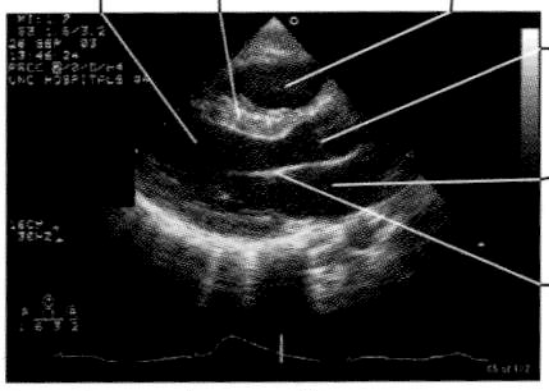

Resting echocardiogram

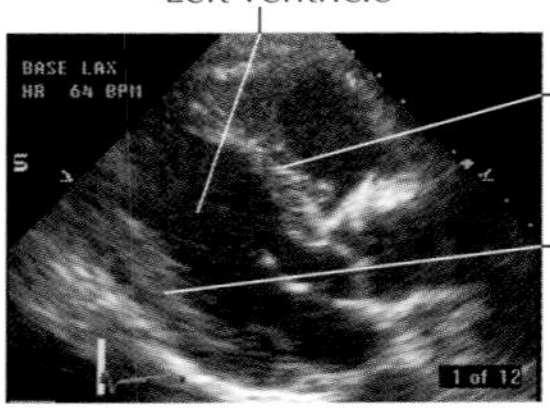

Left ventricle
Anteroseptal wall
Inferoposterior wall

Baseline stress echocardiogram long axis

Exercise echocardiography

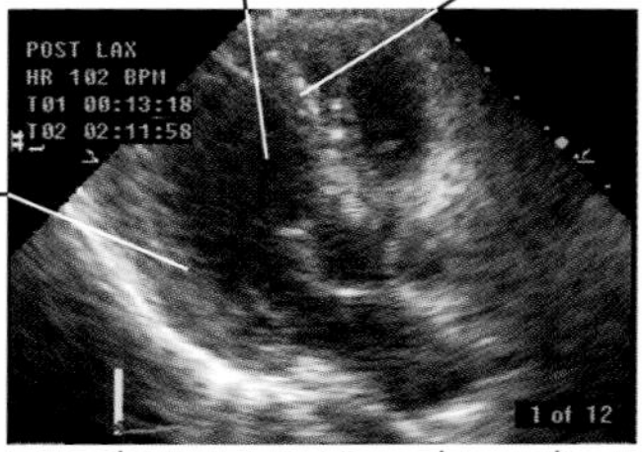

Anteroseptal wall
Left ventricle
Inferoposterior wall

Diastolic postexercise echocardiogram, long axis

Anteroseptal wall
Left ventricle
Inferoposterior wall

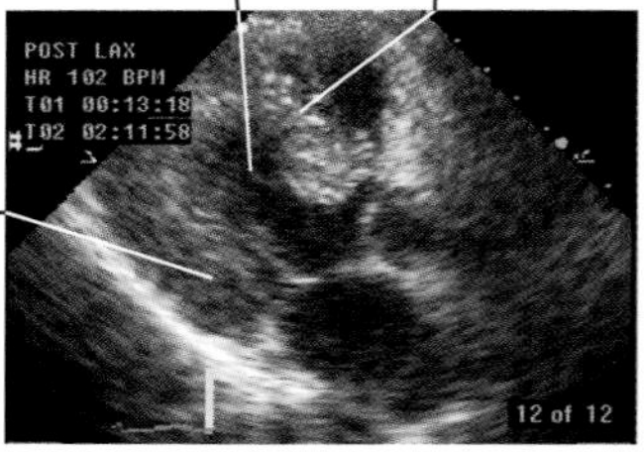

Systolic postexercise echocardiogram, long axis

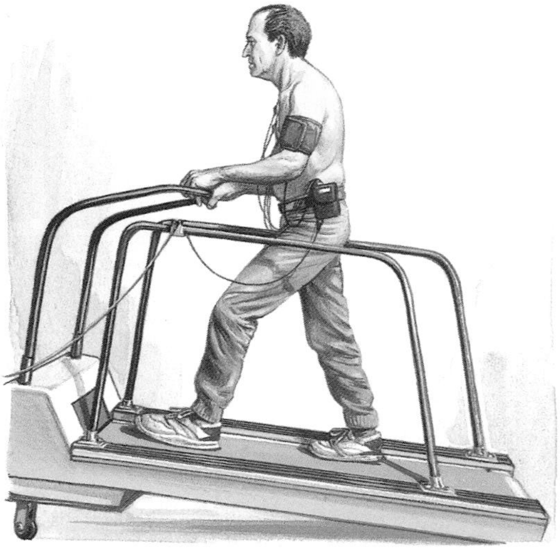

Exercise performed to elicit ischemic signs and postexercise echocardiogram used to evaluate ventricular function, wall motion, and thickness. Often correlated with stress echocardiography

Contrast echocardiography

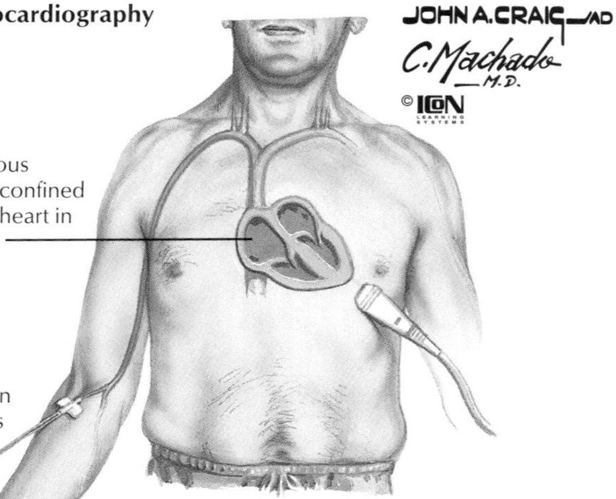

JOHN A. CRAIG—AD
C. Machado
—M.D.
© ICN

Right atrium
Left atrium
Right ventricle
Left ventricle

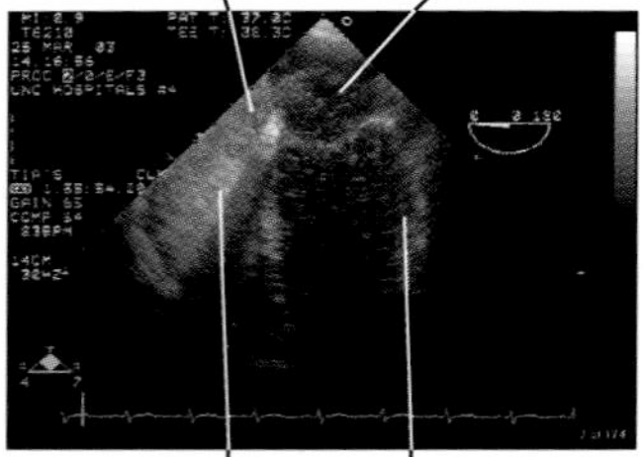

Bubble study in atrial septal defect

Contrast echocardiogram shows right-to-left shunt through atrial septal defect

Peripheral venous contrast agent confined to right side of heart in normal patient

Injection of bolus

Microbubble solution

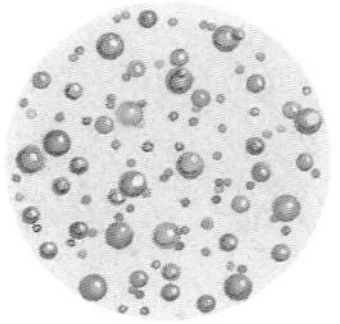

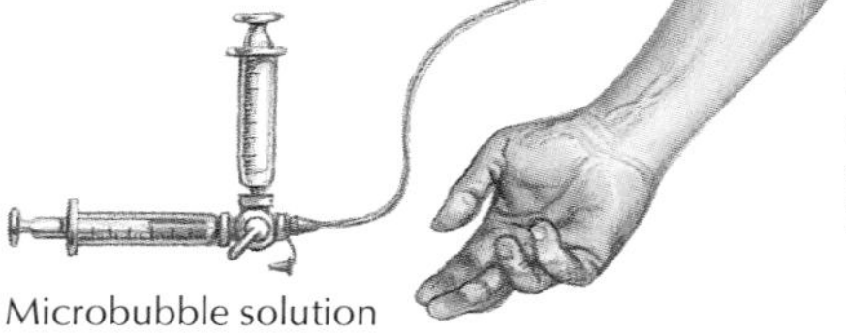

Peripheral venous injection of solution contains acoustically dense microbubbles, affording contrast agent that delineates intracardiac structures and identifies shunts.

fractions is highly accurate with this technique and can be related to long-term prognosis.

Stress (exercise or pharmacologic) radionuclide myocardial perfusion imaging (MPI) in patients with suspected CAD yields a sensitivity of approximately 85 to 90%. When gated SPECT is used, the specificity for excluding CAD is about 90%. Thus, radionuclide imaging is more specific and sensitive in detecting significant CAD than is exercise electrocardiographic testing and (as with exercise echocardiography) has particular value when the resting ECG is abnormal, and when patients are unable to achieve more than 85% of their maximum predicted heart rate because of locomotor or other reasons. The accuracy for diagnosing CAD is probably similar to the accuracy of stress echocardiography, and the choice may depend on which study is performed more often, and reproducibly, at a given center. One advantage of stress MPI is that the number of patients for whom this imaging technique cannot be used is small. In addition, stress radionuclide MPI has a proven role in predicting future cardiac events and, importantly, is able to predict a low mortality and subsequent infarction rate in patients with a totally normal scan. The use of certain radioactive tracers (such as thallium) leads to a high false-positive rate; therefore, technical considerations are paramount when performing and interpreting such scans. In general, the indications for stress MPI are similar to those for stress echocardiography: an intermediate prior probability of disease, an abnormal baseline ECG, or both. Both tests are also useful for patients who cannot exercise adequately, because pharmacologic agents can be used to induce stress.

Magnetic Resonance Imaging

Magnetic resonance imaging (MRI) is an extremely sensitive imaging modality that is superior to other noninvasive imaging investigations in diagnosing congenital heart disease, diseases of the aorta, anomalous coronary arteries, and right ventricular dysplasia (Fig. 6-4). Many surgeons prefer to elucidate cardiac structure prior to repair. The role of MRI has been extended beyond pure anatomic imaging to the evaluation of regional and global cardiac function at

rest and under pharmacologic stress; information such as LV function and myocardial perfusion can be assessed with special contrast agents. MRI can be very useful in assessing myocardial viability because it is possible to visualize wall thickness throughout the left ventricle, allowing an assessment of whether normal wall thickening occurs with systole.

Advances in MRI contrast agents and imaging technology has led to the development of "magnetic resonance coronary angiography" capable of imaging the major coronary arteries, albeit without the diagnostic resolution of coronary angiography. Although MRI is a promising modality, the amount of prognostic information available for stress echocardiography or MPI far exceeds that available for MRI scanning. The use of MRI is also limited because of the cost and the availability of MRI scanners capable of gating the image to the ECG (which is necessary to resolve cardiac structure) and the duration of the study.

Thus, for obtaining anatomic information, most cardiologists advocate transthoracic echocardiography as a first step, followed by either transesophageal echocardiography or MRI if better definition of the cardiac structures is needed. For assessment of CAD, stress electrocardiography would be used as a screen only in individuals with a low prior probability of disease and a normal baseline ECG. Stress echocardiography or MPI should be used for individuals who have an intermediate prior probability of disease, an abnormal baseline ECG, or both or who are taking medications that could nonspecifically alter the ECG during exercise. Patients who are unable to exercise are also well suited for pharmacologic stress testing with either echocardiographic or nuclear imaging. For most individuals with a high prior probability of CAD, coronary angiography should be considered as an initial diagnostic step.

Cardiac Catheterization

Cardiac catheterization, considered the gold standard investigation for patients with CAD, allows the assessment of both coronary artery anatomy and LV function (Fig. 6-5). Historically, cardiac catheterization provided a means of measuring hemodynamic parameters (e.g., pres-

Figure 6-4   Cardiac MRI

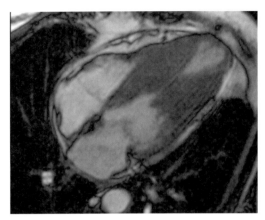

Cardiac MRI in the four-chamber long-axis view demonstrating midventricular variant of hypertrophic cardiomyopathy

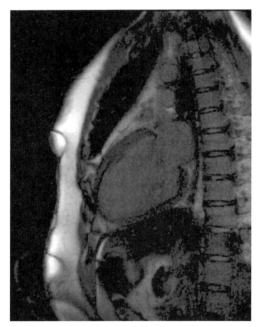

Hyperenhanced cardiac MRI used to detect myocardial viability in a patient with subtotally occluded left anterior descending and RCA and an ejection fraction of 30%. Myocardial scarring shows up as bright contrast in this technique, and this study shows normal myocardial viability despite the presence of multivessel coronary artery disease and left ventricular dysfunction.

sure and oxygen saturation) within various chambers of the heart to assess cardiac anatomy and physiology. Most of these techniques have been superseded by noninvasive tests already described. There are difficult situations, such as the assessment of some valvular lesions or the differentiation of pericardial constriction from myocardial restriction (see chapters 14 and 35), that still often require cardiac catheterization.

Today, the most common use of cardiac catheterization is anatomic delineation of CAD and LV function in anticipation of revascularization (chapter 5). Because of its invasive nature, coronary angiography carries a 0.1% mortality in most laboratories; for this reason, it is often performed after a noninvasive test. However, the sensitivities and specificities of stress echocardiography and MPI are such that a patient whose medical history indicates a high prior probability of CAD would be at risk for a false-negative noninvasive test. For these individuals, coronary angiography should be the initial diagnostic test. Coronary angiography is required before revascularization, by either percutaneous approaches or bypass surgery.

Based on the direct access to the coronary arteries provided by coronary angiography, new techniques have been developed to provide increased accuracy in the diagnosis of coronary heart disease. Intravascular ultrasound provides high-resolution images of the coronary arterial wall and has greater sensitivity in identifying the extent of coronary atherosclerosis than does coronary angiography alone (see chapter 2). In particular, intravascular ultrasound emphasizes the importance of the "burden" of plaque that extends toward the adventitia rather than encroaching on the lumen. Functional information about the physiologic impact of a coronary stenosis is now obtainable through the measurement of blood flow and pressure drop across these lesions with miniaturized pressure and Doppler transducers on the ends of guide wires. These measurements correlate with long-term prognosis and thus provide a means of targeting therapy on physiologic as well as anatomic grounds. Thus, in an individual with compelling symptoms, a noninvasive test diagnostic of myocardial ischemia, or both but with only moderate stenoses by coronary angiography,

Figure 6-5

Left-Sided Heart Catheterization

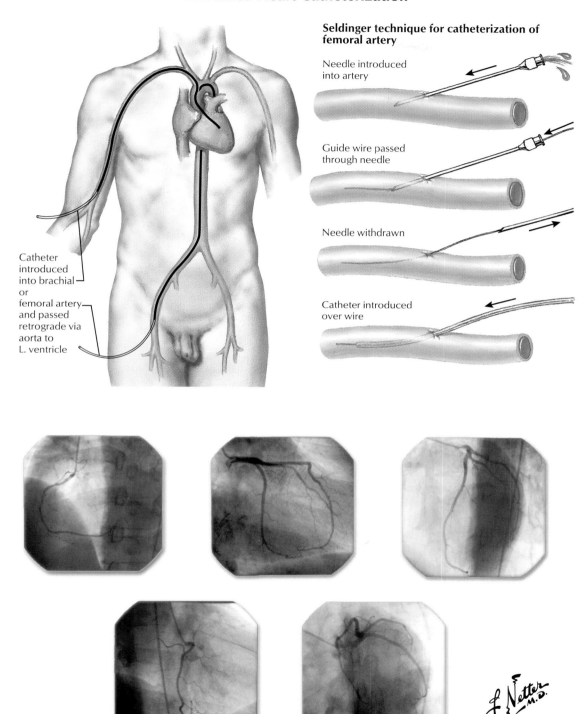

Seldinger technique for catheterization of femoral artery

Needle introduced into artery

Guide wire passed through needle

Needle withdrawn

Catheter introduced over wire

Catheter introduced into brachial or femoral artery and passed retrograde via aorta to L. ventricle

intravascular ultrasound and/or Doppler flow measurements may be indicated to ascertain whether a moderate stenosis by angiography is functionally important and a candidate lesion for revascularization.

Electrophysiology Studies

Although resting electrocardiography and Holter monitoring often provide diagnostic information on the conditions of patients presenting with palpitations or syncope, electrophysiology studies have a role in diagnosing the conditions of patients in which a cardiac etiology is unclear. Invasive stimulation studies are used to diagnose both ventricular and supraventricular arrhythmias and to test the integrity of the conduction system in patients with syncopal episodes (see section IV).

FUTURE DIRECTIONS

A new and extremely important role for diagnostic testing lies in the assessment of myocardial viability, that is, the ability of dysfunctional myocardial tissue to regain function once an adequate blood supply has been restored. In patients with seemingly dead areas of myocardium, the presence of viable regions can support revascularization, based on the potential of these myocardial areas to recover.

Most of the noninvasive tests mentioned in this chapter have been developed to provide measures of viability. Radionuclide (in particular, thallium) uptake has been used to identify areas of myocardial viability. PET scanning is considered the reference standard for measuring viability because it measures myocardial perfusion and metabolism simultaneously. Echocardiography, particularly with and without administration

of low-dose dobutamine, provides a more readily available and cost-effective measure of viability. Contrast echocardiography allows the assessment of microcirculatory integrity with precise anatomic delineation. And, MRI also offers great promise for assessment of viability.

Future diagnostic testing will allow continued integration of anatomic and functional imaging, further improving the ability of clinicians to make the best decisions for their patients.

REFERENCES

Beller GA. Radionuclide perfusion imaging techniques for evaluation of patients with known or suspected coronary artery disease. *Adv Intern Med* 1997;42:139–201.

Beller GA, Zaret BL. Contributions of nuclear cardiology to diagnosis and prognosis of patients with coronary artery disease. *Circulation* 2000;101:1465–1478.

Camici PG. Positron emission tomography and myocardial imaging. *Heart* 2000;83:475–480.

Cheitlin MD, Alpert JS, Armstrong WF, et al. ACC/AHA Guidelines for the Clinical Application of Echocardiography. A report of the American College of Cardiology/American Heart Association Task Force on Practice Guidelines (Committee on Clinical Application of Echocardiography). Developed in collaboration with the American Society of Echocardiography. *Circulation* 1997;95:1686–1744.

Gibbons RJ, Balady GJ, Beasley JW, et al. ACC/AHA Guidelines for Exercise Testing: A report of the American College of Cardiology/American Heart Association Task Force on Practice Guidelines (Committee on Exercise Testing). *J Am Coll Cardiol* 1997;30:260–311.

Kersting-Sommerhoff BA, Diethelm L, Stanger P, et al. Evaluation of complex congenital ventricular anomalies with magnetic resonance imaging. *Am Heart J* 1990;120:133–142.

Pennell DJ, Bogren HG, Keegan J, Firmin DN, Underwood SR. Assessment of coronary artery stenosis by magnetic resonance imaging. *Heart* 1996;75:127–133.

Rasheed Q, Nair R, Sheehan H, Hodgson JM. Correlation of intracoronary ultrasound plaque characteristics in atherosclerotic coronary artery disease patients with clinical variables. *Am J Cardiol* 1994;73:753–758.

Section II

CORONARY HEART DISEASE

Chapter 7

Chronic Coronary Artery Disease

Venu Menon

Advances in pharmacotherapy and revascularization strategies have dramatically improved the short- and long-term outcome for patients with atherosclerotic coronary artery disease (CAD). This improved prognosis, combined with an aging population and epidemics of obesity and type 2 diabetes mellitus, has increased the burden of chronic atherosclerotic heart disease in the developed world. Moreover, recognition of the pandemic of atherosclerotic disease in the developing world exponentially increases the population at risk worldwide.

Atherosclerotic CAD has a heterogeneous clinical presentation. This chapter focuses on chronic **stable** angina. Other clinical presentations of atherosclerotic CAD (acute coronary syndrome, congestive heart failure, sudden cardiac death, and silent ischemia) are described in chapters 8, 12, and 23.

ETIOLOGY AND PATHOGENESIS

In contrast to oxygen extraction by skeletal muscle, oxygen extraction by cardiac tissue is near maximal even at rest (Fig. 7-1). To maintain adequate oxygen supply, an increase in oxygen requirement (increased heart rate, increased wall stress, increased contractility) is accompanied by an increase in coronary blood flow. If a significant underlying coronary epicardial stenosis is present, blood flow at rest is maintained by compensatory dilatation of the coronary bed beyond the stenosis. This diminishes coronary flow reserve and may result in an inability to meet oxygen requirements as myocardial demand increases, creating a supply/demand mismatch. Symptoms of angina arise with a dominant severe fixed stenosis when blood supply to living cardiac tissues is unable to match energy demand. Ischemia is similarly elicited by treadmill or bicycle exercise testing and may be measured as loss of systolic thickening on echocardiography, diminished perfusion on SPECT, ST-segment depression on surface ECG, and angina via clinical history (see chapters 4 and 6).

Increased *vasoreactivity* (vasospasm on a previously narrowed arterial segment) may also result in decreased myocardial blood flow with or without increased demand. Vasoreactivity appears to be responsible for some of the circadian, seasonal, and emotional components associated with angina, and the contributions of stenotic and vasoreactive components may vary in individuals. Plaque rupture or erosion may also result in diminished blood flow from sudden thrombotic narrowing or occlusion of the blood vessel; this is discussed in the section on acute coronary syndromes (see chapter 8).

CLINICAL PRESENTATION

Chronic stable angina is characterized by angina that usually occurs with increased oxygen demand. Symptoms are provoked by exertion, heavy meals, or emotional distress; tend to be reproducible; and usually have been present for a prolonged time. These symptoms most commonly result from fixed coronary stenoses (Fig. 7-2). Chest discomfort is variably described as pressure, tightness, or discomfort over the left precordium. It may radiate along the ulnar aspect of the left arm and is often accompanied by shortness of breath, nausea, and diaphoresis (Fig. 7-3). Symptoms may radiate or be isolated to the throat, jaw, interscapular region, and epigastrium. Radiation below the umbilicus and to the occiput is uncharacteristic, as are symptoms that are well localized to a fingertip, provoked by palpation and movement, or relieved by lying down. Typically, anginal pain lasts for about 5 minutes and is relieved by rest. Relief with use of sublingual nitroglycerin is usually prompt.

DIFFERENTIAL DIAGNOSIS

The quality of chest pain is similar in the setting of acute unstable angina or acute myocar-

Figure 7-1

Chronic Stable Angina

Skeletal Muscle

Cardiac Muscle

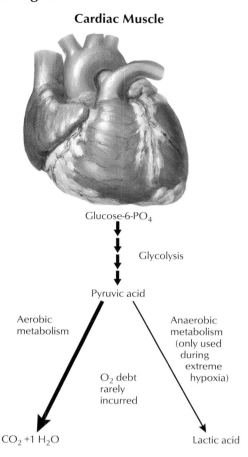

Glucose-6-PO$_4$

Glycolysis

Pyruvic acid

Aerobic metabolism

Anaerobic metabolism (during exercise provides up to 40% of energy)

O$_2$ debt repaid during rest

CO$_2$ +1 H$_2$O

Lactic acid

Glucose-6-PO$_4$

Glycolysis

Pyruvic acid

Aerobic metabolism

Anaerobic metabolism (only used during extreme hypoxia)

O$_2$ debt rarely incurred

CO$_2$ +1 H$_2$O

Lactic acid

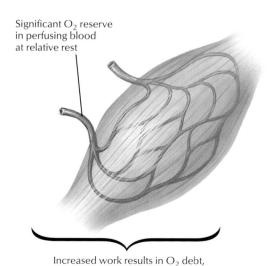

Significant O$_2$ reserve in perfusing blood at relative rest

O$_2$ extraction from perfusing blood nearly maximal at relative rest

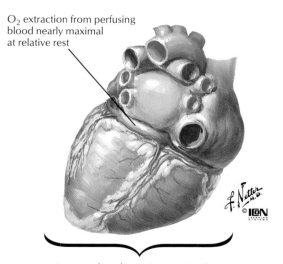

Increased work results in O$_2$ debt, anaerobic metabolism, and increased O$_2$ extraction from blood

Increased work requires greater O$_2$ consumption which must be met by increased blood flow

Figure 7-2

Types and Degrees of Coronary Atherosclerotic Narrowing or Occlusion

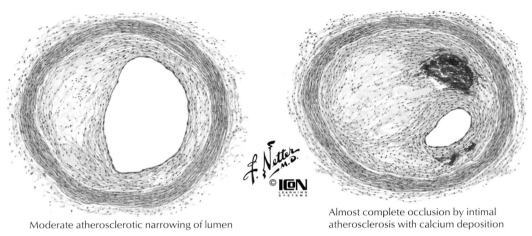

Moderate atherosclerotic narrowing of lumen

Almost complete occlusion by intimal atherosclerosis with calcium deposition

Figure 7-3

Pain of Myocardial Ischemia

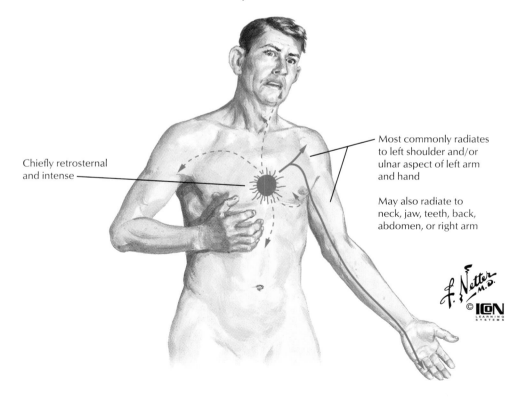

Chiefly retrosternal and intense

Most commonly radiates to left shoulder and/or ulnar aspect of left arm and hand

May also radiate to neck, jaw, teeth, back, abdomen, or right arm

dial infarction (MI). It is usually more intense and prolonged but the difference may be subjective. An important difference is that the pain associated with acute MI is usually unremitting, although it may wax and wane in severity. Angina may occasionally be elicited in the absence of significant epicardial coronary artery stenosis. It may also characterize severe aortic stenosis, hypertrophic cardiomyopathy, and microvascular dysfunction. Other cardiovascular causes of chest pain include pericarditis, aortic dissection, and pulmonary embolism. Clinicians should also attempt to distinguish angina from chest pain arising from a noncardiac etiology. Pleuritis should be considered. Gastrointestinal conditions such as acid reflux, esophageal spasm, peptic ulcer disease, biliary disease, and pancreatitis fall in the differential, and gastroesophageal reflux disease is a particularly common noncardiac cause of anginal-type chest pain. Cervical disk disease, costochondral syndromes, and shingles may also mimic angina. Chest discomfort is also a common manifestation in patients with panic disorder.

DIAGNOSTIC APPROACH

A history suggestive of angina mandates diagnostic and prognostic evaluation. The urgency of treatment is guided by the initial presentation and clinical evaluation. A history of new-onset angina, accelerating angina, angina at a low exertional threshold, and rest angina is considered unstable and the patient should be evaluated immediately. Physical examination during a routine consultation is unlikely to be rewarding, but the clinician should look for clinical evidence of left ventricular (LV) dysfunction (resting tachycardia, laterally displaced apical impulse, an LV S_3, rales, jugular venous distension, positive hepatojugular reflex, pedal edema). In addition to evaluating the status of traditional cardiac risk factors (hypertension, smoking status, hyperlipidemia, diabetes), the consultant should inquire about a history of claudication, stroke, and transient ischemic attack and carefully screen for manifestations of atherosclerotic disease (audible bruits, asymmetrical pulses, palpable aneurysms, ankle–brachial index). The examiner should also look for physical and biochemical signs of the meta-

bolic syndrome (Table 7-1), as well as stigmata of hereditary hyperlipedemic conditions (Fig. 7-4).

The diagnostic approach should be based on the pretest likelihood of disease. Patients with typical angina, multiple risk factors, and/or impaired LV function with a high likelihood of disease should be considered for diagnostic coronary angiography. The few patients with low pretest likelihood of disease should be reassured, without further additional testing. The clinician should, however, emphasize risk reduction with smoking cessation and lifestyle modification. Most patients have an intermediate likelihood of epicardial CAD developing, and stress testing should be planned for further risk stratification (Fig. 7-5). Patients with a normal resting ECG may be referred for standard exercise treadmill testing. Many laboratories initiate evaluation with concomitant nuclear perfusion/stress echo imaging studies due to the incremental physiologic (degree/extent of ischemia, LV function) and prognostic data obtained. This is the approach of choice in persons with pre-excitation, paced rhythms, left bundle branch block, or baseline ST-segment abnormalities or who are taking medications (such as digoxin) that may confound stress ECG interpretation. It should be noted that the inability to perform adequate exercise by itself is a major indicator of adverse prognosis. This subset of patients may be referred for pharmacologic stress testing with use of dipyridamole, adenosine, or dobutamine.

Patients with high-risk nuclear perfusion scans, stress echocardiograms, and exercise tolerance test (ETT) findings, as well as patients with

Table 7-1
Signs of the Metabolic Syndrome

· Abdominal obesity
    Men >102 cm
    Women >88 cm
· BP >130/85 mm Hg
· Fasting glucose >110 mg/dL
· HDL-C
    Men <40mg/dL
    Women <50 mg/dL
· Triglycerides >150 mg/dL

HDL-C indicates high-density lipoprotein cholesterol.

Figure 7-4

Hypercholesterolemic Xanthomatosis

Plain and tuberous xanthoma

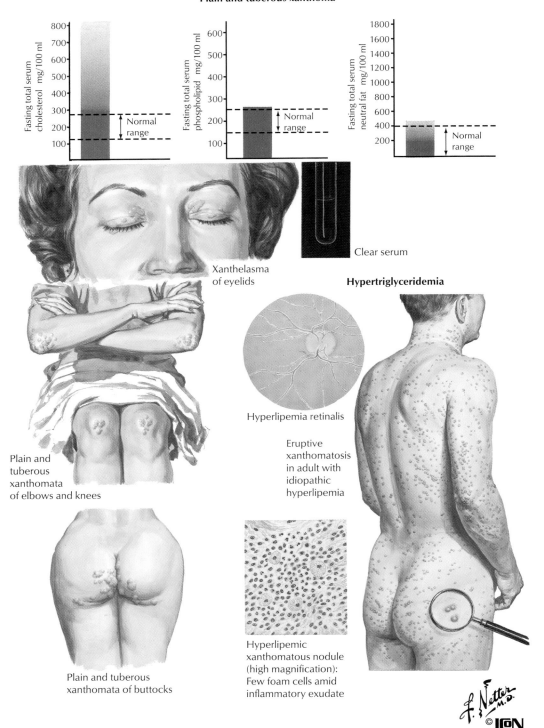

Xanthelasma
of eyelids

Clear serum

Hypertriglyceridemia

Hyperlipemia retinalis

Plain and
tuberous
xanthomata
of elbows and knees

Eruptive
xanthomatosis
in adult with
idiopathic
hyperlipemia

Plain and tuberous
xanthomata of buttocks

Hyperlipemic
xanthomatous nodule
(high magnification):
Few foam cells amid
inflammatory exudate

Figure 7-5

Testing to Detect Myocardial Ischemia

Myocardial Ischemia, Demonstrated by Stress Test

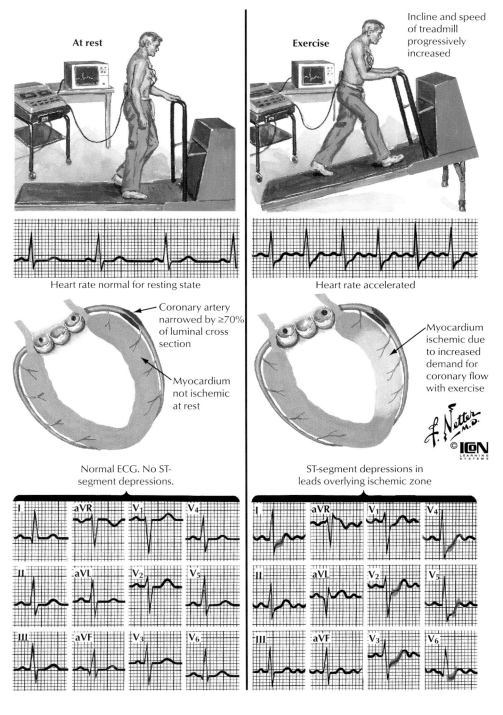

At rest

Exercise

Incline and speed of treadmill progressively increased

Heart rate normal for resting state

Heart rate accelerated

Coronary artery narrowed by ≥70% of luminal cross section

Myocardium not ischemic at rest

Myocardium ischemic due to increased demand for coronary flow with exercise

Normal ECG. No ST-segment depressions.

ST-segment depressions in leads overlying ischemic zone

ischemia with severe LV dysfunction, should be referred for diagnostic coronary angiography. Subjects with severe segmental LV dysfunction and absence of inducible ischemia should be evaluated for viability. The choice and protocol of low-dose dobutamine echocardiography, thallium–dipyridamole imaging, PET, or MRI should be guided by local expertise. Evidence of viability should lead to referral for angiography, with the goal of attempting revascularization whenever feasible. Patients with low-risk scans may be treated medically using risk counseling and adequate follow-up.

MANAGEMENT AND THERAPY

Treatment goals in patients with chronic stable angina are to prolong and improve quality of life. The mitigation of cardiac risk factors with lifestyle alterations and pharmacotherapy to prevent and even reverse progression of atherosclerotic disease helps to achieve these goals (Fig. 7-6).

Smoking cessation should be emphasized and referral to cessation programs should be provided. Patients should be educated about the beneficial effects of physical exercise. High-risk patients should be given a detailed exercise prescription and, in some circumstances, should initiate their exercise in a monitored setting—as provided by cardiovascular rehabilitation programs. The Seventh Joint National Committee on the Prevention, Detection, Evaluation, and Treatment of High Blood Pressure (JNC VII) guidelines direct BP management in hypertensive patients (see chapter 39). People with diabetes should attain tight glucose control; the value of weight reduction must be stressed to appropriate patients. Quality assurance programs should ensure that patients with established atherosclerotic CAD be prescribed proven medical therapy (as described in the following sections on specific pharmacotherapies). Patients should be educated about the early warning signs of MI and stroke, the prompt use of aspirin and nitroglycerin, and access to the emergency medical system.

Antiplatelet Therapy

All patients with atherosclerotic CAD should be treated with antiplatelet therapy. The cost and effectiveness of aspirin makes it the treatment of choice. The Swedish angina pectoris aspirin trial randomized 2035 patients with stable angina to 75 mg aspirin versus placebo. A 33% relative reduction (9% absolute reduction) in cardiovascular events was observed with aspirin therapy. Similarly, a recent collaborative meta-analysis suggested a 34% proportional reduction in nonfatal MI and a 26% reduction in nonfatal MI and death with antiplatelet therapy over placebo in high-risk patients. In patients with a history of MI, antiplatelet therapy prevented 18 nonfatal MIs, 5 nonfatal strokes, and 14 vascular deaths per 1000 patients treated over a mean duration of 2 years. Clopidogrel is an appropriate alternative for patients with a contraindication to aspirin. The concomitant long-term use (up to 12 months) of clopidogrel with aspirin following an acute coronary syndrome and percutaneous intervention is associated with a beneficial outcome. The role of long-term treatment with clopidogrel and aspirin in patients with atherosclerosis is under investigation.

β-Blockade

In the absence of contraindications, all patients with CAD should be prescribed a β-blocker. In the Beta Blocker Heart Attack Trial (BHAT), β-blockade with propanolol reduced the combined end point of recurrent nonfatal reinfarction and fatal coronary heart disease from 13.0% in the placebo group to 10% in the treatment group, a reduction of 23% at 25 months of follow-up. In trials of stable angina, β-blockers were superior to calcium antagonists in reducing episodes of angina. The rates of cardiac death and MI were not significantly different. β-Blockers are also indicated for the majority of patients with Class II–IV heart failure (see chapters 12 and 17).

ACE Inhibitors

All patients with established CAD and LV dysfunction (symptomatic or asymptomatic) should be prescribed an angiotensin-converting enzyme (ACE) inhibitor. In three large postinfarction trials, mortality rate was lower with ACE inhibitors than with placebo, as were the rates of readmission for heart failure and reinfarction and the composite of these events. High-risk patients with preserved LV function also appear to derive benefit. In the Heart Outcomes Prevention Evalua-

Figure 7-6

Cardiac Risk Factors

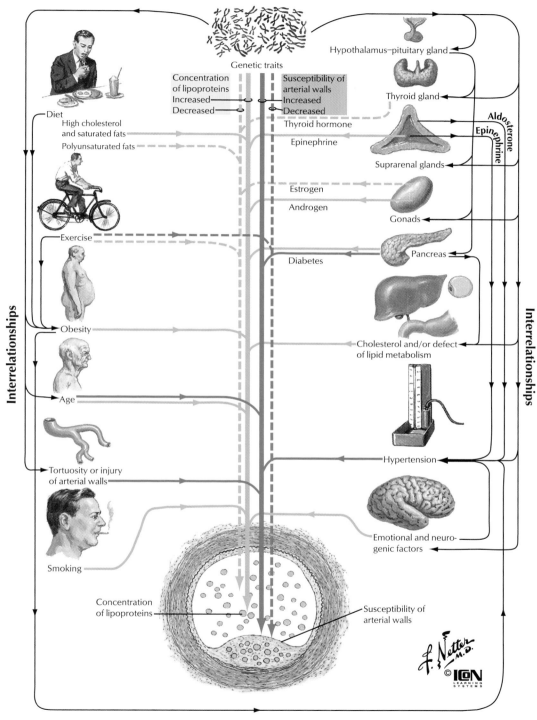

tion study, the use of ramipril in subjects younger than 55 years of age with preserved LV function significantly reduced the primary end points of MI, stroke, and cardiac death. On subgroup analysis, subjects with a history of CAD, MI, cardiovascular disease, cerebrovascular disease, or peripheral vascular disease all derived benefit. Subjects intolerant to ACE-I may be given an angiotensin-II receptor blocker.

Nitrates

Nitrates are endothelium-independent vasodilators that reduce myocardial ischemia and improve coronary blood flow. When used effectively in patients with stable angina, they improve exercise tolerance and increase the anginal threshold. Patients with frequent episodes of angina should be treated with long-acting oral nitrate therapy or with transdermal patches. It is important to ensure a nitrate-free interval. Tachyphylaxis (and loss of nitrate efficacy) occurs in patients without nitrate-free intervals in their treatment regimen. Patients with angina should also be supplied with sublingual pills for breakthrough angina.

Treatment of Hyperlipidemia

Low-density lipoprotein cholesterol (LDL-C) should be the primary target of therapy. Secondary causes of hyperlipidemia, such as diabetes, hypothyroidism, obstructive liver disease, and chronic renal failure, should be considered and managed effectively. Dietary fat should be restricted to 25 to 35% of daily caloric requirement (polyunsaturated fat, 20%; monounsaturated fat, 10%). All patients should receive dietary counseling and instructions for weight reduction and increased physical activity. The current National Cholesterol Education Program (NCEP) guidelines recommend an LDL target of less than 100 mg/dL for patients with established CAD. Pharmacotherapy should be initiated with a statin. Statins decrease LDL-C by 18 to 55%, decrease triglycerides by 7 to 30%, and raise high-density lipoprotein cholesterol (HDL-C) by 5 to 15%. In a meta-analysis combining the results from three secondary and two primary prevention trials, treatment with a statin resulted in a 31% reduction in major coronary events and a 21% reduction in all-cause mortali-

ty rates. Women and elderly individuals derived the same reduction in coronary events as their male and younger counterparts. Subjects with triglyceride levels in the 200- to 499-mg/dL range should be treated with concomitant nicotinic acid or fibrate (a fibric acid derivative) therapy. These HDL-raising drugs may also be used for isolated low HDL levels. A concept of global cardiovascular risk is emerging. Evidence suggests that all patients at cardiovascular risk derive benefit from statin treatment irrespective of their measured lipid profile. However, these findings have not yet been incorporated into healthcare guidelines.

Indications for Revascularization

Percutaneous intervention with adjunctive pharmacotherapy can be successfully performed on the majority of stenotic coronary segments with minimal risk to the patient. This has led to increasing rates of revascularization for chronic CAD, decreasing the number of patients previously treated with medical therapy alone. Revascularization in selected patients increases longevity and improves quality of life. Mortality benefits were initially established by randomized controlled trials that compared medical therapy to coronary artery bypass surgery. Mortality benefits for left main disease, triple-vessel disease with impaired LV function, and two-vessel disease with proximal left anterior descending (LAD) involvement are well established. Early trials comparing percutaneous balloon angioplasty to CABG established the equivalence of angioplasty and CABG in the setting of discrete multivessel disease and preserved LV function. Freedom from angina and target vessel revascularization are considerably greater with CABG, although it is associated with a greater initial risk of procedural mortality, stroke, cognitive dysfunction, and early, transient deterioration in quality of life. Percutaneous intervention, however, is less invasive but requires repeat procedures, mainly due to restenosis. Two recent trials comparing stenting (without the use of glycoprotein [GpIIb/IIIa] inhibitors) with CABG in multivessel disease reported somewhat discordant findings. Although the Arterial Revascularization Trial Study reported similar mortality rates for the two strategies at 1 year, the Surgery or Stent study reported a lower mortality rate with CABG.

It is prudent to refer patients with unprotected left main, diffuse multivessel CAD, diabetes, or severely impaired LV function for CABG. An initial strategy of percutaneous intervention or CABG may be offered to patients with discrete coronary targets and preserved LV function. The heralded conquest of restenosis by drug-eluting stents may increase the threshold for surgical referral in the future. Patients with single- and double-vessel disease and a large ischemic burden, patients with proximal LAD disease, and those with clinical angina refractory to medical therapy should also be offered percutaneous coronary intervention (PCI). Subjects with refractory angina not amenable to revascularization may be considered for transmyocardial revascularization protocols or enhanced external counterpulsation.

FUTURE DIRECTIONS

Accurate noninvasive identification and quantification of atherosclerosis with electron beam CT, intravascular ultrasound, carotid intimal thickness measurements, and endothelial vasoreactivity blurs the traditional distinction between primary and secondary prevention of CAD. Biomarker, genetic and proteonomic research will allow prognostication with increasing accuracy as new therapeutic targets for plaque stabilization and regression are translated from bench to bedside. Treatment for fixed epicardial CAD will be altered by distal protection devices, advances in adjunctive pharmacotherapy, and, perhaps, the much-awaited conquest of restenosis with drug-eluting stents. Advances in angiogenesis and stem cell transfer will potentially revolutionize therapy. A wonderful voyage lies ahead.

REFERENCES

Antithrombotic Trialists Collaboration. Collaborative meta-analysis of randomized trials of antiplatelet therapy for prevention of death, myocardial infarction, and stroke in high risk patients. *BMJ* 2002;324:71–86.

Beta-Blocker Heart Attack Study Group. The beta-blocker heart attack trial. *JAMA* 1981;246:2073–2074.

Flather MD, Yusuf S, Keber L, et al. Long-term ACE-inhibitor therapy in patients with heart failure or left ventricular dysfunction: A systematic overview of data from individual patients. *Lancet* 2000;355;1575–1581.

HOPE investigators. Effects of an angiotensin-converting-enzyme inhibitor, ramipril on cardiovascular events in high-risk patients. *N Engl J Med* 2000;342:145–153.

Meta-analysis of trials comparing beta-blockers, calcium antagonists, and nitrates for stable angina. *JAMA* 1999;281:1927–1936.

Serruys PW, Unger F, Souza JE, et al. Comparison of coronary artery bypass surgery and stenting for the treatment of multivessel disease. *N Engl J Med* 2001;344:1117–1124.

The SoS Investigators. Coronary artery bypass surgery versus percutaneous coronary intervention with stent implantation in patients with multivessel coronary artery disease (the Stent or Surgery trial): A randomized controlled trial. *Lancet* 2002;360:965–970.

Yusuf S, Reddy S, Ounpuu S, Anand S. Global burden of cardiovascular diseases. The epidemiologic transition, risk factors and impact of urbanization. *Circulation* 2001;104:2746-2753.

Chapter 8

Acute Coronary Syndromes

Steven R. Steinhubl

Acute coronary syndromes (ACSs) encompass a wide range of clinical disorders that share a common physiologic derangement: an acute or subacute imbalance between the oxygen demand and supply of the myocardium. The symptoms and eventual diagnosis of a patient presenting with an ACS are dependent on the duration and degree of inadequate oxygenation, making the diagnosis challenging; the outcomes, variable. Unstable angina, non–ST-elevation myocardial infarction (MI), ST-elevation MI, and even sudden cardiac death are potential clinical manifestations of an ACS.

The incidence and potential severity of an ACS makes timely diagnosis and appropriate treatment essential for minimizing morbidity and mortality. Every year in the United States, approximately 2.5 million patients are admitted to a hospital with an ACS, two thirds of whom are eventually diagnosed with unstable angina or non–ST-elevation MI. This chapter focuses on the diagnosis and treatment of patients in the subgroup of ACS called non–ST-elevation ACS. Patients diagnosed with ST-elevation MI are discussed in chapter 9.

ETIOLOGY AND PATHOGENESIS

Several processes can result in an oxygen supply inadequate to meet myocardial demand, the hallmark of an ACS. The principal etiology is the acute formation of a nonobstructive thrombus at the site of a preexisting atherosclerotic coronary plaque, most commonly from plaque rupture and thrombosis (Fig. 8-1). Plaque erosion, characterized by adherence of a thrombus to the plaque surface without an associated disruption of the plaque, is another mechanism of coronary thrombosis. Autopsy series have shown that the prevalence of plaque erosion in ACS is 25 to 40%, with a higher frequency in women than in men.

Atherosclerotic lesions, composed primarily of a lipid-rich core and a fibrous cap, develop in virtually all major arteries. Autopsy and intravascular ultrasound studies have confirmed the presence of coronary atherosclerotic lesions in the majority of asymptomatic individuals older than 20 to 30 years of age. Why some plaques rupture and others do not is not entirely understood, although plaques that are prone to rupture share certain characteristics. The presence of large, eccentric lipid cores and a large percentage of inflammatory macrophages are common findings in fissured or ruptured plaques. The role of inflammatory cells and mediators in the degradation and weakening of the protective fibrous cap has recently been recognized as a critical component in the pathogenesis of an ACS. The majority of lesions rupture at the site of greatest mechanical stress—the shoulder regions where the fibrous cap is adjacent to normal intima—which is also often the site of greatest inflammatory activity. Importantly, neither the size of the plaque nor the degree of luminal obstruction caused by it correlates with the risk of rupture. In fact, nearly two thirds of plaques that subsequently rupture have stenoses of less than 50%, and almost all are less than 70% obstructed—notably, the severity of lesions typically treated with surgical or percutaneous revascularization procedures.

Other less common but important etiologies of an ACS include intense focal spasm of epicardial coronary arteries (Prinzmetal's angina) and conditions in which myocardial ischemia is secondary to a pathologic process extrinsic to the coronary arteries. Examples of the latter include an increase in myocardial oxygen demand secondary to tachycardia or fever and a decrease in myocardial oxygen supply due to systemic hypotension, severe anemia, or hypoxemia. Important differences exist in the pathophysiology and long-term sequelae of non–ST-elevation and ST-elevation MI (Figure 8-2).

Figure 8-1

Atherogenesis: Unstable Plaque Formation

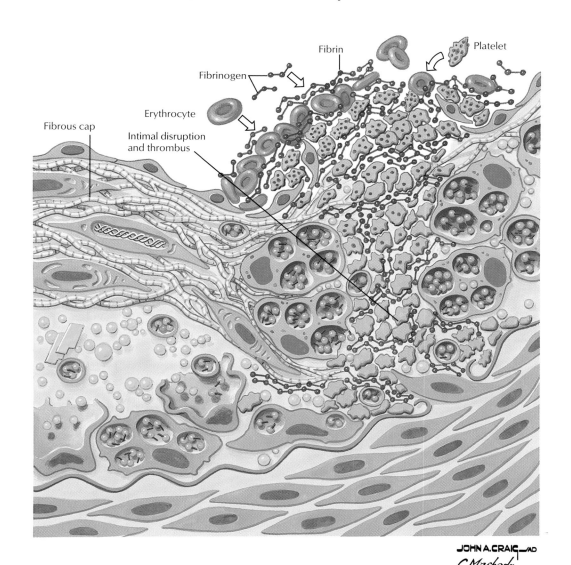

JOHN A. CRAIG—MD
C. Machado—M.D.
©ICN

CLINICAL PRESENTATION

The clinical presentation of ACS encompasses a wide variety of symptoms. In fact, the classic symptom of chest discomfort is absent in up to one third of patients subsequently proven to have MI. The likelihood of an atypical presentation is increased in very young or old patients, in patients with diabetes, and in women. In general, three principal presentations for ACS have been described: (1) angina that commences with a patient at rest, (2) new onset of severe angina (associated with minimal exertion), and (3) a distinct change in the frequency, duration, or threshold of a patient's prior chronic angina pattern.

DIFFERENTIAL DIAGNOSIS

The clinical manifestations of myocardial ischemia can be mimicked by a number of other

Figure 8-2 — Manifestations of Myocardial Infarction

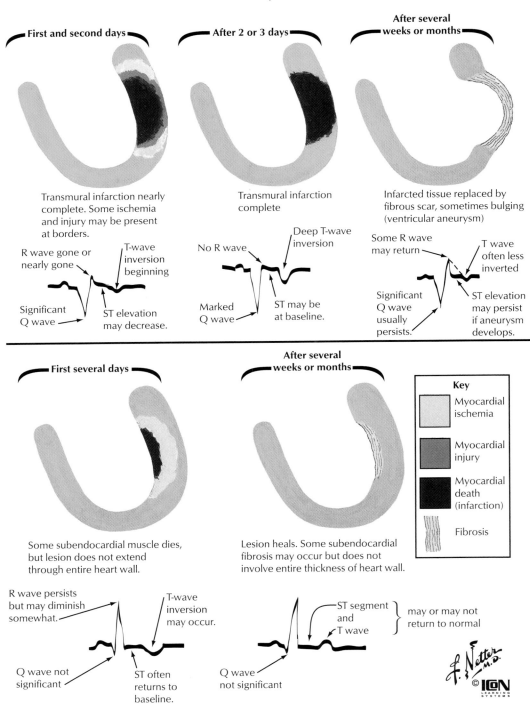

First and second days

Transmural infarction nearly complete. Some ischemia and injury may be present at borders.

R wave gone or nearly gone

T-wave inversion beginning

Significant Q wave

ST elevation may decrease.

After 2 or 3 days

Transmural infarction complete

No R wave

Deep T-wave inversion

Marked Q wave

ST may be at baseline.

After several weeks or months

Infarcted tissue replaced by fibrous scar, sometimes bulging (ventricular aneurysm)

Some R wave may return

T wave often less inverted

Significant Q wave usually persists.

ST elevation may persist if aneurysm develops.

First several days

Some subendocardial muscle dies, but lesion does not extend through entire heart wall.

R wave persists but may diminish somewhat.

T-wave inversion may occur.

Q wave not significant

ST often returns to baseline.

After several weeks or months

Lesion heals. Some subendocardial fibrosis may occur but does not involve entire thickness of heart wall.

ST segment and T wave } may or may not return to normal

Q wave not significant

Key

Myocardial ischemia

Myocardial injury

Myocardial death (infarction)

Fibrosis

processes (see also chapter 1). Musculoskeletal disorders involving the cervical spine, the shoulder, the ribs, and the sternum can manifest as nonspecific chest discomfort. Symptoms from gastrointestinal causes, including esophageal reflux with associated spasm, peptic ulcer disease, and cholecystitis, are often indistinguishable from angina. Intrathoracic processes such as pneumonia, pleurisy, pneumothorax, aortic dissection, and pericarditis can produce chest discomfort. Finally, panic attacks and hyperventilation are neuropsychiatric syndromes that can be mistaken for an ACS.

DIAGNOSTIC APPROACH
History and Physical Examination

Although a careful evaluation of the medical history is a crucial component in determining the diagnosis of a patient with chest pain, medical history alone is an imperfect discriminator of whether a patient is experiencing an ACS because atypical presentations are common. Although the classic symptom of chest discomfort from cardiac angina is described as a pressure or a heaviness, studies show that almost one quarter of patients with chest pain who were eventually diagnosed with myocardial ischemia described chest discomfort as sharp or stabbing. Similarly, 13% of all patients with ACS presented with a pleuritic pain component, and 7% had pain that was reproduced by palpation.

The physical examination in patients with suspected ACS is crucial for ruling out signs of hemodynamic instability and left ventricular (LV) dysfunction, but in the majority of patients, the examination results are normal. Importantly, a thorough physical examination can help to distinguish noncardiac causes of chest discomfort and secondary causes of myocardial ischemia.

Electrocardiogram

The resting ECG is a key component of the proper assessment of a patient with a suspected ACS. ST-segment and T-wave changes are the most reliable electrocardiographic indicators of myocardial ischemia (Fig. 8-2). Twelve-lead electrocardiography, performed when symptoms are present, is particularly valuable; ideally, recordings should be obtained while symptoms are and are not present. When possible, the ECG tracing should be compared with any previous tracings. If transient ST-segment or T-wave changes are identified, the patient probably has acute myocardial ischemia. Importantly, the possibility of an ACS cannot be excluded solely on the basis of a normal ECG in a patient with chest pain. Some studies suggest that 5 to 10% of patients with chest pain and a normal ECG will subsequently be diagnosed with MI or unstable angina.

The ECG is critical not only for the diagnosis of an ACS, but also in providing important prognostic information dependent on the type and magnitude of changes. Patients with ST-segment depression are at highest risk of death during the subsequent 6 months, whereas those with isolated T-wave changes have no more long-term risk than do persons with no ECG changes. In patients with ST-segment depression, as the level of depression and the number of leads with depressions increase, so does the risk of death or the probability of repeat MI.

Biochemical Markers of Myocardial Damage

The biochemical markers of myocardial necrosis, predominately creatine kinase (CK) and its MB isoenzyme (CK-MB), as well as cardiac troponins T and I, are also essential in the diagnosis and prognosis of patients with an ACS. These markers become detectable after myocyte necrosis causes the loss of cell membrane integrity, which eventually allows these intracellular macromolecules to diffuse into the peripheral circulation (Fig. 8-3).

Until recently, CK and CK-MB were the primary biochemical markers used to evaluate patients with chest pain. However, several properties of CK and CK-MB limit their predictive value, including their presence at low levels in the blood under normal conditions, and in noncardiac sources, especially skeletal muscle. Accordingly, cardiac troponins have become the preferred markers of myocardial necrosis. Because cardiac troponins are not generally detected in the blood of healthy individuals and are cardiac specific, they are more sensitive and specific for myocardial necrosis than CK and CK-MB are. Measurement of troponins allows myocardial necrosis to be detected in approximately one third of patients with unstable angina and normal CK-MB levels.

Figure 8-3

Acute Coronary Syndromes

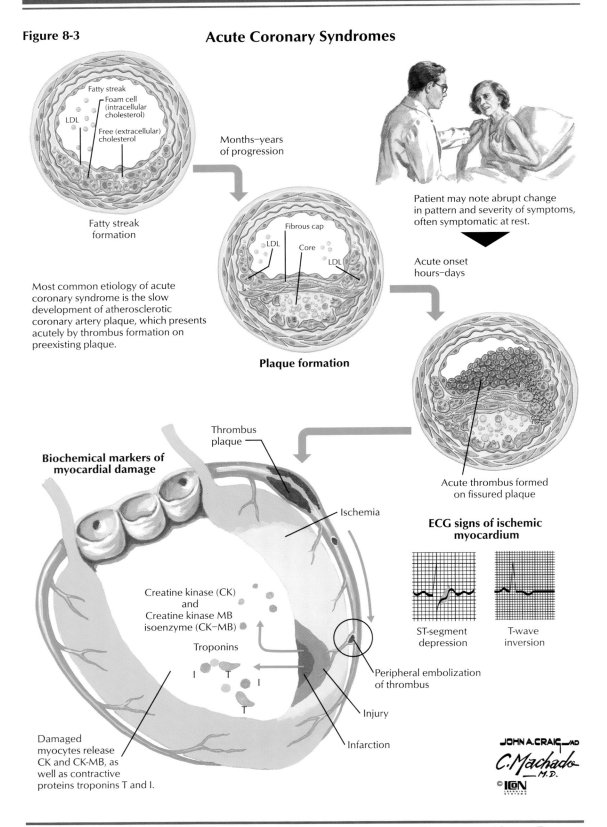

Fatty streak
Foam cell
(intracellular
cholesterol)
LDL
Free (extracellular)
cholesterol

**Fatty streak
formation**

Months–years
of progression

Most common etiology of acute
coronary syndrome is the slow
development of atherosclerotic
coronary artery plaque, which presents
acutely by thrombus formation on
preexisting plaque.

Fibrous cap
LDL   Core
LDL

Plaque formation

Patient may note abrupt change
in pattern and severity of symptoms,
often symptomatic at rest.

Acute onset
hours–days

Acute thrombus formed
on fissured plaque

**Biochemical markers of
myocardial damage**

Thrombus
plaque

Ischemia

Creatine kinase (CK)
and
Creatine kinase MB
isoenzyme (CK–MB)

Troponins

I   T   I

T

Damaged
myocytes release
CK and CK-MB, as
well as contractive
proteins troponins T and I.

Peripheral embolization
of thrombus

Injury

Infarction

**ECG signs of ischemic
myocardium**

ST-segment
depression

T-wave
inversion

JOHN A. CRAIG—AD
C. Machado
—M.D.
© ICON

Because at least 3 to 4 hours are typically necessary after MI to detect an increase in peripheral blood levels of CK-MB or of troponins, serial blood testing during the initial 6 to 12 hours after presentation is needed to safely exclude myocardial damage in patients presenting with chest pain.

MANAGEMENT AND THERAPY
Risk Stratification

The diagnosis of an ACS encompasses a wide spectrum of clinical outcomes; therefore, optimal management is best determined by the patient's risk for an adverse event. In general, this risk can be categorized as the risk that the current acute presentation was caused by a thrombotic event and the long-term risk based on that patient's atherosclerotic disease burden. Currently, the best surrogate for the early thrombotic risk is biomarker—in particular troponin—positivity (Fig. 8-4). Multiple studies have confirmed the prognostic significance of elevated troponin levels and shown a consistent correlation between treatment benefit and troponin status. Other markers of early, thrombotic risk include ST-segment depression, dynamic ST-segment changes, and recurrent chest pain. Risk factors associated with the degree of underlying disease include advanced age, known coronary disease, and history of diabetes or multiple other classic risk factors for coronary disease.

Although multiple, specific criteria and scores for establishing risk have been proposed, none are universally accepted.

Anti-ischemic Agents

Nitrates reduce myocardial oxygen demand primarily by venodilator effects that decrease myocardial preload. They can also dilate coronary arteries and increase collateral flow. All patients with chest pain who are hemodynamically stable should receive serial sublingual nitroglycerin tablets following diagnostic electrocardiography. Early electrocardiography is critical to diagnose dynamic changes and to identify whether right ventricular infarction is present. Nitrates should be used cautiously, or not at all, in patients with right ventricular infarction. If pain is not relieved after electrocardiography and use of other therapies such as β-blockers,

administration of intravenous nitroglycerin should be initiated.

β-Blockers competitively inhibit the effects of circulating catecholamine on cardiac β1 receptors, thereby decreasing myocardial oxygen demand by decreasing heart rate and contractility. β-Blockers should be given early, preferably intravenously, if tolerated. Oral therapy can then be maintained to achieve a resting heart rate of 50 to 60 beats/min. β-Blockers should be used cautiously, if at all, in patients with significant atrioventricular conduction delays, a history of asthma, or acute LV dysfunction. In patients who are intolerant of β-blockers, nondihydropyridine calcium channel blockers can be considered. Dihydropyridine calcium channel blockers should be avoided, especially in patients not receiving a β-blocker because they can cause reflex tachycardia and therefore increase myocardial work and oxygen demand.

Morphine sulfate can be an effective adjunct when other anti-ischemic therapies have not relieved symptoms. Although morphine has some beneficial hemodynamic effects, its primary benefits are analgesia and anxiety reduction. Although these properties are important to calm a patient and decrease associated elevated catecholamine levels, the analgesic effects can mask symptoms of ongoing myocardial ischemia. In a patient who is asymptomatic following morphine administration, if objective evidence suggests ongoing myocardial ischemia, further therapy should not be delayed.

Anticoagulant Drugs

Heparin and low-molecular-weight heparin (LMWH) indirectly inhibit thrombin formation and activity, thereby decreasing thrombus formation and facilitating thrombus resolution. The results of clinical trials comparing the effects of heparin plus aspirin versus aspirin alone have not found a consistent benefit to heparin, but larger trials have not been, and likely will not be, conducted. In general, the addition of full anticoagulation with administration of intravenous heparin and aspirin for the initial treatment of patients with an ACS has been shown to decrease the risk of death and MI by 30 to 40%.

Low-molecular-weight heparin, compared with unfractionated heparin, possesses increased

Figure 8-4

Acute Coronary Syndromes

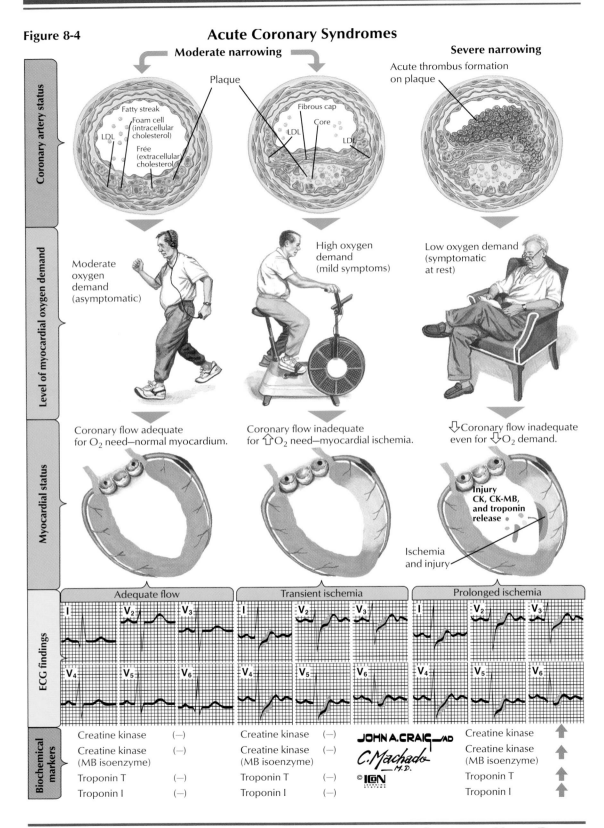

anti–actor Xa activity in relation to anti-factor IIa (antithrombin) activity. LMWH offers several advantages over unfractionated heparin: a more predictable anticoagulant effect so monitoring is not required and subcutaneous administration. Several LMWHs are available that differ somewhat in their anti–factor Xa:IIa activity. How these differences influence the therapeutic benefit of LMWH is unclear, except that enoxaparin is the only LMWH shown to be superior to unfractionated heparin in the treatment of patients with an ACS.

Long-term anticoagulation with use of warfarin, with or without aspirin, has been compared with aspirin alone in several clinical trials. Although the trials have not shown a clear benefit of adding warfarin to aspirin for long-term therapy in patients after admission for a non–ST-elevation ACS, subgroup analysis suggests that if adequate anticoagulation (international normalized ratio >2.0) can be achieved and maintained, the addition of warfarin may be beneficial. At the present time, the routine use of warfarin following non–ST-elevation ACS is not recommended.

ANTIPLATELET AGENTS

Aspirin inhibits the amplification of the platelet activation process by blocking the formation of thromboxane A2 through the irreversible inhibition of platelet cyclooxygenase-1. Multiple placebo-controlled trials, using daily aspirin doses of 75 to 325 mg, have consistently demonstrated a relative decrease in the rate of death and MI: in all studies there is an approximate 50% reduction in patients treated with aspirin versus placebo. Indeed, aspirin therapy provides an acute benefit, and long-term therapy leads to further benefit. Accordingly, aspirin therapy is the cornerstone of antithrombotic therapies in patients with an ACS.

The thienopyridines, primarily clopidogrel, also inhibit the amplification process of platelet activation by irreversibly inhibiting the platelet P2Y12 ADP receptor. Because aspirin and clopidogrel inhibit platelet activation by separate mechanisms, when used together they provide a synergistic antiplatelet effect. The clinical benefit of this combination has been recently demonstrated in the trial Clopidogrel in Unsta-

ble Angina to Prevent Recurrent Ischemic Events (CURE), which enrolled more than 12,500 ACS patients. In this study, combination therapy with clopidogrel and aspirin led to a relative 20% decrease in the combined end point of death, MI, and stroke compared with aspirin alone. This benefit was seen at early time points and continued to increase until the end of follow-up at a mean of 9 months.

Irrespective of the mechanism of platelet activation, platelet aggregation is dependent on platelet–platelet interaction through glycoprotein (GP) IIb/IIIa receptors on the platelet surface and fibrinogen. Several direct antagonists to the platelet GP IIb/IIIa receptor have been developed and studied in ACS patients. Abciximab, tirofiban, and eptifibatide are effective adjunctive agents in patients with an ACS, but primarily in those patients who are troponin positive or undergo a percutaneous coronary intervention (PCI). On the other hand, studies of multiple oral GPIIb/IIIa receptor antagonists showed at least a trend toward an increase in the rate of death and MI, along with a significantly higher bleeding rate, compared with patients treated with aspirin alone. These agents are not indicated in the long-term therapy of patients with ACS.

CORONARY REVASCULARIZATION

Indications for and timing of revascularization of the ACS patient, either through PCI or through coronary artery bypass graft surgery, have been controversial. Early trials (TIMI IIIB and VANQWISH) comparing an invasive approach, which required early angiography and revascularization if indicated, with a more conservative, symptom-driven approach showed little benefit, and even suggested possible harm from use of an invasive strategy. However, recent trials (FRISC II and TACTICS-TIMI 18) have consistently confirmed the benefit of an invasive approach. As with other therapies, the benefit of an invasive approach was primarily realized in those patients at greatest risk, particularly patients with elevated troponins.

FUTURE DIRECTIONS

Dramatic improvements in our understanding of the pathophysiology of ACS and, with it, our treatment of millions of patients have occurred during the last several decades. In the years to come there will be continued improvement in antithrombotic and anti-ischemic therapies, and further research will identify those patients at greatest short- and long-term risk. By improving our ability to identify risk, both for the individual patient and for specific coronary lesions, therapies can be better applied and complications can be further minimized.

REFERENCES

Bertrand ME, Simoons ML, Fox KAA, et al. Management of acute coronary syndromes: Acute coronary syndromes without persistent ST segment elevation. Recommendations of the Task Force of the European Society of Cardiology. *Eur Heart J* 2000;21:1406–1432.

Braunwald E, Antman E, Beasley J, et al. ACC/AHA guideline update for the management of patients with unstable angina and non-ST-segment elevation myocardial infarction: A report of the American College of Cardiology/American Heart Association Task Force on Practice Guidelines (Committee on the Management of Patients with Unstable Angina). 2002. Available at: http://www.acc.org/clinical/guidelines/unstable/unstable.pdf.

Fuster V, Badimon L, Badimon JJ, Chesebro JH. The pathogenesis of coronary artery disease and the acute coronary syndromes. *N Engl J Med* 1992;326:242–250, 310–318.

Libby P. Current concepts of the pathogenesis of acute coronary syndromes. *Circulation* 2001;104:365–372.

Rauch U, Osende JI, Fuster V, Badimon JJ, Fayad Z, Chesebro JH. Thrombus formation on atherosclerotic plaques: Pathogenesis and clinical consequences. *Ann Int Med* 2001;134:224–238.

Yeghiazarians Y, Braunstein JB, Askari A, Stone PH. Unstable angina pectoris. *N Engl J Med* 2000;342:101–114.

Chapter 9
Acute Myocardial Infarction

Christoph Bode and Markus Frey

Acute myocardial infarction (MI) has been described based on findings ranging from clinical presentation to electrocardiographic and/or biochemical findings to pathologic characteristics. Moreover, definitions of MI have varied in different countries. For these reasons a joint committee representing the European Society of Cardiology and the American College of Cardiology developed a consensus statement, published in September 2000, describing diagnostic criteria for MI (included later in chapter).

One of the following criteria (as summarized from *J Am Coll Cardiol* 2000;36:959–969) satisfies the diagnosis for an acute, evolving, or recent MI:

1) Typical rise and gradual fall (troponin) or more rapid rise and fall (CK-MB) of biochemical markers of myocardial necrosis, with at least one of the following:
   a) Ischemic symptoms.
   b) Development of pathologic Q waves on the ECG, ECG changes indicative of ischemia (ST-segment elevation or depression), or coronary artery intervention (e.g., coronary angioplasty).
2) Pathologic findings of an acute MI.

Any one of the following criteria satisfies the diagnosis for an established MI:

1) Development of new pathologic Q waves on serial ECGs. The patient may or may not remember previous symptoms. Biochemical markers of myocardial necrosis may have normalized, depending on the length of time that has passed since the infarct developed.
2) Pathologic findings of a healed or healing MI.

ETIOLOGY AND PATHOGENESIS

The initial event in the formation of an occlusive intracoronary thrombus is the rupture or ulceration of an atherosclerotic plaque. Plaque rupture results in the exposure of circulating platelets to the thrombogenic contents of the plaque, such as fibrillar collagen, von Willebrand factor, vitronectin, fibrinogen, and fibronectin. The adhesion of platelets to the ulcerated plaque, with subsequent platelet activation and aggregation, leads to thrombin generation, conversion of fibrinogen to fibrin, and further activation of platelets, as well as vasoconstriction, due in part to platelet-derived vasoconstrictors. This prothrombotic milieu promotes the propagation and stabilization of an active thrombus that contains platelets, fibrin, thrombin, and erythrocytes, resulting in occlusion of the infarct-related artery.

Upon interruption of antegrade flow in an epicardial coronary artery, the zone of myocardium supplied by that vessel immediately loses its ability to perform contractile work. Abnormal contraction patterns develop: dyssynchrony, hypokinesis, akinesis, and dyskinesis. Myocardial dysfunction in an area of ischemia is typically complemented by hyperkinesis of the remaining normal myocardium, due to acute compensatory mechanisms (including increased sympathetic nervous system activity) and the Frank-Starling mechanism.

CLINICAL PRESENTATION

Typical prodromal symptoms are present in many but not all patients with MI. Of these, chest discomfort, resembling classic angina pectoris but occurring at rest or with less activity than usual is the most common. The intensity of MI pain is variable, usually severe, and in some instances intolerable. The pain is prolonged, usually lasting more than 30 minutes and frequently lasting for hours (see also chapter 1). The discomfort is described as constricting, crushing, oppressing, or compressing. Often, the patient complains of a sensation of a heavy weight on or a squeezing in the chest. The pain is usually retrosternal, frequently spreading to both sides of the anterior chest, with predilection for the left side. Often, the pain radiates down the ulnar aspect of the left arm, producing a sensation in the left wrist, hand, and fingers. In some instances, the pain of an acute MI may begin in the epigastric area and simulate a variety of abdominal disorders. In other patients, MI discomfort radiates to the shoulders, upper extremities, neck, jaw, and even the interscapular region. In patients with preexisting angina pectoris, the pain of infarction usually resembles that of angina. However, it is generally much more severe, lasts longer, and is not relieved by rest and nitroglycerin. In some patients, particularly the elderly, an MI is manifested clinically not by pain but by symptoms of acute left ventricular (LV) failure and chest tightness or by marked weakness or frank syncope. These symptoms may be accompanied by diaphoresis, nausea, and vomiting. More than 50% of patients with ST-segment elevation and severe chest pain experience nausea and vomiting, presumably from the activation of the vagal reflex or from the stimulation of LV receptors as part of the Bezold-Jarisch reflex. These symptoms are more common in patients with an inferior MI than in those with an anterior MI.

Numerous findings may be present in the patient presenting with acute MI. A marked jugular venous distention and waves of tricuspid regurgitation are evident in right ventricular infarction. A third heart sound usually reflects severe LV dysfunction with elevated ventricular filling pressure. Systolic murmurs are commonly audible in patients with an acute MI and result from mitral regurgitation secondary to dysfunction of the mitral valve apparatus (papillary muscle dysfunction, LV dilatation). LV dysfunction may also result in pulmonary edema, hypotension, and decreased peripheral perfusion with cool extremities and mottling.

DIFFERENTIAL DIAGNOSIS

The pain of an acute MI may simulate the pain of acute pericarditis, which is usually associated with some pleuritic features and aggravated by respiratory movements and coughing. Pleural pain is usually a sharp, knife-like, and aggravated in a cyclic fashion by each breath. These features distinguish pleural pain from the deep,

dull, steady pain of an acute MI. Pulmonary embolism generally produces pain laterally in the chest, often is pleuritic, and may be associated with hemoptysis. Pain from acute dissection of the aorta is usually localized in the center of the chest, is extremely severe, persists for many hours, often radiating to the back or the lower extremities, and reaching maximal intensity shortly after onset of the pain. Often, one or more major arterial pulses are absent. Pain arising from the costochondral and chondrosternal articulations is characterized by marked localized tenderness. The pain of an acute MI, particularly of an inferior MI, may also simulate the pain of peptic ulcer disease or stress gastritis.

DIAGNOSTIC APPROACH
Electrocardiographic Findings

The initial ECG of patients with acute chest pain is diagnostic of acute infarction in approximately 50% of patients, abnormal but not diagnostic in approximately 40%, and normal in about 10%. Serial tracings increase the sensitivity to near 95%. A pattern of ST-segment elevation, especially with associated T-wave changes and ST depression in another anatomic distribution ("reciprocal changes"; see chapter 3), and a clinical history of ischemic heart disease are highly suggestive of an acute MI. Evolution of the characteristic ST-segment and T-wave changes coupled with the appearance of Q waves is highly specific for an acute MI (Fig. 9-1). ST-segment depression may reflect subendocardial ischemia, infarction, or reciprocal changes secondary to infarction at a "remote" (opposite) site. Minor, subtle ST-segment depression is common early in an acute MI. Because ST-segment depression is often a nonspecific change, it should be evaluated in light of other clinical and laboratory findings. Many factors limit the ability of ECG to diagnose and localize an MI: the extent of the myocardial injury, the age of the infarct, the location of the infarct (e.g., the 12-lead ECG is relatively insensitive to infarction in the posterolateral region of the left ventricle), conduction defects, previous infarcts or acute pericarditis, changes in electrolyte concentrations, and the administration of cardioactive drugs. General agreement exists on electrocardiographic criteria for recognition of infarction

Figure 9-1

Manifestations of Myocardial Infarction

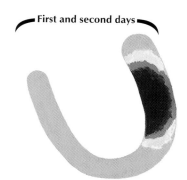

First and second days

Transmural infarction nearly complete. Some ischemia and injury may be present at borders.

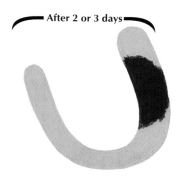

After 2 or 3 days

Transmural infarction complete

of the anterior (Fig. 9-2A) and inferior myocardial walls; there is less agreement on criteria for lateral and posterior infarcts (Fig 9-2B).

Serum Cardiac Markers

Before cardiac markers can be detected in serum, the myocyte cell membrane has to have disintegrated. Because this disintegration process takes time, serum markers are not useful for early detection of an acute MI. Serum markers are, however, proof of an established MI and useful indicators of risk. Serum markers used to diagnose an acute MI are creatine kinase (CK) and CK isoenzymes (CK-MB fraction), myoglobin, and cardiac-specific troponins (troponin I and troponin T). Other serum markers used or proposed for use in an acute MI diagnosis are heart fatty acid–binding proteins, myosin light chain, enolase, lactate dehydrogenase, and myosin light chain.

Traditionally, CK, CK-MB, and lactate dehydrogenase are measured, but additional serum markers have been investigated because of the relatively slow rate of rise above normal for CK. Because noncardiac sources produce significant lactate dehydrogenase, it is rarely used in the diagnosis of MI today. The smaller molecule myoglobin is released quickly from infarcted myocardium but is not cardiac-specific. Therefore, elevations of myoglobin that may be detect-

ed early after the onset of infarction require confirmation with a more cardiac-specific marker, such as troponin I or troponin T. The troponins are the most specific marker in clinical use.

Evidence supports a decisive role of inflammation in the pathogenesis of atherosclerosis and acute coronary syndromes. Acute-phase reactants such as C-reactive protein, serum amyloid A, and fibrinogen are increased in patients with coronary disease, suggesting that inflammation is probably not restricted to the atheromatous plaque. Levels of C-reactive protein provide important short- and long-term prognostic information in patients with unstable angina. Elevated C-reactive protein concentrations have also been associated with increased risk of future cardiac events. *Helicobacter pylori* and *Chlamydia pneumoniae* have been postulated as playing a role in plaque formation and rupture, but controversy continues over whether antigens for these organisms are useful for patients with coronary heart disease.

Other Imaging

In patients with chest pain compatible with an acute MI but with a nondiagnostic ECG, echocardiographic demonstration of a distinct region of disordered contraction can be helpful because this finding supports the diagnosis of myocardial ischemia. In patients with cardiogenic shock,

Figure 9-2

Localization of Anterior Infarcts

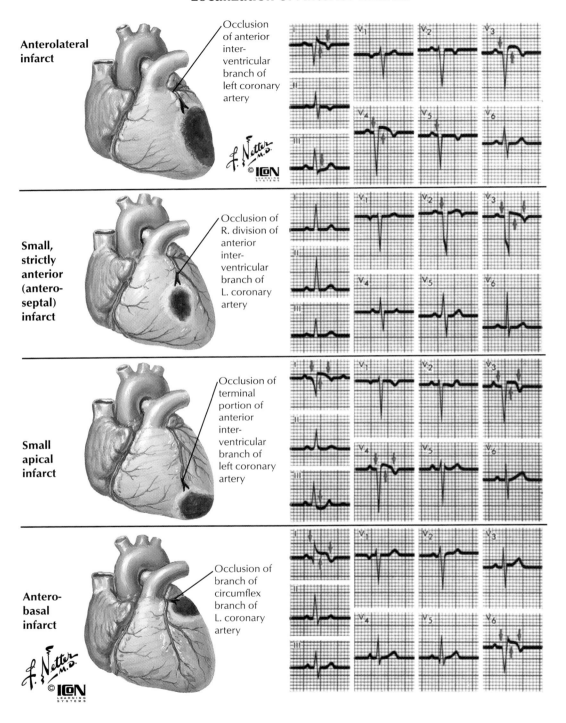

Anterolateral infarct — Occlusion of anterior inter-ventricular branch of left coronary artery

Small, strictly anterior (antero-septal) infarct — Occlusion of R. division of anterior inter-ventricular branch of L. coronary artery

Small apical infarct — Occlusion of terminal portion of anterior inter-ventricular branch of left coronary artery

Antero-basal infarct — Occlusion of branch of circumflex branch of L. coronary artery

A

Figure 9-2 (cont.)

Localization of Posterior Infarcts

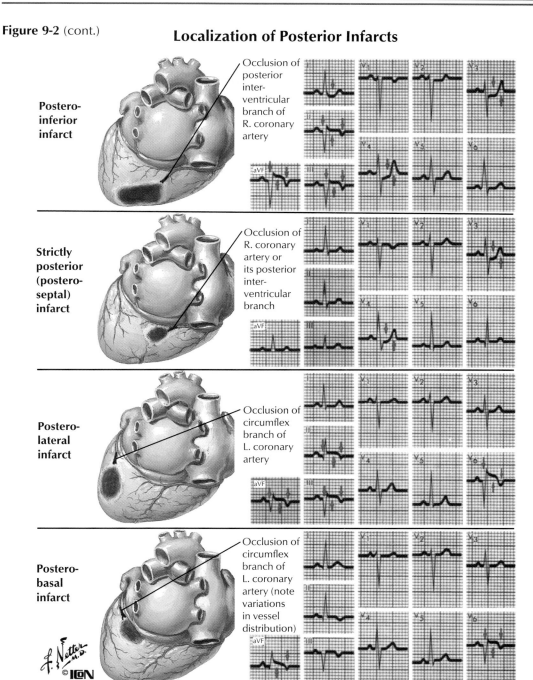

Postero-inferior infarct — Occlusion of posterior inter-ventricular branch of R. coronary artery

Strictly posterior (postero-septal) infarct — Occlusion of R. coronary artery or its posterior inter-ventricular branch

Postero-lateral infarct — Occlusion of circumflex branch of L. coronary artery

Postero-basal infarct — Occlusion of circumflex branch of L. coronary artery (note variations in vessel distribution)

B

echocardiography can be extremely useful in detecting correctable mechanical causes for low cardiac output—for instance, the presence of a new ventricular septum defect or papillary muscle dysfunction—and distinguishing these from global LV dysfunction. Radiographic examination may show signs of LV failure and cardiomegaly. Magnetic resonance imaging can permit the early recognition of an MI and an assessment of the severity of the ischemic insult.

With the emphasis on early reperfusion (see Management and Therapy), the use of MRI is limited in the setting of an acute MI because of the time necessary for these studies.

MANAGEMENT AND THERAPY

Several treatment options lower the mortality rate in an acute MI. These options include early reperfusion (using percutaneous coronary interventions, such as angioplasty; stent placement; or thrombolytic therapy) and administration of aspirin and/or other platelet inhibitors, β-blockers, angiotensin-converting enzyme inhibitors, and statins. Other therapies for acute MI include the use of unfractionated heparin, low-molecular-weight heparin, nitrates, and antiarrhythmic agents; however, the data supporting use of these therapies is less compelling.

Reperfusion is by far the most effective treatment. Until recently, thrombolytic therapy was the best available reperfusion therapy. Thrombolytic therapy is indicated in the case of ST elevation or presumably new left bundle branch block (which obscures the electrocardiographic diagnosis of an MI). Thrombolytic therapy is probably ineffective for normal or nonspecific ECG presentations and possibly harmful for ST-depression presentation in unstable angina and non–ST-elevation MI subgroups. Various thrombolytic agents, including streptokinase, alteplase, and reteplase, are all widely available; their administration does not require specialized facilities or staff; and these agents can be administered with minimal time delay. Numerous large clinical trials have associated the use of thrombolytic therapy with preservation of LV function, limitation of the infarct size, and a highly significant reduction in the mortality rate. This benefit is time-dependent; when administered within 2 hours of symptom onset, fibrinolytic agents are associated with a 30% reduction in the mortality rate; this benefit decreases to an 18% reduction if the fibrinolytic agents are given within 6 hours of symptom onset. Although fibrinolytic agents restore patency in the infarct-related artery in more than 80% of patients within 90 minutes of administration, the failure to achieve complete restoration of normal coronary flow (Thrombolysis in Myocardial Infarction grade 3 flow), which may occur in 45 to 70% of patients, is associated with reduced survival. Even after successful reperfusion, reocclusion occurs in up to 20% of patients and reinfarction in 19%. Therefore, only about 25% of patients treated with thrombolytic therapy achieve the ideal outcome of rapid and sustained normalization of flow in the infarct-related artery. Finally, fibrinolytic therapy is limited by contraindications to its use, which affect up to 30% of patients, and the risk of intracranial hemorrhage.

In recent years, primary angioplasty and stent placement (termed "percutaneous coronary intervention"; PCI) have been shown to be even more efficacious than thrombolytic therapy in the treatment of patients with acute MI. PCI is more effective than thrombolytic therapy because it achieves both higher infarct-related artery patency rates and greater Thrombolysis in Myocardial Infarction grade 3 flow. PCI also has advantages over thrombolytic therapy in terms of the rates of short-term mortality, bleeding complications (including intracranial hemorrhage), and stroke (Figs. 9-3 and 9-4). The benefit of primary angioplasty with regard to the rates of mortality, reinfarction, and recurrent ischemia continues over long-term follow-up. Early intervention has the additional advantage of angiographic definition of the coronary vessels, which allows early risk stratification and identification of patients at particularly high or low risk for recurrent MI or cardiovascular compromise. The use of stents in primary angioplasty adds further benefits, addressing the frequent problem of restenosis and the need for repeat revascularization. The data suggest that mechanical reperfusion is superior to thrombolysis, even if longer transport times to a specialized center must be accepted (Fig. 9-5). Recent studies have suggested that if a patient with acute MI can be transported to a facility with PCI capability within 2 hours, even with the delay in initiation of definitive therapy, patients undergoing PCI (as compared with those undergoing thrombolytic therapy) have improved outcomes.

Hemodynamic Disturbances and Arrhythmias

Left ventricular dysfunction remains the most important predictor of death following MI. In patients with MI, heart failure is characterized by systolic dysfunction or by both systolic and diastolic dysfunction. LV diastolic dysfunction

Figure 9-3   **Acute Coronary Intervention**

Acute coronary intervention reduces mortality from MI, even in critically ill patients. Continuous electrocardiographic and hemodynamic monitoring is performed throughout the procedure and additional hemodynamic support (pharmacologic or with an intra-aortic balloon pump) is available for patients with cardiogenic shock.

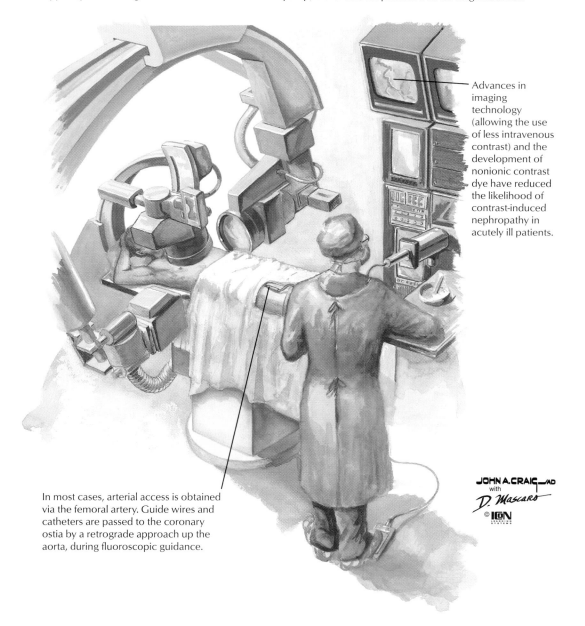

Advances in imaging technology (allowing the use of less intravenous contrast) and the development of nonionic contrast dye have reduced the likelihood of contrast-induced nephropathy in acutely ill patients.

In most cases, arterial access is obtained via the femoral artery. Guide wires and catheters are passed to the coronary ostia by a retrograde approach up the aorta, during fluoroscopic guidance.

JOHN A. CRAIG AD
with
D. Mascaro
© ICN

can lead to pulmonary venous hypertension and pulmonary congestion; systolic dysfunction can result in markedly depressed cardiac output and cardiogenic shock. Mortality rates in patients with acute MI increase with the severity of the hemodynamic deficits.

Mechanical causes of heart failure may occur in an acute MI: free wall rupture, pseudoa-

Figure 9-4   **Acute Myocardial Infarction**

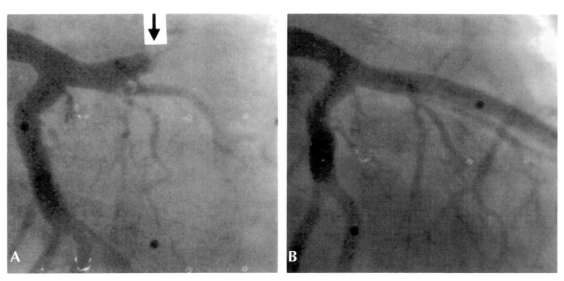

(**A**) Acute myocardial infarction. Occuluded left anterior descending artery (arrow). (**B**)Recanalization of left anterior descending artery after PCI.

neurysm, rupture of the interventricular septum, or rupture of a papillary muscle. Arrhythmias may occur in an MI as a consequence of electrical instability. Sinus bradycardia, sometimes associated with atrioventricular block and hypotension, may reflect augmented vagal activity. Ischemic injury can produce conduction block at any level of the atrioventricular or intraventricular conduction system.

Other complications after an acute MI are recurrent chest discomfort, ischemia, and infarction. Furthermore, pericardial effusion, pericarditis, and Dressler's syndrome may also occur. An LV aneurysm develops in less than 5 to 10% of patients with an MI (especially patients with an anterior MI). The mortality rate is up to six times higher in patients with an LV aneurysm than it is in patients without aneurysms. Death in patients with an LV aneurysm is often sudden and presumably related to ventricular tachyarrhythmias, which frequently occur with aneurysms.

Secondary Prevention

The concept of secondary prevention of reinfarction and death after recovery from an acute MI includes lifestyle modification, cessation of smoking, and control of hypertension and diabetes mellitus. Modification of the lipid profile requires drug therapy (preferably with an HMG CoA reductase inhibitor) in the majority of patients. Several randomized trials with patients with a prior MI have shown that prolonged antiplatelet therapy leads to a 25% reduction in the risk of recurrent infarction, stroke, or vascular death. Indefinite angiotensin-converting enzyme inhibitor therapy is recommended for patients with clinically evident congestive heart failure, a moderate decrease in global ejection fraction, or a large, regional wall motion abnormality. Recent studies have suggested that MI patients with preserved LV function may also benefit from long-term therapy with an angiotensin-converting enzyme inhibitor. Meta-analyses of trials of β-adrenoceptor blockers have shown a 20% reduction in the long-term mortality rate. This reduction is probably due to a combination of an antiarrhythmic effect (prevention of sudden cardiac death) and the prevention of a reinfarction.

Estrogen plus progestin seem to be ineffective for long-term secondary prevention of coronary heart disease in postmenopausal women. Calcium antagonists are not routinely recommended

Figure 9-5 ## ACC/AHA Guidelines for the Management of Patients With Acute Myocardial Infarction

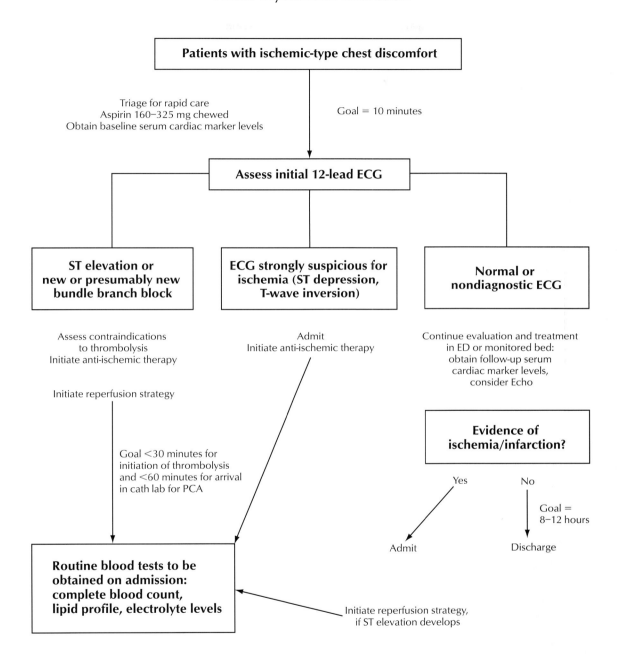

Patients with ischemic-type chest discomfort

Triage for rapid care
Aspirin 160–325 mg chewed
Obtain baseline serum cardiac marker levels

Goal = 10 minutes

Assess initial 12-lead ECG

ST elevation or new or presumably new bundle branch block

ECG strongly suspicious for ischemia (ST depression, T-wave inversion)

Normal or nondiagnostic ECG

Assess contraindications to thrombolysis
Initiate anti-ischemic therapy

Initiate reperfusion strategy

Admit
Initiate anti-ischemic therapy

Continue evaluation and treatment in ED or monitored bed: obtain follow-up serum cardiac marker levels, consider Echo

Goal <30 minutes for initiation of thrombolysis and <60 minutes for arrival in cath lab for PCA

Evidence of ischemia/infarction?

Yes   No

Goal = 8–12 hours

Admit   Discharge

Routine blood tests to be obtained on admission: complete blood count, lipid profile, electrolyte levels

Initiate reperfusion strategy, if ST elevation develops

©1999 by the American College of Cardiology and American Heart Association, Inc.

Reproduced with permission. ACC/AHA Guidelines for the management of patients with acute myocardial infarction: A report on the ACC/AHA Task Force on Practice Guidlines. *J Am Coll Cardiol* 1999:8.

for secondary prevention of infarction, and trials with antiarrhythmics, such as encainide, flecainide, and d-sotalol, following an MI have reported an increased risk of death. Amiodarone may improve survival after an MI in the presence of significant arrhythmias in patients with preserved LV function. Implantable cardioverter defibrillators offer a non-pharmacologic approach for prevention of cardiac arrest from ventricular arrhythmias after an MI. Additional preventive strategies are discussed in section X, Affecting Heart Disease.

FUTURE DIRECTIONS

Patients who survive the initial course of an acute MI are at increased risk because of coronary artery disease and its complications. It is imperative to reduce this risk. For instance, drug-delivering stents (e.g., sirolimus-coated stents) and stem cell therapy with stem cell flow into the infarct area via balloon catheter may offer new strategies in the future, as well as expanding preventive therapies to patients at risk but who have yet to undergo a cardiac event.

REFERENCES

Alpert JS, Thygesen K, Antman E, Bassand J-P. Myocardial infarction redefined—a consensus document of The Joint European Society of Cardiology/American College of Cardiology Committee for the redefinition of myocardial infarction. *J Am Coll Cardiol* 2000;36:959–969.

Braunwald E. Heart Disease. *A Textbook of Cardiovascular Medicine.* 6th ed. Philadelphia: WB Saunders; 2001. Further reading: www.acc.org/clinical/topic/topic.htm#M.

Chapter 10
Percutaneous Coronary Intervention

Bruce R. Brodie and Tift Mann

In the early 1990s, the introduction of coronary stenting revolutionized percutaneous coronary intervention (PCI). Short-term procedural results improved and the incidence of emergency bypass surgery, at 3 to 5% in the 1980s, decreased. Stenting also reduced the frequency of restenosis to 15 to 20% from 30 to 40% with balloon angioplasty. Because of this improvement, the number of PCI procedures increased dramatically in the late 1990s, whereas the volume of coronary bypass surgical procedures remained virtually unchanged (Fig. 10-1).

PERFORMANCE OF PERCUTANEOUS CORONARY INTERVENTION
Procedure and Equipment
Percutaneous coronary intervention is performed in the cardiac catheterization laboratory using the same radiography equipment as used for diagnostic coronary angiography. Access is via the femoral, radial, or brachial artery (Fig. 10-2). The femoral approach is used most frequently because it permits larger catheters to accommodate special devices and requires less technical proficiency. The radial approach has recently increased in popularity as it significantly reduces access site bleeding complications and allows ambulation immediately after PCI. Disadvantages of the transradial approach are the significant learning curve and infrequent asymptomatic radial artery occlusion. The presence of a patent ulnar artery and intact palmar arch (which can be assessed by physical examination) are criteria for use of this technique.

Interventional guide catheters are slightly larger than diagnostic catheters to accommodate balloons, stents, and other devices. After visualization of the coronary artery and target lesion with use of arteriography, a coronary guide wire is advanced across the lesion and positioned in the distal vessel. A small double-lumen catheter with a distal balloon is passed over the guide wire and positioned at the lesion. An inflation device is used to expand the balloon and open the obstruction by fracturing and compressing plaque and stretching the coronary artery. When coronary stenting is performed, as in most cases today, a second balloon catheter containing the stent is passed over the guide wire to the area previously dilated. Balloon inflation expands and deploys the stent (Fig. 10-3). If the stent is not fully deployed, a high-pressure balloon catheter is used to fully expand the stent. Because of recent improvements, it is increasingly common to insert and fully expand the stent using a single-balloon catheter without predilatation.

After PCI, catheters are removed; hemostasis has traditionally been achieved at the access site via manual compression once the activated clotting time has returned to baseline. More recently, the use of "closure devices" at the femoral arteriotomy site has gained popularity. In this circumstance, the femoral arteriotomy site is closed immediately after the procedure, providing immediate hemostasis in suitable patients and allowing earlier ambulation.

Adjunctive Pharmacologic Therapy
All patients undergoing PCI receive aspirin before the procedure and the patient's blood is fully heparinized during the procedure. The activated clotting time (ACT) is maintained at levels appropriate to prevent thrombus formation. Platelet glycoprotein IIb/IIIa inhibitors are commonly used to reduce periprocedural infarction and ischemic events, particularly in acute coronary syndromes. When stents are used, the platelet inhibitor clopidogrel is given before or during the procedure and for 30 days after the procedure until the stent is endothelialized.

Figure 10-1 **Volume of Open Heart and Percutaneous Coronary Intervention (PCI) Procedures in North Carolina 1986–2000**

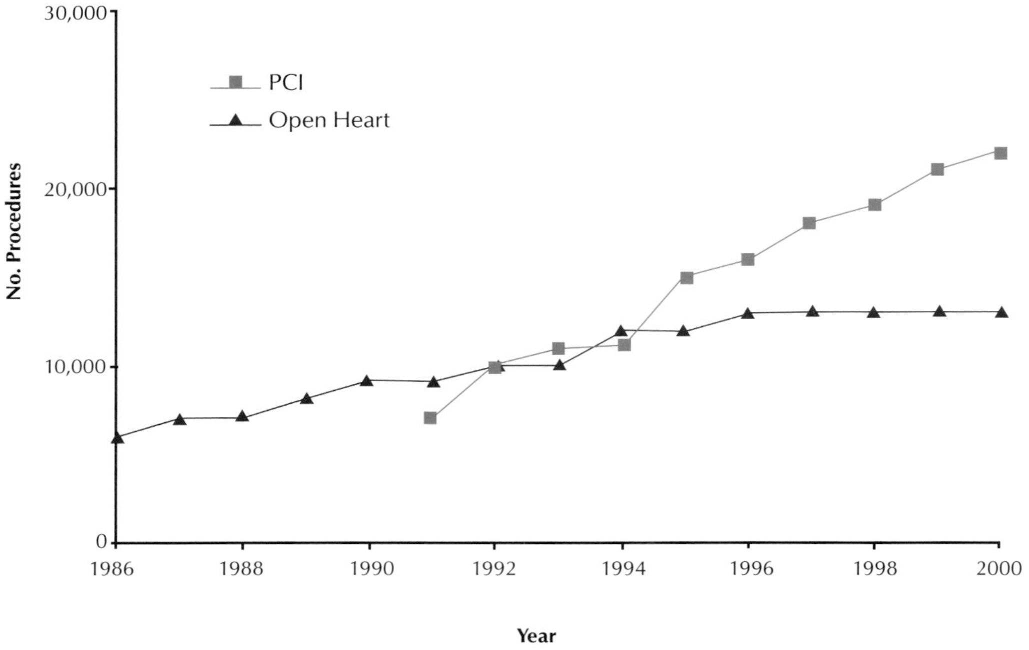

Source: NC Medical Database Commission

Recent studies have suggested additional benefit when clopidogrel is continued for 6 to 9 months after PCI. Intracoronary nitroglycerin, calcium channel blockers, and adenosine may be administered as needed.

Outcomes With Percutaneous Coronary Intervention

With improved technology, availability of stents, and greater operator experience, outcomes of PCI procedures have improved dramatically. With proper patient selection and when performed by experienced operators, procedural success—defined as reduction in the minimal lumen diameter at the lesion site to less than 30% with good flow—can be expected in more than 95% of patients. The American Heart Association (AHA)/American College of Cardiology (ACC) Guidelines for PCI have recommended that PCI be performed only in institutions that do more than 400 PCI procedures per year and by operators who perform more than 75 PCI procedures per year.

Although procedural results with PCI have been excellent, restenosis remains a major limitation. Balloon trauma to the vessel wall induces vascular cell hyperplasia, which may result in a reoccurrence of narrowing of the artery at 3 to 6 months. The need for repeat target vessel revascularization (TVR) occurs in 20 to 30% of patients after balloon angioplasty and in 10 to 15% of patients after coronary stenting. Restenosis after balloon angioplasty can usually be managed with repeat balloon angioplasty or stenting. Restenosis after stenting (in-stent restenosis) is a more difficult problem but can be managed using cutting balloon angioplasty, often combined with local beta or gamma irradiation (brachytherapy). Most recently, "drug-eluting" stents have been approved for use in the United States. These stents are coated with a thin layer of polymer that carries immunosuppressive and antiproliferative agents (sirolimus, tacrolimus, and paclitaxel) that are released over time to prevent the neointimal hyperplasia responsible for restenosis. Early trial results are dramatic and

Figure 10-2

Percutaneous Coronary Intervention:
Vascular Access

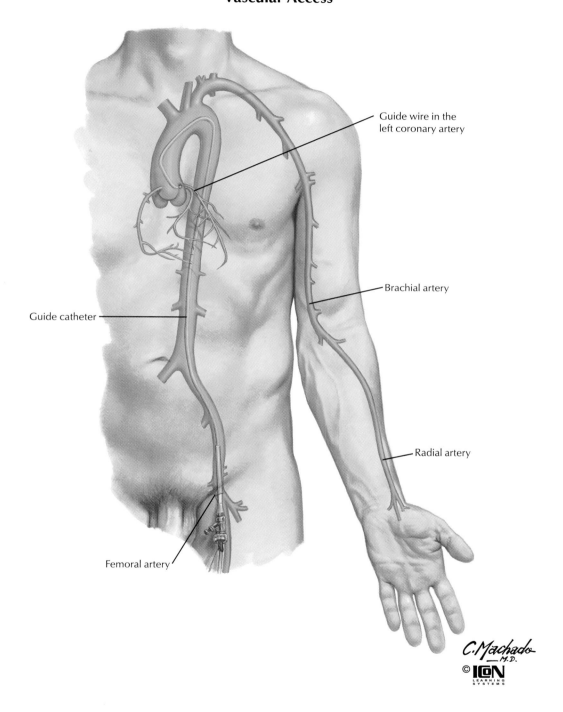

Guide wire in the
left coronary artery

Brachial artery

Guide catheter

Radial artery

Femoral artery

Figure 10-3

Performance of Percutaneous Coronary Intervention:
Stent Deployment

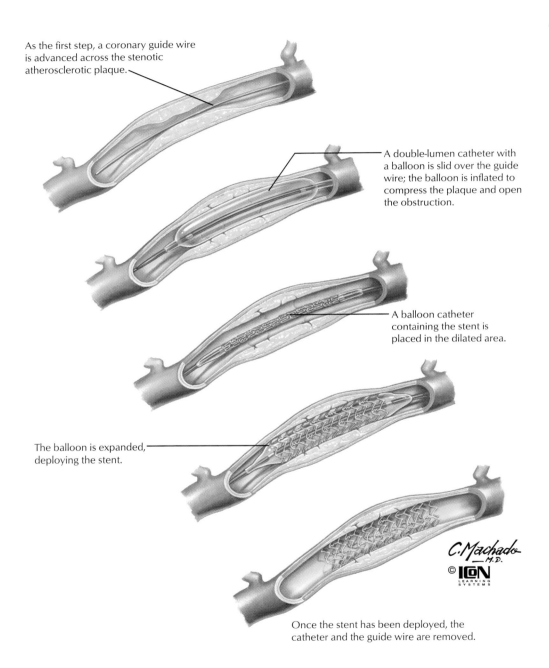

As the first step, a coronary guide wire is advanced across the stenotic atherosclerotic plaque.

A double-lumen catheter with a balloon is slid over the guide wire; the balloon is inflated to compress the plaque and open the obstruction.

A balloon catheter containing the stent is placed in the dilated area.

The balloon is expanded, deploying the stent.

Once the stent has been deployed, the catheter and the guide wire are removed.

show marked reduction in restenosis. If drug-eluting stents prove to be as effective in reducing restenosis as the early trials suggest, the indications and use of stents will increase, as will the number of patients treated with PCI. Despite this advance, it is anticipated that coronary artery surgery will still be required at times for the treatment of refractory restenosis or anytime not suitable for PCI.

Procedural Complications

The most frequent complications with PCI are related to the access site. Bleeding and hematomas occur in 3 to 5% of patients, but can usually be managed conservatively and only occasionally necessitate blood transfusions or surgical intervention. Pseudoaneurysm occurs in less than 1% of patients and can usually be managed with ultrasound-guided compression. Retroperitoneal hemorrhage is rare but may be life threatening, particularly if unrecognized, and may necessitate surgical intervention.

Cardiac complications are surprisingly infrequent. Balloon inflations and stent deployment may result in embolization of atheromatous debris and/or formation of a thrombus in the distal coronary bed. The resultant myocardial infarctions (MIs) are usually small and well tolerated. The use of glycoprotein IIb/IIIa inhibitors reduces MI occurrence in certain clinical situations. Ischemia-induced arrhythmias, including ventricular tachycardia or fibrillation, usually respond to drug therapy and/or cardioversion. PCI-induced coronary artery dissection and/or thrombotic occlusion can result in Q-wave MI, emergency bypass surgery, and occasionally death. Management of coronary dissection with use of stents has greatly reduced these complications. With contemporary PCI performed by experienced operators, the frequency of Q-wave MI is less than 1%; emergency bypass surgery, less than 1%; and mortality, less than 0.5%, after elective PCI.

ADJUNCTIVE DEVICES
Directional Coronary Atherectomy

Directional coronary atherectomy utilizes a high-speed blade to cut plaque, which is then pushed into a flexible nose cone and removed from the artery. This device is technically chal-

lenging to use and has been associated with increased procedural complications. With the advent of stents, it is now only used occasionally as a niche-debulking device.

High-Speed Rotational Atherectomy

High-speed rotational atherectomy (HSRA) uses a diamond-coated burr rotating at high speed to fragment plaque into small particles that are absorbed downstream (Fig. 10-4). It is used primarily to treat heavily calcified, ostial, and bifurcation lesions, and is frequently combined with stenting.

Rheolytic Thrombectomy

Rheolytic thrombectomy uses a unique catheter with a stainless steel tip connected to a hypo-tube, through which high-speed saline is injected. The exit ports are directed back into the main catheter lumen, creating a low-pressure area at the catheter tip that pulls the surrounding thrombus into the catheter. Saline jets then break the thrombus into microparticles and propel them out of the catheter proximal lumen. This device is effective in managing lesions with a large thrombus burden, such as saphenous vein grafts and native arteries in the setting of acute MI.

Distal Protection Devices

Embolization of thrombotic and atherosclerotic debris during balloon inflation and stent deployment remains a serious problem with PCI, especially in degenerated saphenous vein grafts. Various devices have been developed to protect against distal embolization (see also chapter 41). One such device is shown in Fig. 10-5. The guide wire of this device is passed beyond the target lesion and a balloon on the wire distal tip is inflated at low pressure to block distal flow. Atherosclerotic debris, which is embolized during stent deployment, is trapped by the distal balloon and removed with an aspiration catheter. This device has been shown to reduce periprocedural infarction when used with PCI in saphenous vein grafts.

Intravascular Ultrasound

Intravascular ultrasound uses an ultrasonic transducer to visualize the atherosclerotic plaque and vessel wall, providing diagnostic information not available from coronary angiography (see chapter 6). It is used pre-PCI to help select a device and to quantitate lumen and vessel size for sizing stents; it is used post-PCI to assess the adequacy of stent deployment. With technical advances in stent design and deployment, intravascular ultrasound is used less frequently.

Cutting Balloon

The cutting balloon has three cutting blades or atherotomes that cause a controlled dissection and may provide a better opening compared with standard balloon angioplasty. It has been used to treat in-stent restenosis (often combined with brachytherapy), bifurcation and ostial lesions, and small vessels.

Brachytherapy

Brachytherapy uses beta or gamma irradiation applied locally at the target site in the coronary artery immediately after PCI. Brachytherapy reduces restenosis by preventing intimal hyperplasia and is adjunctive therapy for in-stent restenosis.

INDICATIONS

Coronary revascularization with PCI can provide symptomatic relief from angina for patients with obstructive coronary artery disease (CAD) and may improve survival in some patients. Indications for PCI have been outlined in the AHA/ACC guidelines for PCI. The decision to perform PCI involves weighing the likelihood of procedural success and long-term benefits against the benefits of alternative strategies of medical therapy and coronary artery bypass surgery. The likelihood of procedural success and late benefit is highly dependent on lesion and patient selection, as well as operator and institutional experience.

Coronary Lesion Selection

Lesion characteristics associated with the lowest procedural success and highest risk include long lesions (>20 mm), lesions with excessive tortuosity or calcification, extremely angulated segments (>90°), degenerative vein grafts, and chronic total occlusions. Small reference-lumen diameter and most of the aforementioned characteristics predict a higher chance of restenosis and need for repeat target vessel revasculariza-

tion. When such lesion characteristics are present and the likelihood of a favorable outcome with PCI is reduced, other alternatives, such as medical therapy or coronary artery bypass graft (CABG) may become more attractive. The lesion complexity should be considered in deciding whether PCI is the appropriate treatment for the clinical subsets described herein.

Patient Selection

Patients with obstructive CAD who are asymptomatic or have only **mild angina** and who have no or minimal ischemia during stress testing can often be treated medically. However, asymptomatic patients who have significant myocardial ischemia during stress testing and severe obstructive CAD during catheterization are at high risk of cardiovascular morbidity and mortality. This risk can be reduced with revascularization, and PCI may be indicated in these patients.

Most studies have demonstrated that patients with **stable angina** and significant obstructive CAD in one or two vessels have less angina and a better quality of life when treated with PCI versus medical therapy. In patients with stable angina, PCI is generally preferred as the revascularization option if the coronary lesions are suitable. In patients with multivessel disease, CABG and PCI both are options. Several randomized trials (EAST, BARI, ARTS) that compared CABG with PCI in patients with multivessel disease have shown similar survival rates between the two groups but less angina and less need for repeat revascularization in the CABG group. Whether to choose CABG or PCI depends on the presence of comorbid disease that may affect surgical risk; lesion characteristics that may affect PCI outcome; and patient preference, weighing the initial risk and morbidity of open heart surgery against the increased need for repeat revascularization procedures after PCI. Diabetic individuals with multivessel disease have better survival rates with CABG than with PCI and are usually treated best using CABG. Patients with significant left main coronary disease are generally treated using CABG.

Studies in patients with **unstable angina** or **non−ST-segment elevation MI** have shown superior outcomes with PCI using stents and glycoprotein IIb/IIIa inhibitors compared with con-

Figure 10-4

Rotational Atherectomy

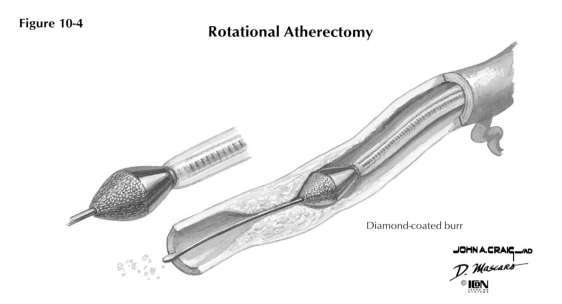

Diamond-coated burr

JOHN A. CRAIG—AD
D. Mascaro
© ICON

servative medical treatment. Consequently, patients with unstable angina and high-risk features or with non–ST-segment elevation MI should undergo early angiography and PCI if severe obstructive CAD is present.

In recent years, primary PCI has become the preferred reperfusion strategy in patients with **ST-segment elevation MI** when facilities and experienced operators are available. Randomized trials have shown that primary PCI is associated with lower mortality rates, fewer episodes of recurrent infarction, and fewer strokes than is thrombolytic therapy. Primary PCI has special advantages in elderly patients, in patients with cardiogenic shock, and in patients ineligible for thrombolytic therapy. Rescue PTCA (emergent PTCA after ineffective thrombolysis) has improved outcome in patients with anterior MI in the RESCUE Trial. Outcomes using rescue PCI have further improved with the addition of stents and glycoprotein IIb/IIIa inhibitors. Urgent angiography with rescue PCI should now be considered in patients with anterior or large MI in whom thrombolysis was thought to be ineffective. PCI may also be indicated after successful thrombolysis for recurrent infarction, recurrent ischemia, or provocable ischemia. The use of PCI to treat residual stenosis in the infarcted artery several days after thrombolytic therapy in patients without con-

firmed ischemia is commonly practiced in the United States, although no large studies document its benefit.

Development of obstructive saphenous vein graft disease (SVGD) after CABG is an increasingly common problem. Saphenous vein graft disease is characterized by diffuse, friable plaque and, often, a thrombus, both of which have an increased frequency of distal embolization during intervention. Distal protection devices have shown improved outcomes by reducing the frequency of distal embolization and periprocedural infarction, and thrombectomy devices may improve outcomes. Glycoprotein IIb/IIIa inhibitors have not shown a benefit in this situation. Patients with obstructive saphenous vein graft disease, objective evidence of ischemia, and favorable lesions are generally good candidates for PCI, especially if an arterial conduit is preserved. Patients in whom multiple saphenous vein grafts are ineffective, especially with LV dysfunction and no functional arterial graft, are usually best treated with subsequent CABG.

FUTURE DIRECTIONS

Technical developments of PCI during the past 25 years are impressive, yet a number of coronary lesion subsets are still difficult to treat: chronic total occlusions, bifurcation lesions, small vessels, saphenous vein grafts, and thrombotic-

Figure 10-5

Example of a Distal Protection Device
(PercuSurge®)

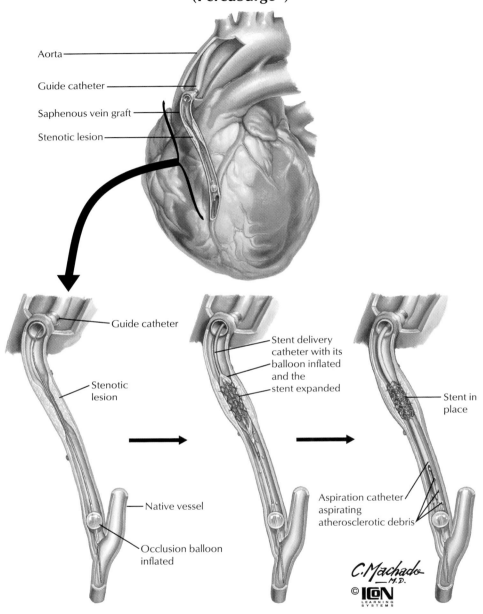

Aorta

Guide catheter

Saphenous vein graft

Stenotic lesion

Guide catheter

Stenotic lesion

Stent delivery catheter with its balloon inflated and the stent expanded

Stent in place

Native vessel

Occlusion balloon inflated

Aspiration catheter aspirating atherosclerotic debris

C. Machado M.D.

© ICON LEARNING SYSTEMS

PercuSurge® Guard Wire (PercuSurge, Inc., Sunnyvale, CA)

containing lesions. Restenosis also remains a major problem and target vessel revascularization is necessary in 10 to 20% of patients, even with stenting.

Trials are evaluating new wires and cutting and ablative devices to facilitate crossing chronic total occlusions. New stents are being designed to specifically address bifurcation lesions and small vessels. New filters are being tested in clinical trials to provide distal protection to prevent distal embolization during saphenous vein graft intervention and during primary PCI in native vessels in the setting of acute MI. Covered stents are being developed to help prevent distal embolization and treat coronary obstruction associated with aneurysmal dilatations. New thrombectomy devices are being tested to better treat thrombotic lesions.

Advances in adjunctive pharmacology are also expected. Low-molecular-weight heparin (enoxaparin) and direct thrombin inhibitors (bivalirudin) both are being tested as replacements for unfractionated heparin with PCI.

The biggest technologic advancement may be the development of drug-eluting stents, and it is anticipated that specific indications for drug-eluting stents will be expanded in the coming years.

REFERENCES

ACC/AHA Guidelines for percutaneous coronary intervention. *J Am Coll Cardiol* 2001;37:2215–2239.

Anderson HV, Shaw RE, Brindis RG, et al. A contemporary overview of percutaneous coronary interventions: The American College of Cardiology–National Cardiovascular Data Registry (ACC-NCDR). *J Am Coll Cardiol* 2002;39:1096–1103.

Douglas JS, King SB III. Percutaneous coronary intervention. In: Fuster V, Alexander RW, O'Rourke RA, eds. *Hurst's The Heart*. 10th ed. New York: McGraw–Hill; 2001:1437–1469.

Topol E. *Textbook of Interventional Cardiology*. 3rd ed. Philadelphia: WB Saunders; 1999.

Chapter 11

Coronary Artery Bypass Surgery

Brett C. Sheridan and Michael R. Mill

Chronic angina affects approximately 5.6 million Americans and new angina develops in an additional 350,000 each year. More than 750,000 Americans present for evaluation with unstable angina/acute coronary syndrome each year. Acute and chronic coronary syndromes result from the myocardial cellular demand for oxygen outstripping the coronary artery system ability to supply this essential element for oxidative metabolism. The insufficient coronary flow of nutrients to myocardial cells results in angina and, if prolonged, leads to myocardial cellular death. The most straightforward solution to this interruption of blood flow through coronary arteries is to bring new or additional blood flow through alternative pathways, thus bypassing the obstructed coronary arteries. The development of coronary artery bypass graft (CABG) surgery was the outgrowth of this understanding.

ETIOLOGY AND PATHOGENESIS

With the presence of risk factors for atherosclerosis—including advanced age, genetic predisposition, male sex, hypertension, diabetes mellitus, hyperlipidemia, and cigarette smoking—the thin and sparsely muscled arterial intima increases in thickness and smooth muscle content. This earliest stage of atherosclerosis is caused by proliferation of smooth muscle cells; formation of a tissue matrix of collagen, elastin, and proteoglycan; and the accumulation of intra- and extracellular lipids. The first phase of atherosclerotic lesion formation is focal thickening of the intima, with smooth muscle cells and extracellular matrix. Intracellular lipid deposits also accumulate. In its earliest phase, the lesion formed is referred to as a fatty streak, an accumulation of intracellular and extracellular lipid that is visible in diseased segments of affected arteries. A fibrous plaque results from continued accumulation of fibroblasts covering proliferating smooth muscle cells laden with lipids and cellular debris. The lesion evolves in complexity as ongoing cellular degeneration leads to the ingress of blood constituents and calcification. The necrotic core of the plaque may enlarge and become calcified. Hemorrhage into the plaque may disrupt the smooth fibrous surface, causing thrombogenic ulcerations. Organization of clot on the plaque surface increases protrusion into the arterial lumen, further decreasing blood flow (see also chapter 2).

Just as the rapidity of atherosclerotic lesion formation varies from individual to individual, the presentation of ischemic heart disease also varies. Objective evidence of myocardial ischemia is identified with concurrent coronary angiographic evidence of flow-limiting atherosclerotic lesions. The need for surgical treatment of coronary heart disease usually is a manifestation of either the presentation of an individual with an acute coronary syndrome and multivessel coronary artery disease or the result of debilitating (albeit stable) angina (see chapter 8). Examples of indications for CABG include postinfarction angina, ventricular septal defect, acute mitral regurgitation, free wall rupture, and/or cardiogenic shock in patients admitted to the hospital with acute myocardial infarction (MI). Each of these acute conditions warrants surgical intervention and revascularization.

DIFFERENTIAL DIAGNOSIS

The differential diagnosis of myocardial ischemia includes atherosclerotic obstruction, as well as nonatherosclerotic causes of epicardial coronary artery obstruction. Nonatherosclerotic causes of epicardial coronary obstruction include congenital anomalies, myocardial bridges, vascularities, aortic dissection, granulomas, tumors, scarring from trauma, as well as vasospasm, and embolism. Many of these entities may also be indications for CABG.

Other diseases mimicking angina include esophagitis due to gastrointestinal reflux, peptic ulcer disease, biliary colic, visceral artery ischemia, pericarditis, pleurisy, thoracic aortic dissection, and musculoskeletal disorders.

DIAGNOSTIC APPROACH

Although patients with ischemic heart disease present with a spectrum of clinical urgency, the diagnostic evaluation relies on objective evidence of ischemia and assessment of disease burden and coronary anatomy. The diagnostic approach begins with a complete history and extensive physical examination (see chapter 1). Often, the physical examination fails to assist in the diagnosis for chronic ischemic heart disease. Many patients with chronic ischemic heart disease have no physical findings related to the disease or, if present, findings are not specific for CAD. Because coronary atherosclerosis is the most common heart disease in industrialized nations, any physical finding suggestive of heart disease should raise the suspicion of chronic ischemic heart disease.

Diagnostic evaluation includes multiple approaches. Laboratory studies are conducted for cardiac risk factors such as diabetes mellitus, hyperlipidemia, and hyperthyroidism. The ECG allows documentation of ischemia during chest pain or after exercise testing. A stress test may be used to detect CAD or assess the functional importance of coronary lesions. The test results are positive if the patient has signs or symptoms of angina pectoris with typical ischemic ECG changes. The specificity of the stress test may improve with thallium injection during exercise. Other ways of assessing myocardial perfusion or stress testing include pharmacologic stressing using the synthetic catecholamine dobutamine, which mimics exercise or other vasodilator drugs, such as dipyridamole and adenosine that produce profound vasodilatation, increased heart rate, and stroke volume, thereby increasing myocardial oxygen demand. Wall-motion abnormalities may be assessed in a stable state with transthoracic echocardiography or in a stress state under increased myocardial demand using an intravenous infusion of the catecholamine, dobutamine. MRI can also assess myocardial perfusion and ventricular wall motion during pharmacologic stress (see chapters 4–6).

The gold standard for evaluating coronary anatomy to determine the suitability for surgical revascularization is coronary angiography. It evaluates epicardial coronary vessels for coronary atherosclerosis, including disease location and severity. Experimental studies suggest that lesions that reduce the cross-sectional area of the coronary artery by 70% or more (50% in diameter) significantly limit flow, especially during periods of increased myocardial oxygen demand. If such lesions are detected, they are considered to be compatible with symptoms or other signs of myocardial ischemia. Coronary angiography is, however, imprecise. The cross-sectional area of the coronary artery at the point of atherosclerotic lesion must be estimated from two-dimensional diameter measurements and in several planes. When compared with autopsy findings, stenosis severity is usually found to have been underestimated by coronary angiography. In addition, coronary angiography does not consider that lesions in series in a coronary artery may incrementally reduce the flow to distal beds by more than is accounted for by any single lesion. Therefore, a series of apparently insignificant lesions may reduce myocardial blood flow substantially.

In choosing a diagnostic approach, noninvasive stress testing is performed first in the evaluation of a patient with suspected coronary atherosclerosis, as long as the patient has not presented with an unstable coronary syndrome. In patients with stable angina, or post-MI, the risk of stress testing is low, compared with coronary angiography. Mortality rates for stress testing average 1 per 10,000 patients compared with 1 per 1,000 for coronary angiography. The physiologic demonstration of myocardial ischemia and its extent form the basis of the therapeutic approach, irrespective of coronary anatomy. Mildly symptomatic patients who have small areas of ischemia at intense exercise levels have an excellent prognosis and are usually treated medically, particularly if left ventricular function is normal or near normal. Knowledge of the coronary anatomy is not necessary to make this therapeutic decision. In general, therefore, a noninvasive technique should be used to detect myocardial ischemia and its extent before considering coronary angiography.

Patients with profound symptoms of myocardial ischemia during minimal exertion are more likely to have severe diffuse multivessel coronary atherosclerosis or left-sided main obstruction of the coronary arteries. The likelihood that revascularization will be required is extremely high and coronary angiography should be performed as soon as possible. Patients with severe unstable angina should undergo coronary angiography directly because of a potential increased risk by stress testing. Patients with angina or evidence of ischemia in the early post-MI period are considered to be unstable angina patients and should also undergo coronary angiography rather than stress testing. Other indications for coronary angiography include situations in which noninvasive testing will be inaccurate, such as for many patients with left bundle branch block on ECG or for patients who are unable to exercise and who are difficult to image noninvasively.

MANAGEMENT AND THERAPY

With an indication for surgical myocardial revascularization, the management evolves into an issue of timing (emergent, urgent, or elective) and surgical approach (traditional revascularization with cardioplegic arrest and cardiopulmonary bypass [CPB] support versus off-pump CABG [OPCABG]) (Table 11-1; Fig. 11-1). Considerations on whether to proceed with percutaneous revascularization or surgical revascularization are discussed in chapter 10. The decision to proceed with CABG emergently is made at the time of coronary angiography confirming the diagnosis of occlusive CAD with hemodynamic instability and/or ongoing myocardial ischemia despite intensive medical treatment and placement of an intraaortic balloon pump. Urgent procedures are performed during the same hospital admission secondary to unstable symptoms and severely obstructed coronary anatomy. Those patients with stable angina patterns, hemodynamic stability, and less threatening coronary anatomy may undergo elective CABG.

The gold standard for CABG is complete myocardial revascularization and this distinguishes CABG from percutaneous coronary revascularization approaches. CABG is traditionally performed with an arrested, still heart with circulatory support utilizing CPB. This approach allows for careful selection of diseased vessels with precise anastomosis of grafts to coronary vessels as small as 1.5 mm in diameter. One widely used CPB system uses a roller pump, a membrane oxygenator, and an open reservoir. Because numerous detrimental effects of CPB

Table 11-1
The Indications for Coronary Artery Bypass Surgery

· Left main coronary disease
· Triple-vessel disease with normal or diminished ejection fraction
· Two-vessel disease with involvement of the proximal left-sided anterior descending coronary artery, with normal or diminished ejection fraction
· Unstable (crescendo) angina
· Post–myocardial infarction angina
· Acute coronary occlusion after percutaneous coronary intervention
· Persistent symptoms despite maximal medical therapy
· Coronary artery disease and the need for heart surgery for other indications (i.e., valve replacement surgery)
· Mechanical complications of acute myocardial infarction
    Ventricular septal defect
    Acute mitral regurgitation
    Free-wall rupture
    Cardiogenic shock

Data from Smith HC, Gersh BJ. Indications for revascularization. In: Edmund LH, ed. *Cardiac Surgery in the Adult*. New York: McGraw-Hill; 1997:441–445.

are clearly time dependent, surgery is conducted as expeditiously as possible to limit the duration of extracorporeal circulation. When CPB time is minimized, outcomes for conventional CABG versus OPCABG are virtually identical.

Technical details are critical in optimizing outcomes and, for this reason, are described herein. With use of a traditional surgical revascularization technique, an aortic cross-clamp is placed on the ascending aorta, initiating myocardial ischemia. To minimize myocardial injury, myocardial protection with hypothermia (systemic and topical) and cardioplegia is used. Blood and crystalloid cardioplegia both are used, with indications for each determined by the presence or absence of acute ischemia and surgeon preference. Antegrade and retrograde hypothermic (4°C) oxygenated blood cardioplegia is induced. Hypothermic systemic perfusion provides enhanced right-sided ventricular protection as retrograde cardioplegia via the coronary sinus may provide limited delivery to the right ventricle. These data become clinically relevant in patients with impaired right-sided ventricular function, proximal right coronary artery occlusion, or pro-

Figure 11-1   ## Off-Pump Coronary Artery Bypass Grafting (OPCABG)

A limited median sternotomy is performed.

After opening the pericardial sac, the target coronary artery is dissected from surrounding tissue and held by sutures. During temporary interruption of blood flow through the coronary artery, the anastomosis is performed without cardiopulmonary bypass as long as myocardial function remains stable.

Sutures with Silastic tapes

Lines of the retraction sutures

Left anterior descending (LAD) branch of the left coronary artery exposed and incised on the site of the anastomosis

Local immobilization at the anastomosis is achieved by the use of a stabilizer.

Arm of the stabilizer

Hoses of the suction device of the stabilizer are connected to a vacuum pump.

The type of stabilizer shown here is attached to the epicardium by means of small suction cups.

Detail of the suction cups of the stabilizer

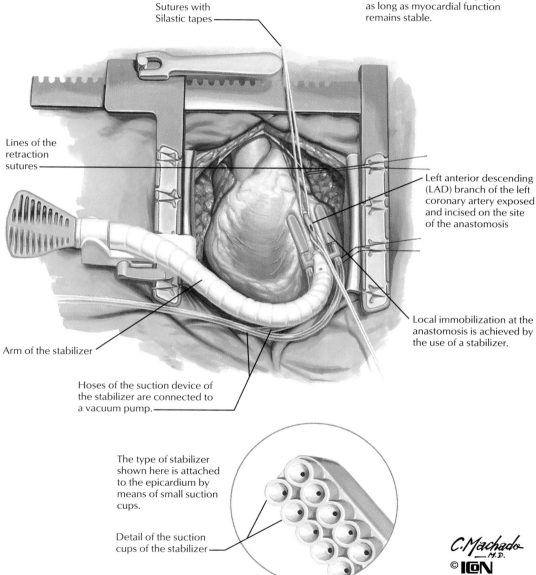

Silastic, Dow Corning, Midland, MI

longed ischemic times, or when right-sided ventricular metabolic demand is increased. A left ventricular (LV) vent is utilized only if the ventricle distends during CPB because ventricular stretch impairs postoperative ventricular function. Approximately 100 ml of crystalloid cardioplegia solution at 4°C are delivered through each graft to the myocardium following completion of anastomoses. Cardioplegic redosing via the aortic root or coronary sinus is performed every 20 minutes throughout the cross-clamp period and is accompanied by strict vigilance to topical cooling, which ensures adequate maintenance of tissue hypothermia during the cross-clamp period.

After cross-clamp application and inducement of cardioplegia, distal anastomoses are performed first. The vessels on the inferior surface of the heart are grafted initially (right coronary artery, posterior descending artery, LV branch); then, proceeding in a counterclockwise direction, the posterior marginals, the mid marginals, the anterior marginals, the ramus–intermedius, the diagonals, and, last, the left-sided anterior descending artery. The internal mammary artery anastomosis to the left anterior descending artery (or alternately, to the most important distal target) is performed last. In the absence of an atherosclerotic aorta, the aortic cross-clamp is removed and a partial occluding clamp is placed on the ascending aorta, and aortotomies are cut and enlarged with a 4-mm punch. If the ascending aorta has substantial disease, embolic risk is minimized by performing the proximal graft anastomosis using a single aortic cross-clamp. Stainless steel washers (which can be visualized by fluoroscopy) are placed on the proximal graft anastomotic sites to assist with later catheterizations. Once proximal and distal anastomoses are completed, the aorta and grafts are de-aired with subsequent removal of the aortic clamp. This initiates myocardial reperfusion and preparations are made for weaning the patient from CPB.

The heart is allowed to reperfuse in an unloaded beating state as electrolyte, acid–base, and hematocrit values are corrected and inotropic agents are started, if indicated. In general, the need for inotropic agents is determined by preoperative or intraoperative factors. Preoperative factors include advanced age, low ejection fraction, high pulmonary artery pressures, high LV end-diastolic pressure, or high central venous pressures. Intraoperative factors that prompt the need for inotropic assistance include incomplete revascularization, severe distal disease, prolonged CPB or cross-clamp times, poor myocardial protection, and poor LV contractility seen by visual inspection after cross-clamp removal. Intraoperative transesophageal echocardiography proves to be helpful in determining the need for inotropic agents after weaning from CPB.

An alternative approach is a beating heart technique in which stabilizing devices are placed on the targeted coronary artery (Fig. 11-1, lower). The coronary artery is briefly occluded (10–20 minutes) or intracoronary shunts are used to allow anastomosis of the graft to the coronary artery distal to the atherosclerotic obstruction. The targeted coronary artery is stabilized and blood pressure is aggressively controlled with volume and inotropic agents delivered during anesthesia. Although hemodynamically and technically more challenging, this procedure allows for pulsatile antegrade flow through the coronary artery and systemic circulation without the added insults of hypothermia, CPB, and the obligatory proinflammatory blood–artificial surface interface.

Minimally invasive surgery is another less widely adapted technique. In brief, this approach incorporates the concept of OPCABG with a limited access incision. A limited left-sided anterolateral thoracotomy is performed through the fourth intercostal space without resection or dissection of the ribs. After opening of the pericardial sac, the target coronary artery is dissected from surrounding tissue and held by sutures at a short distance proximal and distal to the anastomosis that was snared over a piece of pericardium for temporary interruption of blood flow. The anastomosis is performed without CPB as long as myocardial function remains stable. Local immobilization at the anastomosis site is achieved with a stabilizer. This procedure has less utility as minimal exposure limits options with hemodynamic instability and multivessel disease. It is generally limited to single-territory myocardial revascularization because all grafting must be based on the internal thoracic artery.

Figure 11-2

Remote-Access Minimally Invasive
Coronary Artery Bypass Grafting

Images collected by the microcameras inside the chest are transmitted to the computer and displayed on the monitor, for other members of the surgical team.

Sitting a few feet from the patient, the surgeon remotely controls the surgical instruments.

Computer console

Instruments and cameras are inserted into the patient's body via small incisions between the ribs and are remotely controlled by the surgeon.

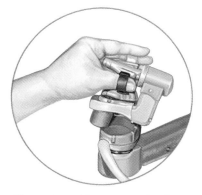

The motions of the surgeon's hand at the console are transmitted to the surgical instruments. Software algorithms filter unwanted motions, including imperceptible tremors of the hands.

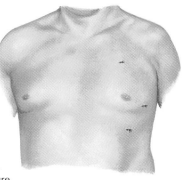

Postsurgical appearance of the patient's chest. Three small sutured incisions are the only sequelae for most patients who undergo this procedure.

C. Machado
—M.D.

© ICN
LEARNING
SYSTEMS

FUTURE DIRECTIONS

Off-pump CABG has reputed advantages in smaller, single-institution prospective series, as well as in retrospective analysis of larger thoracic surgery databases. The advantages of OPCABG appear to include fewer neurological, pulmonary, and renal sequelae. Although the absence of circulatory support with CPB is the prevailing explanation for less end-organ injury, the absence of global ischemia–reperfusion may also play a role in this phenomenon. The potential disadvantage of OPCABG is incomplete myocardial revascularization or compromised distal conduit–coronary anastomosis due to the obligatory movement of a beating heart technique. The ongoing National Institutes of Health (NIH)–sponsored, multicenter, prospective controlled trial evaluating traditional CABG versus OPCABG, will address both questions.

With a rapidly growing incidence of heart failure in the population and a limited number of donors for heart transplantation, techniques to improve LV function in the context of myocardial revascularization have evolved. Surgical restoration of normal LV shape and volume post-MI has gained widespread appeal. The NIH is sponsoring a multicenter, prospective, randomized trial to examine the influence of LV endoaneurysmorrhaphy and CABG on morbidity and mortality rates compared with the influence of medical treatment or CABG alone.

Advances in robotic technology, off-pump multivessel techniques, and closed-chest CPB systems have prompted the exploratory use of remote CABG techniques (Fig. 11-2). One study compared percutaneous intervention to limited-access beating-heart mini-thoracotomy single-vessel coronary revascularization for proximal left-sided anterior CAD. The results proved to be favorable for this hybrid surgical, less invasive approach. The ultimate goal for robotic CABG is complete multivessel revascularization using an off-pump approach without the requirement for sternotomy or even mini-thoracotomy. This requires that conduit harvesting, conduit preparation, target vessel preparation, control, and anastomosis are all performed remotely from a master control unit. Although two-vessel CABG has been successfully performed with this approach in Europe, limitations remain. New technologies in facilitated anastomotic devices, integrated real-time imaging, and guidance control systems will be mandatory to realize the vision of robotic multivessel CABG.

REFERENCES

Barner HB. Techniques of myocardial revascularization. In: Edmunds LH, ed. *Cardiac Surgery in the Adult.* New York: McGraw Hill; 1997.

Diegeler A, Thiele H, Falk V, et al. Comparison of stenting with minimally invasive bypass surgery for stenosis of the left anterior descending coronary artery. *N Engl J Med* 2002;347:561–566.

Dogan S, Aybek T, Andressen E, et al. Totally endoscopic coronary artery bypass grafting on cardiopulmonary bypass with robotically enhanced telemanipulation: A report of 45 cases. *J Thorac Cardiovasc Surg* 2002;123:1125–1131.

Dor V. The endoventricular circular patch plasty ("Dor procedure") in ischemic akinetic dilated ventricles. *Heart Fail Rev* 2001;6:187–193.

Favaloro RG. Saphenous vein autograft replacement of severe segmental coronary artery occlusion. *Ann Thorac Surg* 1968;5:334–339.

Johnson WD, Flemma RJ, Lepley DJ, et al. Extended treatment of severe coronary artery disease: A total surgical approach. *Ann Surg* 1969;170:460–470.

Ross R, Glomset JA. Atherosclerosis and the arterial smooth muscle cell. *Science* 1973;180:1332–1339.

Section III
MYOCARDIAL DISEASES AND CARDIOMYOPATHY

Chapter 12

Dilated Cardiomyopathy

Kirkwood F. Adams, Jr, and Stephanie H. Dunlap

Dilated cardiomyopathy is the most common subset of the myocardial diseases known as cardiomyopathies. To unify the classification of cardiomyopathies, the World Health Organization developed nomenclature that divides the disease process into three categories based on anatomic and physiologic findings: dilated, hypertrophic, and restrictive. Dilated cardiomyopathy, this chapter's focus, is characterized by enlargement of one or both ventricles accompanied by systolic and diastolic contractile dysfunction. The myocardial muscle disease causing contractile dysfunction may be primary, arising within the cardiomyocytes, or secondary to associated systemic diseases.

ETIOLOGY

In the United States and all industrialized countries, the most common form of dilated cardiomyopathy is termed *ischemic* and it reflects left ventricular (LV) dilatation following myocardial infarction (MI). Although the process begins with LV dysfunction, it may subsequently cause pressure overload of the right ventricle and right ventricular dysfunction. The next largest category of causes of dilated cardiomyopathy fall into the category of *idiopathic*, where no definitive cause can be found. Idiopathic cardiomyopathies likely include those resulting from viral causes and some of the specific forms of heart muscle disease, listed in Table 12-1, that were not recognized until the end stage when dilatation is irreversible. **Familial cardiomyopathy** also appears to be a major part of the spectrum of dilated cardiomyopathy. Of patients diagnosed with idiopathic cardiomyopathy, approximately 25% have a familial component.

A significant number of patients with dilated cardiomyopathy have diabetes. Although systolic dysfunction in people with diabetes was attributed solely to coronary artery disease and MI, some studies suggest that myocardial muscle dysfunction occurs in the absence of ischemic heart disease. Hypertension is common in diabetic individuals and may contribute to the development of diabetic cardiomyopathy. Animal studies suggest that, unless hypertension is present, systolic dysfunction is mild or absent despite the presence of diabetes.

Alcohol abuse is an important cause of dilated cardiomyopathy that can be easily missed but that may be reversible if detected early and if alcohol ingestion ceases. Typically, the patient with **alcoholic cardiomyopathy** may not have the characteristics commonly associated with patients who abuse alcohol because the cardiomyopathic presentation tends to occur prior to the development of end-stage liver disease. For instance, in these individuals, hepatic damage is typically absent, unless passive congestion is severe. Other objective and psychosocial characteristics associated with alcohol abuse also may not be present. Alcoholic cardiomyopathy is not seen in the absence of heavy and sustained alcohol ingestion; one definition suggests that a daily intake of 75 g or more for at least 2 years is necessary. Animal studies support the notion that alcohol has a direct toxic effect: a variety of biochemical and molecular abnormalities has been described in the cardiomyocytes of animals with alcoholic cardiomyopathy. As is the case in all "toxin-related" causes of dilated cardiomyopathy, alcohol can act in synergy with other toxins (e.g., radiation, chemotherapy), with the end-result that cardiomyopathy develops at an early stage of the disease process.

Peripartum cardiomyopathy is a serious complication of pregnancy. Although the classic depiction is as a postpartum phenomenon, this form of dilated cardiomyopathy also occurs in the later stages of pregnancy. The broad spectrum of clinical severity in peripartum cardiomyopathy requires that it be differentiated from toxemia of pregnancy, in which myocardial involvement is part of a systemic disease and

Table 12-1
Differential Diagnosis of Dilated Cardiomyopathy

Etiology	Evaluation Needed
Acromegaly	History of change in jaw, hand, or foot size
Alcoholic cardiomyopathy	Documented abuse
Atrioventricular shunt	Consider especially in setting of nonperitoneal dialysis
Beriberi	Thiamine deficiency
Chemotherapy	History of exposure to doxorubicin or cyclophosphamide
Cocaine	Screen for drug use
Collagen vascular disease	ANA, RF
Diabetic	Hemoglobin A1c
Hyperesinophilic heart disease	CBC with differential
Familial	In familial CM, early death (age <50 y)may result from SCD or CHF
Heavy metals	Exposure to lead, arsenic, cobalt
Hemochromatosis	Iron, TIBC
Hemoglobinopathies	Hemoglobin electrophoresis
HIV	Screen for virus
Lyme disease	Screen with immunoassay for *B. burgdorferi* (active infection) or for antibodies to *B. burgdorferi* (prior exposure)
Myocarditis	Troponin, endomyocardial biopsy
Nutritional deficiencies	Thiamine
Peripartum CM	Timing of heart failure relative to pregnancy
Sarcoidosis	Thallium perfusion imaging
Tobacco	Smoking history
Thyrotoxicosis	TSH, T4

ANA indicates antinuclear antibody; CBC, complete blood count; CM, cardiomyopathy; FH, familial hypercholesterolemia; RF, rheumatoid factor; TIBC total iron-binding capacity; TSH, thyroid-stimulating hormone.

often resolves rapidly in the weeks or months after delivery. Women diagnosed with peripartum cardiomyopathy should be advised not to become pregnant, even if objective evidence of myocardial dysfunction has improved.

The role of **myocarditis** in dilated cardiomyopathy remains controversial, with some series reporting significant positive findings on endomyocardial biopsy. Several different chemotherapeutic agents have been associated with the development of dilated cardiomyopathy, the most common being anthracyclines. Onset of the cardiomyopathy is dose dependent and is more frequent after a total dose of 400 mg/m^2.

There are several additional possible causes of cardiomyopathy. **Hypertension** in the absence of ischemic heart disease appears to cause, primarily, diastolic heart failure but may still be associated with severe systolic dysfunction and dilated cardiomyopathy (Fig. 12-1). Cardiomyopathy is a well-recognized complication of **HIV infection**, apparently due to myocarditis from HIV infection of the myocardium. Although cardiac involvement may be clinically silent, symptomatic heart failure may be seen in 10% or more of patients. **Cocaine abuse** has emerged as an important occult cause of LV systolic dysfunction. Cardiomyopathy is part of the late spectrum of cardiac abnormalities secondary to cocaine ingestion and may present without the typical episodes of MI. **Lyme disease**, caused by the spirochete *Borrelia burgdorferi*, may be complicated by cardiac involvement typically presenting with varying degrees of atrioventricular (AV) block, which may produce transient severe symptoms but rarely requires permanent pacing. **Sarcoid** is considered to produce restrictive cardiomyopathy but may also evolve into dilated cardiomyopathy with severe systolic dysfunction.

PATHOGENESIS
Cardiac Remodeling

Cardiac remodeling plays a major part in the pathophysiology of progressive heart failure. Although initially compensatory, remodeling is ultimately a maladaptive response to contractile dysfunction and increased LV volume (Fig. 12-2). Histologically, cardiac remodeling is characterized by significant elongation of cardiomyocytes with less dramatic changes in width, resulting in eccentric hypertrophy. Anatomically, these changes produce dilatation of the left ventricle with a dramatic increase in chamber size relative to wall thickness, resulting in progressive cardiomyocyte dysfunction. Cardiac remodeling is a complex process, ultimately involving changes in gene expression in cardiomyocytes, resulting in substantial changes in cardiomyocyte structure and function. Regardless of the origin of the remodeling, dilatation of the left ventricle is an adverse prognostic factor, independent of impairments of systolic function, which also portends an adverse prognosis. Of the numerous factors that contribute to the cardiac remodeling

process (see chapter 17), neurohormonal activation, particularly involving the sympathetic and renin–angiotensin–aldosterone system, is of specific importance because of its central role and the potential for interrupting maladaptive processes by pharmacologic intervention.

Toxicity of Sympathetic Activation

Major disturbances in autonomic nervous system function are recognized in patients with heart failure. Parasympathetic tone, normally predominant, is reduced with LV dysfunction. Sympathetic activation, in contrast, is common even in asymptomatic systolic dysfunction. Early investigators viewed these changes as a favorable adaptation for the failing heart. Vagal activity has inhibitory effects on heart rate and function that would not help compensate for contractile dysfunction, whereas sympathetic activation results in immediate improvement in all aspects of cardiac function. Heart rate increases, improving cardiac output, and contractility is augmented by the direct positive inotropic effect of norepinephrine. In addition, norepinephrine was known to contribute to cardiac enlargement (by promoting eccentric hypertrophy), and early studies suggested that sympathetic activation improved diastolic function.

Based on these findings, it was suggested that sympathetic activation was beneficial in patients with heart failure. However, epidemiologic and basic laboratory experiments in the 1980s showed an adverse association between sympathetic activation and survival. Plasma norepinephrine, a reasonable approximation of sympathetic activation, was found to positively correlate with increased mortality rate in patients with dilated cardiomyopathy. Studies in animal models of dilated cardiomyopathy indicated that chronic activation of the sympathetic system resulted in decreased production of cyclic AMP in response to adrenergic stimulation. The same finding was present in the failing myocardium of patients undergoing transplantation. Down-regulation of receptor number and function, selective for the β_1 receptor, accounted for this finding. Further studies confirmed that the neurohormone norepinephrine harms the myocardium by promoting apoptosis or programmed cell death. Apoptosis appears to

Figure 12-1

Hypertension and Cardiomyopathy

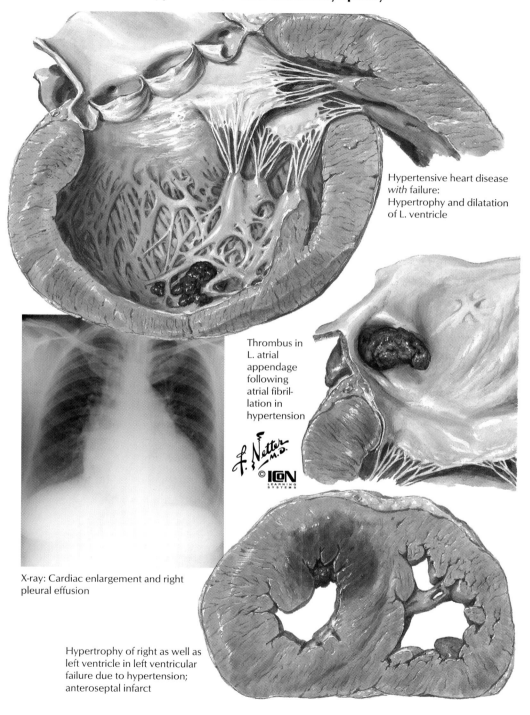

Hypertensive heart disease *with* failure: Hypertrophy and dilatation of L. ventricle

Thrombus in L. atrial appendage following atrial fibrillation in hypertension

X-ray: Cardiac enlargement and right pleural effusion

Hypertrophy of right as well as left ventricle in left ventricular failure due to hypertension; anteroseptal infarct

Figure 12-2

Cardiac Remodeling Secondary to Volume Overload

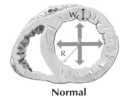

Normal

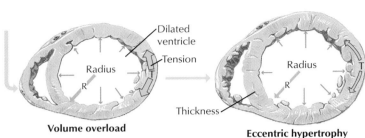

Dilated
ventricle

Radius

Tension

Radius

Thickness

Volume overload

Eccentric hypertrophy

Elevated pressure (P) or volume causes proportionate increases in wall thickness (W) and chamber radius (R); wall tension (T) increases.

Eccentric hypertrophy

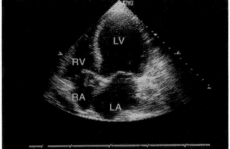

LA indicates left atrium; LV, left ventricle;
RA, right atrium; RV, right ventricle.

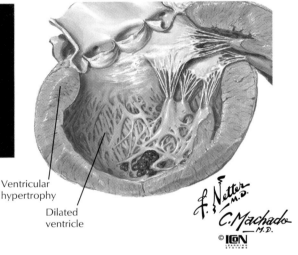

Ventricular
hypertrophy

Dilated
ventricle

contribute significantly to cardiomyocyte loss during progressive heart failure, causes down-regulation of intrinsic contractile mechanisms and aggravates cardiac remodeling by promoting eccentric hypertrophy. Moreover, numerous studies in which patients with dilated cardiomyopathy and CHF were treated with catecholamines (principally dobutamine) demonstrated increased mortality rates in those treated.

Renin–Angiotensin–Aldosterone System

Maladaptive changes in cardiomyocytes similar to those seen with excessive sympathetic activity are induced by activation of the renin–angiotensin–aldosterone system. Increased

tissue and circulating levels of angiotensin II are now recognized to have deleterious effects on cardiac myocytes. Decreased perfusion pressure appears to be a major signal for the juxta-glomerular cells to secret renin, stimulating production of angiotensin I and its subsequent conversion to angiotensin II. Conversion occurs by angiotensin-converting enzyme (ACE) in the lungs and several enzymes in the myocardium, including chymase, cathepsin G, and CAGE. Angiotensin II has adverse effects in heart failure in addition to adverse remodeling. Increased peripheral vasoconstriction, stimulation of aldosterone production, increased circulating catecholamines (particularly norepinephrine), retention of sodium and water by both direct and indirect effects, and increased bradykinin degradation all worsen systolic function and symptoms of CHF. These findings led to the initial study of ACE inhibitors in patients with CHF and their status as a mainstay in the treatment of patients with dilated cardiomyopathy.

Aldosterone has also emerged as an important deleterious neurohormone in heart failure and LV dysfunction. Aldosterone levels are primarily elevated in these states by two mechanisms: increased production by the adrenal glands secondary to stimulation by renin, angiotensin II, and dietary sodium restriction; and decreased hepatic clearance resulting from decreased hepatic blood flow. Increased production of aldosterone causes sodium and water retention and secretion of potassium, which worsens fluid balance and promotes hypokalemia. Adverse effects of aldosterone beyond those on fluid balance include myocardial and vascular fibrosis, baroreceptor dysfunction, and prevention of myocardial norepinephrine uptake. Pharmacologic aldosterone inhibition contributes an additive benefit in patients with severe CHF.

CLINICAL PRESENTATION

The signs and symptoms of dilated cardiomyopathy are not specific but rather reflect the classic presentation of CHF. Patients may present with either left-sided symptoms or primarily symptoms of right-sided CHF (Fig. 12-3). Embolic disease, such as stroke, is a well-recognized complication of dilated cardiomyopathy and may be the presenting manifestation in some patients.

DIFFERENTIAL DIAGNOSIS

Most cases of CHF seen in community practice originate from ischemic heart disease or hypertension complicated by diabetes or primary valvular heart disease. Once these causes of LV systolic dysfunction have been excluded, rarer causes of dilated cardiomyopathy should be investigated. The medical history can identify specific forms of cardiac muscle dysfunction, such as toxicity from chemotherapy and peripartum cardiomyopathy. Selected laboratory tests can be helpful: HIV testing can exclude this etiology; determination of iron and iron binding

can exclude hemochromatosis; and immunoassays can confirm current or prior Lyme disease.

DIAGNOSTIC APPROACH

In patients with dilated cardiomyopathy, the importance of assessment of cardiac structure and function cannot be overemphasized. ECG is important in the initial evaluation of patients suspected to have dilated cardiomyopathy not only because one can detect evidence of previous MI (Fig. 12-4), but also because various other abnormalities are common, especially conduction abnormalities, including left bundle branch block, atrial and ventricular arrhythmia, and evidence of LV hypertrophy.

Accurate assessment of LV ejection fraction (EF), end-diastolic volume, and diastolic function by radionuclide ventriculography or echocardiography are critical to the evaluation of cardiac function and permit detection of cardiac disease and subsequent classification of cardiomyopathy.

MANAGEMENT AND THERAPY

Therapy for symptomatic dilated cardiomyopathy is similar to that for CHF from any cause (discussed in more detail in chapters 17 and 18). β-Blockers and ACE inhibitors are indicated in patients with symptomatic LV systolic dysfunction, a characteristic of dilated cardiomyopathy. The potential for dramatic improvement in LV systolic function, even with severe depression of LVEF, is well established with β-blockade in CHF patients and is even more likely in patients with dilated cardiomyopathy. Anticoagulation with use of warfarin is often necessary because many patients have initial presentations that include embolic events or atrial fibrillation. The use of warfarin in patients with dilated cardiomyopathy but without known embolic events is controversial. Some clinicians routinely institute anticoagulation in patients whose activity is severely limited or who have chronic edema or a markedly dilated left ventricle. Rapid advances in the pharmacologic management of patients with dilated cardiomyopathy appear likely to change the outlook for many patients. Because the therapies described herein may result in improved ventricular function, it is important to reassess cardiac function some months after optimization of drug therapy. If substantial improvements

Figure 12-3

Right-Sided Heart Failure in a Patient With Dilated Cardiomyopathy

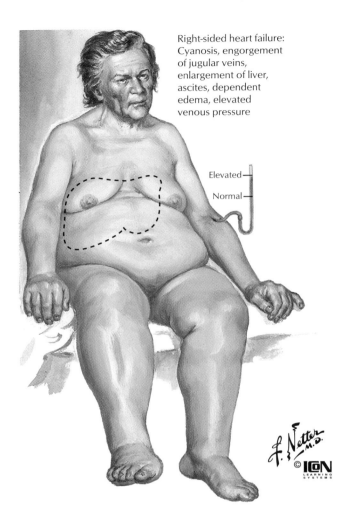

Right-sided heart failure:
Cyanosis, engorgement
of jugular veins,
enlargement of liver,
ascites, dependent
edema, elevated
venous pressure

Elevated —

Normal —

in ventricular function are observed, it is often possible to reduce diuretic therapy and discontinue the use of digitalis. Although current clinical trial data do not specifically address the issue of pharmacotherapy in patients with improved ventricular function, the standard of care today is to continue therapy with ACE inhibitors, β-blockers, and aspirin indefinitely.

FUTURE DIRECTIONS

Dilated cardiomyopathy may be asymptomatic with even profound LV dysfunction. In fact, screening studies indicate that asympto-matic LV dysfunction is several more times common than clinically apparent LV dysfunction. Investigation is being directed toward early detection of these patients and new screening methods, such as determination of plasma B-type natriuretic peptide (BNP or PRO-BNP). The therapeutic approach to these patients remains undefined, but the prevailing thought is that initiation of therapy with ACE inhibitors and β-blockers will delay the onset of overt congestive failure and reduce long-term risk. As more sophisticated knowledge of the genes involved in dilated cardiomyopathy

Figure 12-4

Dilated Cardiomyopathy
After Myocardial Infarction

Ventricular Aneurysm

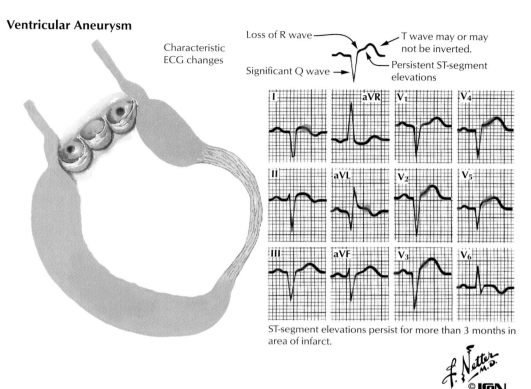

Characteristic ECG changes

Loss of R wave

T wave may or may not be inverted.

Significant Q wave

Persistent ST-segment elevations

ST-segment elevations persist for more than 3 months in area of infarct.

evolves (see also chapter 62), it is likely that early detection will involve identification of genes and clusters of polymorphisms that result in or contribute to the pathogenesis of dilated cardiomyopathy. Earlier diagnosis, coupled with advances in pharmacologic therapy, will likely result in an improved prognosis for patients with dilated cardiomyopathy.

REFERENCES

Barbaro G, Lipshultz SE. Pathogenesis of HIV-associated cardiomyopathy. Review. Annals of the New York Academy of Sciences 2001;946:57-81.

Dunlap SH, Sueta CA, Tomasko L, Adams KF. Association of body mass, gender and race with heart failure primarily due to hypertension. J Am Coll Cardiol 1999;34:1602–1608.

Francis GS, Johnson TH, Ziesche S, Berg M, Boosalis P, Cohn JN. Marked spontaneous improvement in ejection fraction in patients with congestive heart failure. Am J Med 1990;89:303–307.

Goodwin JF, Gordon H, Hollman A, et al. Clinical aspects of cardiomyopathy. BMJ 1961;1:69–79.

Ikeda Y, Ross J Jr. Models of dilated cardiomyopathy in the mouse and the hamster. Curr Opin Cardiol 2000;15:197–201.

Pearson GD, Veille JC, Rahimtoola S, et al. Peripartum cardiomyopathy: National Heart, Lung, and Blood Institute and Office of Rare Diseases (National Institutes of Health) workshop recommendations and review. JAMA 2000; 283:1183–1188.

Spector KS. Diabetic cardiomyopathy. Review. Clin Cardiol 1998;21:885–887.

WHO/ISFC: Report of the WHO/ISFC Task Force on the definition and classification of cardiomyopathies. Br Heart J 1980;44:672–673.

Chapter 13

Hypertrophic Cardiomyopathy

Parag Kale and Richard A. Walsh

Hypertrophic cardiomyopathy (HCM) is the accepted term for a condition associated with unexplained myocardial hypertrophy. HCM is distinct from myocardial hypertrophy that develops in response to known triggers such as hypertension (Fig. 13-1). The cardinal microscopic feature of HCM is myocytes–myofibril disarray occupying 20% or more of at least one ventricular tissue block.

The annual mortality rates from HCM are approximately 6% in patients diagnosed as children and 3% in patients diagnosed as adults. Patients who are older at diagnosis are often symptomatic but, in general, demonstrate slower progression of the disease and a more favorable prognosis. However, the 1-year mortality rate dramatically rises in older patients presenting with New York Heart Association (NYHA) class III and IV congestive heart failure. Other adverse prognostic indicators are a history of atrial fibrillation or hypertension, use of digoxin and diuretics, and ECG evidence of MI. Syncope and a family history of sudden death are most predictive of sudden death. By contrast, hemodynamic parameters do not indicate an adverse prognosis.

ETIOLOGY AND PATHOGENESIS

Various terms have been used to describe the pathophysiology of HCM. These include: hypertrophic obstructive cardiomyopathy (HOMCM), idiopathic hypertrophic subaortic stenosis (IHSS), asymmetric septal hypertrophy (ASH), and muscular subaortic stenosis—all based on the misconception that outflow tract obstruction was the key pathologic determinant of the phenotype (Fig. 13-2).

It is now accepted that, despite the presence or absence of outflow tract obstruction, the principal abnormality is impaired ventricular compliance as a consequence of inappropriate myocardial hypertrophy. The nonobstructive form of HCM accounts for about 75% of cases.

Epidemiology

Hypertrophic cardiomyopathy is inherited in an autosomal dominant pattern in 50 to 75% of cases. Its prevalence is thought to be 1 per 500 in the US population and higher in black individuals. Three age peaks of presentation have been proposed: adolescence, the early 40s, and the early 60s. The clinical presentation of HCM (syncope, sudden cardiac death, severe effort-related chest discomfort, or dyspnea) tend to be most dramatic when HCM presents in adolescence, and more dramatic when the presentation is in the 40s than in the 60s. There is a male predominance in younger patients, whereas there may be an equal or higher prevalence in females in the older population. Clinical presentation with dyspnea, atrial fibrillation, and hypertension is more common in elderly individuals. Echocardiographic differences in two series highlight ovoid LV shape in elderly persons as opposed to reversed septal curvature with a crescent-shaped cavity in persons 40 years or younger. Posterior septal movement, as opposed to systolic anterior motion of the mitral valve, may contribute to higher outflow velocities in elderly individuals. ECG findings of Q waves in the anterior and lateral leads are often seen in the younger group. The genetic basis for HCM is addressed in a separate section in chapter 62, Genetics in CVD, and therefore this chapter focuses on the clinical aspects.

CLINICAL PRESENTATION

Some patients with HCM are asymptomatic and the diagnosis is made after sudden death. The most common symptoms are dyspnea, chest pain, and syncope. Dyspnea is usually exertional and has been reported in more than 90% of patients with HCM. Angina occurs in 75% of patients and MI has been documented in 15% of cases at autopsy. Syncope occurs in about 50% of patients. There is no relation between the

Figure 13-1   ## Heart Disease in Hypertension

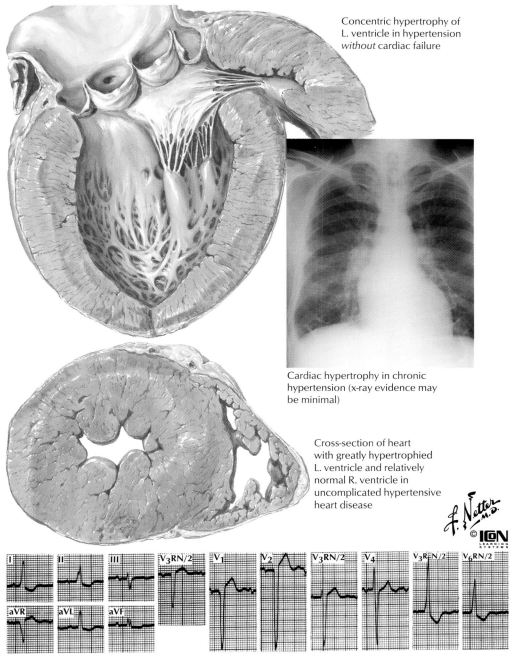

Concentric hypertrophy of
L. ventricle in hypertension
without cardiac failure

Cardiac hypertrophy in chronic
hypertension (x-ray evidence may
be minimal)

Cross-section of heart
with greatly hypertrophied
L. ventricle and relatively
normal R. ventricle in
uncomplicated hypertensive
heart disease

Electrocardiographic evidence of L. ventricular hypertrophy may or may not be present (tall R waves in V_4, V_5, and V_6; deep S waves in V_3R, V_1, V_2, III, and aVR; depressed ST and inverted T in V_5, V_6, I, II, aVL, and aVF)

outflow tract gradient severity and syncopal symptoms, suggesting that the etiology of syncope in HCM is most likely arrhythmic.

Clinical Syndromes/Variants

Apical hypertrophy is a rare manifestation of HCM, usually presenting in a more benign fash-

Figure 13-2   ## Anomalies of the Left Ventricular Outflow Tract

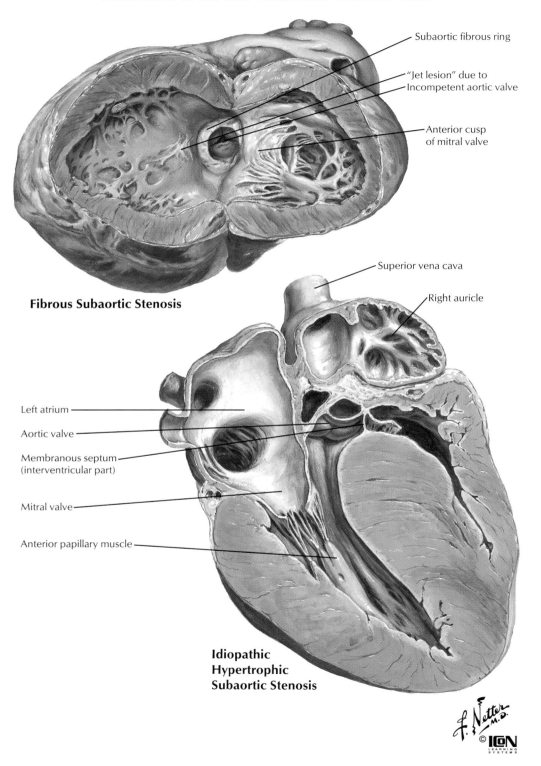

Subaortic fibrous ring

"Jet lesion" due to
Incompetent aortic valve

Anterior cusp
of mitral valve

Fibrous Subaortic Stenosis

Superior vena cava

Right auricle

Left atrium

Aortic valve

Membranous septum
(interventricular part)

Mitral valve

Anterior papillary muscle

**Idiopathic
Hypertrophic
Subaortic Stenosis**

ion. The diagnosis is often suggested by very characteristic ECG findings—typically the ECG shows giant negative T waves in the precordial leads. The configuration of the left ventricle is different than that of the usual form of HCM. In patients with apical hypertrophy, an end-diastolic left ventriculogram in the right anterior oblique projection has a characteristic "spade-like" appearance, so called because the LV cavity in this projection resembled the spade in a deck of playing cards. Patients with *Costello syndrome* have HCM and mental and growth retardation, possibly related to advanced parental age and autosomal dominant inheritance. Distinctive craniofacial findings, resembling those of lysosomal storage disorders, are also present. Other features of this syndrome include acanthosis nigricans, verrucous papillomata of the nose, hyperextensibility of the digits, and soft skin with excess wrinkling over the dorsum of the hands and deep creases on the palms and soles.

DIFFERENTIAL DIAGNOSIS

Left ventricular hypertrophy—mimicking HCM—may also be present in patients with preserved LV systolic function, long-standing systemic hypertension (Fig. 13-3), outflow obstruction secondary to valvular heart disease, such as aortic stenosis or coarctation of the aorta, and infiltrative disorders of the myocardium. At times, distinguishing these conditions from HCM clinically, or even by echocardiography, can be very difficult. Tips to making this diagnostic distinction include the following: 1) In patients with aortic stenosis, the gradient is fixed, unlike in patients with HCM in which the gradient is dynamic and can fluctuate with each beat. 2) The pattern of hypertrophy seen in patients with hypertension is concentric as opposed to the pattern seen in patients with HCM, which is distinctive, as described later in this chapter.

DIAGNOSTIC APPROACH
Physical Examination

The **carotid impulse** of the patient with the obstructive form of HCM is rapid in upstroke, bifid, and followed by a prominent dicrotic notch. This "spike-and-dome" pulse pattern is caused by

rapid ventricular emptying secondary to increased LV contractility, followed by abrupt flow reduction secondary to systolic anterior motion of the mitral valve, causing partial occlusion of the outflow tract. The **jugular venous pulse** in sinus rhythm is characterized by prominent a waves. The **outflow murmur** characteristically is systolic and heard best along the left sternal border without radiation to the carotid arteries. Because the outflow tract gradient is dynamic, the murmur can be altered by various physical and pharmacologic maneuvers (see chapter 1); it increases with amyl nitrate, Valsalva maneuvers, and upright posture and decreases with administration of phenylephrine, squatting, and isometric handgrip.

Mitral regurgitation occurs in almost all patients with obstructive HCM. The mechanism is systolic anterior motion of the mitral valve and incomplete coaptation of the leaflets. There is also a direct relation between the pressure gradient and the severity of mitral regurgitation. Mitral regurgitation in nonobstructive HCM is usually mild and occurs in approximately 30% of patients.

Atrial fibrillation is the most common arrhythmia seen with HCM. Paroxysmal and then persistent atrial fibrillation occurs in at least 20% of patients. Its incidence increases with age. Sequelae commonly associated with atrial fibrillation include embolic phenomena and precipitation of heart failure. The latter is especially true when onset is before 50 years of age in patients with obstructive HCM. Patients with HCM may also experience syncope or presyncope with the onset of rapid atrial fibrillation.

Heart failure symptoms can mainly be attributed to diastolic LV dysfunction because of impaired LV relaxation and wall stiffness. Other contributory factors are outflow obstruction, atrial fibrillation, and myocardial ischemia. LV systolic function may deteriorate in patients with end-stage HCM, leading to severe symptoms of heart failure.

Electrocardiography

The most common abnormalities seen in patients with HCM are ST-segment and T-wave abnormalities. LV hypertrophy is also common, with QRS complexes usually tallest in the mid precordial leads.

Figure 13-3

Left Ventricular Hypertrophy

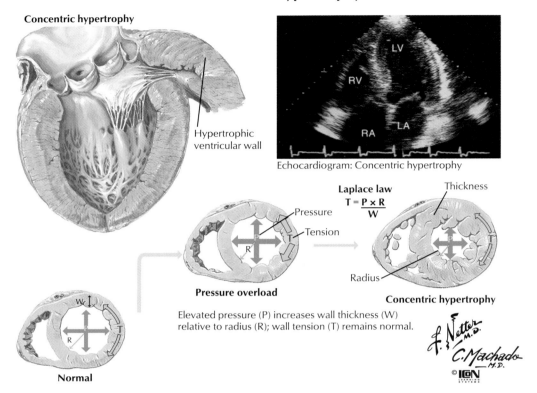

Concentric hypertrophy

Hypertrophic ventricular wall

Echocardiogram: Concentric hypertrophy

Laplace law

$$T = \frac{P \times R}{W}$$

Pressure

Tension

Thickness

Radius

Pressure overload

Concentric hypertrophy

Elevated pressure (P) increases wall thickness (W) relative to radius (R); wall tension (T) remains normal.

Normal

Echocardiography

Now accepted as the imaging study of choice, echocardiography confirms the diagnosis of HCM. Various patterns of LV hypertrophy have been identified. Concentric hypertrophy occurs because of left ventricle pressure overload, as in patients with aortic stenosis. Eccentric hypertrophy usually is a result of left ventricle volume overload, as in mitral or aortic regurgitation (Fig. 13-3). Septal thickening at least 1.5 times the posterior wall thickness in diastole is a diagnostic criterion for HCM. A "ground-glass" or "speckled" appearance may be seen in portions of the hypertrophied myocardium. Anteriorly, the outflow tract of the left ventricle is constituted by the septum and, posteriorly, by the mitral valve anterior leaflet. The leaflets may be enlarged and produce a pressure gradient secondary to abnormal **systolic anterior motion** of the anterior leaflet. Mitral regurgitation is usually noted in association with the outflow gradient.

Cardiac Catheterization

Characteristic hemodynamic findings have been described in HCM patients with outflow tract gradients, including augmented LV systolic contraction immediately after a premature ventricular complex. A decrease in the aortic pulse pressure is often noted in the postpremature ventricular contraction beat (Braunwald sign).

Exercise and HCM

Although the most common cause of death in athletes is trauma, cardiovascular conditions rank second, and HCM constitutes 80% of this subset. HCM gained widespread public recognition after postmortem diagnosis in athletes who died suddenly while engaged in competitive sports. Most athletes with HCM are asymptomatic and, therefore, difficult to diagnose without imaging studies. Although expert opinion varies somewhat, in general, an individual with typical HCM should not engage in competitive sports.

Athletes with a genetic predisposition should undergo serial echocardiography every 12 to 18 months until age 18 because phenotypic expression may not occur until later in adolescence or in adult life when physical maturation is complete. There is no evidence to justify routinely precluding genotype positive–phenotype negative individuals of any age from most activities or employment.

MANAGEMENT AND THERAPY

Medical Management

Conventional therapy focuses on management of symptoms with use of negatively inotropic drugs, such as β-blockers and verapamil, with the idea that this approach will improve diastolic function in HCM. Initial treatment considerations are usually independent of the presence of a gradient.

β-Blockers are usually the first-choice drug and have a salutary effect on symptoms. Verapamil may be considered when β-blockers are ineffective. Alternatively, addition of disopyramide may be effective in decreasing outflow gradient and improving symptoms and exercise tolerance. Endocarditis prophylaxis before dental procedures and surgery is indicated in patients with significant outflow tract gradients and mitral regurgitation.

Treatment of Erectile Dysfunction in Patients With HCM

Sildenafil citrate is commonly used in the treatment of erectile dysfunction. There is very little information regarding its safety in patients with HCM. Two case reports indicate potential negative effects of the use of sildenafil in these patients. One adverse effect is atrial fibrillation, possibly caused by drug-induced arterial vasodilatation producing an increased gradient across the LV outflow tract, with resultant acute increase in LV end-diastolic pressure and left atrial hypertension. Another report was of decreased SBP after administration of sildenafil, possibly due to a marked reduction in LV dimensions, associated with increases in the ejection fraction and subaortic gradient.

Permanent Pacing

The enthusiasm for permanent pacing in all patients with HCM (to reduce LV outflow track obstruction) has diminished over recent years.

The decreased outflow obstruction and reduction in gradient after RV pacing is complicated by significant decreases in stroke volume and aortic pressure. Synchronized atrial and RV apical stimulation reduce subaortic gradients substantially (by 43% in one study) without altering aortic pressure or cardiac output. An optimum AV interval during dual-chamber pacing can be determined by maintenance of early RV apical activation and optimal LV filling pressures. In some patients, this approach has proven useful.

Pacing has not been shown to affect mortality rates in patients who are at various levels of risk for sudden arrhythmic death. There may be a substantial placebo effect because there is poor correlation between reduction in outflow tract gradients and symptoms. Therefore, permanent pacing is a consideration for the elderly individual subgroup as an alternative to surgical or ablative approaches. In this and other settings, permanent pacing may offer benefit to some patients.

Implantable Cardioverter Defibrillator Therapy

The ICD can be highly effective in the prevention of sudden death and, therefore, prolongs the survival of the high-risk patient with HCM (Table 13-1). Sudden cardiac death or aborted cardiac arrests may occur in patients who have little functional impairment. Marked LV hypertrophy alone may not justify prophylactic ICD use. However, marked LV hypertrophy plus an additional risk factor (e.g., family history of sudden death, syncope, chest pain, nonsustained ventricular tachycardia, failure of systolic blood pressure to increase with exercise) may identify a subset that would benefit from prophylactic implantation of an ICD.

Alcohol Ablation of the Septum

In this procedure, approximately 1 to 4 mL of absolute alcohol is injected selectively into the septal perforator branch of the LAD artery via a percutaneous catheter. The resultant MI reduces the thickness of the proximal septum. Thus, the outflow tract dimension is increased; the gradient, reduced. Although considered an alternative to surgery, this procedure is associated with complications such as high-grade AV block, coronary dissection, and anterior wall MI.

Table 13-1
Predictors of the High-Risk Subgroup of HCM

- Prior cardiac arrest
- Sustained ventricular tachycardia
- Family history of sudden or premature HCM-related death
- Nonsustained ventricular tachycardia found on surveillance Holter monitoring
- Syncope–presyncope thought not to be neurocardiogenic in origin
- Left ventricular outflow gradient ≥50 mm Hg
- Substantial LVH (wall thickness ≥20 mm)
- Left atrial enlargement (>45 mm)
- Hypotensive BP response to exercise

HCM indicates hypertrophic cardiomyopathy; LVH, left ventricular hypertrophy.

Additionally, the resultant scar is a substrate for potentially lethal ventricular tachyarrythmia, and no randomized controlled studies have rigorously evaluated the benefit of this procedure. Therefore, surgery, which has equivalent morbidity and mortality rates, remains the gold standard. The results of ongoing trials of septal ablation will clarify the role of this approach in the treatment of patients with HCM.

Surgical Therapy

Subaortic ventricular myotomy was first performed on two patients in 1961, with subsequent reduction in outflow tract gradient and clinical improvement. In general, surgery is considered when debilitating symptoms persist despite maximal pharmacologic therapy. Myocardium from the proximal septum just beyond the mitral leaflets is resected to reduce the outflow gradient. This operation has many advantages: low mortality rate (<2%), reduced symptoms, improved functional capacity, and durable results; symptomatic improvement persists for 5 or more years after surgery in 70% of patients. Occasionally, mitral valve surgery may also be necessary for associated severe mitral regurgitation.

Heart Transplantation

Heart transplatation is an option for end-stage HCM patients with deterioration in LV systolic function who exhibit debilitating symptoms and in whom heart failure develops. Patients with nonobstructive HCM whose symptoms are refractory to pharmacologic therapy are also candidates for transplantation.

FUTURE DIRECTIONS

None of the existing pharmacologic therapies for HCM induces a regression of hypertrophy and fibrosis or reduces mortality rate. Interestingly, simvastatin has been shown to induce regression of cardiac hypertrophy and fibrosis, as well as improve LV filling pressures in a transgenic rabbit model. A clinical trial is needed to study the benefit of statins and other pharmacologic approaches in humans with HCM.

With the rapid growth of molecular genetics, new genetic forms are increasingly being identified. Genetic testing may provide insight into better risk stratification and identification of individuals with HCM or their family members, who are at risk for sudden death.

Newer devices with combined functions of dual-chamber pacing, antitachycardia overdrive pacing, defibrillation, and event recording are likely to play important roles in alleviating symptoms, preventing sudden death, and providing information about the causes of sudden death in patients with HCM.

REFERENCES

Awan GM, Calderon E, Dawood G, Alpert MA. Acute symptomatic atrial fibrillation after sildenafil citrate therapy in a patient with HOCM. *Am J Med Sci* 2000;320:69–71.

Jeanrenaud X, Goy JJ, Kappenberger L. Effects of dual chamber pacing in hypertrophic obstructive cardiomyopathy. *Lancet* 1992;339:1318–1323.

Johnson JP, Golabi M, et al. Costello syndrome: Phenotype, natural history, differential diagnosis, and possible cause. *J Pediatr* 1998;133:441–448.

Maron BJ. Hypertrophic cardiomyopathy a systematic review. *JAMA* 2002;287:1308–1320.

Maron BJ, Mitchell JH. Revised eligibility recommendations for competitive athletes with cardiovascular abnormalities. *JACC* 1994; 24:848–850.

Stauffer JC, et al. Subaortic obstruction after sildenafil in a patient with HCM. *N Engl J Med* 1999; 341:700–701.

Ten Berg JM, Suttorp MJ, Knaepen PJ, et al. Hypertrophic obstructive cardiomyopathy: Initial results and long term follow-up after morrow septal myectomy. *Circulation* 1994;90:1781.

Zieman SJ, Fortuin NJ. Hypertrophic and restrictive cardiomyopathies in the elderly. *Cardiol Clin* 1999;17:159–172.

Chapter 14

Restrictive Cardiomyopathy

Thomas M. Bashore

Cardiomyopathies are generally classified into three forms: dilated, hypertrophic, and restrictive. The restrictive form is the least common endomyocardial disease and is characterized by variable degrees of diastolic dysfunction out of proportion to systolic dysfunction. Restrictive cardiomyopathy is often confused with constrictive pericarditis, and differentiating between them presents an ongoing challenge. Both may coexist, increasing the diagnostic complexity. Because constrictive pericarditis is eminently more treatable than restrictive cardiomyopathy, the distinction is critical.

Restrictive cardiomyopathy was originally described in 1961 as **constrictive cardiomyopathy**. The term was later changed to the more accurate term, *restrictive cardiomyopathy*, which describes a stiff myocardium usually resulting from an infiltrative process. Diastolic heart failure is now recognized to be a common process, often affecting the elderly and those with hypertension and increased systemic arterial stiffness. Some of these patients are also described as having a **restrictive cardiomyopathy**.

ETIOLOGY AND PATHOGENESIS

A variety of disease states produce the clinical manifestation of a restrictive cardiomyopathic process (Table 14-1). Myocardial fibrosis, myocardial infiltration by specific proteins, endomyocardial scarring, and cardiac muscle hypertrophy all may present as diastolic dysfunction.

Noninfiltrative Causes

Idiopathic restrictive cardiomyopathy is associated with patchy endomyocardial fibrosis, increased cardiac mass, and enlarged atria (Fig. 14-1). It is more common in older adults but may be seen in children. A familial component may be present. In adults, 5-year survival is about 64%; mortality may be higher in children. Occasionally, it is accompanied by skeletal muscle myopathy. Idiopathic restrictive cardiomyopathy is also found in families with no skeletal muscle involvement and as an autosomal dominant disorder in patients with Noonan's syndrome. Conduction system disease such as atrioventricular (AV) block may precede clinical myocardial dysfunction.

Infiltrative Causes

Clinically, the most common variety of restrictive cardiomyopathy is that due to **amyloidosis**, resulting from the deposition of fibrils formed by several mechanisms (Fig. 14-1, middle). Primary **amyloidosis** is caused by the deposition of an amyloid protein composed of portions of immunoglobulin light chain (designated **AL** for **light chain–associated amyloidosis**) produced by a monoclonal population of plasma cells. This may be the consequence of multiple myeloma but it is also found in patients without multiple myeloma. **Secondary amyloidosis** is caused by the production of a nonimmunoglobulin protein and termed **AA** (for **amyloid-associated**). **Familial amyloidosis** is an inherited autosomal dominant trait resulting from a variant prealbumin protein, transthyretin. More than 50 point mutations have been described, and familial amyloidosis may present as a cardiomyopathy, a progressive neuropathy, or a nephropathy. **Senile systemic amyloidosis** is produced by an atrial natriuretic-like protein or transthyretin. Its frequency increases with age. It is four times more common in blacks than in whites. Scattered amyloid deposits in the aorta or the atria are almost universally found in individuals older than 80 years. Regardless of the specific etiology, often the LV chamber is normal or small. The greater the myocardial thickness, the more amyloid present and the worse the prognosis.

In amyloidosis secondary to immunocyte dyscrasias, cardiac involvement is common and the most frequent cause of death. In amyloidosis secondary to other diseases, cardiac involvement is much less common, often only manifesting as smaller perivascular deposits that do

Figure 14-1

Idiopathic and Infiltrative Causes
of Restrictive Cardiomyopathy

Idiopathic cardiomyopathy

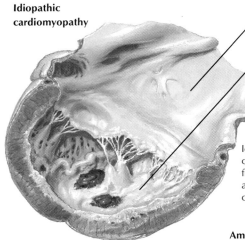

Atrial enlargement

Patchy endocardial fibrosis

"Notching" of right apex

Idiopathic restrictive cardiomyopathy characterized by patchy endocardial fibrosis, increased cardiac mass, and atrial enlargement; may exhibit familial component and distal skeletal muscle myopathy

Amyloidosis

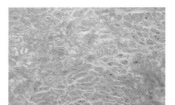

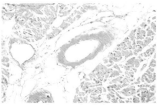

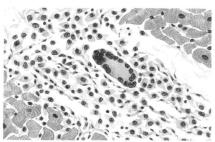

Focal deposition of amyloid around muscle cells of heart with dead myocardial fibers

Perivascular amyloid deposits in myocardium (×40)

Amyloidosis is most common form of restrictive cardiomyopathy. Characterized by deposition of amyloid protein throughout the myocardium, causing thickening and diastolic dysfunction

Thickened myocardium

Sarcoidosis

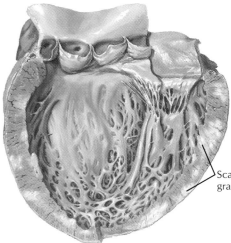

Granuloma with giant cell in heart wall

Scattered sarcoid granulomas in myocardium

Sarcoidosis exhibits myocardial involvement in a small percentage of patients with the systemic disease. Granulomas in myocardium lead to diastolic dysfunction, CHF, heart block, ventricular arrhythmias, and sudden cardiac death.

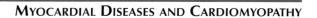

Table 14-1
Classification of Common and Uncommon Types of Restrictive Cardiomyopathy

Common

Noninfiltrative
    Idiopathic restrictive cardiomyopathy

Infiltrative
    Amyloidosis
    Sarcoidosis

Endomyocardial
    Endomyocardial fibrosis
    Radiation fibrosis
    Anthracycline toxicity

Uncommon

Noninfiltrative
    Familial cardiomyopathy
    Hypertrophic cardiomyopathy
    Scleroderma
    Pseudoxanthoma elasticum
    Diabetic cardiomyopathy

Infiltrative
    Gaucher's disease
    Hurler's syndrome
    Fatty infiltration

Storage Diseases
    Hemochromatosis
    Fabry's disease
    Glycogen storage disease

Endomyocardial
    Hypereosinophilic syndrome
    Carcinoid heart disease
    Metastatic cancers
    Drug-induced fibrosis
        Serotonin, methysergide, ergotamine,
        mercurial agents, busulfan

With permission from Kushwaha SS, Fallon JT, Fuster V. Restrictive cardiomyopathy. *N Engl J Med* 1997;336:267–276. ©Copyright Massachusetts Medical Society. All rights reserved.

not cause diastolic dysfunction. About one in four individuals with familial amyloidosis has overt cardiac involvement, with neurologic and renal dysfunction more often dominating the clinical picture. Senile amyloidosis is rarely responsible for cardiac dysfunction.

Sarcoidosis is a granulomatous disease of unknown cause (Fig. 14-1, lower). Of the multiple organ systems commonly involved, including the heart, the most important is usually the lungs, where this involvement manifests as diffuse scarring, pulmonary hypertension, and cor pulmonale. Myocardial involvement causes a restrictive or dilated cardiomyopathy in less than 5% of systemic sarcoidosis patients. More commonly, focal involvement may result in heart block, congestive failure, ventricular arrhythmias, or sudden cardiac death. The noncaseating granulomas have a propensity for involving the interventricular septum (hence the high incidence of heart block) and the left ventricular (LV) free wall. The scattered nature of granulomas contributes to the failure of right ventricular (RV) biopsies to detect the disease in about half the patients.

Endomyocardial Causes
Endomyocardial fibrosis (sometimes known as **Becker's disease**) occurs most commonly in Africa, especially in Uganda and Nigeria (Fig. 14-2, upper). In equatorial Africa, it is responsible for 10 to 20% of deaths from heart disease. Pericardial effusions are common and may be large. Fibrous endocardial lesions are frequently noted in the ventricular inflow tracts and often involve the AV valves, resulting in valvular regurgitation. The involved myocardium demonstrates a thick layer of collagen tissue overlying a layer of loosely arranged connective tissue. Fibrous and granulomatous tissue may extend into the myocardium. Either or both ventricles may be involved and, when the disease process is extensive, papillary muscles and chordae may be matted with a mass of thrombus and tissue, filling the cavity. Clinical manifestations depend on involvement of the right ventricle, the left ventricle, or both. **Eosinophilic endocarditis** (**Löffler's endocarditis**) is likely a manifestation of this same process (Fig. 14-2, lower). Both diseases may be associated with eosinophilia. Epidemiologic evidence suggests Löffler's endocarditis is related to worm (helminth) infestation. Patients with **Churg-Strauss syndrome** (asthma, eosinophilia, neuropathy, pulmonary infiltrates, paranasal sinus abnormalities, and/or extravascular eosinophils) may also develop endomyocardial fibrosis. The intracytoplasmic granular content of activated eosinophils may be toxic to the myocardial and endothelial cells, resulting in the damage observed.

Figure 14-2

Endomyocardial Causes
of Restrictive Cardiomyopathy

Becker's disease

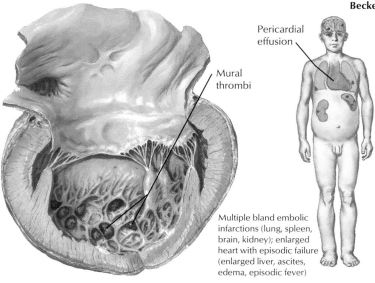

Mural thrombi

Pericardial effusion

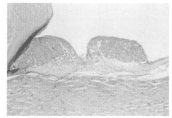

Verrucous lesions on thickened, edematous endocardium

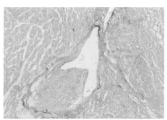

Multiple bland embolic infarctions (lung, spleen, brain, kidney); enlarged heart with episodic failure (enlarged liver, ascites, edema, episodic fever)

Hyalinized polypoid protrusion into lumen of subendocardial vein

Endomyocardial fibrosis (Becker's disease) occurs most commonly in Africa. Pericardial effusions are common. Fibrous endocardial lesions often involve AV valves. Myocardium shows a thick layer of collagen over loose connective tissue. Mural thrombi are common.

Löeffler's endocarditis

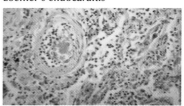

Acute eosinophilic endarteritis in lung; similar lesions occur in small vessels of brain, kidney, and other organs.

Multiple embolic infarcts (lung, brain, spleen, kidney) and diffuse arteriolitis

Brain

Heart enlarged

Liver enlarged

Ascites

Edema

Leukocytosis, eosinophilia

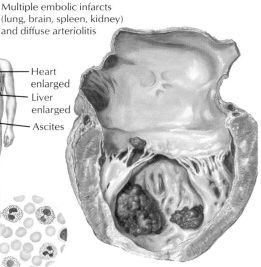

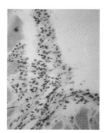

Acute eosinophilic and neutrophilic infiltration of subendocardium

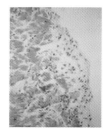

Eosinophilic infiltration and early myocardial damage

Löeffler's endocarditis (eosinophilic endocarditis) likely a manifestation of same condition as Becker's disease; both may be associated with eosinophilia and may be associated with a helminthic infestation.

Greatly enlarged heart: Extensive fibrosis of endocardium and subendocardial myocardium with extension through entire thickness of heart wall and involvement of papillary muscles, chordae tendineae, and valve cusps; mural thrombi

Radiation therapy may result in long-lasting injury to the capillary endothelial cells, leading to cell death, capillary rupture, and microthrombi. Cardiac complications usually occur many years after the initial insult and can vary widely, with constrictive pericarditis the most common manifestation. Pericarditis with effusion, coronary artery fibrosis (especially ostial) with myocardial infarction, valvular stenosis or regurgitation, conduction system disease, and myocardial fibrosis may result from excessive radiation exposure. The severity of cardiac involvement is proportional to the radiation dose (more common at doses greater than 45 Gy) and to the mass of myocardium exposed. Separating the effects of radiation from the consequences of chemotherapy is not always possible. Cardiac radiation exposure is most common following therapy for Hodgkin's disease or breast cancer.

Although acute toxicity from **anthracyclines** does occur, cardiac toxicity usually is delayed and results in a dilated cardiomyopathy. Early manifestations of primarily diastolic dysfunction may herald the cardiotoxicity. There is a nonlinear increase in cardiotoxicity as the cumulative dose increases, with a 7% incidence with doxorubicin doses over 550 mg/m^2. Cytotoxicity from anthracylines appears to be due to inhibition of an enzyme necessary for DNA repair and to generation of free radicals that damage cell membranes, in part by lipid peroxidation. The heart may not detoxify the free radicals because only a small amount of catalase, needed to convert hydrogen peroxide to water, is present. The anthracyclines also chelate iron and generate tissue-damaging hydroxyl radicals locally. Therefore, dexrazoxane, a drug that hydrolyzes to form a carboxylamine capable of removing the iron from the anthracycline-iron complex, is often used as a cardioprotectant in patients receiving anthracyclines. Measures of diastolic dysfunction appear to precede the systolic dysfunction and help in detecting the early onset of anthracycline-induced chronic cardiomyopathy. Other **toxic drugs** are implicated in the development of myocardial fibrosis, including methysergide, ergotamine, mercurial agents, and busulfan.

Other Causes

Less common causes of restrictive cardiomyopathy include certain inherited diseases. The most prominent is **Fabry's disease**, an X-linked recessive disorder caused by deficiency of the lysosomal enzyme α-galactosidase. The accumulation of lysosomal glycolipids in cardiac tissue results in a severe restrictive cardiomyopathy. There may also be valvular involvement. Clinically, the skin, the kidneys, and the lungs may be involved.

Other inherited diseases are more rarely seen. In **Gaucher's disease** (characterized by a deficiency of the enzyme β-glucosidase, with accumulation of cerebrosides in various organs), there may be both myocardial dysfunction and hemorrhagic pericardial effusion. In **Hurler's syndrome**, a deposition of mucopolysaccharide in the myocardium can cause a restrictive process. The cardiac valves and the coronary arteries may be involved. **Hemochromatosis**, arising from an inherited (autosomal recessive) or acquired etiologies, is characterized by iron deposition in many organs, including the heart. Myocardial damage may result from direct tissue damage by the free iron moiety, not from the infiltration of iron.

Carcinoid heart disease primarily affects the right heart and is characterized by fibrous plaque that virtually coats the tricuspid and pulmonic valves and the RV endocardium. Valvular stenosis and regurgitation result, and RV dysfunction is common. The cardiac involvement correlates with serotonin levels.

CLINICAL PRESENTATION

Patients with restrictive cardiomyopathy present with congestion and low output symptoms. Dyspnea, paroxysmal nocturnal dyspnea, orthopnea, peripheral edema, ascites, and overall fatigue and weakness are common. Angina can be a presenting symptom if coronary arteries are involved. Atrial fibrillation is common, and heart block may be particularly evident in patients with amyloidosis or sarcoidosis. Up to one third of patients may present with thromboembolic complications. Unlike in a dilated cardiomyopathy, right-sided heart failure is often more prominent than left-sided heart failure early in the course of restrictive cardiomyopathy.

RESTRICTIVE CARDIOMYOPATHY

DIFFERENTIAL DIAGNOSIS

Most patients present with right heart failure out of proportion to left heart failure and have normal or near-normal cardiac size on examination and chest x-ray. The differential diagnosis of restrictive cardiomyopathy includes constrictive pericarditis, chronic RV infarction, RV dysfunction from RV pressure or (less likely) RV volume overload, intrinsic RV myocardial disease, or tricuspid valve disease. Results of the examination and echocardiography usually narrow the differential diagnosis to restrictive cardiomyopathy and constrictive pericarditis, which affect hemodynamics differently.

Normal Hemodynamics

Intracardiac pressures are a reflection of the contraction and relaxation of individual cardiac structures and the changes imparted to them by the pleural and pericardial pressures (Fig. 14-3). Changes in either pleural or the pericardial pressures can be reflected in the intracardiac pressure. With inspiration, the intrapleural pressures drop and the abdominal cavity pressure increases. Blood flow through the right side of the heart increases, whereas blood return to the left side of the heart decreases slightly. The fall in the intrapleural pressures with inspiration also results in an increase in the transmural aortic root pressure, effectively increasing the impedance to LV ejection. The reverse occurs during expiration. Normally, inspiration lowers the right atrial and the systolic RV pressures slightly more than it lowers the left heart pressures. In severe lung disease, such as asthma, left heart filling is more profoundly affected, in that these changes are exaggerated. The very negative inspiratory intrapleural pressures and very positive expiratory pressures result in marked swings in LV filling. A paradoxical pulse (fall in systemic pressure with inspiration) may thus result from lung disease alone.

The normal atrial and ventricular waveforms are shown on the left in Figure 14-4. With atrial contraction, the atria become smaller and the atrial pressures rise (a wave). With the onset of ventricular contraction, the AV valves bulge toward the atria and a small c wave is inscribed. As ventricular contraction continues, the AV annular ring is pulled into the ventricular cavity and the atria go into their diastole, resulting in enlarging the atria and a decrease in the atrial pressures (x descent). Passive filling of the atria during ventricular systole produces a slow rise in the atrial pressures (the v wave) until the AV valves reopen at the peak of the v wave, and the pressure then falls rapidly as the ventricles actively relax (the y descent). Passive filling of the ventricles continues while the AV valves are open until atrial contraction again occurs, and the cycle repeats.

Following ventricular systole, ventricular diastole can be divided into an initial active phase (a brief period when the ventricle fills about halfway) and a passive filling phase. The nadir or lowest diastolic pressure during ventricular diastole occurs during the early active relaxation phase (suction effect).

Constrictive Pericarditis

Constrictive pericarditis (Fig. 14-4, middle) and restrictive cardiomyopathy (Fig. 14-4, lower) alter the normal intracardiac pressures in several ways as described in the figures. Please refer to chapter 36, which covers these and expected respiratory changes with cardiac flow in detail.

Because the atrial and ventricular septi are unaffected by the pericardial process, changes in filling on the right side can affect left-sided filling by way of chamber interdependence. With inspiration, blood is drawn through the right ventricle into the lungs. Some septal shift toward the left ventricle may thus occur. When the hemodynamics of ventricular pressures are assessed simultaneously, the normal inspiratory decrease in the ventricular systolic pressures is altered because the increase in RV filling causes the RV systolic pressure to rise with inspiration, whereas the LV systolic pressure falls (discordance of RV–LV pressure). This finding is particularly useful in differentiating constrictive pericarditis from restrictive cardiomyopathy.

Restrictive Cardiomyopathy

In restrictive cardiomyopathy, the atrial pressures are high and there is early and rapid diastolic filling similar to the filling seen in constrictive pericarditis. The diastolic pressures of the left heart, however, are higher than those of the right heart throughout the respiratory cycle, with pulmonary hypertension and RV systolic

Figure 14-3

Normal Cardiac Blood Flow
During Inspiration and Expiration

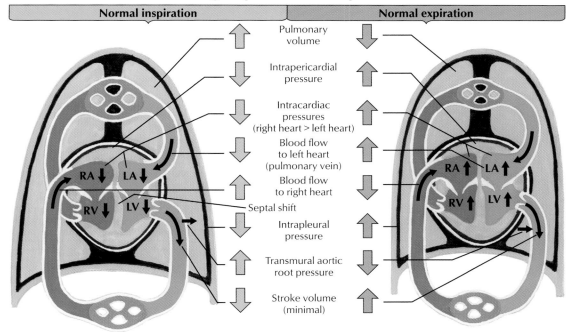

| Normal inspiration | Normal expiration |

Pulmonary volume

Intrapericardial pressure

Intracardiac pressures (right heart > left heart)

Blood flow to left heart (pulmonary vein)

Blood flow to right heart

Septal shift

Intrapleural pressure

Transmural aortic root pressure

Stroke volume (minimal)

On inspiration, intrapleural pressure drops and abdominal pressure increases with increased blood flow through the right heart and slight decrease in flow to left heart. Increased aortic root transmural pressure adds a minor amount of LV afterload.

On expiration, intrapleural pressure increases and abdominal pressure decreases with decreased blood flow through the right heart and increase in flow to left heart.

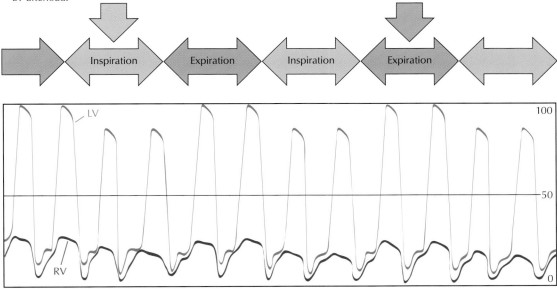

Inspiration   Expiration   Inspiration   Expiration

Simultaneous measurement of RV and LV systolic pressure reveals a concordant decrease in pressure in both chambers during inspiration, with a similar concordant increase in pressure in both ventricles during expiration. Pressure changes are exaggerated for emphasis.

JOHN A. CRAIG—AD
©ICON

Figure 14-4 Comparisons of Normal and Pathologic Intracardiac Pressures

Normal

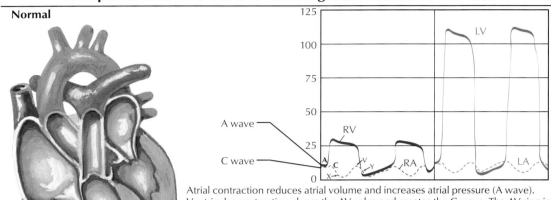

Atrial contraction reduces atrial volume and increases atrial pressure (A wave). Ventricular contraction closes the AV valve and creates the C wave. The AV ring is pulled into atria, and atrial relaxation ensues with pressure decrease (x descent). Passive atrial filling causes V wave until AV valves open and pressure drops rapidly (y descent) while ventricles relax. Following ventricular systole, an active and passive diastolic filling phase follows, with ventricular pressure lowest in active phase.

Constrictive pericarditis

Thickened constrictive pericardium

Normal Myocardium

Equalization of diastolic pressures

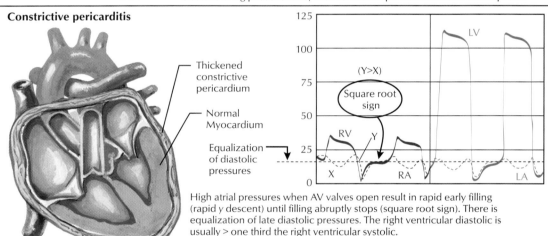

High atrial pressures when AV valves open result in rapid early filling (rapid y descent) until filling abruptly stops (square root sign). There is equalization of late diastolic pressures. The right ventricular diastolic is usually > one third the right ventricular systolic.

Restrictive cardiomyopathy

LVEDP > RVEDP

Elevated right ventricular systolic pressure

Abnormal myocardium

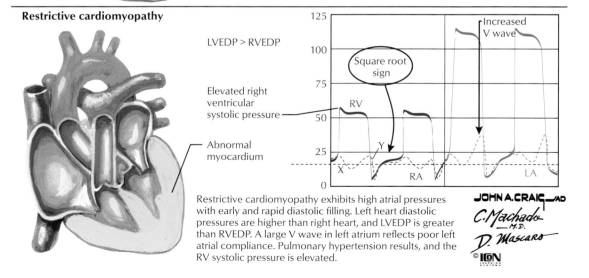

Restrictive cardiomyopathy exhibits high atrial pressures with early and rapid diastolic filling. Left heart diastolic pressures are higher than right heart, and LVEDP is greater than RVEDP. A large V wave in left atrium reflects poor left atrial compliance. Pulmonary hypertension results, and the RV systolic pressure is elevated.

JOHN A. CRAIG—MD
C. Machado—M.D.
D. Mascaro
© ICN

hypertension as common findings (Fig. 14-4). The elevation of the RV systolic pressure means that the RV end-diastolic pressure will not be greater than one third of the RV systolic pressure (unlike in constrictive pericarditis). In a patient with myocardial restriction but a normal pericardium, the normal inspiratory decrease in all intracardiac pressures is expected. Hence, there is no inherent change in the driving pressure across the pulmonary veins into the left atrium and the left ventricle and LV filling are barely affected by the change in inspiratory negative pressure. The normal concordant fall in the RV and LV systolic pressures occurs. These findings help to differentiate constrictive pericarditis from myocardial restriction in the clinical setting.

DIAGNOSTIC APPROACH (Table 14-2)
Electrocardiography

The ECG in patients with restrictive cardiomyopathy is often abnormal but usually nonspecific. Low voltage may be a prominent feature, especially in amyloidosis. The QRS pattern often simulates myocardial infarction with poor R wave progression in the precordial leads or a pseudoinfarction pattern in the inferior leads. If pulmonary hypertension is present, evidence of RV hypertrophy may be noted. Interatrial conduction delays (notched P waves) and evidence of atrial enlargement are also common. AV heart block is common in sarcoidosis and less common in amyloidosis. Atrial arrhythmias, especially fibrillation, are common, although rarely a presenting symptom; sick sinus syndrome is also common. Ventricular tachyarrhythmias are frequent with disease progression and in amyloidosis may be a harbinger of sudden cardiac death.

Blood Tests

Patients presenting with a restrictive cardiomyopathy should be screened for all systemic diseases that may be contributory. Often blood tests are unrevealing. There are no specific markers, but a complete blood count with differential helps exclude anemia and eosinophilia. The sedimentation rate is usually reduced in patients with right heart failure, and an elevated sedimentation rate may suggest an inflammatory process such as sarcoidosis. Although only rarely helpful, an angiotensin-converting en-

zyme level may also be elevated in sarcoidosis. If signs of systemic illness, such as multiple myeloma, are present, measures of serum and urine electrophoresis in search of a monoclonal gammopathy are appropriate. Renal failure should be excluded, because it may suggest Fabry's disease or renal involvement from another systemic process. Hemochromatosis is characterized by an elevated plasma iron level, a normal or low total iron-binding capacity, elevated serum ferritin, high saturation of transferrin, and urinary iron. Carcinoid syndrome is associated with high levels of circulating serotonin and urinary 5-hydroxy-indoleacetic acid. Endemic forms of endomyocardial fibrosis have been related to high levels of cerium and low levels of magnesium.

Chest X-ray

The chest x-ray in most restrictive cardiomyopathies reveals a normal heart size and enlarged atria. With pulmonary hypertension, an enlarged right ventricle may be seen. Pericardial calcium is usually not present. Mediastinal nodes may be prominent if sarcoidosis is a consideration. Diastolic heart failure should be suspected in all patients with a relatively normal heart size and pulmonary edema.

Echocardiography

Echocardiography is usually revealing and frequently diagnostic. Ventricular Doppler filling patterns can be assessed, and changes in the patterns with respiration recorded. Pulmonary venous and hepatic venous flow patterns in concert with mitral flow patterns provide additional information. Transesophageal echocardiography is usually not necessary.

The classic restrictive cardiomyopathy two-dimensional echocardiographic image includes severe biatrial enlargement and thickened LV walls, often with a speckled or unusual myocardial texture. There is often thickening of the interatrial septum. There is no ventricular septal bounce or shifting with inspiration, which might be seen in constrictive pericarditis. Patients with endomyocardial fibrosis usually have involvement of the ventricular apices and the subvalvular apparatus. In endomyocardial fibrosis, the ventricles may be virtually obliterated by the collagen tissue.

Table 14-2
Differential Diagnosis of Restrictive Cardiomyopathy
Versus Constrictive Pericarditis

Examination Procedure	Restrictive Cardiomyopathy	Constrictive Pericarditis
Physical Examination	Kussmaul's sign occasionally present Paradoxical pulse absent Apical impulse prominent S_3 and S_4 present Regurgitant murmurs common	Kussmaul's sign common Paradoxical pulse may be present Apical impulse retracts or absent Pericardial knock may be present Regurgitant murmurs rare
Chest X-ray	Enlarged atria Pulmonary edema at times	Normal heart size Occasional pericardial calcium
ECG	Low voltage Atrial hypertrophic P waves Conduction disease common Atrial fibrillation common	Occasional low voltage P waves reflect interatrial conduction delay Conduction defects rare
Echocardiography	Small cavity with large atria Increased wall thickness. Sparkling texture Thickened cardiac valves at times Septal notch rarely seen Little septal movement with inspiration Thickened atrial septum <15% inspiratory decrease in MV velocity In PV: D>S (S/D ratio <1) TV flow with inspiration: 　Mild decrease in E wave 　No change in peak TR velocity	Mild or no atrial enlargement Normal wall thickness Abrupt septal notch in early diastole Septal movement to left ventricular with inspiration >25% inspiratory decrease in MV velocity In PV: S>D In PV: inspiratory decrease in S and D waves TV flow with inspiration: 　Decreased inflow E wave 　Increased peak TR velocity
Cardiac Catheterization	LVEDP – RVEDP >5 mm Hg Pulmonary hypertension Dip and plateau in RA and RV common RVEDP <1/3 RV systolic Late inspiratory RV/LV systolic pressure in phase (concordant) Paradoxical pulse rare	Equalization of pressures LVEDP – RVEDP <5 mm Hg PA systolic rarely >40 mm Hg Dip and plateau in RA and RV common RVEDP >1/3 RV systolic Late inspiratory RV/LV systolic pressure discordant Paradoxical pulse more common
CT/MRI	LA enlargement, LV hypertrophy, thickened atrial septum	Occasionally thickened pericardium or calcium

LA indicates left atrial; LV, left ventricular; LVEDP, left ventricular end-diastolic pressure; MRI, magnetic resonance imaging; MV, mitral valve; PA, pulmonary arterial; PV, pulmonary vein; RA, right atrial; RV, right ventricular; RVEDP, right ventricular end-diastolic pressure; TR, tricuspid regurgitant; TV, tricuspid valve.

Doppler filling patterns, especially during respiration, help differentiate constrictive pericarditis from restrictive cardiomyopathy (Table 14-2). Normal Doppler echocardiographic patterns and definitions are shown in Figure 14-6. The time from aortic valve closure to mitral valve opening represents the isovolumic relaxation time. If the left atrial pressure is high and the end-systolic aortic pressure normal, this interval shortens. This may occur in both constrictive pericarditis and restrictive cardiomyopathy. Once the mitral valve opens, the filling rate in both diseases is rapid (elevated E wave). The E wave acceleration time is the time from the opening of the mitral valve to the peak flow; the time from the peak flow to diastasis is the deceleration time. In both constriction and restriction, because the LV pressures rise quickly, rapid filling is limited and the deceleration time shortens from normal. Normal atrial contraction results in an A-wave, reflecting the acceleration of blood flow into the left ventricle; the A-wave velocity may be increased in diastolic dysfunction. The tricuspid flow pattern reflects right-sided filling and usually mirrors the mitral flow pattern.

The Doppler pulmonary venous flow pattern reveals the filling of the left atrium from the pulmonary veins. Normally, the left atrium fills during ventricular systole in concert with atrial diastole and while the mitral ring is being pulled toward the left ventricle. The left atrium fills again during ventricular diastole while the mitral valve is open to the ventricle. Normally, about an equal amount of left atrial filling occurs during ventricular diastole as ventricular systole (S = D). When the atrial kick occurs, some reversal of flow is normally seen in the pulmonary vein because of the rapid rise in the left atrial pressure. Relative to the transducer, hepatic flow is negative but is similar to pulmonary venous flow. The flow reversal pattern in the hepatic veins during atrial systole—and during the c wave when the tricuspid valve bulges into the atrium at the onset of ventricular systole—is usually more prominent than that in the pulmonary veins.

Figure 14-6 (bottom) shows the mitral pattern of impaired early relaxation and contrasts the findings seen with impaired LV compliance. The E-wave velocity is normally greater than the A-wave velocity, but if early relaxation is impaired, the rate of initial filling (E wave) is reduced, the isovolumic relaxation time and the mitral deceleration time increased, and there is reversal of the E/A ratio. The pulmonary venous flow is similarly blunted in ventricular diastole, and ventricular systolic filling of the left atrium from the pulmonary vein is greater than the diastolic filling. The S/D ratio is therefore greater than 1.

As described above, in restrictive cardiomyopathy, the issue is not impaired early LV filling,

but abnormal LV compliance and restricted late filling. Since the left ventricle fills mostly in early diastole, the E wave is more prominent, and the time to fill the ventricle is reduced (a shortened isovolumic relaxation time). Because of the rising LV diastolic pressures, the deceleration time is faster, and the contribution from the atrial kick to the late flow velocities is reduced (the E is much more prominent than the A). The pulmonary venous pattern reflects this, with rapid flow during early ventricular diastole and little flow into the stiff left atrium during ventricular systole. Thus, the S/D ratio of the pulmonary venous flow pattern is much less than 1. Hepatic venous flow patterns again resemble the pulmonary venous flow.

Because similar diastolic flow patterns may occur in constrictive pericarditis, patterns during inspiration are the key to differentiating constriction from restriction. There is usually little respiratory change in the mitral and pulmonary venous flow patterns in restrictive cardiomyopathy, but there is a significant (>25%) inspiratory drop in the maximal velocity of these flow patterns in constriction. The increased inspiratory filling of the right ventricle with constrictive pericarditis results in the increased RV pressure described above, and that increased pressure can be recorded in the tricuspid regurgitant jet velocity with inspiration. In restriction, the RV systolic pressure usually falls with inspiration.

Making the distinction even more difficult, pericardial constriction and restrictive cardiomyopathy may occur together, and atrial fibrillation often confuses the Doppler patterns. It is estimated that equivocal echocardiographic patterns are present in up to one third of the patients with possible constrictive pericarditis. Doppler myocardial velocity gradients may help with the distinction, but cannot always ensure a diagnosis.

Cardiac Nuclear Imaging

First-pass and multigated radionuclide angiography can provide ventricular volume data and a time-activity curve reflecting the ventricular volumetric changes of each heartbeat. Because of beat-to-beat variations and difficulties with describing late filling parameters, diastolic radionuclide angiographic information is confined primarily to early filling measurements. Diastolic

Figure 14-6

Doppler Flow Studies: Comparison
of Mitral and Pulmonary Vein Flow Velocities

Normal mitral flow velocity studies*

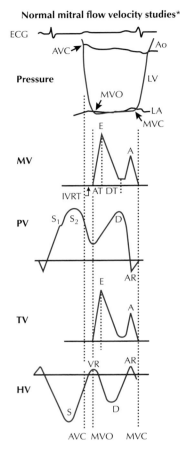

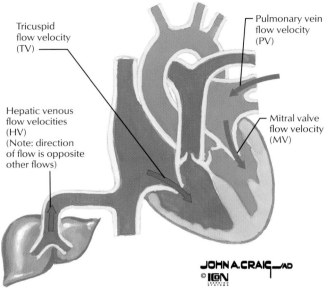

JOHN A. CRAIG—MD
©ICN

ECG provides cycle timing, and "pressure" panel represents aortic (Ao), left ven-tricular (LV), and left atrial (LA) pressures. Mitral valve flow pattern (MV) is con-trasted with pulmonary vein (PV), tricuspid valve (TV), and hepatic venous (HV) flow velocities. The time from aortic valve closure (AVC) to opening of mitral valve (MVO) defines the isovolumetric relaxation time (IVRT) and reflects active myxocardial relaxation. The MV Doppler pattern reflects early filling (E wave), with Doppler its acceleration time (AT) and deceleration time (DT). Following a dia-stasis period, atrial contraction creates the A-wave velocities. PV velocities re-flect flow into the LA, with systolic flow (S) occurring during ventricular sys-tole (atrial relaxation and mitral ring descent into LV) and again during ven-tri-cular diastole (D) while mitral valve is open. Reversal of flow (AR) occurs during atrial systole; tricuspid flows are similar to mitral. Hepatic flow velocities are similar to PV except direction is away from transducer (negative) and there is some flow reversal seen during early ventricular systole (C wave) and during atrial systole.

Mitral and pulmonary venous Doppler flow patterns in diastolic dysfunction and restrictive cardiomyopathy

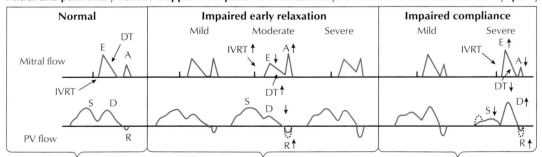

Note: Normal E > A and normal isovolumetric relaxation time (IVRT); DT = deceleration time of E wave; PV systolic velocity (S) about equal to diastolic (D); Some flow reversal (R) during atrial systole

Note: Varying degrees of impaired relaxation with prolongation of IVRT and DT, reduced E wave and increased A wave and PV flow reversal; systolic is greater than diastolic pulmonary flow because of impaired early filling in diastole.

Note: Varying degrees of reduced LV compliance with E wave much greater than A wave. Reduced DT due to rapid rise in LV diastole pressure, increased PV flow reversal, and more PV flow in early diastole than in systole because the LV filling occurs primarily in early diastole.

*Modified with permission from Klein AL, Scalia GM. Disease of the pericardium, restrictive cardiomyopathy and diastolic dysfunction. In: Topol EJ, ed. *Comprehensive Cardiovascular Medicine*. Philadelphia: Lippincott–Raven; 1998:669–716.

filling can be described with early filling parameters (peak filling rate, time to peak filling rate, first third filling time) with some accuracy, but these same data are similar to the data from echocardiography/Doppler studies and are not widely used clinically. The dissociation between systolic and diastolic function can be well demonstrated using nuclear imaging and may be useful in patients in whom echocardiography/Doppler studies are difficult or nondiagnostic.

In patients with amyloidosis, technetium 99m pyrophosphate myocardial imaging may be abnormally positive and indium-labeled antimyosin antibody scans can also be abnormal. In patients with familial cardiac amyloid polyneuropathy, metaiodobenzylguanidine (MIBG) scintigraphy assessments for sympathetic denervation have been proposed, but are only occasionally of use because of low specificity. Segmental perfusion defects are occasionally seen with perfusion imaging (thallium 201 or technetium 99m sestamibi) in sarcoidosis; gallium 67 scans may also localize inflammation in this disorder.

Computed Tomography and Magnetic Resonance Imaging

Cardiac anatomic features and their relationship to the lungs are best described by CT and magnetic resonance imaging (MRI). Pericardial thickening is poorly described by echocardiography, but both CT and MRI can detect pericardial thickening of 2 mm or more. However, a normal pericardium does not exclude constrictive pericarditis. A thickened interatrial septum suggests amyloidosis.

Cardiac Catheterization and Endomyocardial Biopsy

Because of confusion created by the noninvasive tests, cardiac catheterization is important in distinguishing between restrictive cardiomyopathy and constrictive pericarditis. Although many of the subtle findings listed herein can be helpful in determining whether restriction or constriction is more likely, more often than not, only some of these findings can be documented.

The relationship between right and left heart filling pressures during inspiration is key to understanding the hemodynamics (Table 14-2).

A **right heart only** procedure is **inadequate** for differentiating constriction from restriction: simultaneous ventricular pressure measurements are often critical to the diagnosis because the right heart pressure waveforms may be similar in both disease states. Kussmaul's sign (lack of fall of the right atrial pressure with inspiration) may be seen in both diseases. Pericardial thickening can be demonstrated at cardiac catheterization by an anterior–posterior right atrial angiogram with the presence of a shadow between the atrial wall and the lung fields noted, or by careful observation of a **peel** over the coronary arteries during coronary angiography. In constriction, portions of the coronary arteries may be encased in the pericardium and can seem to be **frozen** because they do not move with the rest of the beating heart. Unfortunately these findings are the exception rather than the rule in patients with pericardial constriction.

In restrictive cardiomyopathy, the LV end-diastolic pressure should be more than 5 mm Hg higher than the RV end-diastolic pressure at all phases of respiration, and pulmonary hypertension is present (Fig. 14-4). Hence, the RV end-diastolic pressure should be less than a third of the RV systolic pressure despite an elevated RV end-diastolic pressure. Unfortunately, lung disease may also be present in the same patient, and other causes of pulmonary hypertension may make this criterion less specific. The pulmonary vascular resistance is normal or near normal in both constrictive pericarditis and restrictive cardiomyopathy unless there is associated lung disease. Elevated pulmonary resistance implies that the left heart may not be solely responsible for the observed pulmonary hypertension. A prominent left atrial (or pulmonary capillary wedge) v wave may be present in restriction because of abnormal left atrial compliance and may or may not be associated with mitral valve regurgitation. An elevated v wave is unlikely in the pulmonary wedge tracing in constriction. The ventricular systolic pressures should be tracked together with inspiration, and both should fall in restrictive disease. The late inspiratory RV systolic pressure may actually rise in constrictive pericarditis.

Endomyocardial biopsy is often of limited value in dilated cardiomyopathy, but it may be helpful in restrictive cardiomyopathy. In cardiac amyloidosis, histochemical staining helps distinguish the primary AL type (kappa or lambda immunoglobulin light chains) from the less common AA (nonimmunoglobulin protein A) or secondary amyloidosis. Senile cardiac amyloidosis may have extensive or minor deposits, and its prevalence increases with age. Sarcoidosis is spotty and may be missed by percutaneous biopsy. Fabry's disease is distinctive, with deposition of glycolipid in the affected lysosomes, and the diagnosis is often first detected on myocardial biopsy. Other diseases that result in a restrictive process cause myocardial fibrosis of a general nature, with interstitial fibrosis, loss of myofibrils, and vacuolation of cytoplasm. Myocardial biopsy is often not diagnostic in these circumstances.

MANAGEMENT AND THERAPY
Diastolic Heart Failure

The treatment of diastolic heart failure centers on reducing symptoms and assessing whether therapy can be directed at the underlying process (Table 14-3). When diastolic pressures are elevated, diuretics are used to treat pulmonary and systemic congestion. However, the stiff ventricle is dependent on adequate preload, and the overzealous use of diuretics can result in hypotension. Increased bowel edema may reduce the absorption of furosemide, so it should initially be given intravenously. Oral torsemide is often the preferred diuretic when bowel edema is present. Spironolactone is a useful adjunct, especially if liver congestion and ascites are present. Maintenance of slow heart rates improves diastolic time and allows for adequate diastolic filling. β-Blockers can improve rate control. Calcium channel blockers are used routinely and can help control the ventricular rate in atrial fibrillation, thereby improving cardiac function. Calcium channel blockers may also improve myocardial diastolic relaxation. Sinus rhythm should be maintained if possible, because the atrial contribution to output may be significant in diastolic dysfunction. Angiotensin-converting enzyme inhibitors may also improve myocardial relaxation and are often useful despite relatively normal ventricular systolic function. Angiotensin receptor blockers have also been reported to provide symptomatic relief and can be used in concert with ACE inhibitors.

Table 14-3
Therapy in Restrictive Cardiomyopathy

General

Diuretics (furosemide, torsemide)
Spironolactone
Slow heart rate
    In sinus rhythm: β-blockers
    Antiarrhythmics to maintain sinus rhythm if possible
    In atrial fibrillation: β-blockers, calcium channel blockers
Improve diastolic relaxation
    Calcium channel blockers
    β-blockers
    ACE inhibitors and possibly ACE receptor blockers
Control systemic blood pressure
Avoid digitalis preparations
Anticoagulation
Cardiac transplantation

Specific

Amyloidosis
    Alkylating agents
    Interferon (?)
    Steroids
    Colchicine
Hypereosinophilic syndrome
    Steroids
    Hydroxyurea
Sarcoidosis
    Steroids and other anti-inflammatories
    Pacemaker if heart block present
Hemochromatosis
    Phlebotomy
    Desferrioxamine
    Liver transplantation
Fabry's disease
    α -Galactosidase enzyme replacement
Carcinoid syndrome
    Somatostatin analogs
    Serotonin antagonists
    α-Adrenergic blockers
    Surgical valve replacement

ACE indicates angiotensin-converting enzyme.

Systemic blood pressure control is important to reduce the cardiac workload and decrease any stimulus for further LV hypertrophy. However, hypotension is usually a more difficult clinical problem than hypertension in restrictive cardiomyopathy. Digoxin may result in increased arrhythmias, especially in patients with amyloidosis, and should generally not be used.

The use of the Doppler flow pattern may tailor therapy. For instance, fusion of the mitral inflow E and A waves implies inadequate diastolic time; therefore, heart rate reduction is needed. A pseudonormal or restrictive pattern (E>A) implies high diastolic filling pressures and the need for further angiotensin-converting enzyme inhibitors, calcium blockers, and diuretics. If the PR interval is prolonged, dual chamber pacing may maximize the relationship of the atrial kick to ventricular contraction. Anticoagulation with warfarin is often recommended to reduce the risk of atrial appendage thrombi, especially in patients with continuous or paroxysmal atrial fibrillation (see also chapter 19).

Gradually, medical therapy tends to fail. Cardiac transplantation in selected patients may be the only option. Unfortunately, following cardiac transplantation, amyloidosis has been reported to recur in the transplanted heart, suggesting that cardiac transplantation is not appropriate for patients with amyloidosis.

Specific Therapy

Therapy directed at the underlying cause of the restrictive process is limited. The prognosis for primary amyloidosis is poor, with a median survival time of about 2 years despite the use of alkylating agents and other approaches. Interferon has been tried with little success, although the combination of steroids and interferon shows some promise. Combination therapy with melphalan, prednisone, and colchicine may relieve some of the noncardiac and renal aspects of the disease. Liver transplantation may be an option in familial amyloidosis, because the circulating transthyretin that causes the disorder is manufactured in the liver.

Corticosteroids and hydroxyurea are used in the early stages of the hypereosinophilic syndrome. There has been some success with interferon in this disease. Surgery can debride the fibrous plaque, and valve replacement may be indicated.

Corticosteroids and other inflammatory agents are used in sarcoidosis. Heart block can be treated with permanent pacing; implantable defibrillators help patients susceptible to severe ventricular tachyarrhythmias.

Hemochromatosis is generally managed by phlebotomy, chelating agents such as desferrioxamine, or both. Heart transplantation and combined heart-liver transplantation have been used.

Fabry's disease can now be treated with intermittent intravenous infusion of the enzyme α-galactosidase A, although the results with regard to cardiac improvement are preliminary.

Carcinoid syndrome is treated with somatostatin analogues, serotonin antagonists, and α-adrenergic blockers. Surgical valve replacement is an option, especially in patients under 65 years of age.

FUTURE DIRECTIONS

The definition of diastolic heart failure needs to be further standardized. Abnormalities of active relaxation and compliance of the ventricles are often dissociated from systolic dysfunction. Diastolic dysfunction may precede systolic dysfunction in many diseases, especially diseases with concentric hypertrophy, such as aortic stenosis and systemic hypertension. The prevalence of normal systolic function and diastolic dysfunction in heart failure studies varies from 14 to 75%, depending on how these are defined. Abnormalities of early diastolic relaxation clearly differ from those of late diastolic compliance.

Clinically, the elderly present with diastolic dysfunction more commonly than do younger individuals. Despite this, the prognosis in patients with diastolic dysfunction is far better than it is in patients with systolic dysfunction, unless an infiltrative process is present.

Diastolic dysfunction need not be present with even profound systolic dysfunction. Many patients who have a poor LV ejection fraction suffer no symptoms of congestion for many years. Only when diastolic dysfunction manifests do congestive symptoms emerge.

Diastolic dysfunction from a restrictive cardiomyopathy suggests that a definable etiology is present, although it is often difficult to identify. Early detection might improve the dismal outcome, so sensitive tests continue to be sought. Several noninvasive modalities are being investigated, including Doppler tissue imaging, which records the motion of the mitral annulus or the interventricular septum to form a pattern similar to that of the mitral inflow. Doppler tissue imaging appears to be particularly useful in patients with mitral valve disease. Three-dimensional echocardiography allows for multiple planes to be reconstructed from a single beat and may also be useful in diagnosis, prognosis, and evaluation of the effectiveness of therapeutic interventions. Exercise measures of diastolic function may be possible that demonstrate early abnormalities not evident at rest. Cardiac MRI is perhaps the most promising new imaging modality, with improved imaging of all the cardiac chambers. MRI may help distinguish those with epicardial restriction from those with pericardial constriction and better identify patients for whom pericardial stripping may help. It also may provide better definitions of tissue characteristics and thus allow more precise diagnoses in infiltrative disorders.

Therapy remains the greatest challenge. Although some advances have been made in symptomatic treatment, until satisfactory therapy is available for diseases such as amyloidosis, the outlook for most patients with restrictive cardiomyopathy will remain grim.

REFERENCES

Asher CR, Klein AL. Diastolic heart failure: Restrictive cardiomyopathy, constrictive pericarditis, and cardiac tamponade: Clinical and echocardiographic evaluation. *Cardiol Rev* 2002;10:218–229.

Frank H, Globits S. Magnetic resonance imaging evaluation of myocardial and pericardial disease. *J Magn Reson Imaging* 1999;10:617–626.

Klein AL, Scalia GM. Disease of the pericardium, restrictive cardiomyopathy and diastolic dysfunction. In: Topol EJ, ed. *Comprehensive Cardiovascular Medicine*. Philadelphia: Lippincott-Raven; 1998:669–716.

Kushwaha SS, Fallon JT, Fuster V. Restrictive cardiomyopathy. *N Engl J Med* 1997;336:267–276.

Nishimura RA. Constrictive pericarditis in the modern era: A diagnostic dilemma. *Heart* 2001;86:619–623.

Palka P, Lange A, Donnelly JE, Nihoyannopoulos P. Differentiation between restrictive cardiomyopathy and constrictive pericarditis by early diastolic doppler myocardial velocity gradient at the posterior wall. *Circulation* 2000;102:655–662.

Spodick DH. Combined restrictive cardiomyopathy and constrictive pericarditis. Circulation 1996;93:616.

Spodick DH. Restrictive cardiomyopathy. *N Engl J Med* 1997;336:1917–1918.

Chapter 15

Hereditary Cardiomyopathies

José Ortiz and Richard A. Walsh

The definition of cardiomyopathies was previously restricted to disorders intrinsic to the myocardium and for which no other primary cause was evident. It included myocardial processes, most of which have an underlying genetic alteration, but excluded myocardial pathology secondary to hypertension, valvular disease, coronary artery disease, inflammatory processes, or other disorders. The World Health Organization/International Society and Federation of Cardiology Task Force on the Definition and Classification of the Cardiomyopathies has expanded the definition of cardiomyopathies, and its use today includes myocardial damage regardless of etiology. Cardiomyopathies intrinsic to the myocardium form the basis of this chapter.

There are five categories of cardiomyopathic heart disease, based on morphologic and hemodynamic characteristics: dilated cardiomyopathy (DCM), hypertrophic cardiomyopathy (HCM), restrictive cardiomyopathy, arrhythmogenic right ventricular (RV) cardiomyopathy, and nonclassifiable cardiomyopathies (such as noncompaction and mitochondrial cardiomyopathy).

Numerous genetic mutations, either de novo, or with a clear familial transmission, are associated with each of these categories of cardiomyopathy. A familial cause has been found in about 50% of patients with HCM, 35% with DCM, and 30% with arrhythmogenic RV cardiomyopathy (ARVC) (Tables 15-1, 15-2, and 15-3). As yet, no specific genetic mutations have been found in restrictive cardiomyopathy, but their pedigree analysis points portend the eventual assignment of genetic abnormalities to this classification as well.

Evidence of a gene defect associated with an intrinsic heart muscle disease was first published in 1990. The discovery of the mutation in the gene encoding for β-myosin heavy chain (Table 15-1; Fig. 15-1), with resultant familial hypertrophic cardiomyopathy, was followed by discoveries of gene mutations for the entire spectrum of cardiomyopathies. This chapter focuses on the breadth of mutations that affect the myocardium, whereas chapter 62 addresses the general topic of genetics in cardiovascular diseases.

ETIOLOGY AND PATHOGENESIS
Familial Dilated Cardiomyopathy
The phenotype for familial DCM is divided into three groups (Table 15-2; Fig. 15-1), two that are based on the type of genetic transmission and the Barth syndrome (previously included among "X-linked" cardiomyopathies), which is considered a third group because of its peculiar mitochondrial involvement.

Autosomal Dominant Transmission

Autosomal dominant transmission accounts for most cases of familial DCM, which may present either as heart failure or as a conduction abnormality. Ten genetic loci have been mapped for cardiomyopathy without conduction system disease. Seven of these genes are known: *actin* (chromosome 15q14), *desmin* (chromosome 2q35), *α-sarcoglycan* (chromosome 5q33), *β-sarcoglycan* (chromosome 4q12), *cardiac troponin T* (chromosome 1q32), *β-myosin heavy chain* (*βMHC*; chromosome 14q11), and *α-tropomyosin* (chromosome 15q2) (see Table 15-1). (Mutations in the *α-tropomyosin* gene are associated with familial hypertrophic cardiomyopathies.) Actin, a sarcomeric protein, leads to DCM if the mutation affects its binding to dystrophin (at the sarcolemma level) or to HCM if the mutation affects the myosin-binding region. Mutations of the *βMHC* and of *cardiac troponin T* genes are thought to produce DCM by causing reduced force generation by the sarcomere. In particular, the *βMHC* mutation disrupts interactions between *actin* and *myosin* or a hinge area within *myosin* that transmits movement; the mutations in *cardiac troponin T* decrease the power of

Figure 15-1

Interaction of Affected Proteins in
DCM, HCM, and ARVC (Cardiac Muscle Cell)

In red, the defective proteins that are related to the cause of DCM, HCM, and ARVC

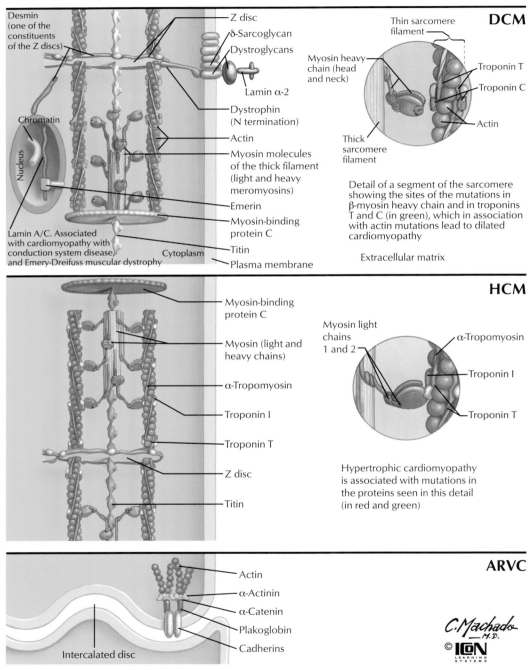

DCM

Desmin (one of the constituents of the Z discs)

Chromatin

Nucleus

Lamin A/C. Associated with cardiomyopathy with conduction system disease, and Emery-Dreifuss muscular dystrophy

Cytoplasm

Z disc
δ-Sarcoglycan
Dystroglycans

Lamin α-2

Dystrophin (N termination)

Actin

Myosin molecules of the thick filament (light and heavy meromyosins)

Emerin

Myosin-binding protein C

Titin
Plasma membrane

Thin sarcomere filament

Myosin heavy chain (head and neck)

Troponin T

Troponin C

Actin

Thick sarcomere filament

Detail of a segment of the sarcomere showing the sites of the mutations in β-myosin heavy chain and in troponins T and C (in green), which in association with actin mutations lead to dilated cardiomyopathy

Extracellular matrix

HCM

Myosin-binding protein C

Myosin (light and heavy chains)

α-Tropomyosin

Troponin I

Troponin T

Z disc

Titin

Myosin light chains 1 and 2

α-Tropomyosin

Troponin I

Troponin T

Hypertrophic cardiomyopathy is associated with mutations in the proteins seen in this detail (in red and green)

ARVC

Actin
α-Actinin
α-Catenin
Plakoglobin
Cadherins

Intercalated disc

C.Machado M.D.

© ICON LEARNING SYSTEMS

Table 15-1
Gene Defects Associated With Hypertrophic Cardiomyopathy

Gene Product	Chromosome	Risk of Frequent Sudden Death	FHC	Remarks
Myofilaments				
β-Myosin heavy chain	14q11·2-12	High (R403Q, R453C, R719W)	Yes	Degree of hypertrophy correlates with risk of sudden death
Myosin light chain-1	3p21	Low	Yes	Papillary muscle thickening, rare cases
Myosin light chain-2	12q23-24.3	Low	Yes	Papillary muscle thickening, rare cases
Thin-filament proteins				
Troponin T	1q3	High (Int15G1_A, ΔE160, R92Q, 179N)	Yes	High risk of sudden death, mild or absent hypertrophy; 13 different mutations reported on the cTnT gene
Troponin I	19q13.4	High (ΔK183)	Yes	Apical variant of HCM, occasionally DCM-like features in elderly patients
Actin	15q14	Low	Yes	Some mutations might also cause primary DCM
α-Tropomyosin	15q22	High (V95A)	Yes	Usually favorable prognosis, high phenotypic variability
Other defects associated with FHC				
Myosin-binding protein C	11p11.2	Low	Yes	Benign clinical course, progressive hypertrophy with rather late onset
Titin	Spontaneous	Not applicable	Yes	Only one patient reported
Other defects associated with HCM				
AMP-activated protein kinase γ2	7q3	Low	No	Associated with Wolff-Parkinson-White syndrome
α-Myosin heavy chain	Spontaneous	Low	No	Late onset, rare

DCM indicates dilated cardiomyopathy; FHC, familial hypertrophic cardiomyopath; HCM, hypertrophic cardiomyopathy. Reprinted with permission from Elsevier (*The Lancet* 2001;358:1629).

contraction by reducing the ionic interactions between cardiac *troponins T* and *C*. The *α-tropomyosin* mutation interferes with the integrity of the thin filaments. Other mutations are involved either with the stability of the sarcomere, or the sarcolemma, or with signal transduction.

Cardiomyopathy with conduction system disease is associated with five mapped loci and

Table 15-2
Gene Defects Associated With Dilated Cardiomyopathy

Gene Product	Chromosome	Skeletal Involvement	Frequent Sudden Death or Rapid Progressive Heart Failure	Remarks	Mutations of the Same Gene Cause Primary MD
DCM with mainly LV dysfunction					
Troponin T	1q3	Not reported	SD, HF (Δk210)	Early-onset ventricular dilation	HCM
δ-Sarcoglycan	5q33-q34	None/sub-clinical	SD, HF (Δk238)	Early-onset ventricular dilation	Limb girdle MD 2F
β-Sarcoglycan	4q12	May be severe	HF	May be the initiating deficiency and lead to multiple defects in sarco-glycan expressions	Limb girdle MD 2E
βMHC	14q11·2-12	None	HF (S532P, F764L)	Early-onset ventricular dilation	HCM
Actin	15q14	Not reported		Defect located in *dystrophin*-binding region	HCM
NK	1q32	Not reported		First to second decade, incomplete penetrance	
NK	2q31	None	HF	Native American family, incomplete penetrance	
NK	9q13-22	None		Large Italian family, incomplete penetrance	
NK	10q21-23	Not reported		Mitral valve prolapse, occasionally sudden death	
DCM with early conduction disease					
Lamin A/C	1q21·3	None/ mild	SD	Frequently in DCM with conduction abnormalities	Emery-Dreifuss MD, limb girdle MD 2B
Desmin	2q35	None/ severe		Syncope, can develop severe skeletal myopathy	*Desmin* myopathy
NK	2q14-q22	Not reported		Frequently ventricular tachycardia	
NK	3p22-25	Not reported		Associated with sick sinus syndrome and stroke	
NK	6q23	Severe		Associated with adult-onset limb girdle MD	
DCM with sensorineural hearing loss					
NK	6q23-24	None		Associated with juvenile sensorineural hearing loss	
tRNA-Lys	Mitochondrial DNA	Mild	Involvement of organs with high oxidative metabolism: heart, cochlea, brain, skeletal muscle		
DCM with rapid progression in young men					
Dystrophin	Xp21	Mild	HF	Rapid progression to end stage heart failure	Becker's and Duchenne's MD
Tafazzin	Xq28	Mild	HF	Usually fatal in infancy, rare survival to adulthood	Barth syndrome, endocardial fibroelastosis

DCM indicates dilated cardiomyopathy; HCM, hypertrophic cardiomyopathy; HF, heart failure; LV, left ventricular; MD, muscular dystrophy; MHC, myosin heavy chain; NK, not known; SD, sudden death.
Reprinted with permission from Elsevier (*The Lancet* 2001;358:1629).

Table 15-3
Gene Defects Associated With Arrhythmogenic Right Ventricular Cardiomyopathy

Gene Product	Chromosome	Inheritance	Remarks
Plakoglobin	17q21	Autosomal recessive	Associated with palmoplantar keratoderma and woolly hair (Naxos disease)
Desmoplakin	6p23-p24	Autosomal recessive	Associated with palmoplantar keratoderma and woolly hair (Naxos disease)
Ryanodine receptor	1q42	Autosomal dominant	Identification of four different mutations in independent families
NK	2q32	Autosomal dominant	
NK	3p23	Autosomal dominant	
NK	10p12-p14	Autosomal dominant	
NK	14q12	Autosomal dominant	
NK	14q23	Autosomal dominant	

NK indicates not known.
Reprinted with permission from Elsevier (*The Lancet* 2001;358:1629).

one identified gene, *lamin A/C*, on chromosome 1q21, which encodes a nuclear envelope intermediate filament protein. This mutation also causes Emery-Dreifuss muscular dystrophy.

X-Linked Transmission

Characterized by elevated amounts of serum creatine kinase muscle isoforms, the disease-causing gene of X-linked transmission leads to a severe reduction or absence of dystrophin, a cytoskeletal protein, in the heart. This gene is responsible for Duchenne's and Becker's muscular dystrophies as well. The mutations cluster in the 5' portion of the gene affecting the N-terminal actin-binding region of the dystrophin protein.

Mitochondrial Inheritance (Barth Syndrome)

Seen most often in male infants, mitochondrial inheritance (Barth syndrome) also follows an X-linked genetic transmission but is considered a separate category because it is characterized by abnormal mitochondrial function, neutropenia, and 3-methylglutaconic aciduria. The responsible gene was found to encode for the protein tafazzin; although the role of tafazzin is unknown, its mutation results in many clinical disorders, including DCM, hypertrophic DCM, endocardial fibro-

elastosis, and left ventricular (LV) noncompaction, with or without Barth syndrome features. There are also reports linking abnormalities of energy production and mitochondrial DNA mutations to cardiomyopathies. In at least two families, HCMs that have evolved to severe DCMs have been linked to *tRNA-Lys* defects.

Hypertrophic Cardiomyopathy

Familial hypertrophic cardiomyopathy with autosomal dominant inheritance encompasses most of the cases of HCM (see Table 15-1; Fig. 15-1). The first gene for familial hypertrophic cardiomyopathy was mapped to chromosome 14q11.2-14q12. Familial hypertrophic cardiomyopathy can be caused by mutations in nine different genes encoding sarcomere proteins expressed in cardiac muscle.

Left Ventricular Noncompaction

Two inheritance patterns of LV noncompaction have been described: One is an X-linked form, seen in males. The mutation has been localized to the gene G4.5, which encodes *tafazzin*, as described previously in the section Mitochondrial Inheritance (Barth syndrome). The other inheritance pattern is a dystrophin-associated protein gene mutation. The gene *α-dystrobrevin*, which maps to the chromosome 18q12, has structural properties as well as nitric oxide signaling functions. Its deletion causes cardiomyopathy in mutant mice, supporting its deletion as a cause of ventricular dysfunction.

Arrhythmogenic Right Ventricular Dysplasia

Arrhythmogenic RV dysplasia presents as a familial disease in at least 30% of patients (see Table 15-3; Fig. 15-1). It is mostly inherited in an autosomal dominant fashion, and mutations in *plakoglobin* (chromosome 17q21), *desmoplakin* (chromosome 6p23-p24), and *ryanodine* (chromosome 1q42) have been found.

CLINICAL PRESENTATION

Patients with hereditary cardiomyopathy have a spectrum of clinical manifestations, from the asymptomatic patient discovered during the screening of a patient's relatives to the patient presenting with sudden cardiac death or heart failure. Many patients, regardless of the type of cardiomyopathy, present with classic heart failure symptoms, such as dyspnea, orthopnea, paroxysmal nocturnal dyspnea, angina, syncope, edema, evidence of low cardiac output (fatigue, weakness, exercise intolerance), and conduction abnormalities. Symptoms depend on the degree of ventricular dysfunction, valvular involvement, and cardiac arrhythmias (if present), and the cardiac chamber involved. Presentation, clinical course, and prognosis also vary according to the altered gene and the mutation responsible for the disease. Less understood variables may affect genetic background and alter the clinical course of the disease.

Hypertrophic cardiomyopathy deserves special consideration because sudden death may be the initial presentation in a young, otherwise healthy patient. As seen in Table 15-1, the risk of sudden death correlates reasonably well with the type of genetic mutation and the degree of LV outflow obstruction and hypertrophy (see also chapters 13 and 23). Studies linking the incidence of sudden deaths in athletes have shown different results according to the country of origin of the patient population. This is a consequence of the relative frequency of the various genotypes that affect the likelihood of sudden death. Atrial fibrillation, considered by some to be a sign of disease progression, may develop. Atrial fibrillation may add to treatment difficulties by predisposing the patient to stroke and worsening CHF caused by the hard-to-control ventricular response, the impact on diastolic filling, or both. Patients may also progress to a dilated phase, in which symptoms are similar to those of patients with DCM.

Patients with genetically determined DCM most commonly present with symptoms between the ages of 18 and 50 years. Genetically determined DCM occurs more frequently in men than in women and in black individuals than in white individuals. Without cardiac transplantation, about 50% of patients die within 5 years of the date of diagnosis. As with acquired cardiomyopathy, patients succumb to progressive heart failure or sudden death from ventricular tachyarrhythmias. Although beyond the scope of this chapter, DCM can also be associated with genetic systemic disorders such as glycogen storage disorders, mucopolysaccharidosis, neuromuscular disorders, and fatty acid disorders. In patients with any of these disorders, symptoms related to the systemic disorder are also present.

Patients with DCM may present with conduction system disease. For these patients, the age at death is usually in the third decade of life. The cardiomyopathy is disproportionate to the electrical abnormality, which may have started as mild conduction disease and progressed to complete heart block over several years.

Patients with LV noncompaction have deep trabeculations in the LV endocardium and hypertrophy, dilation, or both can develop. Patients may also have septal defects, a pulmonic stenosis, or a hypoplastic left ventricle.

Patients with arrhythmogenic RV dysplasia usually have a progressive replacement of the RV myocardium with fibrofatty tissue. Patients present with significant arrhythmias of RV origin, ranging from premature beats to sustained ventricular fibrillation and sudden death.

DIFFERENTIAL DIAGNOSIS AND DIAGNOSTIC APPROACH

Patients with a significant family history of cardiomyopathy usually do not represent a diagnostic dilemma, and genetic workup should be requested promptly after the onset of symptoms. Diagnosis starts with a well-focused history, an appropriate physical examination, and ECG, usually followed by an echocardiography and a right and left heart catheterization. Myocardial biopsy should be performed whenever an inflammatory or viral cardiomyopathy is suspected. Even in cases in which a clear familial inheritance is well documented, the initial workup should exclude secondary causes of cardiomyopathies, such as coronary artery disease and hypertension, which may act alone or in combination with the genetic disorder. All patients with DCM should undergo a complete neuromuscular evaluation to exclude an associated muscular pathology; conversely, patients with any type of muscular dystrophy should undergo a cardiac evaluation to assess for the presence of a concomitant cardiomyopathy.

MANAGEMENT AND THERAPY

Specific treatments for familial cardiomyopathy are not available, and much of the supportive management is based on heart failure therapy. The main goals of therapy are to halt/reverse the progressive ventricular functional deterioration and to prevent sudden cardiac death. β-Blockers and angiotensin-converting enzyme inhibitors are considered the cornerstone of treatment and should be given at the maximum doses tolerated. Patients intolerant of angiotensin-converting enzyme inhibitors may benefit from angiotensin receptor blocker therapy. Other heart failure medications may be indicated, depending on the type of cardiomyopathy. For example, although positive inotropic agents are very useful for patients with acutely decompensated cardiomyopathy who are not responding to less aggressive therapy, they are contraindicated in patients with HCM and normal systolic function (or hyperkinesis). Similarly, diuretic agents should be used cautiously in HCM because patients with HCM are preload dependent and even relative volume depletion can further impair their already altered diastolic function.

For moderate to severe heart failure, the aldosterone antagonist spironolactone has decreased morbidity and mortality. For patients with severe conduction abnormalities, especially left bundle branch block, biventricular pacing (also know as resynchronization therapy) may help to relieve symptoms. Because of the fairly recent introduction of biventricular pacing, data on its effect on mortality are lacking. Improvement in functional mitral regurgitation and the freedom to use β-blockade without the risk of bradycardia may be two of the most important benefits of this minimally invasive procedure.

Because sudden cardiac death is so prevalent in patients with cardiomyopathy, multiple antiarrhythmic agents have been used, with little success in preventing sudden cardiac death. Of all the drugs, only amiodarone has shown a marginal decrease in sudden cardiac death in ischemic cardiomyopathies. More recently, it has been demonstrated that the use of implantable cardioverter defibrillators provides an even further mortality benefit, in particular when used for secondary prevention. Because of their extremely low predictive value, diagnostic electrophysiology studies help little in the decision of whether to use an implantable cardioverter defibrillator, especially in patients with DCM.

Lifestyle modifications such as a regular physical exercise program have been shown to improve well-being and endothelial function and should be encouraged. Surgical options (prior to heart transplantation) may improve the quality of life and even reduce mortality rate. Despite the usually complicated early postoperative period, high-risk surgeries such as mitral valve repair or replacement can be performed. Partial ventriculectomies, aneurysm resections, latissimus dorsi cardiomyoplasty, and other surgeries have been performed with mixed results.

Finally, patients may become refractory to standard management and require more aggressive means, including ventricular assist devices (as a bridge to recovery/transplantation) and, eventually, cardiac transplantation.

Specific therapies for patients with DCM and HCM are discussed in chapters 12 and 13, respectively. Periodic screening of family members is indicated and strongly encouraged; there is not an obvious "cutoff" time beyond which further vigilance is not needed. First-degree relatives of DCM patients, even relatives with no apparent findings at initial screening, should be rescreened every 3 to 5 years. The medical history of every new patient should include a detailed cardiac family history on at least first- and second-degree relatives, and examination, ECG, and echocardiography should follow this for all relatives. Particular attention should be paid to those relatives with abnormal findings that do not necessarily fit the criteria for cardiomyopathy (such as bundle branch block or LV enlargement with normal LV systolic function). Relatives with these abnormal findings may have a high risk of development of cardiomyopathy. The presence of isolated LV enlargement may be a key indicator or an early stage of disease. When LV enlargement is discovered in a relative, further screening should be performed every 1 to 3 years, depending on the degree of dilation. Because of the variable degree of phenotypic expression and the severity of outcomes, it is advisable for families to receive genetic counseling from a specialist.

FUTURE DIRECTIONS

Early data suggest that novel therapies may provide benefit for patients with cardiomyopathies. The use of immunoadsorption to remove cardiodepressant antibodies from the plasma of patients with DCM may result in early hemodynamic improvement. This technique appears to be advantageous in patients with high levels of β-receptor antibodies. Treatment with carvedilol or long-acting metoprolol may induce a significant change in myocardial gene expression in patients with DCM. The European Study of Epidemiology and Treatment of Cardiac Inflammatory Diseases is an ongoing investigation that evaluates antiviral agents, immunoglobulins, anticytokines (in particular those directed against tumor necrosis factor α (TNF-α), IL-6, and endothelin) and gene therapy. It is expected to contribute significantly to the understanding of cardiomyopathy.

To understand the pathologic variability, researchers are exploring the possible role as genetic modifiers of angiotensin I–converting enzymes and β-blockers. Finally, ongoing, large, multicenter registries and international studies (e.g., the Eurogene Heart Failure Study) are attempting to establish and refine the understanding of the prevalence and the significance of the different known mutations.

REFERENCES

Arbustini E, Morbini P, Pilotto A. Familial dilated cardiomyopathy: From clinical presentation to molecular genetics. *Eur Heart J 2000*; 21:1825–1832.

Crispell KA, Hanson EL, Coates K, et al. Periodic rescreening is indicated for family members at risk of developing familial dilated cardiomyopathy. *J Am Coll Cardiol* 2002;39: 1503–1507.

Davies, MJ. The cardiomyopathies: An overview. *Heart* 2000;83:469–474.

Franz WM, Müller OJ, Katus HA. Cardiomyopathies: From genetics to the prospect of treatment. *Lancet* 2001; 358:1627–1637.

Kamisago M, Sharma SD, DePalma SR, et al. Mutations in sarcomere protein genes as a cause of dilated cardiomyopathy. *N Engl J Med* 2000;343:1688–1696.

Lowes BD, Gilbert EM, Abraham WT, et al. Myocardial gene expression in dilated cardiomyopathy treated with beta blocking agents. *N Engl J Med* 2002;346:1357–1365.

Maisch B, Ristic AD, Hufnagel G, et al. Dilated cardiomyopathies as a cause of congestive heart failure. *Herz* 2002;27:113–134.

Towbin, JA, Bowles NE. The failing heart. *Nature* 2002;415:227–233.

Chapter 16

Myocarditis

Paresh K. Patel and Daniel J. Lenihan

Myocarditis is inflammation of the myocardium and may include involvement of the myocytes, the interstitium, and/or the vasculature. The etiology of the inflammatory response may be infection, pharmacologic agents, toxicity, hypersensitivity, physical damage, or systemic disease. The clinical course of myocarditis is as diverse as its etiologies. Most patients have a subclinical, self-limited course, but myocarditis may also have fulminant, acute or chronic presentations. The burden of this condition is difficult to determine, in part because of its diversity and the elusiveness of diagnosis. However, new knowledge in immunology and molecular analyses has made a causal link between chronic effects of viral myocarditis and dilated cardiomyopathy more evident. Research investigating novel treatments for dilated cardiomyopathy and congestive heart failure has focused on immunomodulating therapy partly based on this knowledge. Further elucidation of the pathogenesis of myocarditis will likely affect the management of left ventricular (LV) dysfunction and heart failure.

ETIOLOGY AND PATHOGENESIS

In North America and Europe, it is likely that the majority of cases of myocarditis result from viruses. Many viruses have been associated with myocarditis (Table 16-1). Enteroviruses, such as coxsackie B, have been implicated from serologic evidence as the most common cause of viral myocarditis. However, the application of direct molecular techniques to endomyocardial biopsies, and perhaps changing epidemiology, have led to the increasing recognition of adenoviruses and hepatitis C as etiologic agents. In HIV infection, there is often evidence of myocarditis when cardiac decompensation occurs, although it is unclear whether HIV or opportunistic infections are responsible.

The mechanisms of myocardial injury in viral myocarditis remain under investigation. The initial phase of injury likely depends on viral attachment to myocytes and direct cell damage by the virus, resulting in myocyte necrosis. The identification of a common membrane receptor for adenoviruses and coxsackieviruses correlates with the preponderance of these viruses as causative agents. Host immune response to the virus may play a dominant role in myocardial injury. Animal models have shown that after the initial phase of entry and proliferation of the virus in the myocyte cytoplasm, inflammatory cells (including natural killer cells and macrophages) infiltrate with subsequent release

Table 16-1
Selected Etiologies of Myocarditis*

Infectious

Viral (coxsackievirus, HIV, hepatitis C, Parvovirus, Epstein-Barr virus)

Bacterial (meningococcus, *Corynebacterium diphtheriae*)

Protozoal (*Trypanosoma cruzi*)

Spirochetal (*Borrelia burgdorferi*)

Rickettsial (*Rickettsia rickettsii*)

Parasitic (*Trichinella spiralis, Echinococcus granulosus*)

Fungal (*Aspergillus, Cryptococcus*)

Inflammatory Diseases

Sarcoidosis

Giant cell myocarditis

Scleroderma

Systemic lupus erythematosis

Hypersensitivity reactions

Serum sickness (antibiotics, tetanus toxoid, acetazolamide, phenytoin)

Toxic Exposures

Cocaine

Anthracyclines

*Examples are shown in each category, but this is not an all-inclusive list.

of proinflammatory cytokines. T lymphocytes are activated through classic cell-mediated immunity. Cytotoxic T cells recognize viral protein fragments on the cell surface in a major histocompatibility complex–restricted manner. Molecular mimicry can occur when antigens intrinsic to the myocyte cross-react with viral peptides, inducing persistent T-cell activation. Cytokines, including tumor necrosis factor, IL-1, IL-2, and interferon γ have important roles in the development of chronic inflammatory disease. These cytokines can cause myocyte damage resulting in fewer contractile units and thus exerting a negative inotropic effect. Humoral immunity appears to have less of an impact on the pathogenesis of myocarditis than does cellular immunity. Nevertheless, autoantibodies to myocyte components are often found in patients with myocarditis, although most studies measuring autoantibody levels were in patients with idiopathic dilated cardiomyopathy.

Although it is rare, bacterial infections can produce focal or diffuse myopericarditis primarily through hematogenous spread from endogenous sources (Fig. 16-1). Probably the earliest recognized cause of myocarditis was **diphtheria**. Up to 20% of diphtheria cases have cardiac involvement, and myocarditis is the leading cause of death with this infection. The toxin produced by the diphtheria bacillus injures myocardial cells (Fig. 16-2). In South and Central America, the most common cause of infectious myocarditis is the protozoan *Trypanosoma cruzi* (**Chagas disease**).

Sarcoidosis, a systemic granulomatous disorder of unknown etiology, involves the myocardium in at least 20% of cases. Cardiac involvement ranges from a few scattered lesions to extensive involvement (Fig. 16-3). As a result, endomyocardial biopsy may be diagnostic but is frequently unreliable in confirming myocarditis. **Giant cell myocarditis** is a rare but highly lethal form of myocarditis of suspected immune or autoimmune etiology that may be associated with other inflammatory conditions such as Crohn's disease. These forms of myocarditis may respond to immunosuppression, although results can be variable. Peripartum cardiomyopathy has been associated with a greater than 50% rate of myocarditis on endomyocardial biopsy, although the etiology remains unknown.

Hypersensitivity reactions resulting in myo-

Table 16-2
Clinical Presentations of Myocarditis

· Unexplained fever or viral syndrome
· Asymptomatic LV dysfunction
· Symptomatic LV dysfunction
· Acutely decompensated heart failure
· Acute MI with normal coronaries
· Sudden cardiac death
· Arrhythmias

LV, indicates, left ventricular; MI, myocardial infarction.

carditis are characterized by eosinophilia and a perivascular infiltration of the myocardium by eosinophils and leukocytes. Any drug may cause hypersensitivity myocarditis, but clinically this condition is rarely recognized. Therefore, a high index of suspicion should be maintained.

Direct myocardial toxins are an important cause of myocarditis. Cocaine use, for instance, produces myocyte necrosis—mostly from profound sympathetic overstimulation. Anthracyclines are direct myocardial toxins with a dose-dependent effect that can profoundly affect the heart even at low doses.

CLINICAL PRESENTATION

The clinical course of a patient with myocarditis is variable and the disease is self-limited in up to 40% of patients (Table 16-2). Some patients have a defined prodromal viral illness with fever and arthralgia. Often cardiac symptoms are nonspecific and include fatigue, dyspnea, and chest pain with pleuritic features. Other patients present more acutely with progressive cardiac decompensation from heart failure and necessitate intensive support. The presentation of patients with focal myocarditis may mimic that of acute myocardial infarction (MI) but with normal coronary arteries. Patients may present with symptoms of arrhythmia, including palpitations or syncope. Sudden death may occur with myocarditis and is presumed to be secondary to arrhythmia because even focal inflammation in the cardiac conduction system can be significant. Chronic immune-mediated myocardial injury, or persistent myocyte viral gene expression, may cause progressive dilatation and resultant LV dysfunction after the resolution of a clinically apparent or subclinical illness.

Figure 16-1

Septic Myocarditis

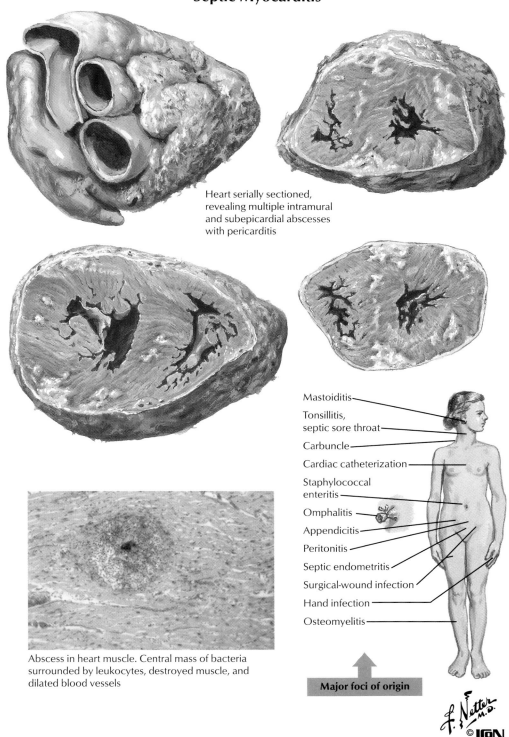

Heart serially sectioned, revealing multiple intramural and subepicardial abscesses with pericarditis

Mastoiditis
Tonsillitis, septic sore throat
Carbuncle
Cardiac catheterization
Staphylococcal enteritis
Omphalitis
Appendicitis
Peritonitis
Septic endometritis
Surgical-wound infection
Hand infection
Osteomyelitis

Major foci of origin

Abscess in heart muscle. Central mass of bacteria surrounded by leukocytes, destroyed muscle, and dilated blood vessels

Figure 16-2   ## Diphtheritic and Viral Myocarditis

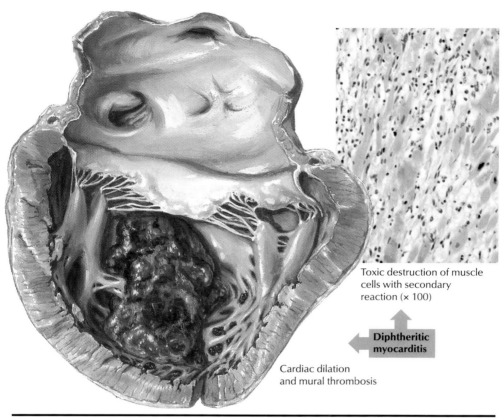

Toxic destruction of muscle
cells with secondary
reaction (× 100)

**Diphtheritic
myocarditis**

Cardiac dilation
and mural thrombosis

Viral myocarditis

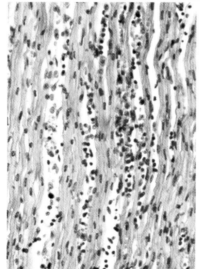

Coxsackie group B virus infection. Diffuse
and patchy interstitial edema; cellular
infiltration with only moderate muscle
fiber destruction (× 100)

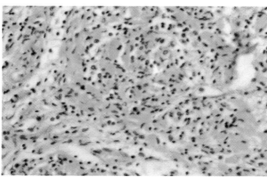

Diffuse cellular infiltration of bundle of His and right and left
bundle branches (× 100)

Figure 16-3

Myocarditis in Sarcoidosis and Scleroderma

Sarcoidosis

Brain + (15%)

Eyes ++ (20%)

Nasal and pharyngeal mucosa, tonsils + (10%)

Salivary glands + (1%)

Lymph nodes ++++ (80%)

Lungs ++++ (80%)

Heart ++ (20%)

Liver ++++ (70%)

Spleen ++++ (70%)

Skin ++ (30%)

Bones ++ (30%)

Relative frequency of organ involvement in sarcoidosis

Perivascular infiltration, chiefly of histiocytes in cardiac interstitium

Granuloma with giant cell in heart wall

Scleroderma

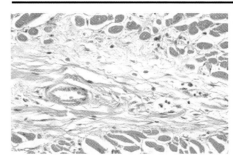

Extensive fibrosis between and around cardiac muscle fibers and in arterial wall, with only moderate lymphocytic and histiocytic infiltration

Physical findings in mild cases of infectious myocarditis may include low-grade fever, and a pericardial friction rub may be audible. Physical features of the underlying etiology, such as erythema nodosum (sarcoidosis) and erythema chronica migrans (Lyme disease), can be important clues in determining the cause of myocarditis and should be elicited. If congestive heart failure is evident, there may be a third heart sound, jugular venous distension, or evidence of pulmonary edema. Sinus tachycardia is usually prominent and out of proportion to temperature elevation.

DIFFERENTIAL DIAGNOSIS

The differential diagnosis of myocarditis depends mainly on the presentation of the illness. Many illnesses are potentially implicated with or causal of myocarditis (Tables 16-1 and 16-2). In terms of other causes of LV dysfunction or congestive heart failure, the more common causes include long-standing hypertension, coronary artery disease, valvular heart disease, or inherited cardiomyopathy. Myocarditis, with evidence of LV dysfunction, is typically a diagnosis of exclusion after the other myriad causes of the clinical presentation have been considered.

DIAGNOSTIC APPROACH

Few reliable diagnostic tests are available for myocarditis; therefore, clinical suspicion is vital (Table 16-3). CK−MB fraction and cardiac troponin I and troponin T concentrations are often increased, confirming the presence of myocardial cell injury. There may be evidence of a systemic infection with an increased white blood cell count and sedimentation rate. Blood cultures may confirm a bacterial etiology, but in viral infections, this is frequently not possible. Acute and convalescent titers for viruses (such as coxsackie B and Epstein-Barr) may provide some evidence of recent infection, especially if there is a two- to fourfold increase in neutralizing antibody

Table 16-3
Diagnostic Testing Useful to Establish the Diagnosis of Myocarditis

· Cardiac markers (CK-MB and troponins)

· Serologic tests for viral, spirochetal, or parasitic etiologies

· Blood cultures (for infectious causes)

· Markers of inflammation or underlying inflammatory disease (erythrocyte sedimentation rate, antinuclear antibodies, ACE level)

· Echocardiography

· Endomyocardial biopsy

· Cardiac catheterization

· Nuclear and magnetic resonance imaging

ACE indicates angiotensin-converting enzym; CK, creatine kinase.

titers to a virus (or spirochetes in the case of Lyme disease). Other laboratory testing may confirm a systemic immunologic disease associated with myocarditis, such as sarcoidosis (ACE level) or connective tissue diseases (antinuclear antibodies). Typical ECG findings include nonspecific ST-segment and T-wave abnormalities, atrial and ventricular arrhythmias, AV blocks, widened QRS complexes from intraventricular conduction delays, and, rarely, Q waves. Intraventricular conduction abnormalities are associated with disease that is more diffuse and may predict a poorer prognosis. Some patients with myocarditis may present with classic ECG findings of MI but have normal coronary arteries. Radiographic findings are also nonspecific but may confirm the presence of cardiomegaly or pulmonary edema in a patient with severe heart failure. Echocardiography is useful to assess the global and regional LV function, as well as diastolic dysfunction. Echocardiography can also demonstrate findings resulting from myocarditis, including increased wall thickness, ventricular thrombi, and valvular abnormalities, in addition to pericardial involvement. Cardiac catheterization may exclude the presence of coronary disease or confirm the hemodynamic disturbances of heart failure. Nuclear imaging techniques, such as antimyosin antibody scanning, can identify myocardial inflammation but are not widely available. MRI may detect tissue alterations associated with myocarditis, but no large-scale study has been reported and, therefore, the reliability of this test is not established.

The only gold standard to confirm myocarditis is endomyocardial biopsy. This method has a small, defined risk to the patient, as well as disparities in interpretation. An expert panel of cardiac pathologists formulated the Dallas criteria to standardize the histologic diagnosis of myocarditis on endomyocardial biopsy. They concluded that the histologic hallmark of myocarditis is an inflammatory myocardial infiltrate with associated evidence of myocytolysis. *Borderline myocarditis* was defined as an inflammatory infiltrate without clear evidence of myocyte necrosis. The positive predictive value of endomyocardial biopsy using these criteria is low (10%); however, it can be marginally increased with more samples. These criteria probably underestimate the true incidence of myocarditis. Because there can be sampling error, interobserver variability in interpretation, or patchy infiltrate, a negative result does not exclude the diagnosis of myocarditis. Confirming the presence of the viral genome by polymerase chain reaction or in situ hybridization is a relatively new development that has the potential to significantly improve diagnosis and assessment of prognosis.

MANAGEMENT AND THERAPY
Nonpharmacologic Therapy
The treatment of a patient with myocarditis is largely supportive. Activity should be restricted to bed rest or a minimal level until active myocarditis is resolved because exercise increases myocardial damage in animals with myocarditis. Athletes should refrain from sports for a 6-month period until heart size and function have returned to normal. Those with arrhythmia should refrain from athletic activities until arrhythmia resolves. Salt restriction (typically emphasized in the management of heart failure) should be recommended for this population, especially in patients with LV dysfunction. In the rare cases that progress to severe heart failure, supportive care may include an LV-assist device or even transplantation. All unnecessary medications should be eliminated because of the potential that one may be responsible for a hypersensitivity reaction resulting in myocarditis.

Pharmacologic Therapy
The etiology established in a patient with myocarditis dictates the specific treatment plan. For instance, in myocarditis caused by diphtheria, antitoxin should be administered as rapidly as possible. In the treatment of Lyme myocarditis, antibiotic therapy is used, although its efficacy is not established. Efforts at treatment of Chagas disease have focused on vector control and immunoprophylaxis.

Patients with dilated cardiomyopathy secondary to myocarditis are treated with the conventional therapy for LV dysfunction: ACE inhibitors, β blockers, diuretics for volume overload, spironolactone for severe heart failure, and digoxin if symptoms persist. During the acute phase of myocarditis, digoxin should be used with caution because of increased sensitivity to digitalis toxicity.

Because the long-term effects of viral myocarditis are believed to be due, in part, to immune-mediated mechanisms, immunosuppressive therapy has been studied. The multicenter, NIH-sponsored Myocarditis Treatment Trial evaluated the role of immunosuppressive therapy using prednisone with either cyclosporine or azathioprine in those with endomyocardial biopsy–proven myocarditis and an LVEF less than 45%. There was no significant change in LVEF at 28 weeks and no survival difference between those treated with immunosuppression and controls in this prospectively randomized study. Smaller studies evaluating the role of intravenous immunoglobulins (IVIGs) provided mixed results in myocarditis, but a large-scale randomized study failed to demonstrate a significant effect. Hence, until evidence is presented with randomized placebo-controlled studies of IVIG in the treatment of acute myocarditis, IVIG should be considered only when the likelihood of benefit is greater, such as in systemic autoimmune disease or biopsy-proven myocarditis with decompensation.

FUTURE DIRECTIONS
Future therapy for myocarditis will likely be directed at the specific mechanisms of myocardial injury. The common pathway for many causes of myocarditis is the host immune response, so antiviral drugs and virus-specific vaccines are treatments of possible future benefit.

Immune-modulating therapy for heart failure is being considered, and these treatments may have a role in myocarditis or even idiopathic dilated cardiomyopathy. Proinflammatory cytokines may contribute to disease progression in heart failure by their direct toxic effects on the heart. Several studies suggest that tumor necrosis factor, a cytokine with negative inotropic properties, is potentially an important therapeutic target for heart failure patients, especially those with more severe decompensation. Inhibitors of tumor necrosis factor have been investigated in treating heart failure from LV dysfunction and have shown promising results, but larger scale studies did not clearly demonstrate benefit. Other forms of immunomodulating therapy, including plasma exchange and immunoabsorption, are being actively investigated and may prove to be a useful adjunct to established therapy.

REFERENCES

Feldman AM, McNamara D. Myocarditis. *N Engl J Med* 2000;343:1388–1398.

Gullastad L, Halfdan A, Fjeld J, et al. Immunomodulating therapy with intravenous immunoglobulin in patients with chronic heart failure. *Circulation* 2001;103:220–225.

Lange LG, Schreiner GF. Immune mechanisms of cardiac disease. *N Engl J Med* 1994;330:1129–1135.

Liu PP, Mason JW. Advances in the understanding of myocarditis. *Circulation* 2001;104:1076–1082.

Mason JW, O'Connell JB, Herskowitz A, et al. A clinical trial of immunosuppressive therapy for myocarditis. *N Engl J Med* 1995;335:269–275.

McNamara D, Holubkov R, Starling RC, et al. Controlled trial of intravenous immune globulin in recent-onset dilated cardiomyopathy. *Circulation* 2001;103:2254–2259.

O'Connell JB, Renlund DG. Myocarditis and specific cardiomyopathies. In: Alexander RW, Schlant RC, Fuster V, eds. *Hurst's: The Heart*. 9th ed. New York: McGraw-Hill;1998:2089–2108.

Wynne J, Braunwald E. The cardiomyopathies and myocarditides: Toxic, chemical, and physical damage to the heart. In: Braunwald E, ed. *Heart Disease*. 4th ed. Philadelphia: WB Saunders; 1992:1425–1450.

Chapter 17

Management of Congestive Heart Failure

Carla A. Sueta and Kirkwood F. Adams, Jr

Congestive heart failure (CHF) is a clinical syndrome resulting from any structural or functional cardiac disorder that impairs the ability of the ventricle to fill or eject blood. Systolic dysfunction is the inability of the ventricle to empty normally, manifested by a reduced ejection fraction (EF) and usually accompanied by ventricular dilatation. Diastolic dysfunction is the inability of the ventricle to fill normally without a compensatory increase in left atrial pressure. Ventricular size and contraction are normal. Diastolic dysfunction accounts for 40 to 50% of CHF cases and is more common in older patients, especially women. Studies suggest similar prognosis for both types of heart failure. Although considered mutually exclusive in the past, it is now clear that systolic and diastolic dysfunction coexist in patients with reduced LVEF.

Congestive heart failure affects 4.9 million Americans, with 550,000 new cases diagnosed each year. The incidence of CHF increases significantly with age, affects 10% of people older than 65 years of age, and is the most common cause of hospital admission in that age group. Improved survival rate after MI and subsequent development of heart failure contributes to the incidence of this syndrome. Despite therapeutic advances, the mortality rate from CHF remains high: 50% at 5 years, with nearly 300,000 patients dying each year. Undertreatment and suboptimal risk factor modification may contribute to the continued high morbidity and mortality rates and are opportunities to positively influence this disease. The annual healthcare cost of CHF has been estimated to be approximately $24.3 billion, with approximately $3 billion spent each year on drug therapy.

Prevention and early detection of CHF is essential. Risk factors for CHF include hypertension, CAD, diabetes mellitus, obesity, a history of cardiotoxic drug therapy, alcohol or cocaine abuse, and family history of cardiomyopathy. Clinical trials have shown that treatment of hypertension, CAD, vascular disease, hyperlipidemia, and diabetes results in a significant reduction in the development of CHF.

ETIOLOGY AND PATHOGENESIS

Although the clinical syndrome of CHF may result from disorders of the pericardium, the myocardium, the endocardium, or the great vessels, most patients have an impairment of LV myocardial function. CAD accounts for one half to two thirds of CHF cases. Hypertension is also a common cause, particularly in black women and older women. The most frequent cause of initially unexplained CHF is idiopathic cardiomyopathy. Other causes include a history of myocarditis, diabetes, alcohol abuse, cocaine use, cardiotoxic drug therapy (doxorubicin, trastuzumab), HIV infection, thyroid disease, valvular disease, peripartum cardiomyopathy, connective tissue disease, and arrhythmias; a family history of cardiomyopathy (including dilated and hypertrophic cardiomyopathy); a history of infiltrative diseases (hemochromatosis, amyloid, sarcoid); and a history of pericardial disease. Anemia or thiamine deficiency can cause high output CHF.

Systolic heart failure results in a reduction in cardiac output regardless of cause, which the kidneys perceive as hypovolemia. Activation of the renin–angiotensin–aldosterone system causes salt and water retention, producing an increase in preload, allowing the Frank-Starling mechanism to maintain cardiac output at the expense of elevated LV diastolic and left atrial pressures. Subsequently, pulmonary congestion and edema develop. Decreased blood pressure from decreasing cardiac output also triggers activation of the sympathetic nervous system and the renin–angiotensin–aldosterone system, creating systemic vasoconstriction. Other vaso-constrictors are stimulated as well, including vasopressin and endothelin. While attempting to maintain organ perfusion, vasoconstriction contributes to increased afterload and worsening CHF. Additionally, sympathetic nervous system activation can precipitate ventricular arrhythmias that may result in sudden death. Although initially compensatory, prolonged neurohormonal activation is detrimental. Cardiac dysfunction triggers remodeling, a process involving dilatation and hypertrophy that changes ventricle geometry, which further increases preload, afterload, and wall stress; produces mitral regurgitation; and leads to worsening cardiac performance. Angiotensin-converting enzyme inhibitors (ACE-I) and β-blockers can attenuate or even reverse remodeling.

Causes of diastolic heart failure include myocardial ischemia, with or without epicardial coronary disease; myocardial fibrosis; pressure overload hypertrophy; genetic hypertrophy; infiltrative cardiomyopathies; or constrictive pericarditis. Diastolic dysfunction occurs as a result of three pathophysiologic mechanisms. First, slowed or incomplete LV relaxation affects early filling. This may shift the LV diastolic pressure–volume relation upward, resulting in increased pressure relative to volume throughout diastole. Thus, even small increases in volume caused by mild sodium and volume overload can result in pulmonary congestion. Second, increased wall thickness increases chamber stiffness, precluding a normal increase in end-diastolic volume during exercise. Consequently, stroke volume fails to increase, manifested as exercise intolerance. Finally, accumulation of interstitial collagen, commonly seen in hypertrophy and following MI, increases myocardial stiffness and, subsequently, diastolic pressure.

CLINICAL PRESENTATION

The cardinal manifestations of CHF are dyspnea and fatigue—which may limit exercise tolerance—and fluid retention, that is, pulmonary congestion and peripheral edema. The symptoms of dyspnea and fatigue may be difficult to elicit due to patient restriction of activity and perception of acceptable age-related functional loss. Patients with severe systolic dysfunction who are already being treated medically may present with symp-toms of low cardiac output, including profound fatigue, narrow pulse pressure, tachycardia, oliguria, and the absence of fluid overload.

Patients should be queried about the following symptoms: dyspnea on exertion, orthopnea, paroxysmal nocturnal dyspnea, cough, chest discomfort, palpitations, syncope or near syncope, fatigue, nausea, abdominal pain, nocturia, oliguria, confusion, insomnia, and depression. The following signs should be assessed: weight change; blood pressure; pulse; jugular venous distension; presence of audible rales, wheezing, and pleural effusion; a displaced point of maximum intensity (PMI); a right ventricular heave, presence of an audible S_3 or S_4; and the presence of audible murmurs, hepatomegaly, low-volume pulses, and peripheral edema.

DIFFERENTIAL DIAGNOSIS

Dyspnea and exercise intolerance can be attributed to many causes other than CHF, including lung disease, pulmonary emboli, pulmonary hypertension, thyroid disease, arrhythmias, anemia, deconditioning, obesity, and cognitive disorders. Renal disease, cirrhosis, and malnutrition can also cause signs of volume overload. All of these causes may mimic CHF and make definitive diagnosis difficult. The assay for B-type natriuretic peptide, secreted predominantly by the left ventricle in response to ventricular volume expansion and overload, is a promising diagnostic test that demonstrates high sensitivity, specificity, and negative predictive values for diagnosis of symptomatic CHF.

DIAGNOSTIC APPROACH
Type and Degree of LV Dysfunction

Systolic and diastolic CHF are indistinguishable by history, physical examination, or chest radiography (Fig. 17-1). Therefore, all patients with suspected heart failure require assessment of LV function. Echocardiography is the most commonly available, noninvasive method utilized in patients with suspected CHF. Echocardiography allows simultaneous assessment of EF, valve function, and hypertrophy, and has the advantage of providing structural information (e.g., valvular heart disease) that may help elucidate the underlying cause of CHF. Radionuclide ventriculography provides a more precise measurement

Figure 17-1   ## Left-Sided Heart Failure and Pulmonary Congestion

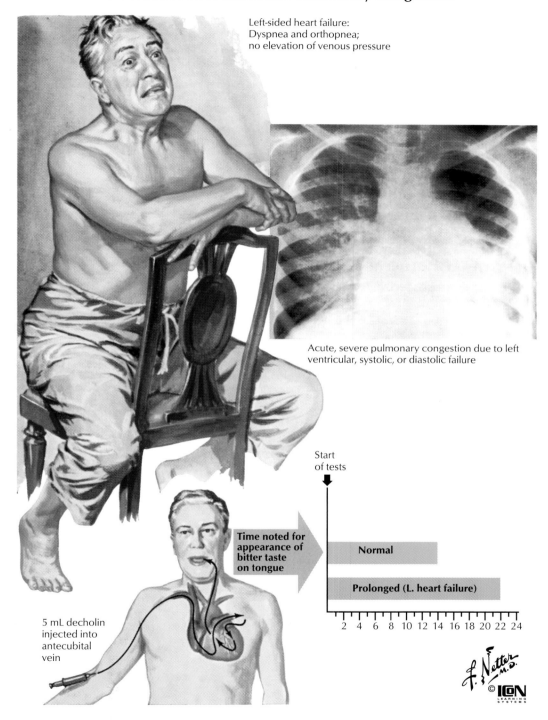

Left-sided heart failure:
Dyspnea and orthopnea;
no elevation of venous pressure

Acute, severe pulmonary congestion due to left
ventricular, systolic, or diastolic failure

Start
of tests

Time noted for
appearance of
bitter taste
on tongue

Normal

Prolonged (L. heart failure)

2 4 6 8 10 12 14 16 18 20 22 24

5 mL decholin
injected into
antecubital
vein

of volumes and EF and is preferred by some for this reason. Radionuclide ventriculography is the method of choice for obese patients and those with significant lung disease in whom imaging by echocardiography may be difficult. Thus, both of these methods provide more accurate and quantitative assessment of LV function than do physiologic studies such as injection of decholin (Fig. 17-1) or indicator dyes that were mainstays prior to the development of echocardiography and radionuclide ventriulography.

Systolic dysfunction is defined as an EF generally less than 0.40 or moderate-severe dysfunction. Abnormalities in LV filling may be detected by noninvasive measurements, but they are not sensitive. A rigorous definition for diastolic dysfunction is not established. Diastolic dysfunction is largely a diagnosis of exclusion; it applies to patients with typical symptoms and signs of CHF but a normal EF and no valvular abnormalities.

Etiology

Prognosis, degree of reversibility, and management strategies differ among etiologies. Poor prognostic indicators include ischemic etiology, age, being of male gender, decreased EF, hyponatremia, and New York Heart Association (NYHA) Functional Classification. Ischemic heart disease must be excluded in every patient by use of cardiac catheterization or noninvasively by exercise–pharmacologic stress testing with imaging by echocardiography or nuclear methods (sestamibi or thallium). Focal wall motion abnormalities do not always represent ischemic heart disease and, conversely, global hypokinesis does not rule out ischemic disease. The demonstration, in multiple large, prospectively randomized studies, that bypass surgery improves symptoms and survival rate in patients with CHF, angina and CAD who have an EF greater than 0.35 emphasizes the importance of evaluating patients with CHF for the presence of CAD. Observational studies suggest that patients with an EF less than 0.35 who have reversible ischemia may also have an improved prognosis with revascularization, but definitive trials are lacking.

The routine laboratory evaluation listed in Table 17-1 should be performed in all patients with CHF and may help establish etiology. Serum ferritin and transferrin saturation should be checked if hemochromatosis is suspected. HIV testing should be performed in high-risk patients.

New York Heart Association Classification

Determination of the NYHA class—useful for prognosis, medical management, and evaluation of response to treatment—can be made by referring to Table 17-2.

MANAGEMENT AND THERAPY

The paradigm for the management of established CHF has shifted from treating symptoms to a combined approach of symptom relief and preventing progression of the disease.
· Precipitating factors must be addressed: dietary noncompliance, ischemia, uncontrolled hypertension, atrial fibrillation, hypoxemia, thyroid disease, anemia, and medical nonadherence

Table 17-1
Routine Laboratory Evaluation

· Chest radiograph
· ECG
· Electrolytes, including calcium and magnesium
· Total protein, albumin, BUN, and creatine
· Liver function tests
· Lipid panel
· CBC
· Urinalysis
· Thyroid function tests
· BNP or PRO-BNP

BNP indicates B-type natiuretic peptide; BUN, blood urea nitrogen; CBC, complete blood count; PRO-BNP, pro–B-type natiuretic peptide.

Table 17-2
NYHA Functional Classification

Class	Description
Class I	Symptoms at exertion levels similar to normal individuals
Class II	Symptoms with ordinary exertion
Class III	Symptoms with minimal activity
Class IV	Symptoms at rest

With permission from The Criteria Committee of the New York Heart Association. *Diseases of the Heart and Blood Vessels: Nomenclature and Criteria for Diagnosis.* 6th ed. Boston: Little Brown; 1964.

Table 17-3
Target Doses Shown to Provide a Mortality Rate Benefit

Drug	Starting Dose	Target Dose	Comments
ACE-I			
Enalapril	2.5 mg bid	10 mg bid	
Captopril	6.25 mg tid	50 mg tid	Affected by food
Ramipril	1.25–2.5 mg qd	10 mg qd	
Lisinopril	2.5–5 mg qd	20 mg qd	
Quinapril	10 mg bid	20 mg bid	
Fosinopril	5–10 mg qd	20 mg qd	
Trandolapril	1 mg qd	4 mg qd	
β-Blockers			
Carvedilol	3.125 mg bid	25–50 mg bid	>85 kg, 50 mg bid
Bisoprolol	2.5 mg qd	10 mg qd	
Metoprolol XL	12.5–25 mg qd	200 mg qd	
Metoprolol	6.25 mg bid	75–100 mg bid	

ACE indicates angiotensin-converting enzyme; bid, two times/day; tid, three times/day; qd, every day.

(which may be due to inability to purchase prescribed medications).

· Revascularization should be considered in ischemic patients with evidence of residual viable but at-risk myocardium.

· Optimization of pharmacologic therapy is essential.

Systolic Dysfunction

Medications That Improve Survival

All patients with systolic dysfunction should receive an ACE-I. An angiotensin II receptor blocker (ARB), or a combination of nitrates and hydralazine may be substituted in the minority of patients intolerant of ACE-I agents.

ACE-I therapy is the treatment of choice; it improves survival and quality of life and reduces hospital admission rates in NYHA class II, III, and IV patients, as well as in post-MI patients. It also delays progression of CHF in asymptomatic patients. Target doses shown to provide a mortality rate benefit are listed in Table 17-3. Contraindications include moderate–severe aortic stenosis, renal artery stenosis, angioedema, and hyperkalemia more than 5.5 mEq/dL. Caution should be used in patients with hypotension (SBP, <80 mm Hg) or a serum creatinine concentration more than 3 mg/dL. If patients do not tolerate an ACE-I due to angioedema or intractable cough, an ARB should be prescribed. The effects of ACE-Is and ARBs on renal function are equivalent. In patients with significant renal dysfunction (i.e., potassium concentration, >5.5 mEq/dL) the combination of isosorbide (40 mg four times daily) and hydralazine (75 mg four times daily) is an alternative that improves mortality rate, though it is not as effective as ACE-I therapy.

The controversy about aspirin attenuating the effect of ACE-Is has not been tested by prospective randomized trials. Therefore, all patients with CAD should receive aspirin unless it is contraindicated.

β-Blockers should be added in all stable, euvolemic patients with systolic dysfunction, beginning with a low dose and increasing the dose every 2 to 4 weeks. In patients already receiving an ACE-I, β-blockers improve EF and survival rate, which includes a reduction in sudden death, and reduce hospital admission rates. Contraindications to β-blocker therapy include severe reactive airway disease, β-agonist therapy, severe bradycardia, or advanced heart block (unless a pacemaker is placed). Side effects are more common with the first few doses. Fatigue, weight gain, and diarrhea are transient. Target doses shown to improve prognosis are listed in

Table 17-3. Although target doses should be the goal, low doses are beneficial, and these drugs should not be discontinued if target doses are not achieved.

β-Blockers should not be initiated or their concentration increased in patients who exhibit volume overload; instead, diuretics should first be administered. Diuretics are recommended in patients who are beginning β-blocker therapy to compensate for possible fluid retention.

Spironolactone can be added to therapy in patients with class III or IV CHF. A mortality rate benefit was demonstrated in one trial in patients receiving 12.5 to 50 mg every day. However, only 10% of patients were receiving a β-blocker. Enrollment in that study was limited to those patients with a serum creatinine concentration less than 2.5 mg/dL. Potassium concentrations generally increases during spironolactone therapy, especially in patients with diabetes, so monitoring is necessary.

Additional Medications

Diuretics, prescribed in most patients to alleviate fluid overload, activate the renin–angiotensin system, so the minimal effective dose should be used. In patients with severe CHF, combination therapy can be utilized, for example, a loop diuretic and hydrochlorothiazide or metolazone. Potassium and magnesium concentrations must be monitored.

Digoxin reduces hospital admission, improves symptoms, and should be considered in all patients with systolic dysfunction who remain symptomatic despite ACE-I and β-blocker therapy. Low but detectable serum concentrations (<0.9 ng/dL) appear to provide the same benefits as higher levels. The usual daily dosage is 0.125 mg every day.

Nitrates reduce preload and are prescribed as antianginal agents. Systemic and pulmonary vasodilatation occur at higher doses. Nitrate intolerance can be prevented by increasing the dose in the short-term setting and allowing a nitrate-free interval of at least 8 hours during long-term treatment.

The newer **calcium channel blockers**, felodipine and amlodipine, may be used to treat hypertension and angina unresponsive to ACE-I and β-blockers. Nifedipine, verapamil, and diltiazem should not be used in these patients because of their negative effect on contractility.

The use of **intravenous medications** may be required for optimal management of acute decompensation or refractory CHF due to systolic dysfunction. Continuous furosemide infusion results in steady diuresis. Hydrochlorothiazide (50 mg two times daily), chlorothiazide (500 mg maximum dose), and renal-dose dopamine ($2–3\ \mu g \cdot kg^{-1} \cdot min^{-1}$) may be helpful in patients with CHF that is refractory to other therapies. Nitroglycerin therapy is particularly effective in the setting of acute MI with pulmonary edema. Intravenous sodium nitroprusside is a more powerful afterload-reducing agent than nitroglycerin and can be used in severe CHF (often in combination with dopamine or dobutamine). Arterial pressure and/or Swan-Ganz monitoring is usually necessary in patients being treated with intravenous nitroprusside. Dobutamine ($5–8\ \mu g \cdot kg^{-1} \cdot min^{-1}$) is an inotropic agent with a short half-life. It is well tolerated and useful for treatment of patients with systolic dysfunction and acute exacerbation of CHF. Milrinone, a phosphodiesterase inhibitor, is a vasodilator and the inotropic agent of choice in patients already receiving a β-blocker. Milrinone is not indicated in most patients with acute decompensated heart failure who present with volume overload. Hypotension can be prevented by ensuring that patients are not volume depleted and by starting at a low dose, 0.1 or $0.2\ \mu g \cdot kg^{-1} \cdot min^{-1}$, without a loading bolus. Neseritide, recombinant human brain natriuretic peptide, is a diuretic and a vasodilator and is more effective in reducing wedge pressure than intravenous nitroglycerin in acutely congested patients. Patients should be carefully monitored for hypotension, which is dose dependent but less likely with a bolus of 2 μg/kg followed by a maintenance infusion of $0.01\ \mu g \cdot kg^{-1} \cdot min^{-1}$.

Swan-Ganz monitoring should be considered in patients with uncertain volume status, low-output syndrome, or systemic hypotension (SBP, <90 mm Hg) especially before administration of vasodilators.

Devices

The use of implantable cardioverter defibrillators (ICDs) is indicated in patients who have survived cardiac arrest. Their use has been shown to reduce mortality rates in patients with a history of MI and an EF of 0.30 or less, or a history of MI and an EF of 0.35 or less, and nonsustained ventricular tachycardia who are inducible by electrophysiologic testing. Patients with unexplained syncope are at high risk and should be evaluated aggressively with use of electrophysiologic testing. Biventricular pacemakers also can improve quality of life and reduce hospital admission in NYHA class III or IV patients with a prolonged QRS (>130 ms) and an EF of 0.35 or less. However, the effect on mortality rate is unknown. LV assist devices (see also chapter 18) are used as a bridge to cardiac transplantation and have been shown to prolong life in patients who are not transplant candidates.

Diastolic Dysfunction:
Preserved Ejection Fraction

There are no completed randomized trials indicating which (or whether) pharmacologic therapy improves survival rates in patients with diastolic dysfunction. Because pulmonary congestion (in the absence of systolic dysfunction) is a major problem in these patients, agents such as diuretics and nitrates that reduce preload are effective in relieving symptoms and rarely cause hypotension. Nitrates are also used to treat ischemia. ACE-I, calcium channel blockers, ARB, and β-blockers have been shown to cause regression of LV hypertrophy and may, as such, slow (or even reverse) the progression of diastolic dysfunction. Calcium channel blockers, particularly verapamil, improve ventricular relaxation. Agents that decrease heart rate and, therefore, increase diastolic filling time, including verapamil, diltiazem, and β-blockers, are also beneficial. Atrial contraction contributes up to 50% of ventricular filling in patients with diastolic dysfunction; hence, the loss of atrial systole in atrial fibrillation can result in acute decompensation. Cardioversion and treatment with antiarrhythmic agents are options that should be considered in patients with diastolic dysfunction and atrial fibrillation. Dual-chamber pacemakers in patients with a junctional rhythm or a heart block unresponsive to adjustment of medication has been shown to be helpful in small studies.

Additional Management Strategies

Additional management strategies include the following:

· Treatment of comorbid disease, including aggressive management of hyperlipidemia, hypertension, and diabetes, should be part of routine care.
· Nonpharmacologic strategies include daily exercise, salt intake less than 2 to 2.5 g/day, fluid restriction, daily weighing, and evaluation for sleep apnea. Weight loss and discontinuation of alcohol should be encouraged. Smoking cessation counseling with nicotine replacement and addition of bupropion, if indicated, should be implemented.
· Education of the patient and family about the symptoms and signs of the disease, prognosis, medications and about when to contact a health professional is an essential component to management.
· Referral to a heart failure specialist is appropriate if patients remain severely limited while on an optimized medical regimen or do not tolerate increased dosages, are transplant candidates (refractory CHF with full medical management, LVEF less than 0.20, high 1-year mortality rate, no significant comorbid disease, age younger than 65 years, compliant, psychologically stable with good social support), or are candidates for clinical trials.

FUTURE DIRECTIONS

Research in many areas shows promise for diagnosis and treatment of CHF. Blockers of metalloproteinases that mediate tissue remodeling are in development. A randomized trial on the long-term effects of exercise training is ongoing. The efficacy of nocturnal oxygen and devices that provide continuous positive airway pressure are being studied in CHF patients with sleep apnea. Anemia is associated with worsening symptoms and prognosis in patients with CHF. Small studies have demonstrated the beneficial effects of its treatment; larger trials are ongoing. Artificial ventricular assistance with totally implantable systems is being investigated as destination therapy. Enhanced external counterpulsation, which mimics the effects of the intraaortic balloon pump, is undergoing evaluation in clinical trials for chronic CHF. The first human pilot study of myoblast cell transplantation showed beneficial cardiovascular effects, but the risk of ventricular arrhythmia was high, necessitating future studies to include ICD therapy. Gene therapy is advancing, with improvements in vector technology and cardiac gene delivery and understanding of molecular pathogenesis. Finally, disease prevention by early detection and aggressive modification of risk factors will continue to have an enormous impact on cardiovascular disease leading to CHF.

REFERENCES

Adams KF, Dunlap SH, Sueta CA, et al. Relation between gender, etiology and survival in patients with symptomatic heart failure. *J Am Coll Cardiol* 1996;28:1781–1788.

Adams KF, Gheorghiade M, Uretsky BF, Patterson JH, Schwartz TA, Young JB. Clinical benefits of low serum digoxin concentrations in heart failure. *J Am Coll Cardiol* 2001;39:946–953.

Cuffe MS, Califf RM, Adams KF, et al, for the Outcomes of a Prospective Trial of Intravenous Milrinone for Exacerbations of Chronic Heart Failure (OPTIME-CHF) Investigators. Short-term, intravenous milrinone for acute exacerbations of chronic heart failure: A randomized controlled trial. *JAMA* 2002;287:1541–1547.

Heart Failure Society of America. HFSA guidelines for management of patients with heart failure caused by left ventricular systolic dysfunction—Pharmacologic approaches. *J Cardiac Failure* 1999;5:357–382. www.hfsa.org.

Hunt SA, Baker DW, Chin MH, et al. ACC/AHA guidelines for the evaluation and management of chronic heart failure in the adult. *Circulation* 2001;104:2996–3007 www.americanheart.org.

Sueta CA, Chowdhury M, Boccuzzi SJ, et al. Analysis of the degree of undertreatment of hyperlipidemia and congestive heart failure secondary to coronary artery disease. *Am J Cardiol* 1999;83:1303–1307.

Chapter 18
Cardiac Transplantation

Michael R. Mill and Brett C. Sheridan

Cardiac transplantation developed as an outgrowth of research into heart preservation to allow safe open-heart surgery. In 1961, Shumway and Lower published their seminal article describing the technique of orthotopic cardiac transplantation in a canine model, with successful functioning of the transplanted heart for several days. While Shumway was preparing to begin a human clinical trial of cardiac transplantation, Christiaan Barnard, a South African surgeon who had worked in the United States, learning the techniques of immunosuppression and surgical transplantation, shocked the world in December 1967 by performing the first human-to-human heart transplant in Capetown. His patient lived for 18 days before succumbing to infectious complications. Shumway performed the first successful cardiac transplantation in the United States in January 1968, beginning what has become the longest ongoing program of cardiac transplantation in the world.

Activity in cardiac transplantation exploded after these initial successes. However, a dismal initial 1-year survival rate of 22% led most programs to abandon the procedure. Early transplant patients died of both immune rejection of the transplanted heart and infectious complications.

Two major developments allowed surgeons and those caring for cardiac transplant patients to balance more successfully the complications of graft rejection versus systemic infection. The development in 1971 of the cardiac bioptome by Caves, combined with Billingham's pathologic grading system for rejection, removed much of the treatment guesswork and permitted accurate diagnosis of rejection and rational treatment strategies for maintenance immunosuppression and rejection. Cardiac transplantation improved rapidly again with the introduction of cyclosporine A in 1980. This interleukin-2 (IL-2) inhibitor dramatically reduced the incidence of rejection.

More recently, further investigation into the basic mechanisms of transplant rejection resulted in triple-drug immunosuppressive regimens that used smaller doses of prednisone, azathioprine, and cyclosporine, allowing better rejection control with fewer infectious complications and adverse effects from these powerful immunosuppressive agents. Newer agents, especially tacrolimus, mycophenolate mofetil, and sirolimus, are also now part of the antirejection armamentarium, and drugs continue to be developed.

INDICATIONS

Cardiac transplantation is indicated for patients with end-stage heart disease who are not amenable to standard medical or surgical therapy. As other therapeutic approaches have improved—from coronary artery bypass grafting (chapter 11) to percutaneous interventions (chapter 10) to advances in medical therapy for congestive heart failure (chapters 12 and 17)—patients who need transplantation are generally older and more sick, and have multiple comorbidities. In addition, the spectrum of individuals considered for cardiac transplantation today has been broadened to include elderly patients, children, and newborns. The most common indications for cardiac transplantations in the adult population are dilated cardiomyopathies and end-stage coronary artery disease (CAD). The etiologies of dilated cardiomyopathies are varied. Most are idiopathic, but some are related to viral illnesses, chronic alcohol abuse, or familial or postpartum cardiomyopathies (see chapter 12). Patients with CAD have generally sustained multiple heart attacks and undergone revascularization procedures. A minority of transplants are performed in patients with valvular heart disease, graft vasculopathy, and other less common indications. Because of the high incidence of malignant ventricular arrhythmias in this population, many patients awaiting transplantation also have implantable cardioverter–defibrillators. In children, the leading diagnoses are dilated cardiomyopathies and congenital heart disease.

Potential transplant patients undergo an intensive screening process by a multidisciplinary team of cardiothoracic surgeons, cardiologists, transplant coordinators, social workers, dieticians, physical therapists, psychologists/psychiatrists, and financial counselors. The screening ensures not only that the patient needs the transplant, but also that he or she is physically and mentally able to comply with the rigorous post-transplantation medical regimen and has the appropriate social supports to undergo transplantation successfully.

DONORS

Transplant donors are individuals who are brain dead but continue to have adequate cardiac function to temporarily support other organ function. Most die of catastrophic intracranial events or trauma. The hearts are carefully evaluated with respect to cause of death, need for cardiopulmonary resuscitation, and use of inotropic support; they undergo electrocardiography and echocardiography to ensure adequate ventricular and valvular function. In men aged older than 45 years, women aged older than 55 years, and patients with other risk factors for CAD, cardiac catheterization and coronary angiography are frequently performed. Donors undergo thorough serologic testing to rule out transmissible diseases, and their medical and social histories are evaluated.

DONOR–RECIPIENT MATCHING

Patients accepted for transplantation are placed on a national waiting list maintained by the United Network for Organ Sharing (UNOS). UNOS has a contract with the US government to act as the organ procurement and transplantation network. Patients are placed on the waiting list by size, ABO blood type, medical urgency status, and waiting time. When a suitable donor is identified, UNOS generates a list that ranks potential recipients by distance from the donor hospital (to minimize the organ ischemic time during travel and implantation), size, ABO type, medical urgency, and waiting time. An organ is then offered to a prospective recipient's transplant center. If the transplant physicians believe that the organ is suitable for their patient,

arrangements are made to procure the organ and perform the transplantation. On occasion, a potential recipient is precluded from transplantation because of ongoing infection or another potentially reversible contraindication. If the initial center does not accept the organ, it is offered sequentially to all patients on the local list, followed by patients in ever-enlarging geographic circles until the nation is covered. Given the number of patients actively awaiting transplantation, the majority of hearts are placed within their local or regional areas. Other available organs are likewise matched with potential recipients.

DONOR PROCEDURE

After all the organs are placed, procurement surgeons arrive at the donor hospital, and a coordinated procedure allows simultaneous procurement of all useable organs, often including the heart, lungs, liver, kidneys, and pancreas and occasionally including the small intestine. The heart explant procedure depends on whether the heart alone will be used or whether the lungs will also be used separately or as a combined heart–lung transplant. After initial dissection of the aorta and superior and inferior vena cavae, placement of a cardioplegia cannula in the ascending aorta, and completion of the other teams' initial dissections, the donor is systemically heparinized. The superior vena cava is tied off, the left atrial (LA) appendage is amputated, and the inferior vena cava is partially transected to decompress the heart and prevent ventricular distention. The aorta is then cross-clamped, and cardioplegia is infused while the heart is lavaged with ice-cold saline (Fig. 18-1).

Simultaneously, the other organs are flushed with their own preservative solutions and lavaged with cold saline. After completing the cardioplegia infusion, the superior and inferior vena cavae are transected. If only the heart is to be used, the pulmonary veins and pulmonary arteries are divided at the pericardium, and the aorta is divided. If the lungs are to be used, the left atrium is divided at the midatrial level, leaving enough cuff of the left atrium for cardiac implantation and cuffs around the pulmonary veins for lung implantation. The pulmonary trunk is divided at its bifurcation to leave enough length on the pulmonary arteries for the lung

Figure 18-1

Technique of Orthotopic Biatrial Cardiac Transplantation I

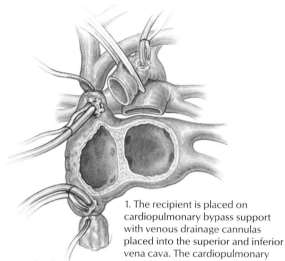

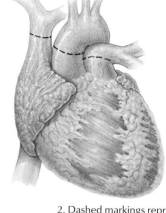

1. The recipient is placed on cardiopulmonary bypass support with venous drainage cannulas placed into the superior and inferior vena cava. The cardiopulmonary bypass circuit returns oxygenated blood with controlled perfusion into the ascending aorta through a cannula placed distal to the aortic cross clamp. Cardiopulmonay bypass provides systemic perfusion allowing excision of the recipient heart retaining the posterior cuff of the right and left atrium as well as the ascending aorta and main pulmonary artery.

2. Dashed markings represent excision lines for removal of the donor heart.

3. The donor heart is excised across the pulmonary veins, followed by preparation for transplantation by opening the posterior wall of the left atrium.

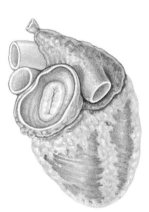

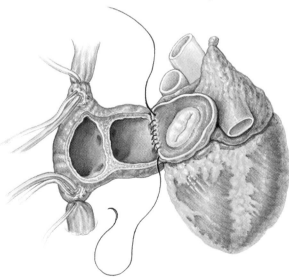

4. View of the donor mitral valve through the surgically opened left atrial posterior wall.

5. Initiation of cardiac implantation with anastamosis of left atrium of recipient to donor using a continuous mono-filament suture line

S. Moon, M.S.
© ICON
LEARNING SYSTEMS

implantation. If a combined heart–lung transplant is planned, the two organs are resected en bloc by dividing the cavae, aorta, and trachea and dissecting the heart–lung block from its mediastinal attachments. The organs are then stored in ice-cold saline in multiple layers of plastic bags to ensure sterility, and they are packed in an ice-filled cooler for transportation to the transplanting center.

TRANSPLANTATION

The standard surgical procedure has changed little from that developed by Shumway and Lower. Although variations have been described, none is consistently superior. Occasionally, abnormal anatomy warrants alteration to the basic procedure.

The operation is performed through a standard median sternotomy using cardiopulmonary bypass with aortic and bicaval cannulation. The initial dissection and cannulation are performed while the heart is being transported to the recipient hospital. When the new heart arrives, cardiopulmonary bypass is instituted at moderate systemic hypothermia (approximately 32°C), and caval tapes are secured around the caval cannulas. The aorta is cross-clamped and then divided just above the level of the aortic valve. The pulmonary trunk is divided above its respective valve, and the atria are divided at the midatrial level, with removal of the atrial appendages and preservation of the posterior atrial cuffs containing the pulmonary veins on the left and the cavae on the right. The donor heart is prepared by freeing the pulmonary artery from the aorta and the roof of the left atrium. The pulmonary venous orifices are interconnected to create a cuff for the LA anastomosis. Excess LA tissue can be removed to create a better size match for this anastomosis. The oval fossa of the donor heart is examined for a patent foremen ovale. If identified, it is closed. The LA anastomosis is then fashioned with a suture in a continuous running fashion. The suture line is begun at the base of the donor LA appendage, just above the recipient left superior pulmonary vein. It is continued clockwise until the interatrial septum is encountered (Fig. 18-2). The other arm of the suture is then sewn in a counterclockwise fashion over the roof of the left atri-

um, along the atrial septum, and is tied to the initial suture. An IV line with a macro drip chamber is placed into the left atrium through the LA appendage, and ice-cold saline is run through this line to aid in myocardial hypothermia and in deairing of the left side of the heart. The donor right atrium is opened from the orifice of the inferior vena cava through the right atrial appendage and then sewn to the recipient atrial cuff. This is begun at the midpoint of the atrial septum and runs clockwise past the inferior caval cannula. Sewing continues with the other end of the suture, running counterclockwise, until closure is complete and the suture is tied. Next, the donor and recipient pulmonary trunks are cut to appropriate lengths. The recipient pulmonary artery is explored digitally and with a suction catheter to rule out occult pulmonary emboli. The pulmonary trunks are then anastomosed end to end with a running suture. This suture is not tied until after the cross clamp is removed to allow for deairing of the right side of the heart. Systemic rewarming is begun, and the donor and recipient aortas are trimmed and anastomosed with a running suture. Frequently, one end of the aorta needs spatulation to accommodate a size difference. The heart is deaired, the suture line is secured, the patient is placed in a steep Trendelenburg position, and the cross clamp is released, thus ending the donor heart ischemic time. Some surgeons administer a "hot shot" of warm blood substrate–enhanced cardioplegia before releasing the cross clamp. During rewarming and reperfusion, the right side of the heart is deaired, the caval tapes are removed, and the pulmonary artery suture line is secured. The "cold line" is removed, and the LA appendage is repaired. The donor superior vena cava is oversewn. With rewarming and reperfusion, a spontaneous normal sinus rhythm usually develops. If not, atrial and ventricular pacing wires are placed, and temporary atrioventricular sequential pacing is initiated at a rate of 100 beats/min. After the onset of forceful ventricular contractions and completion of deairing maneuvers, inotropic support is begun, initially consisting of dobutamine or dopamine at 5 to 10 $\mu g \cdot kg^{-1} \cdot min^{-1}$. If the heart rate is less than 100 beats/min, isoproterenol is used to increase the heart rate to

Figure 18-2

Technique of Orthotopic Biatrial Cardiac Transplantation II

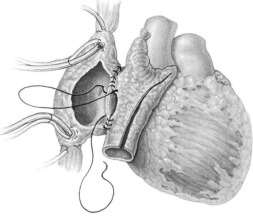

6. The left atrial anastamosis is completed, and the donor right atrium is opened from the inferior vena cava extending to the right atrial appendage.

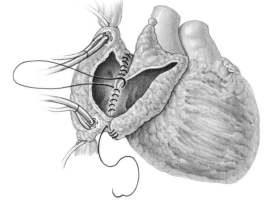

7. The right atrial cuff of the donor is anastomosed to the recipient right atrial cuff directly over the left atrial suture line reinforcing the edge of the interatrial septum.

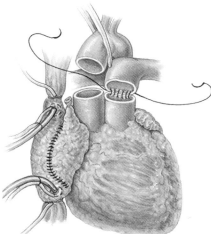

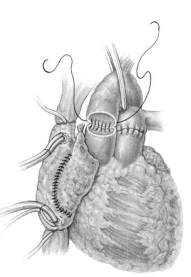

10. Completed biatrial orthotopic cardiac transplant with separation from cardiopulmonary bypass and removal of cannulas.

S. Moon, M.S.
©ICN

8. The right atrial suture line is completed on the free wall, and the retained main pulmonary artery is anastomosed to the donor pulmonary artery in end-to-end fashion.

9. The fourth and final anastamosis aligns the ascending aorta of donor and recipient in end-to-end fashion.

approximately 120 beats/min instead of temporary pacing. Depending on the donor heart ischemic time and size, the recipient's pulmonary vascular resistance, and the preoperative use of antiarrhythmic drugs (especially amiodarone), additional inotropic support or vasoconstrictive agents are sometimes necessary. The patient is then weaned from cardiopulmonary bypass. Heparin is reversed with protamine sulfate, and the heart is decannulated. After ensuring adequate hemostasis, chest drains are placed, and the sternotomy is closed.

POSTOPERATIVE MANAGEMENT

The initial postoperative treatment of cardiac transplant recipients is similar to that of open-heart surgery patients, especially in terms of fluid and electrolyte management, ventilator care and weaning, and pain control. The major differences include isolation precautions because of the increased infection risk and immunosuppression to prevent rejection. Multiple protocols for transplant immunosuppression and rejection monitoring exist. Most rely on initial triple-drug immunosuppression with an IL-2 blocker (cyclosporine or tacrolimus), a purine synthesis inhibitor (azathioprine or mycophenolate mofetil), and prednisone. The doses of IL-2 blockers are monitored and adjusted based on daily serum concentrations, the standard doses of purine synthesis inhibitors are decreased if leukopenia or pancytopenia develops, and steroids are tapered by schedule in the absence of rejection. Most programs use a protocol of endomyocardial biopsies, supplemented when indicated by echocardiography, right-sided heart catheterization, or both to diagnose rejection and monitor response to therapy. With significant rejection or hemodynamic compromise, patients are treated with bolus steroids (IV methylprednisolone, 1 g/d for 3 days). If this is ineffective or if a pattern of recurrent rejection develops in the patient, other protocols are used. During follow-up examinations, patients are monitored for the development of arrhythmias, immunosuppressive side effects, and signs and symptoms of infection. Routine electrocardiograms often show two p waves: one from the recipient right atria and one from the donor right atria. This can be misdiagnosed as atrial fibrillation or premature atrial contractions. The correct diagnosis is established by confirming that one set of p waves (from the donor) is synchronous with the QRS complex. Routine radiography of the chest is vital to detect new infiltrates that most commonly represent preclinical pneumonias or early malignancies. Aggressive evaluation of these infiltrates is mandatory because immunosuppressive agents increase the risks of infection and can accelerate the growth of malignancies. Early detection and treatment can mean the difference between survival and death. Chronic renal insufficiency is a common adverse effect of long-term IL-2 blocker use and can be ameliorated by dose modulation. Likewise, chronic hypertension is common because of the use of IL-2 blockers and steroids and can necessitate multiple agents to control. Hyperlipidemia occurs with both agents also, and evidence suggests all transplant patients should be routinely treated with statins. IL-2 blockers and steroids are also diabetogenic and usually necessitate aggressive therapy with insulin for adequate control. The frequency of endomyocardial biopsies gradually decreases in the absence of rejection; by 1 year, they are only performed with clinical suspicion of rejection or as part of the annual examination.

RESULTS

Data on more than 61,000 cardiac transplant procedures from 200 centers (all centers in the United States; mandatory for UNOS membership and voluntary for international centers) have been collected and analyzed by the International Society of Heart and Lung Transplantation and UNOS since 1983. The 1-, 5-, and 10-year survival rates are approximately 90%, 70%, and 50%, respectively. The youngest patient to survive a transplant was 1 day old; the oldest was 78 years old. The longest surviving transplant recipient has lived more than 26 years with his original donor heart. Approximately 90% of patients who are alive have no functional limitations, and many have returned to full-time work. In the early years after transplantation, rejection and infection are the most common causes of death. Later, graft vasculopathy, infection, and malignancies become more common. Patients are particularly susceptible to posttransplantation lymphoproliferative disease, a form of lymphoma believed related to Epstein-Barr virus. These patients are also subject to the common malignancies that affect their age-matched cohorts.

Graft vasculopathy occurs in many cardiac transplant recipients. *Graft vasculopathy* is a type of CAD that seems to be related to chronic humoral rejection. It is similar to native CAD in that subintimal lipid-laden plaques develop, narrowing the coronary luminal diameter. It differs in its propensity to be concentric and involves the entire length of the coronary arteries. Because of this diffuse pattern, the usual treatments for CAD, percutaneous intervention or surgical revascularization, are not effective. Patients present with silent myocardial infarctions because the denervated heart does not produce anginal pain, or overt heart failure. The only reliable treatment is repeat transplantation. Of interest, the patient's underlying cause of end-stage cardiac disease (e.g., CAD) has no bearing on the development of graft vasculopathy. To detect this potentially silent killer, patients undergo routine annual examinations, which include history, physical examination, extensive laboratory evaluation, echocardiography, cardiac catheterization, and coronary angiography. The detection of wall motion abnormalities, depressed ventricular function, and/or CAD guides intervention.

MECHANICAL CARDIAC ASSIST DEVICES

Many mechanical assist devices have been developed, but this discussion is limited to those with US FDA approval for use as a bridge to transplantation or as destination therapy. The *Thoratec ventricular assist device* (VAD) is a paracorporeal instrument that can be used as a right, left, or biventricular assist device. It is connected by inflow cannulas to the right atrium, left ventricular (LV) apex, or both and outflow cannulas to the pulmonary trunk and/or aorta. These cannulas exit the skin in the epigastrium, are connected to one or more pneumatically driven pumps containing mechanical inflow and outflow valves, and lie on the patient's abdomen. Although patients can be ambulated with this device and have been supported in excess of 1 year before transplantation, its paracorporeal position limits its applicability to postcardiotomy support or as a bridge to transplantation. Its advantages are the ability to support either or both ventricles, the wide range of patient sizes that can be supported because the pumps do not have to be placed inside the patient, and the ability to be removed easily when used as a bridge to recovery.

The *Novacor Left Ventricular Assist System* (LVAS) is an electrically driven, implantable device that can fully sustain systemic circulation and adapt to increased cardiac output needs with exercise. The inflow cannula connects to the LV apex, and the outflow cannula connects to the aorta. The pump is implanted in an abdominal wall pocket, and a single transcutaneous cable exits the right epigastrium and connects to the wearable external driver, which controls the pump, transmits electrical energy to the pump, and allows for volume compensation for the implanted ventricle. The patient can be fully mobile while wearing the portable controller and two rechargeable batteries. Although this device is only approved as a bridge to transplantation in the United States, it has been used as an alternative to transplantation, or destination therapy, in Europe, where patients have been supported for more than 4 years with their original pump.

The Thoratec Heartmate left ventricular assist device is also an implantable electrical device with cannulation and pump implantation, similar to the Novacor LVAS. Although it is capable of complete and adaptable support, long-term durability remains a problem. Many patients have been supported more than 1 year with this device. Its notable feature is a "flocked" surface lining the pump chamber that promotes formation of a pseudointima, which reduces the need for anticoagulation and is associated with fewer neurologic events than the other devices. It has been approved as a bridge to transplantation since 1998, and received US FDA approval in 2003 for use as destination therapy in patients with intractable stage IV heart failure who are not candidates for transplantation. These and other devices remain in development in the quest for a safe and durable mechanical replacement for the human heart.

FUTURE DIRECTIONS

Cardiac transplantation is an established, safe, durable, and reliable therapy for patients with end-stage heart disease. Its application is limited only by an inadequate supply of donor organs, mandating careful selection of recipients to ensure the best results in the use of this scarce resource. As care for these complex patients improves, mid- and long-term survival continue to increase and morbidity continues to decrease. Future activities will emphasize expansion of the donor pool, improving results and developing a suitable alternative to human donors, whether xenotransplants or mechanical hearts. The development of better immunosuppressive agents will decrease adverse effects and rejection. This might also pave the way to xenotransplantation (cross-species transplantation), although most research suggests it will be best accomplished with concurrent genetic research to develop genetically engineered animals that are minimally immunogenic. The most advanced current model is that of transgenic pigs with "humanized" components of the major histocompatibility complex. Other genetic research to induce tolerance in the recipient could conceivably allow long-term decreases if not complete discontinuation of immunosuppressive medications.

Alternatives to transplantation exist, but their widespread application remains several years away. Several models of implantable VADs and total artificial hearts are in development. Some have been used clinically in limited trials, with promising results. The long-term application of these devices will necessitate advances in miniaturization, biocompatible blood surfaces, improved battery design and transcutaneous energy transfer technology, and the development of durable components to withstand years of wear. Given the epidemic of heart failure, research interest and clinical activity will continue and it is likely that the future will hold significant advances.

REFERENCES

Baumgartner WA, Reitz BA, Achuff SC, eds. *Heart and Heart-Lung Transplantation*. Philadelphia: W.B. Saunders; 1990.

Billingham ME, Cary NRB, Hammond ME, et al. A working formulation for the standardization of nomenclature in the diagnosis of heart and lung rejection: Heart Rejection Study Group. *J Heart Transplant* 1990;9:587.

Hertz, MI, Taylor DO, Trulock EP, et al. The Registry of the International Society for Heart and Lung Transplantation: Nineteenth Official Report-2002. *J Heart Lung Transplant* 2002;21:950–970.

Hood KA, Zarembski DG. Mycophenolate mofetil: A unique immunosuppressive agent. *Am J Health Syst Pharm* 1997;54:285.

Kelly PA, Burckart GJ, Venkatarmanan R. Tacrolimus: A new immunosuppressive agent. *Am J Health Syst Pharm* 1995;52:1521.

Shumway SJ, Shumway NE, eds. *Thoracic Transplantation*. Cambridge, Mass: Blackwell Science; 1995.

Stuart FP, Abecassis MM, Kaufman DB. *Organ Transplantation*. Georgetown, Tex: Landes Bioscience; 2000.

United Network for Organ Sharing. Available at: http://www.unos.org.

Section IV
CARDIAC RHYTHM ABNORMALITIES

Chapter 19

Atrial Fibrillation

Richard G. Sheahan and Marschall S. Runge

Atrial fibrillation, the most common arrhythmia in adults and the elderly, occurs in response to a myriad of conditions. The irregular pulse found with mitral valve disease, described as *delirium cordis*, results from atrial fibrillation. With the decreasing prevalence of rheumatic fever, other causes of atrial fibrillation far surpass mitral valve disease. Moreover, it is understood that patients with atrial fibrillation have substantially increased morbidity and mortality.

The prevalence of atrial fibrillation is increasing worldwide, particularly as populations age. Atrial fibrillation is uncommon in infants and children and becomes increasingly common with age. Of adults under 55 years of age, less than 0.1% have atrial fibrillation, whereas 4% of individuals over 60 years of age and approximately 10% of those over 80 years of age have atrial fibrillation. It is estimated that more than 2 million US adults have atrial fibrillation; by the midpoint of the 21st century, that number may exceed 5.5 million, with more than 50% being older than 80 years. Patients with atrial fibrillation have a 1.5- to 2.0-fold increased mortality risk, compared with age- and disease-matched controls, and a markedly increased risk of embolic events and congestive heart failure (CHF), according to data from the Framingham Study.

ETIOLOGY AND PATHOGENESIS

Many factors predispose the heart to atrial fibrillation (Table 19-1; Fig. 19-1), including structural abnormalities (such as valvular heart disease), systolic or diastolic dysfunction, CHF, hypertension, diabetes, and myocardial infarction. Other conditions associated with an increased prevalence of atrial fibrillation include acute or chronic alcohol ingestion, hyper- or hypothyroidism, and alterations in vagal or sympathetic tone. Of patients with atrial fibrillation, less than 10% are classified as having *lone atrial fibrillation*, that is, no clinical, electrocardiographic, or echocardiographic evidence of structural heart disease and none of the predisposing factors cited above.

No single electrical mechanism causes atrial fibrillation. Early investigators proposed multiple reentrant waves (or **wavelets**) to indicate that these small multiple waves initiate in the atrium, spreading and coalescing to form small circuits of reentrant electrical activity. The short and variable wavelengths of these activities preclude organized atrial electrical activity and result in atrial fibrillation. It has been found that rapid, repetitive impulse generation by atrial myocytes located near the orifice of the pulmonary veins stimulates atrial fibrillation. Moreoever, atrial

Table 19-1
Underlying Etiologies of Atrial Fibrillation

Cardiac

· Mitral valvular heart disease
· Systolic or diastolic dysfunction
· Congestive heart failure
· Hypertension
· Diabetes
· Myocardial infarction
· Hypertrophic cardiomyopathy
· Pericarditis
· Wolff-Parkinson-White syndrome
· Sick sinus syndrome
· Congenital heart disease
· Post coronary artery bypass surgery

Noncardiac

· Acute or chronic alcohol ingestion (holiday heart syndrome)
· Hyper- or hypothyroidism
· Alterations in vagal or sympathetic tone
· Pulmonary embolism
· Sepsis
· Chronic obstructive pulmonary disease
· Lone atrial fibrillation

Figure 19-1

Atrial Fibrillation

Abnormal repetitive impulses (wavelets)

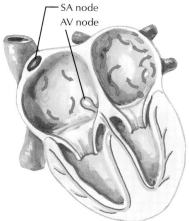

SA node
AV node

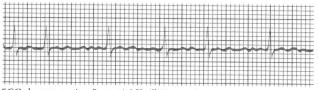

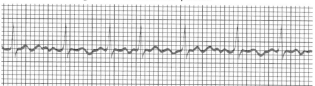

ECG demonstrating fine atrial fibrillation pattern

ECG demonstrating coarse atrial fibrillation pattern

No single mechanism causes atrial fibrillation. Small, multiple re-entrant wavelets may coalesce to form small atrial circuits. Rapid repetitive impulses generated by myocytes located in left atrium near pulmonary vein orifices stimulate atrial fibrillation.

Causes and associated conditions

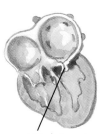

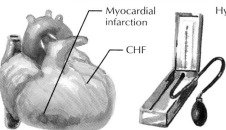

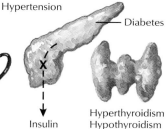

Mitral stenosis

Myocardial infarction

CHF

Hypertension

Diabetes

Insulin

Hyperthyroidism
Hypothyroidism

Acute or chronic alcohol use

Electrical intervention options

Cardioversion

Dual chamber pacing (may include implantable defibrillator)

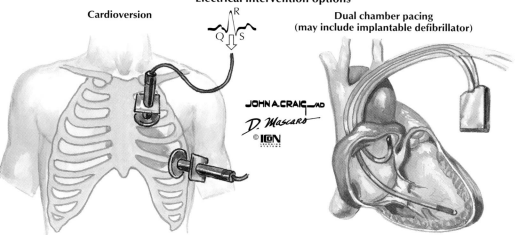

JOHN A. CRAIG—AD
D. Mascaro
© ICN

Emergent cardioversion is considered in two circumstances: (1) when onset of atrial fibrillation results in hemodynamic instability in a previously stable patient (manifest as hypotension, angina/myocardial ischemia, or rapid onset of CHF) or (2) when patient with borderline hemodynamic status suddenly develops atrial fibrillation. Elective cardioversion is indicated unless severe circumstances.

Permanent dual chamber pacing should be considered in those with bradycardia and paroxysmal atrial fibrillation (to help maintain sinus rhythm) or in patients with persistent atrial fibrillation in whom use of AV-node-suppressing drugs (to prevent rapid ventricular response) results in significant bradycardia at rest

fibrillation begets atrial fibrillation. Anatomic remodeling, disruption of electrical circuits, and cellular damage and fibrosis result from permanent atrial fibrillation, decreasing the likelihood of a return to normal sinus rhythm.

CLINICAL PRESENTATION

The clinical presentation of patients with atrial fibrillation varies. Some patients are asymptomatic. The diagnosis of atrial fibrillation may be made on a regular annual examination or as an incidental finding during the evaluation of a patient being seen for a different (sometimes related) illness. Others note sensations that reflect the irregularity of the rhythm, often indistinguishable from frequent ventricular or atrial premature contractions. These symptoms may range from noticeable but not bothersome to nerve-racking. Occasionally, a patient presents for evaluation of **bradycardia** diagnosed by the patient or someone who recorded a slow radial pulse rate (that underestimates the true heart rate). Still others present with symptoms reflecting decreased cardiac output, which occurs when atrial fibrillation replaces normal sinus rhythm; these symptoms range from fatigue to shortness of breath at rest and/or with activity, to chest pain. Severe symptoms and physical examination findings of CHF occasionally are found in patients with new-onset atrial fibrillation.

DIAGNOSTIC APPROACH

The history, physical examination, electrocardiogram, and a variety of laboratory and cardiovascular tests are commonly employed in the initial evaluation of atrial fibrillation. Upon presentation, most patients can be classified into one of four categories, as recommended by a joint task force of the American College of Cardiology, the American Heart Association, and the European Society of Cardiology: paroxysmal, persistent, permanent, or lone atrial fibrillation. Treatment differs among the four groups.

1. *Paroxysmal atrial fibrillation* is described as episodes of atrial fibrillation that last less than a week (and often less than 24 hours), self-terminate, and are usually recurrent.
2. *Persistent atrial fibrillation* lasts more than a week, does not self-terminate, and may recur after cardioversion.

3. *Permanent atrial fibrillation* is diagnosed if atrial fibrillation has lasted more than a year, has been refractory to cardioversion, or both.
4. *Lone atrial fibrillation* can be paroxysmal, persistent, or permanent atrial fibrillation in the absence of structural heart disease.

In addition to classifying the atrial fibrillation, the history and physical examination should focus on clues to the underlying etiology. Symptoms and examination findings relevant to the conditions that predispose to atrial fibrillation (Table 19-1) should be sought. It is important to seek evidence for complications of atrial fibrillation including presyncopal symptoms (especially with initiation or termination of atrial fibrillation), decreased cardiac output, and thromboembolism (including transient ischemic attacks, evidence of peripheral embolization, or both). An ophthalmoscopic examination may reveal retinal artery embolism in some patients with atrial fibrillation. Patients at highest risk for atrial fibrillation with rapid ventricular response, including those with accessory pathways (Wolff-Parkinson-White syndrome) or dilated cardiomyopathy, can present with frank syncope or even sudden cardiac death.

The ECG can confirm atrial fibrillation, heart rate, and the presence of underlying structural heart disease; such as chamber enlargement, (hypertrophy), prior myocardial infarction, and conduction abnormalities. The transthoracic echocardiogram is an essential part of a complete evaluation, particularly in patients being considered for cardioversion. Underlying structural contributors to atrial fibrillation and left atrial size, a predictor of short- and long-term success in cardioversion, should be examined by echocardiography. Transesophageal echocardiography is indicated in some settings to document, before cardioversion, the presence or absence of thrombi in the left atrium or the left atrial appendage. Laboratory testing should be performed to evaluate thyroid status and screen for electrolyte abnormalities. Additional testing may include functional assessment for coronary heart disease (exercise or pharmacologic stress testing with or without imaging) and even coronary angiography. Electrophysiology studies are not indicated as part of the initial evaluation but are indicated when radiofrequency ablation of potential atrial fibrillation sites is being considered. An electrophysiology study may also be considered for younger patients with a history of supraventricular tachycardia and a regular rhythm, which has now become more irregular. In this setting, the supraventricular tachycardia may be the trigger for the initiation of atrial fibrillation. Although uncommon, this is an example of tachycardia-induced tachycardia. In this circumstance, radiofrequency ablation of the supraventricular tachycardia mechanism leads to prevention of the atrial fibrillation.

MANAGEMENT AND THERAPY

Treatment of atrial fibrillation mainly depends on symptoms and the etiology of the atrial fibrillation (Tables 19-2, 19-3, and 19-4). Are the symptoms related to atrial fibrillation tolerable or intolerable to the patient? Has atrial fibrillation resulted in an unfavorable hemodynamic picture that may have long-term consequences? Have embolic events occurred, and what is the long-term risk for thromboembolism? Consideration of important issues related to each of these areas can help guide treatment options.

Four major issues must be considered in determining the treatment of atrial fibrillation: conversion from atrial fibrillation to normal sinus rhythm, maintenance of normal sinus rhythm, rate control in patients with permanent atrial fibrillation, and prevention of thromboembolic complications (Fig. 19-2). These four issues are discussed with special emphasis on controversial factors.

Cardioversion

Cardioversion for atrial fibrillation should be considered in two settings. In patients who present acutely with hemodynamically unstable atrial fibrillation, immediate cardioversion may be indicated. Remember the **sinus tachycardia** concept: atrial fibrillation with a rapid ventricular response may be triggered by an underlying cause. Initially, this cause should be sought and, if necessary, addressed. Other causes of hypotension and tachycardia should be excluded, including hypovolemia, septic shock, acute hemorrhage, profound anemia, and acute myocardial infarction leading to cardiogenic shock. Usually, patients who are hypotensive

Table 19-2
Long-Term Management of Paroxysmal Atrial Fibrillation

· Confirm Diagnosis: ECG, Holter, or loop recorder

· Anticoagulation: assess risk factors

· Echocardiogram: assess LV function, LV hypertrophy, LA dimensions

· Assess Comorbidities
    Coronary artery disease/angina: rate
    Congestive heart failure: rate and exacerbations
    Hypertension: with LV hypertrophy, consider avoiding Class I agents
    Tachy-brady syndrome
        EF >40%: consider dual chamber pacemaker with atrial fibrillation suppression software that decreases atrial fibrillation burden
        EF <35%: consider implantable cardioverter defibrillator that combines atrial overdrive pacing and atrial defibrillation
    Renal function: review renally excreted rhythm and rate control medications

· Quality of Life Assessment: review limitations on physical activity since onset of atrial fibrillation

· Asymptomatic Without Limitations on Physical Activity
    Holter monitor to exclude persistently elevated heart rates during paroxysmal atrial fibrillation
    Any average hourly rate >95 beats/min, rate control β-blockers, calcium channel blockers
    Consider antiarrhythmic agents for patients with CHF

· Symptomatic
    Structurally abnormal LV
    Dofetilide
    Amiodarone
    Structurally normal LV
    Dofetilide
    Amiodarone
    Sotalol
    Propafenone
    Flecainide

· Failed or Poorly Tolerated Antiarrhythmics: ablation with pulmonary vein isolation

CHF indicates congestive heart failure; EF, ejection fraction; LA, left atrium; LV left ventricular.

from atrial fibrillation with a rapid ventricular rate also have underlying cardiovascular disease. After reversible factors have been addressed, these patients should undergo elec-

Figure 19-2

Complications of Atrial Fibrillation

Hemodynamic deterioration in existing CHF

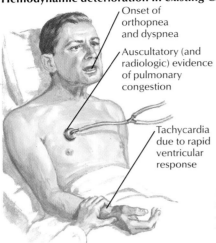

Onset of orthopnea and dyspnea

Auscultatory (and radiologic) evidence of pulmonary congestion

Tachycardia due to rapid ventricular response

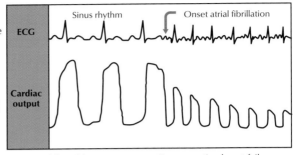

Sinus rhythm   Onset atrial fibrillation

ECG

Cardiac output

Patients with stable or asymptomatic congestive heart failure may show marked worsening if atrial fibrillation (AF) ensues. Loss of atrial contraction and rapid ventricular heart rate decreases cardiac output and increases congestive symptoms.

Thromboembolic complications

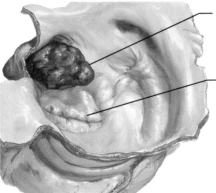

Thrombi commonly originate in the left atrial appendage in atrial fibrillation patients

Mitral stenosis

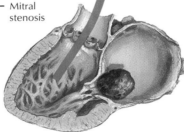

Emboli

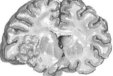

Embolic sites

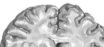

Cerebral infarction

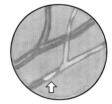

Retinal emboli

Example of left atrial thrombus in patient with atrial fibrillation due to mitral stenosis

High incidence of atrial thrombi in AF patients with increased risk of peripheral embolization warrants consideration of anticoagulation unless contraindicated

Other peripheral sites include spleen, kidney, mesenteric vessels

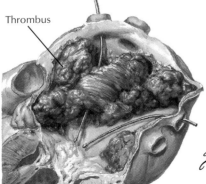

Thrombus

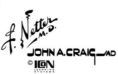

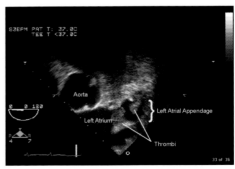

Thrombus may be quite large and fill most of atrium (probes in "open" channels)

Transesophageal echocardiographic findings in a patient with atrial fibrillation, showing thrombi in the left atrial appendage and main left atrium

Table 19-3
Long-Term Management of Persistent Atrial Fibrillation

· Confirm Diagnosis: ECG
· Anticoagulation: assess risk factors
· Echocardiogram: assess LV function, LV hypertrophy, LA dimensions
· Assessment of Comorbidities
    Coronary artery disease/angina: rate
    Congestive heart failure
· Rate and Exacerbations
    Hypertension: with LV hypertrophy, consider avoiding Class I agents
    Tachy-brady syndrome
      EF >40%: consider dual chamber pacemaker with atrial fibrillation suppression software that decreases atrial fibrillation burden
      EF <35%: consider implantable cardioverter defibrillator that combines atrial overdrive pacing and atrial defibrillation
    Renal function: review renally excreted rhythm and rate control medications
· Quality of Life Assessment: review limitations on physical activity since onset of atrial fibrillation
· Asymptomatic Without Limitations on Physical Activity
    Holter monitor to exclude persistently elevated heart rates during persistent atrial fibrillation
    Any average hourly rate >95 beats/min, rate control β-blockers, calcium channel blockers
    Consider antiarrhythmic agents for patients with CHF
· Symptomatic
    Clearly <24–48 hours:
      proceed with IV heparin and cardioversion
    >48 hours or unclear onset:
      IV heparin, transesophageal echocardiogram and cardioversion
      Or
      IV heparin until warfarin in the target INR 2.0–3.0 for 3–4 weeks
· Synchronized Biphasic DC Cardioversion
    May need ibutilide to facilitate cardioversion
    Structurally abnormal LV with ≥2 episodes
      Dofetilide
      Amiodarone
    Structurally normal LV with ≥2 episodes
      Dofetilide
      Amiodarone
      Sotalol
      Propafenone
      Flecainide
    Failed or poorly tolerated antiarrhythmics: ablation with pulmonary vein isolation

CHF indicates congestive heart failure; EF, ejection fraction; LA, left atrium; LV, left ventricular.

Table 19-4
Long-Term Management of Permanent Atrial Fibrillation

· Confirm Diagnosis: ECG
· Anticoagulation: assess risk factors
· Echocardiogram: assess LV function, LV hypertrophy, LA dimensions
· Assessment of Comorbidities
    Coronary artery disease/angina: rate
    Congestive heart failure
· Rate and Exacerbations
    Hypertension: with LV hypertrophy, consider avoiding Class I agents
    Tachy-brady syndrome
      EF >40%: consider single chamber pacemaker with rate regulation suppression software that decreases rapid ventricular responses
      EF <35%: consider implantable cardioverter defibrillator
    Renal function: review renally excreted rhythm and rate control medications
· Quality of Life Assessment: review limitations on physical activity since onset of atrial fibrillation
· Rate Control
    Directed by Holter monitor to exclude persistently elevated heart rates during activities of daily living
    Any average hourly rate >95 beats/min, rate control β-blockers, calcium channel blockers
    Digoxin as a second agent or for inactive patients
· Annual Echocardiography and Holter Monitor: to avoid tachycardia-induced cardiomyopathy
· Rapid Ventricular Response Despite Maximally Tolerated Rate Control Agents: AV node ablation and biventricular pacemaker

EF indicates ejection fraction; LA, left atrium; LV, left ventricular.

trical cardioversion immediately. Rate control with intravenous short-acting β-blockers (esmolol) or calcium channel blockers (diltiazem) can be considered, but in the setting of marked hypotension, these should be cautiously initiated. However, because there is no atrial contraction in atrial fibrillation, the left ventricle fills passively. Therefore, in patients with a rapid ventricular response, slowing of the ventricular rate allows a more prolonged diastolic filling time and thus may improve cardiac output. In hemodynamically stable patients with myocardial ischemia, either intravenous β-blockers (including esmolol or metoprolol) or calcium channel blockers (diltiazem or verapamil) can be used safely before cardioversion. Neither β-blockers nor calcium channel blockers are effective agents for cardioversion, although spontaneous cardioversion may occur when the heart rate is slowed pharmacologically. There is a growing indication for certain type III antiarrhythmic drugs in the urgent treatment of atrial fibrillation. Intravenous ibutilide and amiodarone are safe in this setting, when used with proper monitoring. In some circumstances, Class IA agents (intravenous procainamide principally) are recommended in the acute setting, but the advent of ibutilide and amiodarone have largely displaced their use.

The second setting in which cardioversion is considered for atrial fibrillation is in symptomatic (or sometimes even asymptomatic) but stable patients. In this setting, before cardioversion, it is essential to consider the need for anticoagulation (see Anticoagulation in Atrial Fibrillation). In general, in uncomplicated cases when the duration of atrial fibrillation is clearly less than 24 hours, anticoagulation is not required before cardioversion. When the duration of atrial fibrillation is more than 48 hours, it is generally recommended that the patient be started on IV heparin. Differences of opinion exist on whether to anticoagulate patients who have been in atrial fibrillation for 24 to 48 hours. The more conservative approach (which we adhere to) is to anticoagulate, the same as for patients in whom the duration of atrial fibrillation has been more than 48 hours. An alternative approach uses transesophageal echocardiography to screen for thrombi in the atria or the atrial appendages and proceed with cardioversion if no thrombi are present. In this case, anticoagulation with warfarin (INR 2.0–3.0) is initiated at the time of cardioversion and for at least 1 month afterward. These issues are discussed in the following subsections.

Rhythm Control

The selection of electrical versus pharmacologic cardioversion is often an individualized decision based on the patient's history and predisposing factors for atrial fibrillation. For instance, patients with paroxysmal or persistent atrial fibrillation are likely to require antifibrillatory medication to maintain sinus rhythm. Obvi-

ously, these patients need to be maintained on anticoagulants prior to chemical cardioversion. The pharmacologic choices for cardioversion are principally amiodarone, sotalol, and dofetilide. All have advantages and disadvantages. For patients with paroxysmal atrial fibrillation, amiodarone can safely be initiated in the outpatient setting and is probably the most effective antifibrillatory agent. Even at the low doses used for atrial fibrillation prophylaxis (~200 mg/day), the side effect profile of amiodarone requires semiannual screening for thyroid and hepatic dysfunction and for the rare occurrence of diminishing pulmonary function from early pulmonary fibrosis. Sotalol is also effective and can be particularly beneficial in patients who require β-blockade for other reasons, but sotalol should be initiated in an inpatient setting because of unpredictable QT prolongation in some individuals. Dofetilide is a very promising agent, but its use also requires 3 days of telemetry monitoring for QT prolongation and torsades de pointes. The initial dofetilide dosage is based on renal function. Subsequent doses are determined by QT response to the previous dose until a steady state is reached.

The decision to use medications to maintain normal sinus rhythm is common. Indeed, less than one third of patients who are successfully cardioverted maintain normal sinus rhythm for more than a year without antifibrillatory therapy. Many predictors of the potential need for antifibrillatory therapy are known. Sometimes the use of β-blockers can blunt adrenergic drive sufficiently to prevent recurrence of atrial fibrillation, although this is the exception. Many cardiologists favor an initial trial of electrical cardioversion alone in low-risk patients with atrial fibrillation, reasoning that the third of patients who do not require antifibrillatory therapy will be spared the expense and the associated risks. In patients who have an increased risk of recurrent atrial fibrillation, or who have had a second electrical cardioversion, use of the medications discussed above (and in Tables 19-2 and 19-3) is generally indicated for maintenance of normal sinus rhythm. However, this practice has come into question and is discussed below, in the section Rate Versus Rhythm Control.

Rate Control

Many patients with permanent atrial fibrillation are not successfully treated with cardioversion or antiarrhythmic agents, are unwilling to undergo cardioversion, are unable to tolerate antiarrhythmic agents, and/or have factors that predict that treatment will fail and are minimally symptomatic except at rapid heart rates. For them (Table 19-4), pharmacologic rate control should be considered. β-Blockers, calcium channel blockers, or both can often control rapid heart rates with or without digoxin. Digoxin is particularly useful in controlling atrioventricular (AV) conduction in patients who are minimally active or bedridden from comorbidities. However, because there is considerable overlap between atrial fibrillation and conduction abnormalities including sinus node dysfunction (**sick sinus syndrome**), an appropriate balance between tachycardia and bradycardia may be difficult to obtain. These patients may require a permanent pacemaker to prevent bradycardic episodes while being treated with β-blockers, calcium channel blockers, or antifibrillatory medications for tachycardia. Although the initial promise of permanent dual chamber pacing (or even atrial pacing alone) to prevent atrial fibrillation has not been fulfilled, in patients with episodic atrial fibrillation, dual chamber pacing with an atrial fibrillation suppression algorithm should be considered when a pacemaker is indicated. Use of ventricular pacing is likely to convert episodic atrial fibrillation into permanent atrial fibrillation. Another special case, discussed (see Atrioventricular Node Ablation and Permanent Pacing), is the patient whose rapid ventricular response is resistant to pharmacologic control or for whom the pharmacologic approach results in intolerable side effects.

Anticoagulation in Atrial Fibrillation

Anticoagulation considerations include anticoagulation during restoration of normal sinus rhythm, chronic anticoagulation, and cessation and restoration of anticoagulation for patients with atrial fibrillation who are undergoing surgical procedures. Consensus panels from the American College of Cardiology, the American Heart Association, the European Society of Cardiology, and the American College of Chest Physicians have concurred on the use of anticoagulation therapy in the pericardioversion period. In patients with atrial fibrillation of unknown duration, valvular heart disease, evidence of left ventricular dysfunction, or prior thromboembolism or for whom cardioversion is entirely elective, therapeutic anticoagulation with warfarin (with an INR of 2.0–3.0) for 3 to 4 weeks before cardioversion is strongly recommended. Anticoagulation should be continued at the same level for at least 4 weeks after cardioversion. An alternative approach is to assess for atrial or atrial appendage thrombi by transesophageal echocardiography. Lacking thrombi, or **a low flow state** (also referred to as increased spontaneous echocardiographic contrast), the patient can be safely cardioverted without antecedent anticoagulation with warfarin, although heparin or low molecular weight heparin should be initiated before cardioversion. These patients do require anticoagulation for 4 to 6 weeks after cardioversion.

Long-term anticoagulation with warfarin is advocated in patients in several settings. Because many patients have recurrent atrial fibrillation, some episodes of which may not be recognized, anticoagulation is indicated. Other symptomatic patients may also experience asymptomatic episodes of atrial fibrillation that predispose to embolic events, even when they are in sinus rhythm. Finally, in patients with permanent atrial fibrillation, five large prospectively randomized studies demonstrated that warfarin reduced the risk of stroke by 45 to 82%. Patients with hypertension, diabetes, CHF, a previous embolic event, or age older than 75 years require anticoagulation with warfarin. The use of aspirin remains controversial for patients at low risk for stroke (lone atrial fibrillation) or for patients with increased risk of bleeding in whom warfarin may be contraindicated.

SPECIAL ISSUES

Because atrial fibrillation represents a diverse group of etiologies and risks, several special issues merit further discussion.

Lone Atrial Fibrillation

By definition, *lone atrial fibrillation* occurs in individuals less than 60 years of age who lack evidence of other cardiovascular diseases including structural heart disease, hypertension,

Figure 19-3

Surgical Management of Atrial Fibrillation

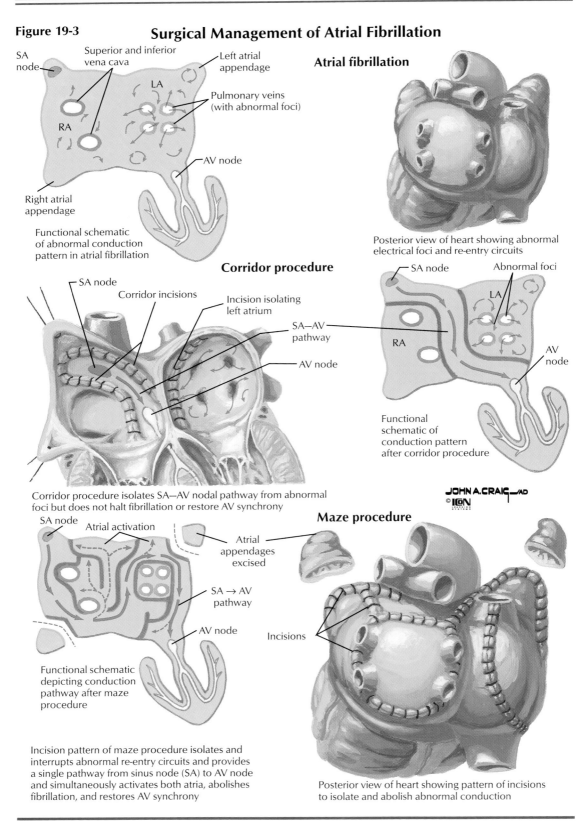

SA node

Superior and inferior vena cava

Left atrial appendage

LA

RA

Pulmonary veins (with abnormal foci)

AV node

Right atrial appendage

Functional schematic of abnormal conduction pattern in atrial fibrillation

Atrial fibrillation

Posterior view of heart showing abnormal electrical foci and re-entry circuits

Corridor procedure

SA node

Corridor incisions

Incision isolating left atrium

SA—AV pathway

AV node

SA node

Abnormal foci

LA

RA

AV node

Functional schematic of conduction pattern after corridor procedure

Corridor procedure isolates SA—AV nodal pathway from abnormal foci but does not halt fibrillation or restore AV synchrony

JOHN A. CRAIG—AD
©ICON

Maze procedure

SA node

Atrial activation

Atrial appendages excised

SA → AV pathway

AV node

Incisions

Functional schematic depicting conduction pathway after maze procedure

Incision pattern of maze procedure isolates and interrupts abnormal re-entry circuits and provides a single pathway from sinus node (SA) to AV node and simultaneously activates both atria, abolishes fibrillation, and restores AV synchrony

Posterior view of heart showing pattern of incisions to isolate and abolish abnormal conduction

or diabetes. This definition has been refined with the use of echocardiography to confirm the lack of structural heart disease, even including mild mitral valve regurgitation, left atrial enlargement, and left ventricular hypertrophy. The general experience in patients with lone atrial fibrillation is that their risk of stroke is low, anticoagulation is unnecessary for stroke prophylaxis, and further treatment for atrial fibrillation is probably also not necessary. As lone atrial fibrillation has become more clearly defined, this trend holds. Questions that remain include: How often should individuals carrying the diagnosis of lone atrial fibrillation have echocardiography to be certain that structural abnormalities are still absent and should patients with lone atrial fibrillation be given aspirin? There are no studies that answer these questions. In general, patients with lone atrial fibrillation should be seen at least annually to document that stroke risk factors including hypertension and diabetes are still absent, and echocardiography and Holter monitoring should be performed annually to ascertain that there is no evidence of tachycardia-induced cardiomyopathy. The results of studies are mixed on the role of aspirin in patients with lone atrial fibrillation, and there is no consensus for its use. However, given the strong epidemiologic data on the role of low-dose aspirin (81–325 mg/day) in healthy individuals in lessening the risk of stroke and myocardial infarction, low-dose aspirin can be recommended in patients with lone atrial fibrillation. Those aged older than 60 and younger than 75 years should be prescribed aspirin.

Nonpharmacologic Approaches to Preventing Atrial Fibrillation

Surgical and percutaneous approaches exist for the treatment of atrial fibrillation (Tables 19-2, 19-3, and 19-4; Fig. 19-3). The best studied surgical approaches are the corridor and maze procedures. In the *corridor procedure*, a corridor of atrial tissue is surgically isolated between the sinus and the AV nodes from the rest of the atria, providing chronotrophic rate control and demonstrating an increased ability to maintain normal sinus rhythm. In the *maze procedure*, small incisions are made to effectively interrupt reentrant atrial arrhythmias and prevent sustained atrial fibrillation, while providing one

pathway from the sinus node to the AV node and simultaneously activating the right and left atria. The concept behind both of these procedures is maintenance of normal sinus rhythm and atrial systole. Although both procedures are effective, they both require open surgery, usually require continued anticoagulation, and are complicated by the frequent need for permanent pacing, and, hence, are indicated only for a small portion of patients with atrial fibrillation, principally those with a planned cardiac surgical procedure for other reasons (coronary or valvular heart disease). An alternate approach, radiofrequency catheter ablation of atrial fibrillation, isolates foci of early depolarizing atrial cells in the cuffs of the pulmonary veins and has had increasing success but a significant incidence of recurrent atrial fibrillation (from other sites) and of pulmonary vein stenosis. The use of advanced mapping techniques will undoubtedly improve the efficacy of radiofrequency catheter ablation, which still is recommended in cases where pharmacotherapy and other approaches are unsuitable.

Frequently because of coexistent sinus node dysfunction, tachy-brady syndrome, or excessive bradycardia caused by medications, a permanent pacemaker is indicated. For patients with paroxysmal or persistent atrial fibrillation (Tables 19-2 and 19-3), a pacemaker that combines atrial suppression software should be considered. These pacemakers prevent atrial oversensing by pacing faster than the underlying atrial rhythm. In clinical trials, these pacemakers reduced atrial fibrillation burden by up to 25%. Dual chamber pacemakers are superior to ventricular pacemakers in preventing the development of atrial fibrillation.

Rate Versus Rhythm Control

On the basis of hemodynamic studies, it has been assumed that patients with normal sinus rhythm fare better than do those with atrial fibrillation but well-controlled ventricular rates. Two studies call into question this conventional wisdom. In both, rhythm control did not provide a survival advantage over rate control in terms of symptoms, risks of stroke, or other morbidities. The groups were highly selected and minimally symptomatic and there was considerable crossover, such that a significant portion of the **rate control** group was actually in normal sinus rhythm at the conclusion of the studies, creating a significant, negative impact on the power of the study. In addition, patients at higher risk for hemodynamic compromise were largely excluded from these studies. Although we await a final answer to the debate on rate versus rhythm control, these studies clearly demonstrate that rate control is a more viable option than it was previously considered to be.

Atrioventricular Node Ablation and Permanent Pacing

Consistent with the idea that rhythm control is a useful approach, several studies demonstrated remarkable symptom reduction in patients with atrial fibrillation and refractory rapid ventricular response by making these patients **pacemaker-dependent**. In essence, the patient undergoes radiofrequency catheter ablation of the AV node and implantation of a permanent pacemaker. Depending on the likelihood of restoring normal sinus rhythm, a dual chamber pacemaker may be used, or in cases where that likelihood is low, a single-chamber ventricular pacemaker is implanted. Studies support the rationale that the rapid ventricular response resulting from atrial fibrillation can be effectively eliminated for selected patients. There may also be a reversal of tachycardia-induced cardiomyopathy, with improvement in left ventricular ejection fraction. Uniformly for patients with permanent atrial fibrillation, quality of life scores and exercise tolerance improve and rehospitalization and resource utilization decrease following AV node ablation and permanent pacemaker placement. Recent reports indicate that biventricular pacing is superior to RV pacing.

Congestive Heart Failure

Atrial fibrillation occurs in 15 to 30% of patients with CHF. Atrial fibrillation leads to hemodynamic deterioration and rehospitalization with worsening of symptoms in patients with existing heart failure. The rapid heart rate and loss of atrial contraction can precipitate an exacerbation of CHF in patients with asymptomatic stable left ventricular dysfunction. These changes can be reversed with rate control or reversion to sinus rhythm. It appears that patients with more severe CHF (New York Heart Association class III

and IV) and atrial fibrillation have higher all-cause mortality and pump failure deaths. In patients with milder forms of CHF (New York Heart Association class I and II), though, atrial fibrillation was not associated with an increase in mortality or rehospitalization. Class I antiarrhythmic agents are independently associated with an increased mortality in patients with CHF and atrial fibrillation and should be avoided. Amiodarone and dofetilide are safe for patients with CHF. Optimal pharmacologic therapy may play a favorable role in influencing the outcomes for these patients. Even in patients at highest risk with atrial fibrillation and severe CHF, it has not been shown that maintenance of sinus rhythm with antiarrhythmic agents improves survival.

Implantable Atrial Defibrillation

Between 20 and 30% of patients have a coexisting atrial fibrillation at the time of placement of an implantable cardioverter defibrillator. Seventeen months after placement of an implantable cardioverter defibrillator, up to 45% of patients have atrial fibrillation. The latest implantable cardioverter defibrillators also incorporate atrial conversion therapy, which includes atrial overdrive antitachycardia pacing, atrial high frequency burst pacing, and atrial defibrillation. These devices are safe and efficacious. Therefore, an implantable cardioverter defibrillator with atrial therapies should be considered for patients with atrial fibrillation or the potential to develop atrial fibrillation.

Coronary Artery Bypass Surgery

Atrial fibrillation is frequently seen in patients after CABG surgery. Up to 40% of patients are estimated to develop atrial fibrillation, usually beginning after postoperative day 1 and lengthening the hospital stay. Older patients and those who have β-blockers withdrawn before surgery are more likely to develop atrial fibrillation. Use of β-blockers or amiodarone preoperatively decreases the frequency of postoperative atrial fibrillation. Interestingly, atrial fibrillation is a transient phenomenon; most patients are in sinus rhythm when discharged. Only a minority, less than 5%, are in atrial fibrillation 30 days after surgery.

Ablation has been performed during CABG in patients undergoing mitral valve surgery. The four pulmonary veins are isolated with either radiofrequency ablation or cryoablation. In some circumstances, the ablation line has been extended to the mitral valve annulus, with reportedly fewer episodes of recurrence of atrial fibrillation. Early studies showing sinus rhythm maintenance have been encouraging, even in patients with permanent atrial fibrillation before surgery.

FUTURE DIRECTIONS

Advances in the treatment of atrial fibrillation hold promise. Newer antifibrillatory agents are in development, such as azimilide, as are anticoagulants that will be easier to administer and safer than warfarin. Exciting nonpharmacologic therapies are undergoing testing and early clinical use, including implantable atrial defibrillators (with the rationale that early conversion of atrial fibrillation to normal sinus rhythm facilitates maintenance of normal sinus rhythm), newer mapping, and more sophisticated percutaneous approaches. Eventually, it may be possible to cure atrial fibrillation, much as radiofrequency catheter ablation can now cure supraventricular tachycardias in many and maintain normal sinus rhythm in most. Another approach, still experimental, is the percutaneous left atrial appendage transcatheter occlusion device. It is implanted and designed to seal the left atrial appendage and prevent development of atrial thrombi in the appendage. This may be an attractive strategy for patients who cannot or will not take warfarin or for patients who have embolic episodes while taking warfarin. Early clinical data suggest that this device can be safely used in humans. However, there are no clinical studies of long-term safety or efficacy.

REFERENCES

Atrial Fibrillation Investigators. Risk factors for stroke and efficacy of antithrombotic therapy in atrial fibrillation: analysis of pooled data from five randomized controlled trials. *Arch Intern Med* 1994;154:1449–1457.

Fitzpatrick AP, Kourouyan HD, Siu A, et al. Quality of life and outcomes after radiofrequency His-bundle catheter ablation and permanent pacemaker implantation: Impact of treatment in paroxysmal and established atrial fibrillation. *Am Heart J* 1996;131:499–507.

Fuster V, Ryden LE, Asinger RW, et al. ACC/AHA/ESC guidelines for the management of patients with atrial fibrillation: Executive summary. A report of the American College of Cardiology/American Heart Association Task Force on Practice Guidelines and the European Society of Cardiology Committee for Practice Guidelines and Policy Conferences (Committee to develop guidelines for the management of patients with atrial fibrillation). Developed in collaboration with the North American Society of Pacing and Electrophysiology. *Eur Heart J* 2001;22:1852–1923.

Haissaguerre M, Jais P, Shah DC, et al. Spontaneous initiation of atrial fibrillation by ectopic beats originating in the pulmonary veins. *N Engl J Med* 1998;339:659–666.

Klein AL, Grimm RA, Murray RD, et al, for the Assessment of Cardioversion Using Transesophageal Echocardiography Investigators. Use of transesophageal echocardiography to guide cardioversion in patients with atrial fibrillation. *N Engl J Med* 2001;344:1411–1420.

Kober L, Bloch Thomsen PE, Moller M, et al. Effect of dofetilide in patients with recent myocardial infarction and left-ventricular dysfunction: A randomised trial. *Lancet* 2000;356:2052–2058.

Sheahan RG. Left atrial thrombus, transient ischemic attack, and atrial fibrillation: Does left atrial thrombus predict? Does absence protect? *Am Heart J* 2003;145:582–585.

Wyse DG, Waldo AL, DiMarco JP, et al, for the Atrial Fibrillation Follow-up Investigation of Rhythm Management (AFFIRM) Investigators. A comparison of rate control and rhythm control in patients with atrial fibrillation. *N Engl J Med* 2002;347:1825–1833.

Chapter 20
Ventricular Tachycardia

Richard G. Sheahan

Ventricular tachycardia (VT) refers to wide complex rhythms that originate from the ventricle. Of all patients who present with wide complex tachycardias, more than 80% have VT as a diagnosis. VT is usually found in patients with underlying structural heart disease, predominantly coronary artery disease (CAD) and myocardial ischemia. However, it has been increasingly recognized that specific congenital or hereditary cardiac abnormalities predispose to VT in many situations. In patients with known coronary or congenital heart disease and a wide complex tachycardia, the diagnosis is VT in up to 95% of cases. Because the treatment of VT varies depending on its underlying mechanism, this chapter will separately examine the known causes of VT and their therapies (Fig. 20-1). VT plays an important role in syncope and sudden cardiac death, and the evaluation and treatment of VT in these settings are discussed in Chapters 20 and 23.

ETIOLOGY AND PATHOGENESIS

Ventricular tachycardia is the commonest cause of a wide complex tachycardia; other causes include supraventricular tachycardia (SVT) or atrial fibrillation/flutter with aberrant conduction (left or right bundle branch block), antidromic reentrant tachycardia (antegrade over an accessory pathway), Mahaim fiber tachycardia, and pacemaker-mediated tachycardia. Three key features that favor VT over SVT with aberrant conduction are fusion beats, capture beats, and atrioventricular dissociation. Many other features may be helpful in discerning VT from SVT, but when these key features are present, a confident diagnosis of VT can be made. A resting ECG showing either pre-excitation of Wolff-Parkinson-White syndrome or a dual chamber pacemaker provides further diagnostic information.

DIFFERENTIAL DIAGNOSIS

The diagnosis of VT can be difficult. Findings such as atrioventricular dissociation or fusion beats are diagnostic for VT; however, these are present in only about 5% of cases (see chapter 3). Beyond these certain markers, countless criteria for distinguishing between VT and SVT on the basis of characteristics of the QRS morphology (on the 12-lead ECG) have been proposed. Unfortunately, none of these criteria are foolproof. As suggested above, in patients with known coronary heart disease and wide complex tachycardia, the diagnosis is VT until proven otherwise. The same is true for patients with known congenital heart disease or a hereditary predisposition toward VT. SVT can mimic VT, occurring in individuals with an existing bundle branch block. Aberrant conduction can also produce SVT with a wide QRS complex. Likewise, atrial fibrillation with a rapid ventricular response commonly results in a widened QRS complex. All of these can be difficult to distinguish from VT. Response to therapeutic challenge can be helpful. For instance, a wide complex tachyarrhythmia terminated by adenosine infusion is much more likely to be SVT with aberrant conduction than it is to be VT. Conversely, a wide complex tachyarrhythmia terminated by lidocaine infusion is much more likely to be VT than SVT. Nonetheless, an electrophysiology study (EPS) may be required to confirm the diagnosis of VT versus SVT.

CLINICAL PRESENTATION AND DIAGNOSIS

The hemodynamic consequences of VT depend on many factors, including the VT rate, left ventricular ejection fraction (LVEF), comorbidities, and medications. Exercise-induced VT in a normal heart may be better tolerated than a slow VT in patients with ejection fractions of 10%. Anemia or preexisting orthostatic hypotension and VT may be poorly tolerated. Therefore, patients may present with a range of symptoms:

Figure 20-1

Ventricular Tachycardia

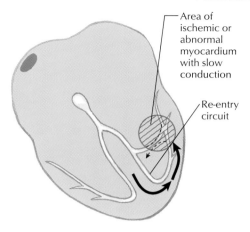

Area of ischemic or abnormal myocardium with slow conduction

Re-entry circuit

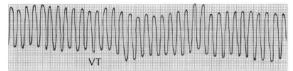

VT

Ventricular tachycardia refers to wide-complex rhythms of ventricular origin. Most originate from abnormal re-entry circuits.

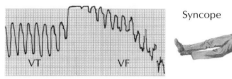

VT　　　VF

Syncope

The two major clinical concerns in ventricular tachycardia are conversion to ventricular fibrillation and syncope due to rapid rate and decreased output

Underlying causes of ventricular tachycardia

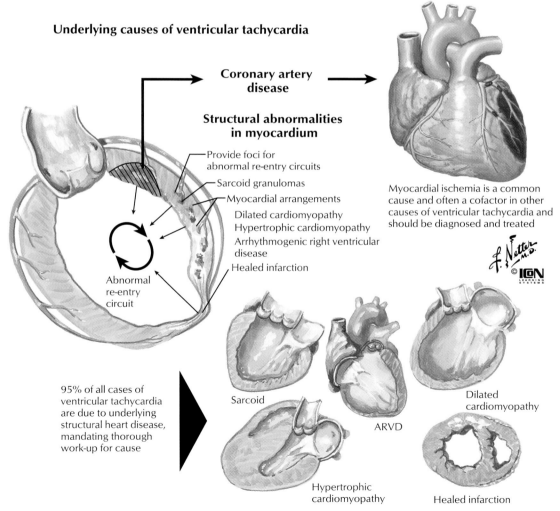

Coronary artery disease

Structural abnormalities in myocardium

Provide foci for abnormal re-entry circuits

Sarcoid granulomas

Myocardial arrangements

Dilated cardiomyopathy
Hypertrophic cardiomyopathy
Arrhythmogenic right ventricular disease

Healed infarction

Abnormal re-entry circuit

Myocardial ischemia is a common cause and often a cofactor in other causes of ventricular tachycardia and should be diagnosed and treated

95% of all cases of ventricular tachycardia are due to underlying structural heart disease, mandating thorough work-up for cause

Sarcoid

ARVD

Dilated cardiomyopathy

Hypertrophic cardiomyopathy

Healed infarction

an awareness of palpitations, dizziness, shortness of breath, chest pain, presyncope, syncope, or sudden cardiac death (SCD). Physical examination easily confirms the diagnosis of tachycardia, with or without hypotension, tachypnea, hypoxia, or signs of pulmonary edema. Occasionally, patients tolerate VT very well, and apart from palpitations and tachycardia, they may have no other physical findings. Electrocardiography can often confirm the diagnosis of VT.

ACUTE MANAGEMENT AND THERAPY

Acute management combines stabilizing the patient and terminating the VT. Urgent blood samples should be obtained for CBC, electrolytes including magnesium, blood urea nitrogen, creatinine, cardiac markers, blood glucose, and toxicology screen. When appropriate, an arterial blood gas measurement should be obtained. If the patient is presyncopal, hypotensive, or in severe respiratory distress from pulmonary edema, the patient should, after appropriate sedation, receive a synchronized external direct current (DC) cardioversion. If the VT is well tolerated, antiarrhythmic agents (such as intravenous amiodarone, intravenous lidocaine, intravenous magnesium, and, in some circumstances, intravenous metoprolol) may be given. If the VT fails to terminate, overdrive pacing with a transvenous right ventricular (RV) lead or a synchronized DC cardioversion should be performed. DC cardioversion should be performed only after the patient has received adequate and appropriate sedation. Later management includes ruling out myocardial infarction and correcting any abnormal blood tests. Subsequent management of the patient with VT depends on the etiology and the absence of reversible causes (Fig. 20-2; Table 20-1).

Monomorphic Ventricular Tachycardia

Monomorphic VT is the commonest wide complex rhythm. It is usually a regular sustained rhythm originating from the ventricles. The mechanism depends on the underlying etiology (Fig. 20-3).

Coronary Artery Disease

Patients who have a healed myocardial infarction without ongoing ischemia may present with VT, even years after the original myocardial infarction. The mechanism of the VT is usually reentry. Viable myocardial tissue survives in the scar and provides an area where slow conduction can occur, critical to the maintenance of a VT reentrant circuit. Ventricular aneurysms are also associated with VT. Patients who present with VT and CAD initially require an ischemic evaluation and, if necessary, revascularization. In patients for whom revascularization is possible, an evaluation of the need for placement of an implantable cardioverter defibrillator (ICD) should be performed following revascularization. An ICD is superior to amiodarone, or other antiarrhythmic agents, in decreasing mortality in patients with VT. These patients should also be given maximally tolerated doses of β-blockers, angiotensin-converting enzyme (ACE) inhibitors, aspirin, and, for the majority of patients, a lipid-lowering agent. In patients who have recurrent VT, antiarrhythmic agents such as amiodarone or sotalol may be used. Alternatively, radiofrequency ablation of the VT circuit can be performed, which can decrease the frequency of VT episodes. For patients who develop coexisting atrial arrhythmias, amiodarone, sotalol, or dofetilide can decrease their frequency.

Dilated Cardiomyopathy

Ventricular tachycardia may occur in patients with dilated cardiomyopathy (DCM). Coexistent CAD must to be excluded. In most cases, patients with DCM and no significant CAD should undergo ICD implantation without further evaluation because EPS is often not useful in these patients. One exception is bundle branch reentrant VT, which manifests as a VT with a left bundle branch block morphology. Bundle branch reentrant VT occurs with His-Purkinje dysfunction and a prolonged HV interval. Retrograde conduction over the left bundle branch activates transseptal conduction, which then activates the right bundle branch, establishing the reentrant circuit. Radiofrequency ablation of the right bundle branch may prevent VT recurrences, although most patients also require ICD plaement.

In general, patients with DCM (especially those with VT) should be treated with the maxi-

Figure 20-2

Management of Ventricular Tachycardia

Acute management

Patient assessment and stabilization

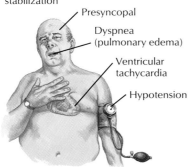

- Presyncopal
- Dyspnea (pulmonary edema)
- Ventricular tachycardia
- Hypotension

Patient status

Ventricular tachycardia well tolerated

Presyncope, hypotension pulmonary edema

IV antiarrhythmic agents
Amiodarone
Magnesium
Metoprolol

DC cardioversion also utilized in cases refractory to medical management

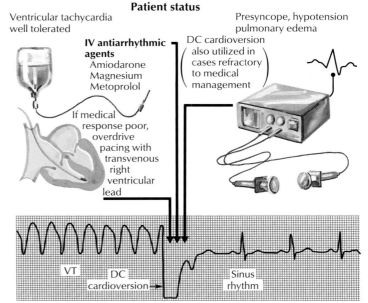

If medical response poor, overdrive pacing with transvenous right ventricular lead

Urgent blood studies

CBC
electrolytes (including magnesium)
BUN, creatinine, cardiac enzymes
Glucose, toxicology screen
blood gases if indicated
(follow-up studies to rule out myocardial infarction)

VT | DC cardioversion → | Sinus rhythm

Primary acute management goal after stabilization of patient is termination of ventricular tachycardia. Treatment modalities based on assessment of patient status.

Long-term management

Long-term management with antiarrhythmics and other pharmacologic agents is often dictated by diagnosis of underlying condition and comorbidities in a given patient

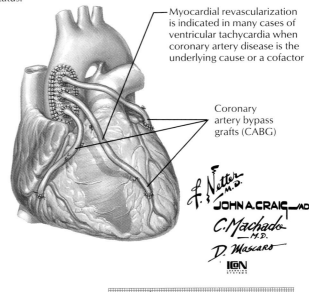

Myocardial revascularization is indicated in many cases of ventricular tachycardia when coronary artery disease is the underlying cause or a cofactor

Coronary artery bypass grafts (CABG)

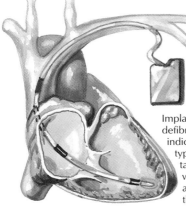

Implantable cardioverter defibrillator (ICD) indicated in many types of ventricular tachycardia, particularly when rate and rhythm are refractory to other therapies

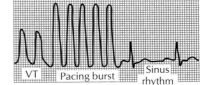

VT | Pacing burst | Sinus rhythm

ECG demonstrating pacing effect on rhythm

Figure 20-3

Ventricular Tachycardia (VT)

Monomorphic VT

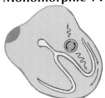

Most common wide complex rhythm, usually a regular sustained rhythm. Re-entry is usual mechanism usually due to structural heart disease.

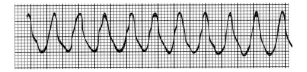

Monomorphic VT with RBBB (BBRVT)

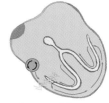

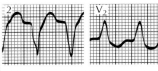

Usually arises from left ventricle focus

Monomorphic VT with LBBB

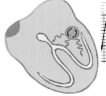

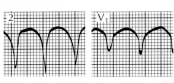

Usually arises in right ventricle or interventricular septum

Bundle branch re-entry VT

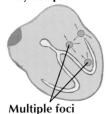

Usually seen in patients with dilated cardiomyopathy. Shows LBBB morphology.

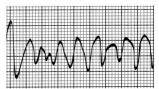

Usually arises in right ventricle

Polymorphic VT

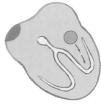

Multiple foci

Wide complex tachycardia with two or more ventricular morphologies. Chaotic electrical activity due to multiple, simultaneous wave fronts.

Normal QT interval

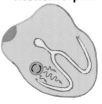

Polymorphic VT occurring with normal QT interval may be due to ischemia and is a cause of sudden cardiac death

Long QT interval

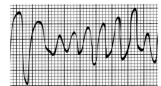

Torsade de pointes is VT with long QT interval. Many have family history of sudden cardiac death.

Accelerated idioventricular rhythm

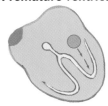

Wide complex rhythm with heart rate ranging between 50–120 beats/min. Usually results after reperfusion as enhanced automaticity of ectopic ventricular focus.

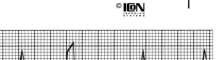

JOHN A.CRAIG—AD
©ICON
LEARNING SYSTEMS

Premature ventricular complexes (PVCs)

PVCs frequently asymptomatic. Some cause palpitations; are usually not significant, but increasing frequency may be marker of significant underlying condition.

Table 20-1
Overview of the Management of Ventricular Tachycardia

Type of Tachycardia	Etiology	Therapy
Monomorphic ventricular tachycardia	CAD	Revascularization, ICD, BB, ACE-I, ± RFA
	DCM	ICD, ± RFA, BB, ACE-I
	HCM	ICD, BB
	Sarcoidosis	ICD, BB
	ARVD	ICD, BB, ± RFA
	RVOT, normal EF	RFA, verapamil,
	Idiopathic LV tachycardia	RFA, verapamil
Nonsustained ventricular tachycardia	CAD, EF >40%	Revascularization, BB, ACE-I
	CAD, EF >35% <40%	Revascularization, EPS, ICD if positive, BB, ACE-I
	CAD, EF <35%	Revascularization, ICD, BB, ACE-I
	DCM >35%	BB, ACE-I
	DCM <35%	ICD, BB ACE-I
	HCM	EPS ± ICD, BB
	Sarcoidosis	EPS ± ICD, BB
	ARVD	EPS ± ICD, BB
	Normal heart	Rule out ischemia BB, RFA
Polymorphic ventricular tachycardia	CAD	Revascularization, B, ACE-I, ± ICD (if EF <35%), amiodarone
	DCM	ICD, BB, ACEI, amiodarone
	HCM	ICD, BB, amiodarone
	Sarcoidosis	ICD, BB, amiodarone
	ARVD	ICD, BB, amiodarone
	Normal heart	Ischemic evaluation, ICD, BB
	Long QT syndrome	ICD, A pacing, BB
Accelerated idioventricular rhythm	CAD, stable hemodynamically	Observe, BB, ACE-I
	CAD, unstable hemodynamically	Atropine, temporary atrial pacing
Premature ventricular complexes	CAD	Revascularization, BB, ACE-I, RFA
	DCM	BB, ACE-I, RFA
	HCM	BB, EPS ± ICD, RFA
	Sarcoidosis	BB, EPS ± ICD, RFA
	ARVD	BB, EPS ± ICD, RFA
	Normal heart	BB, RFA

ACE-I indicates angiotensin-converting enzyme inhibitor; ARVD, arrhythmogenic right ventricular dysplasia; BB, β-blocker; CAD, coronary artery disease; DCM, dilated cardiomyopathy; EF, ejection fraction; EPS, electrophysiology study; HCM, hypertrophic cardiomyopathy; ICD, implantable cardioverter defibrillator; LV, left ventricular; RFA, radiofrequency ablation; RVOT, right ventricular outflow tract.

mum tolerated doses of β-blockers and ACE inhibitors. Amiodarone or sotalol may also help patients with recurrent VT or atrial arrhythmia who have already received ICD therapy. The diagnosis of tachycardia-induced cardiomyopathy should be considered in patients with DCM and persistent atrial arrhythmias. Left ventricular size and function may return to normal or near normal with control of atrial tachyarrhythmias.

Hypertrophic Cardiomyopathy

Ventricular tachycardia in hypertrophic cardiomyopathy requires placement of an ICD. As these patients frequently have coexistent atrial arrhythmias, consideration should be given to placing an ICD that is also capable of atrial overdrive pacing and atrial defibrillation. Where possible, β-blockers should be prescribed. Amiodarone, sotalol, or dofetilide may be helpful in patients with frequent ICD discharges.

Sarcoidosis

Sarcoidosis may infiltrate multiple areas of the myocardium. Sarcoid granulomas in the ventricular myocardium can become foci for abnormal automaticity, or they may disrupt ventricular activation and recovery. This scarring may cause VT recurrences. VT with sarcoidosis requires an ICD and β-blockers.

Arrhythmogenic Right Ventricular Dysplasia

Arrhythmogenic RV dysplasia (ARVD; also referred to as "arrhythmogenic RV cardiomyopathy") is a condition of segmental or diffuse replacement of the RV myocardium with fatty and fibrofatty tissue. The RV free wall is affected initially. Fatty tissue replacement is most severe in areas near the epicardium and mid-myocardium. The disease may progress to the left ventricle. ARVD is inherited as an autosomal dominant condition, and it is estimated that half the patients found to have this disease have a family history of arrhythmogenic RV dysplasia. The remaining cases are new mutations. ARVD is an important cause of SCD. VT in arrhythmogenic RV dysplasia requires an ICD, and ongoing treatment with β-blockers is thought to be helpful for these patients. Because the RV free wall is involved, the ICD lead must be placed in the RV septum to avoid myocardial perforation through the fatty RV wall and potential alterations in the sensing and capture thresholds during the course of this progressive condition. Radiofrequency ablation should be considered for recurrent VT.

Right Ventricular Outflow Tract Ventricular Tachycardia

Right ventricular outflow tract VT is an exercise-induced tachycardia that typically occurs in young patients with structurally normal hearts. The ECG shows a left bundle branch block with a right or normal axis. An automatic or triggered mechanism is likely responsible for this tachycardia. RV outflow tract VT responds not only to adenosine and β-blockers, but it is also one of the rare types of VT that respond to verapamil. SCD rarely occurs in these patients, and for this reason may be treated pharmacologi-

cally. For recurrent episodes, an EPS with radiofrequency ablation should be performed. During EPS, isoproterenol is frequently required to initiate and/or maintain the tachycardia for mapping of the VT origin.

Idioventricular Left Ventricular Tachycardia

Idioventricular left ventricular tachycardia typically occurs in young, predominantly male, patients with structurally normal hearts. SCD is rare. This VT is responsive to intravenous verapamil, the drug of choice. The ECG shows right bundle branch block with left axis morphology. The earliest ventricular activation usually occurs at the left ventricular apex or in the mid–left ventricular septum. During mapping, a discrete electrical potential can often be identified. The arrhythmia is thought to result from a triggered mechanism. If the patient remains symptomatic, in spite of pharmacologic therapy, an EPS and radiofrequency ablation are needed, including mapping of the earliest activation and the identification of a discrete potential.

Nonsustained Ventricular Tachycardia

Nonsustained VT is defined as a wide complex tachycardia between 3 and 30 beats. Some patients are asymptomatic; others may experience hemodynamic consequences of the nonsustained VT. Symptoms include palpitations, dyspnea, chest pain, dizziness, presyncope, or, potentially, syncope. Management of nonsustained VT depends on the etiology of the rhythm. It may act as a marker for SCD and therefore should never be ignored.

For patients with CAD and nonsustained VT, an ischemic evaluation is required and revascularization should be completed. Management depends on the underlying LVEF. For patients with an LVEF of greater than 40%, β-blockers, and ACE inhibitors should be prescribed. For patients with an LVEF of less than 40% but greater than 35%, an EPS should be performed; if VT is induced, an ICD should be placed. β-Blockers and ACE inhibitors should also be prescribed in patients with ischemic cardiomyopathy. For patients with an LVEF of less than 35%, an ICD should be placed, accompanied by long-term treatement with β-blockers and ACE inhibitors (see chapters 12 and 17). The addition of amiodarone can also be considered for patients who have recurrent symptoms without sustained VT.

Patients with a DCM, LVEF of less than 35%, and nonsustained VT, should receive an ICD, β-blockers, and ACE inhibitors. For patients with a DCM and LVEF of greater than 35%, the predictive value of EPS for arrhythmia recurrence is poor. Amiodarone should be considered in patients who have recurrent symptoms without sustained VT.

For patients with hypertrophic cardiomyopathy, sarcoidosis, or arrhythmogenic RV dysplasia, nonsustained VT is a concern. An EPS should be performed, and an ICD should be placed if sustained VT is induced. An ICD should also be considered in patients with syncope and a family history of SCD. β-Blockers and/or amiodarone should also be prescribed.

For patients presenting with nonsustained VT, a structurally normal heart, and a negative ischemic evaluation, β-blockers are the initial therapy of choice. If the patient continues to be symptomatic with frequent palpitations, amiodarone or mapping with radiofrequency ablation should be performed.

Polymorphic Ventricular Tachycardia

Polymorphic VT is a wide complex tachycardia that has two or more ventricular morphologies. Patients presenting with acute myocardial ischemia may have polymorphic VT, and the possibility of ongoing ischemia should be addressed immediately. Electrolytes should be obtained and corrected. These patients are at very high risk for ventricular fibrillation and should be monitored in a coronary care unit. Once revascularization is completed, β-blockers and ACE inhibitors should be started. If the polymorphic VT persists, consideration should be given to implanting an ICD and initiating amiodarone.

In the absence of ischemia, polymorphic VT with DCM, hypertrophic cardiomyopathy, sarcoidosis, or arrhythmogenic RV dysplasia is associated with a poor prognosis. Almost always, ICD implantation and subsequent therapy with a β-blocker is indicated. Amiodarone may also be required.

In a patient with a structurally normal heart and a negative ischemic evaluation, a polymorphic VT should prompt careful evaluation of the underlying ECG to exclude long QT syndrome.

Torsades de pointes is a polymorphic VT that is most commonly found in patients with a prolonged QT interval. Patients should be carefully assessed for metabolic derangements or medications that may prolong the QT interval. In addition, a family history of SCD, other unexplained deaths related to drowning, or single motor vehicle accidents should prompt the placement of an ICD.

For patients with symptomatic long QT syndrome and a family history of SCD, an ICD with atrial pacing capacity should be implanted. The addition of β-blockers should be considered.

Accelerated Idioventricular Rhythm

Accelerated idioventricular rhythm (AIVR) is a wide complex rhythm with a heart rate between 50 and 120 beats/min. Typically, AIVR is an arrhythmia observed after reperfusion therapy of acute myocardial infarction. AIVR results from enhanced automaticity of an abnormal ectopic ventricular focus. This focus discharges earlier than the sinus node. AIVR is generally well tolerated and requires no therapy. If the rhythm is associated with hemodynamic compromise, antiarrhythmic agents are contraindicated. Increasing discharges from the sinus node at a rate faster than the ectopic focus will overcome the AIVR. Therefore, atropine or atrial pacing should be considered. AIVR is not associated with an increased risk for the development of ventricular fibrillation or increased mortality.

Premature Ventricular Complexes

Premature ventricular complexes (PVCs) are frequently asymptomatic, but occasionally patients note palpitations that can be ascribed to the PVCs. Reassurance is generally the treatment of choice. However, PVCs or an increased frequency of PVCs may be a marker for significant underlying conditions such as CAD, congestive heart failure, DCM, or hypertrophic cardiomyopathy, infiltrative conditions, sarcoidosis, and arrhythmogenic RV dysplasia. A normal echocardiogram and a negative stress imaging study should be obtained before reassurance is given that the PVCs are benign. In the symptomatic patient, a clear explanation of the hemodynamic consequences of PVCs should be discussed. Exercise should be encouraged. Some patients respond to a magnesium supplement. For those few individuals who remain symptomatic, a β-blocker is the drug of choice. For patients whose symptoms persist and who have frequent PVCs (>2 to 3 per minute), radiofrequency ablation can be considered. However, mapping can be performed only if the patient has frequent PVCs during the procedure, and thus the use of this approach is limited.

FUTURE DIRECTIONS

Preventing VT is a complex undertaking. Addressing the risk factors underlying CAD, and prompt treatment of acute MI will certainly decrease the numbers of future patients presenting with VT. Techniques with good positive and negative predictive values to identify those at high risk for VT still need development. T-wave alternans may be such a tool. However, the predictive values of such tools have not yet been determined prospectively for large populations. The impact of stem cell research and its effects on the VT substrate will require careful evaluation because it is possible that "new" myocardial cells may be arrhythmogenic. Finally, developments in pharmacogenetics may improve the likelihood of identifying patient populations who would benefit from certain antiarrhythmic agents.

REFERENCES

The Antiarrhythmics versus Implantable Defibrillators (AVID) Investigators. A comparison of antiarrhythmic-drug therapy with implantable defibrillators in patients resuscitated from near-fatal ventricular arrhythmias. *N Engl J Med* 1997;337:1576–1583.

Bardy G. Sudden cardiac death in Heart Failure Trial (SCD-HeFT). Late Breaking Clinical Trials, American College of Cardiology 2004.

Boutitie F, Boissel J-P, Connolly SJ, et al, and the EMIAT and CAMIAT Investigators. Amiodarone Interaction with β-blockers: Analysis of the merged EMIAT (European Myocardial Infarct Amiodarone Trial) and CAMIAT (Canadian Amiodarone Myocardial Infarction Trial) databases. *Circulation* 1999;99:2268–2275.

Buxton AE, Lee KL, Fisher JD, et al. A randomized study of the prevention of sudden death in patients with coronary artery disease. Multicenter Unsustained Tachycardia Trial Investigators. *N Engl J Med* 1999;341:1882–1890.

Maron BJ, Shen WK, Link MS, et al. Efficacy of implantable cardioverter-defibrillators for the prevention of sudden death in patients with hypertrophic cardiomyopathy. *N Engl J Med* 2000;342:365–373.

Moss AJ, Hall WJ, Cannom DS, et al, for the Multicenter Automatic Defibrillator Implantation Trial Investigators. Improved survival with an implanted defibrillator in patients with coronary disease at high risk for ventricular arrhythmia. *N Engl J Med* 1996;335:1933–1940.

Moss AJ, Zareba W, Hall WJ, et al. Prophylactic implantation of a defibrillator in patients with myocardial infarction and reduced ejection fraction. *N Engl J Med* 2002;346:877–883.

Chapter 21

Bradyarrhythmias

Bryon E. Rubery and William E. Sanders, Jr

The **normal resting heart rate** has been arbitrarily defined as 60 to 100 beats/min, and **bradycardia** as a rate less than 60 beats/min. It should be noted that some otherwise healthy individuals have resting heart rates less than 60 beats/min. The greatest variation is found in athletes, who commonly have resting heart rates less than 50 beats/min, primarily from increased parasympathetic tone and decreased basal sympathetic output (Fig. 21-1).

In certain cases, distinguishing between physiologic and pathologic bradycardia is difficult, and true pathology requires correlation of symptoms with the observed rhythm. Neurologic symptoms attributable to pathologic bradycardia include syncope and near-syncope, dizziness, lightheadedness, and confusion, which all result from impaired cerebral perfusion. Fatigue, exercise intolerance, and even congestive failure may occur if cardiac output is significantly compromised.

ETIOLOGY AND PATHOGENESIS

Major components of the conduction system of the heart include the sinus node, the atrioventricular (AV) node, the bundle of His, and the right and left bundle branches. Bradycardia is caused by conditions that alter the automaticity of the sinus node or AV nodal conduction or that interfere with propagation of electrical impulses through the lower conduction system.

Neurally induced bradycardia can result from alternating sympathetic or parasympathetic tone through an effect on the sinus or AV nodes, which are innervated by both nervous systems. Increased parasympathetic tone, mediated by the vagus nerve, decreases automaticity of the sinus node and slows conduction through the AV node. Increased sympathetic tone has the opposite effects; baseline heart rate reflects the balance between these two influences. A variety of physiologic and pathologic states, as well as drugs, affect this balance. Vagal tone is physiologically increased during sleep and more pronounced in athletes. Vomiting, coughing, micturition, defecation, and pressure on the carotid sinus also increase vagal tone, which is considered to be physiologic or pathologic depending on the circumstances. Obstructive sleep apnea increases vagal tone, and bradycardia (sometimes extreme) may occur during apneic episodes.

Many commonly prescribed drugs produce bradycardia. Digoxin increases vagotonic effects at the sinus and AV nodes, whereas clonidine reduces sympathetic tone. β-Blockers have some direct antiarrhythmic effects from membrane-stabilizing properties but act primarily by preventing adrenergic stimulation of β receptors. Calcium channel blockers directly influence the sinus and AV nodes by altering the shape of the action potential. Among antiarrhythmic drugs, sotalol and amiodarone are most likely to produce clinically significant bradycardia. Sotalol has significant β-blocking activity, and amiodarone exhibits both β-blocking and calcium channel–blocking activity. Type I antiarrhythmic drugs generally do not have a significant effect on nondiseased nodal tissue, but they can reduce automaticity and increase block in patients with preexisting conduction system disease.

Other conditions affecting the conduction system include metabolic (hypothyroidism, hypothermia, hypokalemia, and hyperkalemia) and neurologic conditions (partial seizures and increased intracranial pressure).

DIFFERENTIAL DIAGNOSIS
Sinus Node Dysfunction

Sinus node dysfunction, or "sick sinus syndrome," is a common cause of bradycardia that increases in prevalence with age. Sinus node function may be altered by extrinsic causes, such as drugs and vagal tone, or intrinsic factors, such

Figure 21-1

Sinus Bradycardia

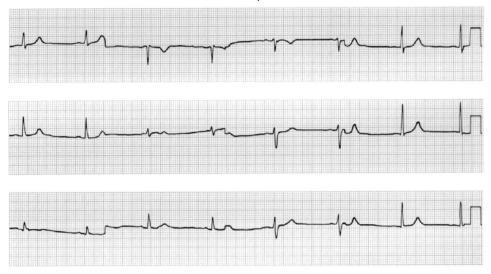

Sinus bradycardia, rate 45. Although rate limits for normal sinus rhythm are traditionally given as 60 to 100/minute, sinus rates below 60 are frequently normal. Physical conditioning, for example, increases stroke volume and usually decreases resting heart rate. Many normal athletes have low resting heart rates, often sinus bradycardia with rates in the 50s and even 40s. This ECG was recorded in a healthy 23-year-old and is a normal variant.

as ischemia or slowly progressive nodal tissue fibrosis. Manifestations of sinus node disease include persistent, inappropriate sinus bradycardia, intermittent sinus arrest, and supraventricular tachyarrhythmias alternating with sinus bradycardia or asystole (the tachy–brady syndrome). Mechanisms include decreased automaticity of sinus nodal tissue and sinoatrial (SA) exit block. In SA exit block, rhythmic depolarization continues to occur, but the impulse is delayed or blocked in the perinodal tissue. Diagnosis by surface ECG is difficult, because external leads do not directly record activity within the sinus node. A P wave is produced only if the sinus nodal impulse succeeds in depolarizing the atria. Intracardiac catheter recordings have confirmed the existence of SA block (as well as the mechanisms responsible for various arrhythmias that represent normal variants; Fig. 21-2).

Atrioventricular Block

First-degree AV block is abnormal prolongation of the PR interval to more than 200 ms. Despite the nomenclature, no "block" occurs; all atrial beats are conducted to the ventricles

(Fig. 21-3). Causes include drug effects, transient ischemia of the AV node, altered conduction after catheter ablation procedures, and its presence in the absence of a defined cause. First-degree AV block is often found in conjunction with higher grades of block, but it does not by itself produce bradycardia. In the absence of organic heart disease, isolated first-degree AV block has a benign prognosis, with no increased risk of progression to higher degrees of block. In rare cases, marked first-degree AV block may produce a pseudopacemaker syndrome from loss of AV synchrony. Marked prolongation of the PR interval delays the ventricular contraction until just before the subsequent atrial contraction, preventing complete atrial and ventricular filling. This results in decreased cardiac output, which corresponds to an increased pulmonary capillary wedge pressure.

In second-degree AV block, intermittent AV conduction occurs, resulting in a combination of conducted and nonconducted beats. Two classic types of second-degree AV block exist: Mobitz type I (Wenckebach's) and type II (Fig. 21-3). **Mobitz type I block** is characterized by pro-

Figure 21-2

Supraventricular Rhythms

A. Normal sinus rhythm

Impulses originate at SA node at normal rate

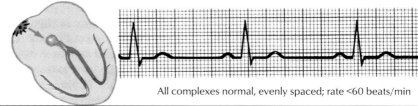

All complexes evenly spaced; rate 60 to 100 beats/min

B. Sinus bradycardia

Impulses originate at SA node at slow rate

All complexes normal, evenly spaced; rate <60 beats/min

C. Sinus tachycardia

Impulses originate at SA node at rapid rate

All complexes normal, evenly spaced; rate >100 beats/min

D. Sinus arrhythmia

Impulses originate at SA node at varying rate

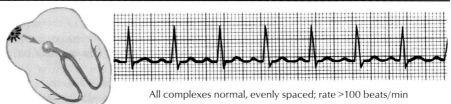

All complexes normal but rhythmically irregular; longest PP or RR interval exceeds shortest by 0.16 seconds or more

E. Nonsinus atrial rhythm

Impulses originate low in atrium; travel retrograde as well as distally

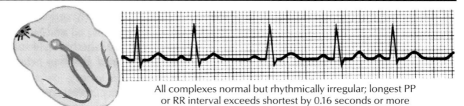

Lead II

P waves inverted in leads II, III, and aVF

F. Wandering atrial pacemaker

Impulses originate from varying points in atria

Variation in P-wave contour, PR interval, PP, and thus RR intervals

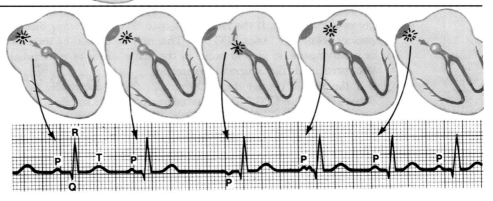

Figure 21-3
Atrioventricular Conduction Variations

Fixed but prolonged PR interval

First-degree AV block

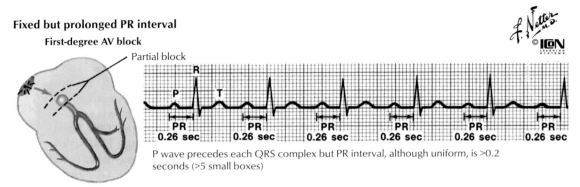

P wave precedes each QRS complex but PR interval, although uniform, is >0.2 seconds (>5 small boxes)

Progressive lengthing of PR interval with intermittent dropped beats

Second-degree AV block: Mobitz I (Wenckebach)

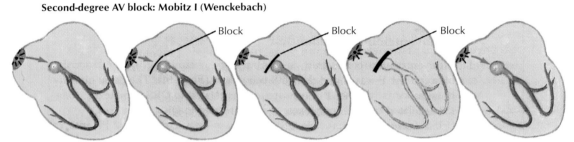

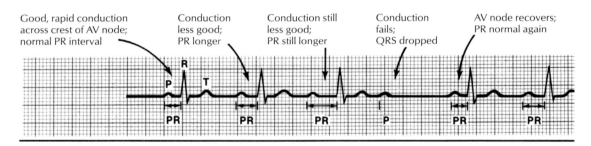

Good, rapid conduction across crest of AV node; normal PR interval

Conduction less good; PR longer

Conduction still less good; PR still longer

Conduction fails; QRS dropped

AV node recovers; PR normal again

Sudden dropped QRS without prior PR lengthing

Second-degree AV block: Mobitz II (non-Wenckebach)

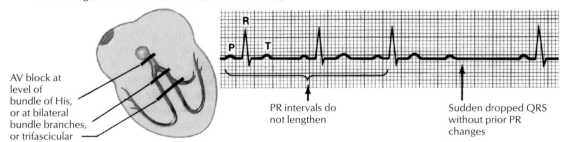

AV block at level of bundle of His, or at bilateral bundle branches, or trifascicular

PR intervals do not lengthen

Sudden dropped QRS without prior PR changes

Figure 21-4   Atrioventricular Conduction Variations

No relation between P waves and QRS complexes: QRS rate slower than P rate

Third-degree (complete) AV block

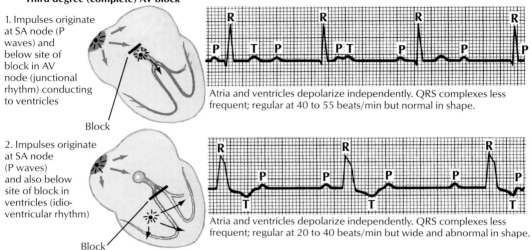

1. Impulses originate at SA node (P waves) and below site of block in AV node (junctional rhythm) conducting to ventricles

Block

Atria and ventricles depolarize independently. QRS complexes less frequent; regular at 40 to 55 beats/min but normal in shape.

2. Impulses originate at SA node (P waves) and also below site of block in ventricles (idioventricular rhythm)

Block

Atria and ventricles depolarize independently. QRS complexes less frequent; regular at 20 to 40 beats/min but wide and abnormal in shape.

Features of two types of atrioventricular block

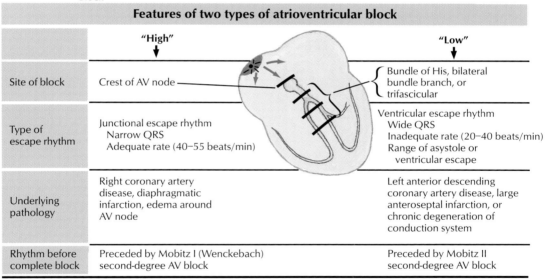

	"High" ↓	"Low" ↓
Site of block	Crest of AV node	Bundle of His, bilateral bundle branch, or trifascicular

Type of escape rhythm	Junctional escape rhythm
	  Narrow QRS
	  Adequate rate (40–55 beats/min)
		Ventricular escape rhythm
		  Wide QRS
		  Inadequate rate (20–40 beats/min)
		  Range of asystole or
		    ventricular escape

Underlying pathology	Right coronary artery disease, diaphragmatic infarction, edema around AV node	Left anterior descending coronary artery disease, large anteroseptal infarction, or chronic degeneration of conduction system
Rhythm before complete block	Preceded by Mobitz I (Wenckebach) second-degree AV block	Preceded by Mobitz II second-degree AV block

No relation between P waves and QRS complexes: QRS rate faster than P rate

AV dissociation

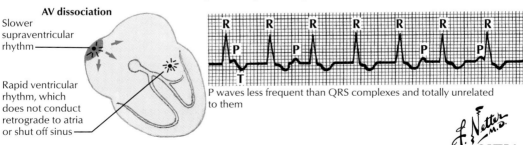

Slower supraventricular rhythm

Rapid ventricular rhythm, which does not conduct retrograde to atria or shut off sinus

P waves less frequent than QRS complexes and totally unrelated to them

gressive lengthening of the PR interval until a P wave fails to conduct, resulting in a "dropped" beat. This pattern strongly suggests that the AV node is the site of block, although some exceptions exist. **Mobitz type II block** demonstrates an "all-or-none" phenomenon; conducted beats maintain a constant PR interval, with no warning before sudden loss of conduction. This pattern indicates disease in the His-Purkinje system, or infranodal block.

The distinction is important, because type II block commonly progresses to complete heart block, whereas type I rarely does. Type I block is also more likely to be transient and due to reversible causes such as drugs, metabolic disturbances, or increased vagal tone. **Advanced AV block** occurs when two or more consecutive P waves are blocked. Advanced AV block can occur with either type I or type II block and may precede progression to complete heart block. Acute inferior myocardial infarction frequently produces bradyarrhythmias, including type I AV block. Increased vagal tone is the main cause, but because the AV node is supplied by the right coronary artery in 90% of people, AV nodal ischemia can also have this effect. Collateral flow from the left coronary circulation usually prevents infarction of the AV node, so progression to complete heart block is rare, or if it occurs, it is usually transient. Anterior myocardial infarction produces type II AV block via necrosis of the interventricular septum. Anterior myocardial infarction has a much higher incidence of progression to complete, often permanent, heart block.

Third-degree AV block, or **complete heart block**, is diagnosed when no atrial impulses are conducted to the ventricles (Fig. 21-4). In this case, AV dissociation occurs as evidenced on the surface ECG by regular P-P and R-R intervals but a continually changing PR interval. The QRS complex may be narrow or wide, depending on the level of the block and the location of the escape pacemaker. Block at the AV node level may produce an escape pacemaker in the bundle of His, which tends to result in escape rhythms in the range of 40 to 55 beats/min, is partially responsive to sympathetic tone and is usually adequate to maintain cardiac output. Conversely, infranodal block results in an escape pacemaker distal to the His bundle, with an inherently unreliable escape rhythm less than 40 beats/min, potentially leading to life-threatening ventricular asystole.

Complete heart block may be congenital or acquired. Congenital heart block may result from grossly abnormal cardiac anatomy with resultant infranodal block, or from AV node dysfunction as a result of the neonatal lupus syndrome. Acquired causes include drug effects, age-related degeneration and fibrosis, ischemia and infarction, infiltrative diseases such as amyloidosis, sarcoidosis, and hemochromatosis, infectious diseases such as Lyme disease, syphilis, and viral myocarditis, and neuromuscular diseases including muscular dystrophy.

Neurocardiogenic Syncope

Carotid sinus hypersensitivity and vasovagal syncope are examples of neurally mediated syncope. In both, sudden excessive vagal tone leads to inappropriate bradycardia, and the cardioinhibitory response, which can include sinus bradycardia, sinus arrest, or AV block. The vasodepressor response results from sudden withdrawal of sympathetic tone, producing a greater than 50 mm Hg decrease in SBP. This can occur even in the absence of bradycardia. The carotid sinus is located on the internal carotid artery, just above the bifurcation of the common carotid. Gentle pressure on the carotid sinus produces a fairly pronounced physiologic increase in vagal tone, even in asymptomatic individuals; up to a 3-second sinus pause is considered normal, but a more pronounced pause (>3 seconds) is abnormal. In affected persons, simply turning the head may produce enough carotid sinus stimulation to result in syncope. Vasovagal syncope results in the same cardioinhibitory and vasodepressor responses but is initiated differently. An emotionally upsetting stimulus such as pain, fright, or the sight of blood triggers an initial increase in sympathetic discharge, leading to peripheral vasodilation and decreased venous return. Forceful ventricular contraction then stimulates cardiac mechanoreceptors, which initiate the neural reflexes mentioned above. The resultant combination of enhanced vagal tone and sudden sympathetic withdrawal causes abrupt hypotension and syncope.

Figure 21-5

AV Block

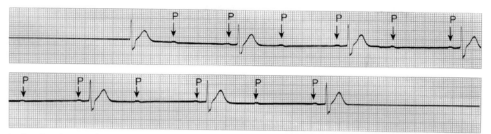

In the situation in which every other P wave is blocked, it is impossible to tell whether the PR interval is progressively increasing (since there is never more than one completed PR interval at a time). Thus, one cannot differentiate between Mobitz I and Mobitz II, and it is unclear whether the site of block is at the crest of the AV node or in the His–Purkinje system. If this differentiation is clinically vital, intracardiac electrophysiologic study is necessary.

DIAGNOSTIC APPROACH

Although invasive electrophysiology studies are useful in evaluating certain tachyarrhythmias, they are infrequently needed for bradyarrhythmias. In many cases, 12-lead ECG results are sufficient to make the diagnosis. When the suspected arrhythmia is intermittent, however, or correlation with symptoms is unclear, long-term recording is necessary. A Holter monitor provides continuous recording of two ECG leads for 24 to 48 hours. Holter monitoring is especially useful for patients with frequent symptoms or arrhythmias during sleep. For patients with less frequent symptoms, a 30-day event monitor is more appropriate. For very infrequent symptoms, an implantable loop recorder may be inserted under the skin of the chest, where it performs as an event monitor for up to 18 months. The patient or a family member activates this device with a magnet.

Interpretation of bradyarrhythmias on ECG is usually straightforward, because sinus node dysfunction and the various forms of AV block are easily recognized. One exception is second-degree AV block with a P:QRS ratio of 2:1 (Fig. 21-5). Conducted beats alternate with nonconducted beats, so progressive PR prolongation cannot be observed. In this situation, it is impossible to differentiate type I from type II block on a single ECG. A very long tracing may eventually demonstrate a 3:1 or greater conduction ratio to make the diagnosis. Certain autonomic maneuvers may also be performed. Carotid sinus massage worsens AV conduction in type I block

whereas atropine improves it. The opposite generally occurs in type II block, although exceptions exist (Fig. 21-6).

Sinoatrial block is also difficult to recognize on a surface ECG. First-degree SA block is never seen, because all impulses are transmitted to the atria. Third-degree SA block is indistinguishable from sinus arrest. Second-degree SA block produces intermittent sinus pauses. Surface ECG may provide clues to the mechanism. Second-degree SA type I block produces grouped beating, with progressively shortening P-P intervals before a sinus pause, which is less than twice the duration of the shortest P-P interval. Type II SA block has a more random distribution of sinus pauses, with pause duration being an exact multiple of the baseline P-P interval.

Complete heart block requires dissociation of P waves and QRS complexes. AV dissociation is not synonymous with AV block, however, because it is possible for a subsidiary pacemaker to capture the ventricles at a faster rate than that generated in the atria. An example is accelerated junctional rhythm without retrograde atrial conduction. While the ventricles are under the control of the junctional pacemaker, the sinus node continues to fire, resulting in the ECG pattern of AV dissociation. The sinus beats are not transmitted to the ventricles because the AV node is refractory to them. If the sinus rate becomes more rapid than the junctional rate, atrial capture resumes, proving that no block is present. For this reason, complete AV block may be diagnosed only when the atrial rate is faster than the ventricular rate.

Figure 21-6

Sinus Arrest and Sinus Block

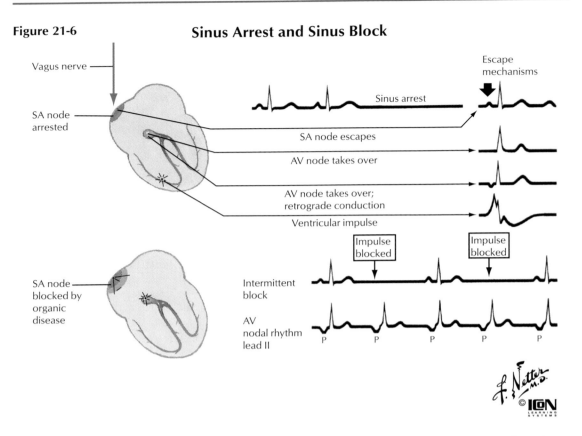

The diagnostic approach to syncope is discussed in chapter 22. For neurocardiogenic syncope, the best method is a careful history and physical examination. Prodromal symptoms and circumstances are especially useful in establishing the diagnosis of vasovagal syncope. Tilt-table testing and ambulatory monitoring may be performed when the history and physical are unrevealing. In patients with ischemic heart disease and syncope, electrophysiologic testing is often needed to rule out dangerous tachyarrhythmias, but in patients with structurally normal hearts the diagnostic yield is low. Further, even if abnormalities are found on provocative testing, it is not always possible to correlate these findings with the symptoms under evaluation. In patients at low risk for life-threatening arrhythmias, long-term ambulatory monitoring may be more useful than provocative testing.

MANAGEMENT AND THERAPY

The primary treatment for symptomatic bradycardias is cardiac pacing. Although medications may be useful in the acute setting, there is no place for long-term medical therapy of bradyarrhythmias. For acute bradycardias from increased vagal tone, atropine is most often used. Isoproterenol may be effective in some cases, but it must be used carefully because it may worsen ischemia and predispose to tachyarrhythmias. Theophylline has been used in sinus node dysfunction but is only marginally effective and limited by a narrow therapeutic index. Indications for permanent pacemaker implantation are discussed in chapter 26. Some conditions, such as inferior myocardial infarction, may require temporary but not permanent pacing.

Ideal treatment of neurocardiogenic syncope has not been established. Trials are studying the efficacy of permanent pacing, including the use of pacemaker algorithms designed specifically for this purpose. ß-blockers are the most effective agents available and prevent the initial sympathetic discharge thought to trigger the neural reflexes in vasovagal syncope. Fludrocortisone, midodrine, and increased dietary salt intake prevent hypovolemia and hypotension. Selective serotonin reuptake inhibitors show some promise, although the mechanism is not fully understood.

FUTURE DIRECTIONS

One of the challenges in the treatment of a patient with symptomatic bradycardia is defining the mechanism responsible for that patient's bradycardia and symptoms. As noted above, some patients with bradycardic syndromes will not experience resolution of symptoms simply with permanent pacing. In addition, modification of pacemaker properties may offer reduced morbidity and even reduced mortality. Some of these issues are addressed in chapter 26, and others are being addressed in ongoing studies on the use of new pacemaker modalities, in combination with pharmacologic therapy.

REFERENCES

Devinsky O. Bradycardia and asystole induced by partial seizures: A case report and literature review. *Neurology* 1997;48:1712–1714.

Gregoratos G, Abrams J, Epstein AE, et al. ACC/AHA/NASPE 2002 guideline update for implantation of cardiac pacemakers and antiarrhythmia devices: Summary article. A report of the American College of Cardiology/American Heart Association Task Force on Practice Guidelines (ACC/AHA/NASPE Committee to Update the 1998 Pacemaker Guidelines). *Circulation* 2002;106:2145–2161.

Gregoratos G, Cheitlin MD, Conill A, et al. ACC/AHA guidelines for implantation of cardiac pacemakers and antiarrhythmia devices: A report of the American College of Cardiology/American Heart Association Task Force on Practice Guidelines (Committee on Pacemaker Implantation). *J Am Coll Cardiol* 1998;31:1175–1209.

Kaushik V. Bradyarrhythmias, temporary and permanent pacing. *Crit Care Med* 2000;28:121–128.

Krahn AD. Use of an extended monitoring strategy in patients with problematic syncope. *Circulation* 1999; 99:406–410.

Mymin D. The natural history of primary first-degree atrioventricular heart block. *N Engl J Med* 1986;315: 1183–1187.

Oakley D. General cardiology: The athlete's heart. *Heart* 2001;86:722–726.

Sheldon R. Pacing to prevent vasovagal syncope. *Cardiol Clin* 2000;8:81–93.

Chapter 22
Cardiac Syncope

Richard G. Sheahan

Syncope is defined as a sudden loss of consciousness associated with an inability to maintain postural tone, followed by spontaneous recovery. Syncope accounts for about 3% of emergency room visits, and 1 to 6% of general hospital admissions. Episodes reoccur in a third of patients. Recurrences have a substantial and deleterious effect on lifestyle, sense of physical well-being, driving, and employment opportunities.

The etiology of syncope can be divided into three broad categories: cardiac, noncardiac, and unknown. In most studies, 75 to 85% of syncopal episodes, for which an etiology is determined, are cardiac in origin. Cardiovascular mechanisms of syncope include hypotension alone, hypotension with tachyarrhythmias, and hypotension with bradyarrhythmias. Hypoperfusion of the cerebral cortexes and the reticular activating system is the final common pathway for the majority of episodes. Interruption of cerebral blood flow for 8 to 10 seconds usually produces loss of consciousness. The severity of symptoms depends on a complex interaction between the hemodynamic consequences of the arrhythmia/hypotension and the underlying cardiac function. The occurrence of syncope during exercise requires urgent evaluation, as this may be the harbinger of severe coronary artery disease or aortic valve disease.

CLINICAL PRESENTATION

The reported symptoms that precede an episode of syncope can offer important diagnostic information. Symptoms such as nausea and vomiting may suggest vagal etiologies, whereas symptoms of shortness of breath, sweating, or chest pain suggest an ischemic etiology. Frequent palpitations may indicate the presence of an underlying arrhythmia. However, not uncommonly, there may be no symptoms that herald a syncopal episode. It is crucial to determine the circumstances of the episode and, specifically, what the patient was doing at the time of the episode. Table 22-1 shows a patient history checklist. Note that features including a prodrome with an aura, long dura-

tion of loss of consciousness, disorientation after the event, slow return to full consciousness, or jerking movements are suggestive of a seizure. Risk factors for coronary artery disease, including premature family history, hypertension, hyperlipidemia, diabetes mellitus, and smoking, should be considered. In some circumstances, psychiatric illnesses should be considered because a psychiatric diagnosis is ultimately made in more than 5% of syncopal patients.

DIFFERENTIAL DIAGNOSIS
Value of Testing in Syncope

Determining the etiology of syncope is frequently difficult and often frustrating. Episodes may be brief and infrequent, or syncope may never recur. The evaluation of the patient in this setting requires analysis of a complete and accurate history and physical examination. Critical positive findings on physical examination may include an ejection systolic murmur of aortic stenosis, or profound orthostatic hypotension. Frequently, a careful physical examination is within normal limits, so testing is required. The goal of testing is ideally to provide a symptom rhythm correlation.

Before determining an approach to further evaluation, it is necessary to understand the limitations and potential information of each test.

Electrocardiography

Frequently, the baseline ECG is normal. During baseline testing, findings of note may include bifascicular block with or without PR prolongation, Mobitz type II second-degree atrioventricular block, complete heart block, Wolff-Parkinson-White syndrome, long QT syndrome,

Table 22-1
Key Questions for the Patient With a History of Syncope

· Activities performed when the episode began
    Exercise
    Position changes
    Postmicturition
    Defecation
    Cough
· Time of day
· Medications
    Insulin
    Other prescription medications
    Over-the-counter medications
    Drugs
    Alcohol
    Time interval after taking medications/insulin
    New medications or changes in dosing of
      medications/insulin
· Any recent febrile illness
· Vomiting or diarrhea
· Anemia
· Recent fractures
· Recent air travel
· Recent trauma
· Near-drowning
· Sight of blood
· Looking upward
· Family history of sudden unexplained death even in
  remote cousins
· Information about the episode
    Presence of pallor, clamminess, or sweating
    Tonic-clonic activity
    Duration of the episode
    Time until patient awoke (from a witness)
    From witnesses: the time it took the patient to
      become fully alert and oriented
· Pulse rate
· Symptoms following the episode
    Palpitations
    Nausea
    Vomiting
    Chest pain
    Shortness of breath
    Sweating
· Pain related to injuries resulting from the syncopal
  episode

Brugada's syndrome, left ventricular hypertrophy suggestive of hypertrophic cardiomyopathy, tachyarrhythmia, acute or old myocardial infarction, and pulmonary embolism. Any of these findings will direct the initial evaluation.

An ECG obtained during an episode may be diagnostic. However, as most patients are asymptomatic after their episode, many will have a normal standard ECG.

Blood Tests

Routine complete blood count, electrolytes (especially potassium and magnesium), blood glucose, serial cardiac enzymes, serum therapeutic levels of medications including digoxin, serum and urine toxicology screen, and alcohol levels may be performed. In a healthy individual, these will be within normal limits.

Risk Factor Assessment for Coronary Artery Disease

If the patient has significant risk factors for coronary artery disease, an ischemic evaluation is needed. Ideally, an exercise imaging study should be performed, and if the study is positive or borderline positive, cardiac catheterization should be performed.

Echocardiography

An assessment of left ventricular ejection fraction including systolic and diastolic function, right ventricular function, valvular abnormalities, hypertrophy, and restrictive processes should be obtained. Prognosis has been closely linked to left ventricular ejection fraction. In a patient with syncope and evidence of a structural abnormality a diagnosis of ventricular tachycardia (see chapter 20) should be considered the cause of syncope until disproven. Although an echocardiogram may detect features consistent with diastolic dysfunction, it is less helpful in excluding an infiltrate process such as sarcoidosis.

Head-up Tilt-Table Test

The head-up tilt-table test is particularly helpful in confirming a diagnosis of neurocardiogenic syncope for patients in whom the exact prodrome and symptom complex are reproduced during the test, in association with hypotension, inappropriate bradycardia, or both. The addition of isoproterenol or nitroglycerin is often required to achieve a positive result. False-positive and false-negative results are common. Other limitations of head-up tilt-table testing include the poor specificity of high-dose isoproterenol protocols and the fact that the day-to-day reproducibility of a positive test is not 100%. Nonethelesss, head-up tilt-table testing can be very useful in identifying patients with a prominent bradycardia response, who may benefit from placement of a permanent pacemaker. An echocardiogram should be performed before a head-up tilt-table test to exclude left ventricular dysfunction, which carries a significantly greater mortality risk. Patients with a diagnosis of neurocardiogenic syncope have a benign prognosis.

Holter Monitoring

The goal of Holter monitoring is to provide a correlation between symptoms and cardiac rhythm. A 24- or 48-hour Holter monitoring is effective in patients who are experiencing symptoms several times a day. The unpredictable frequency of events with months to years separating episodes and the high remission rate limit the potential role of Holter monitoring. Studies that showed symptoms occurring with significant arrhythmias in only 2 to 4% of patients, asymptomatic arrhythmias in 13%, and symptoms without arrhythmia in 17% confirmed the low yield.

Event or Loop Recorders

The goal of longer-term monitoring is to provide a symptom rhythm correlation. The unpredictable frequency of events with months to years separating episodes and a high remission rate limit the potential role of prolonged external monitoring. Although keeping these monitors for 1 to 3 months increases the diagnostic yield, a diagnosis may not be made despite symptom recurrence because of device malfunction, patient noncompliance, or inability to activate the recorder. The current loop recorders have automated detection algorithms, which enhances arrhythmia detection and increases the likelihood of defining arrhythmias responsible for syncopal and presyncopal symptoms.

Cardiac Catheterization

Information that can be obtained from cardiac catheterization, in addition to the presence or absence of flow-limiting coronary artery disease, includes left ventricular end diastolic pressure,

intracavity gradients, valvular gradients, pulmonary artery pressure, anomalous origin of the coronary arteries, or myocardial bridging. All are potentially important in the evaluation of syncope.

Electrophysiology Study

An electrophysiology study can assess for the presence and mechanism of tachycardia (either supraventricular or ventricular), atrioventricular node function, and sinus node function. For patients with inducible arrhythmias, a radiofrequency ablation may be performed simultaneously. However, the diagnostic yield in patients without palpitations and a normal left ventricular function is low. In patients with an ischemic cardiomyopathy, an electrophysiology study can detect those patients who are at a higher risk for subsequent ventricular tachyarrhythmias. An electrophysiology study in patients with dilated cardiomyopathy is less helpful in distinguishing those patients who are at a high risk for sudden cardiac death (see chapter 20). In the event that the EF is less than 35%, an ICD should be placed and an EP study is not required.

Signal-Averaged Electrocardiogram and T-Wave Alternans

Signal-averaged electrocardiography has been proposed as a means to predict which patients are at risk for sudden cardiac death. Although signal-averaged electrocardiogram has a very high negative predictive value, its positive predictive value is very low. For this reason, signal-averaged electrocardiograms have little use in the evaluation of syncope. T-wave alternans is a very promising technology and is being tested prospectively in a substudy of the Sudden Cardiac Death in Heart Failure Trial and the Alternans Before Cardioverter Defibrillator Trial (ABCD). Preliminary reports, which need to be confirmed in larger studies, suggest that T-wave alternans analysis may be the first useful noninvasive test in patients with syncope and ventricular arrhythmias.

Magnetic Resonance Imaging

Magnetic resonance imaging technology is useful in confirming a diagnosis of arrhythmogenic right ventricular cardiomyopathy (also known as "arrhythmogenic right ventricular dysplasia"; see chapter 20) and anomalous origin of the coronary arteries. In the future, magnetic resonance imaging will likely have a more significant role in the diagnosis of other infiltrative cardiomyopathies.

Insertable Loop Recorders

The goal of longer-term monitoring is to correlate symptoms with a rhythm. The unpredictable frequency of events with months to years separating episodes and a high remission rate limit the potential of prolonged external monitoring. For this reason, insertable (implantable) loop recorders have been developed and are currently being studied in patients with syncope but infrequent symptoms. Preliminary studies indicate that, on average, the duration of monitoring necessary to make a diagnosis is greater than 4 months. The current insertable loop recorders have both patient-activated and automatic detection algorithms that enhance arrhythmia detection, particularly in patients who have difficulty activating the device. The use of insertable loop recorders is indicated in patients with infrequent but recurring syncopal episodes.

Procainamide Provocative Test

In patients with a family history of Brugada's syndrome or in whom Brugada's syndrome is suspected, an IV procainamide infusion of 10 mg/kg, should be infused over 10 minutes. A test is considered positive with a negative baseline ECG when the J-wave absolute amplitude is greater than 2 mm in lead V_1 and/or V_2 and/or V_3 with or without right bundle branch block. Monitoring until the ECG returns to baseline is recommended. Serious ventricular arrhythmias may occur during the procainamide infusion (due to QT prolongation), requiring immediate discontinuation. An isoproterenol infusion may be needed to treat the arrhythmias.

DIAGNOSTIC APPROACH

Table 22-2 highlights a diagnostic approach and Figures 22-1 and 22-2 provide a flow diagram for the diagnostic strategy. In patients for whom a diagnosis is made, a history including eyewitness accounts, risk factor assessment and family history of sudden cardiac death, and a thorough physical examination provide the diag-

Table 22-2
Evaluation of a Patient With Syncope

- History and physical examination
    - Family history of sudden death
    - Risk factor assessment for coronary artery disease
    - Medications
    - Blood pressure both arms, lying and standing
- Laboratory: may include complete blood count, electrolytes, blood glucose, serial cardiac enzymes, thyroid-stimulating hormone, digoxin, blood and urine drug screen and alcohol levels
- Electrocardiogram: baseline and during event
- Carotid sinus massage
- Echocardiogram: to document cardiac function and rule out valvular abnormality and cardiomyopathy
- Ischemic evaluation: including stress test with imaging and/or cardiac catheterization
- Ambulatory Holter monitoring
- Head-up tilt-table test
- Patient-activated monitoring device: may include event, loop, or insertable loop recorder
- Procainamide provocative test
- Electrophysiology study

With permission from Sheahan RG. Syncope and arrhythmias: Role of the electrophysiological study. *Am J Med Sci* 2001;322:37–43; and Sheahan RG. *Cardiac Arrhythmias.* Runge MS, Greganti MA, eds. ICON Publishers; 2003.

nosis in 50 to 80%. Confirmatory tests including appropriate therapy should be performed.

If the confirmatory test is negative, routine laboratory tests should be performed. If abnormal tests are detected (e.g., profound anemia or hypoglycemia), these should be corrected.

Step 1

All patients presenting with syncope should have an ECG (Figs. 22-1 and 22-2). Although the initial assessment and evaluation may provide the diagnosis, life-threatening abnormalities may coexist that can be detected on ECG. Young patients presenting with syncope may have a plausible explanation for their syncopal episode. However, one should not accept a plausible explanation in a patient with an abnormal ECG. Further evaluation is always indicated in this case.

If the ECG is abnormal, confirmatory testing and appropriate therapy should be provided. In the patient with a normal ECG but positive risk

Figure 22-1 **Cardiac Syncope: Four-Step Decision Strategy**

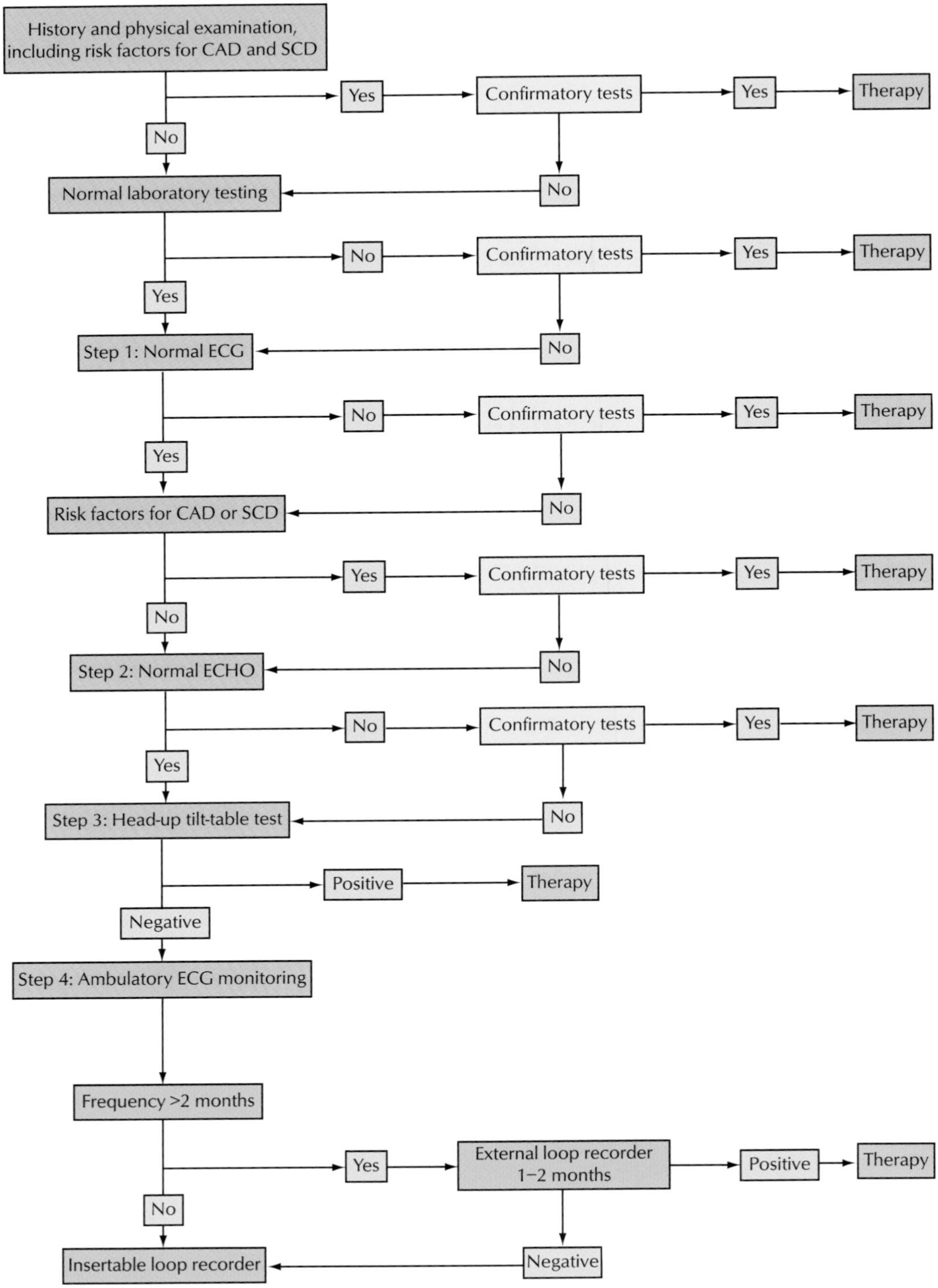

Figure 22-2

Syncope: Four-Step Management Approach

Step 1: Electrocardiogram

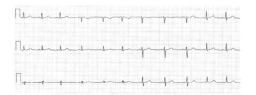

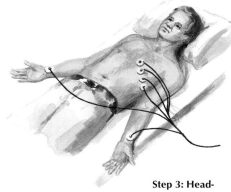

All patients with syncope should undergo electro-cardiography. If ECG abnormal, confirmatory testing and appropriate therapy should be instituted.

Step 2: Echocardiography

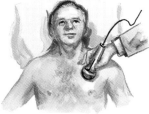

Step 3: Head-up tilt- table test

Should be considered if steps 1 and 2 are negative

In most patients without a diagnosis, a structural evaluation with echo-cardiograph is required.

Step 4: Monitoring for symptom–rhythm correlation

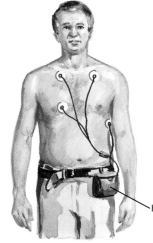

Holter monitor

Positive neurocardiogenic tilt-table test shows drop in BP and heart rate.

Normal tilt-table test shows maintenance of normal BP and heart rate.

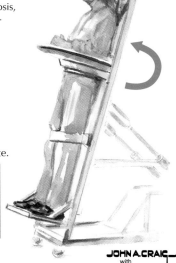

JOHN A. CRAIG—AD
with
D. Mascaro
© ICN

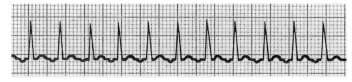

Ambulatory monitoring recommended for patients with negative evaluation; Duration of monitoring dependent on frequency of episodes; For daily symptoms, 48-hour monitor adequate

factors for coronary artery disease or sudden cardiac death, appropriate stress testing with imaging or provocative testing should be considered.

Step 2

In most patients without a diagnosis, a structural evaluation with an echocardiogram is required. Structural abnormalities must be excluded. These include left ventricular dysfunction, hypertrophic cardiomyopathy, right ventricular dysplasia, segmental wall abnormalities, moderate to severe valvular abnormalities, intracardiac tumors, and coronary artery abnormalities associated with Kawasaki disease. Frequently, the echocardiogram is within normal limits. In the event of abnormal findings, appropriate tests should be performed to confirm the diagnosis.

Step 3

A head-up tilt-table test should be considered for patients with a negative evaluation in steps 1 and 2. The tilt-table test helps correlate symptoms with a rhythm. It can also frequently be used to reassure the patient if symptoms are reproduced in association with a benign rhythm abnormality.

Step 4

A symptom and rhythm correlation is the gold standard for diagnosing patients with syncope. Ambulatory ECG monitoring is recommended for patients with a negative evaluation. The type of monitoring depends on the frequency and duration of the episode and the patient's ability to tolerate and activate the recording devices. For patients with episodes on most days, a 48-hour Holter monitor may be appropriate and should detect the episode.

For patients with two or more episodes a month, an external event or loop recorder is appropriate. Over 2 to 3 months, provided the patient stays motivated, an episode should be recorded.

In patients with fewer than two episodes per month, or where an external loop recorder has been unsuccessful in recording the arrhythmia, an insertable loop recorder should be implanted. The patient can activate this device, or the device can be automatically triggered by tachyarrhythmic or bradyarrhythmic events. The device may record multiple episodes. Batteries may function up to 18 months.

FUTURE DIRECTIONS

Improved awareness of potentially lethal ECG findings will improve the management of patients at risk. Persistence is crucial to the evaluation and diagnosis of unexplained syncope. Many patients with a negative evaluation have no further syncopal episodes. However, more have recurrent episodes. The understanding and evaluation of the autonomic system is incomplete and requires more research and development of more sophisticated evaluation techniques. A multidisciplinary approach to syncope may be needed, which should include a psychological evaluation and social worker support. Finally, syncope that is not neurocardiogenic in etiology is associated with an increased mortality. The cause of syncope should always be sought.

REFERENCES

Sheahan RG. Syncope and arrhythmias: Role of the electrophysiology study. *Am J Med Sci* 2001:322:37–43.

Soteriades ES, Evans JC, Larson MG, et al. Incidence and prognosis of syncope. *N Engl J Med* 2002;347:878–885.

Wilde AAM, Antzelevitch C, Borggrefe M, et al. Proposed diagnostic criteria for the Brugada syndrome: Consensus Report. *Circulation* 2002;106:2514–2519.

Chapter 23

Sudden Cardiac Death

Jeff P. Steinhoff, Sanjeev Shah, and Richard G. Sheahan

Sudden cardiac death (SCD) is defined as any death from a cardiac cause occurring within an hour of symptom onset. SCD occurs in 300,000 to 450,000 individuals in the United States annually. SCD has many potential etiologies (Table 23-1). Coronary artery disease and its sequelae (acute ischemia, or prior infarction with an arrhythmogenic scar) are responsible for up to 80% of fatal arrhythmias. Other common etiologies include cardiomyopathy (dilated, infiltrative, or hypertrophic), valvular heart disease, myocarditis, and congenital heart disease. Acute myocardial infarction (MI) is considered the most common inciting event for fatal arrhythmias; other mechanisms, including adverse stressors, have been identified (e.g., physiologic, metabolic, neurochemical, toxic, pharmacologic).

ETIOLOGY AND PATHOGENESIS

The pathogenic electrical event leading to SCD is most likely ventricular tachycardia (VT), followed by ventricular fibrillation (VF) and eventual asystole (Fig. 23-1). One registry found that 75% of cardiac arrests involved VF, with 20% involving asystole and 5% involving pulseless electrical activity. Of course, the inciting arrhythmia (VT) may no longer be present when rescue personnel record the rhythm in a resuscitation attempt. Therefore, much current research is focused on identifying the earliest warning signs for SCD.

Acute Myocardial Infarction

It is thought that MI causes fatal arrhythmias by two distinct mechanisms. The first is VT or VF in the setting of acute ischemia. The second is related to the propensity of islands of surviving myocardial tissue in the myocardial scars to act as foci for the initiation and/or maintenance of ventricular arrhythmias, including VT (see chapter 20). One report showed 60% of deaths associated with acute MI occurred within the first hour and were attributable to a ventricular arrhythmia, particularly VF. The incidence of stable and unstable ventricular rhythms is high in the immediate postinfarction period, with a reported 3 to 39% incidence of VT and a 4 to 20% incidence of VF in longitudinal studies of MI survivors. These studies were conducted primarily in the pre-reperfusion era. Today, because a greater number of MI survivors have received pharmacologic or percutaneous revascularization, it is predicted that postinfarction ventricular arrhythmias may correlate better with overall residual left ventricular (LV) function than with ventricular scars. A meta-analysis of several non–ST-elevation MI trials found the risk of sustained or unstable ventricular arrhythmias

Table 23-1
Etiologies of Sudden Cardiac Death

· Structurally Normal LV Function
    Brugada syndrome
    Long QT syndrome: genetic; acquired
    Commotio cordis
· Structurally Normal LV Function With Ischemia
    Coronary artery disease: injury; tissue hypoxia
    Coronary embolism
    Coronary spasm
· Structurally Abnormal LV Function or Anatomy
    LV hypertrophy
    Cardiomyopathy (dialated alcoholic, hypertensive, or hypertrophic)
    Prior MI (scar)
    Coronary artery anomalies
    Kawasaki disease
    Arrhythmogenic right ventricular dysplasia
    Pre-excitation syndrome, Wolff-Parkinson-White syndrome
    Myocarditis
    Sarcoidosis
    Chagas' disease
    Complete heart block
    Valvular disease
    Congenital heart disease: tetralogy of Fallot; transposition of the arteries; coarctation of the aorta; Ebstein's anomaly; congenitally corrected transposition of the arteries

LV indicates left ventricular; MI, myocardial infarction.

Figure 23-1

Sudden Cardiac Death

Potential etiologies

Mechanism

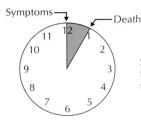

Symptoms — Death

Sudden cardiac death (SCD) defined as any death from a cardiac cause occurring within 1 hour of symptom onset

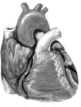

Ischemic heart disease

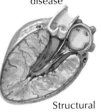

Structural cardiac abnormalities

Molecular or genetic abnormalities

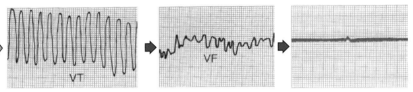

The pathogenic electrical event leading to sudden cardiac death is likely ventricular tachycardia (VT) followed by ventricular fibrillation (VF) and eventually asystole

Ischemic heart disease and SCD

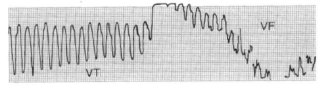

Patients with history of VT–VF episodes or those resuscitated from SCD, especially those with nonsustained VT, have high risk of fatal arrhythmia

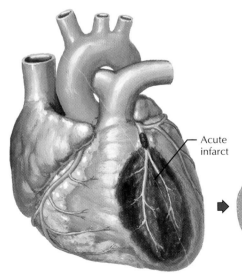

Acute infarct

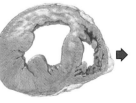

Healed infarct

LVEF <35%

Reduced left ventricular function

Myocardial infarction causes fatal arrhythmias by two distinct mechanisms—the first is VT or VF in ischemic setting (acute MI). The second is propensity of myocardial scars to act as foci for initiation of fatal arrhythmias. CAD accounts for 80% of fatal arrhythmias.

Patients with reduced LV function after MI (LVEF, 35%) are at high risk for fatal arrhythmias

F. Netter M.D.
JOHN A. CRAIG—MD
with E. Hatton
© ICN

(VT/VF) to be 2.1% during the initial hospital admission. Patients with VT and VF had the highest mortality rate (>60%), followed by patients with VF only (>45%), followed by patients with VT only (>30%). During follow-up, patients with peri-infarct VT/VF have a higher subsequent mortality rate compared with patients with an MI without ventricular arrhythmias. The patients in the Global Utilization of Streptokinase and Tissue Plasminogen Activator for Occluded Coronary Arteries Trial, which studied fibrinolytic therapies for ST-elevation MI, demonstrated higher incidences of arrhythmias, specifically, 3.5% for VT, 4.0% for VF, and 2.6% for VT/VF. The rates for in-hospital mortality and 1-year mortality postdischarge were higher among patients with VT and VT/VF than among patients without these arrhythmias, even excluding those in cardiogenic shock. Even patients with VT within the first 48 hours had a higher in-hospital mortality rate.

Ischemic Cardiomyopathy

Patients with resuscitated SCD, nonsustained VT, or reduced LV function after MI are at highest risk for fatal arrhythmias. A prior episode of VT/VF is predictive of a recurrent event, as observed in the Antiarrhythmics Versus Implantable Defibrillators (AVID) Trial. AVID studied patients with an ejection fraction (EF) below 40% (mean, 32%) who were resuscitated from SCD and then randomized to treatment with an implantable cardiac defibrillator (ICD) or pharmacologic therapy of amiodarone or sotalol. A 39% relative reduction in death was observed in patients who received an ICD compared with pharmacologic therapy, with an absolute reduction in the mortality rate of 7%.

In patients with low EFs, nonsustained VT is also predictive of SCD (see also chapter 20). The Multicenter Automatic Defibrillator Implantation Trial showed a 54% reduction in mortality rate in high-risk patients [LVEF <35%, nonsustained VT (3–30 beats), and inducible, but nonsuppressible VT during electrophysiology study] who received an ICD versus those who received conventional antiarrhythmic therapy. This finding was confirmed in the Multicenter Unsustained Tachycardia Trial Investigation, which enrolled patients with nonsustained VT on telemetry and an EF of less than 40%. All patients underwent programmed stimulation (an electrophysiology study), and patients with inducible VT were randomized to either ICD or antiarrhythmic therapy. The patients who received an ICD had better outcomes than did those who were treated with antiarrhythmic agents or those who had a negative electrophysiology study.

Following MI, the presence of a low EF alone is a powerful predictor of SCD. The second Multicenter Automatic Defibrillator Implantation Trial showed a 39% reduction in mortality rate in patients with an EF below 30% (mean EF ~23%) in whom an ICD was implanted; absolute reduction in mortality rate was 5.6%. Optimal pharmacologic therapy for reduced LV function included (as tolerated) β-blockers, angiotensin-converting enzyme inhibitor/angiotensin-receptor blocker, aspirin, and, where appropriate, lipid-lowering agents. A common misconception is that the prognosis in patients with "correctable" causes of SCD is more benign. The AVID registry of more than 4000 patients showed that "correctable" causes of SCD (acute MI, electrolyte imbalance, cocaine or other drug use, or antiarrhythmic drug–induced) carried a 17.8% mortality rate at 16.9 ± 11.5 months of follow-up.

Nonischemic Cardiomyopathy

Sudden cardiac death is also a common occurrence in individuals with structurally abnormal hearts, in the absence of coronary artery disease. This heterogeneous group accounts for 10 to 15% of SCD. The underlying etiologies are varied. Results of studies on the most appropriate therapy for this group are less clear than they are for post-MI patients. It is reported that between 1 and 25% of patients are successfully resuscitated after SCD, depending on where the patient was when SCD occurred and the availability of external cardiac defibrillators. SCD is the major cause of death in patients with nonischemic cardiomyopathy, accounting for up to 72% of deaths in some studies. Most of the fatal arrhythmias are thought to be tachyarrhythmias, mainly monomorphic VT and polymorphic VT/VF. The primary mechanism of polymorphic VT/VF is unknown. Secondary causes include electrolyte abnormalities, often from diuretics, and proarrhythmic effects of medications. Atrial arrhythmias are also common in this group, and therapies directed at suppressing atrial arrhythmias may increase the likelihood of VT. A particular type of monomorphic VT (see chapter 20) from bundle branch reentry is characteristic of nonischemic cardiomyopathy. In bundle branch reentry, a "macro" reentrant circuit involving both bundles, the Purkinje system, and the myocardium can be documented. Preliminary results support the prophylactic use of an ICD in patients with dilated cardiomyopathy and an EF less than 35%.

SYMPTOMS AND RISK OF SUDDEN CARDIAC DEATH

Although mortality increases with decreasing EF and deteriorating New York Heart Association class, the risk of SCD is paradoxically reversed (Table 23-2). In other words, the patients with stable and well-compensated congestive heart failure have a lower overall risk of death, but the deaths in these patients are usually sudden. A meta-analysis pooling patients with nonischemic cardiomyopathy and patients with ischemic cardiomyopathy showed the highest proportion of SCD (50–80%) occurred in patients with New York Heart Association class II symptoms, with an overall annual mortality rate of 5 to 15%. For patients with New York Heart Association class IV symptoms, the mortality rate was much greater, but the proportion of sudden deaths was lower, reflecting a higher incidence of death from "pump failure." The Metoprolol Controlled-release Randomized Intervention Trial in Heart Failure confirmed these data.

STRUCTURAL CONGENITAL ABNORMALITIES

Hypertrophic Cardiomyopathy

The most common example of a congenital structural cardiac abnormality with an associated increased risk of SCD is hypertrophic cardiomyopathy (HCM), an autosomal dominant disease estimated to affect 1 in 500 adults. Many genetic abnormalities can result in the similar hypertrophic phenotypes, a fact further confused by the variable penetrance in affected individuals (see chapters 15 and 62). The overall risk of SCD in patients with HCM is estimated at 1 to 4% per year, but within subgroups of patients with this disease, the risk of SCD varies substantially. General-

Table 23-2
Sudden Death by New York Heart Association Functional Class

NYHA Class	Annual Mortality	Sudden Death
II	5–15%	50–80%
III	20–50%	30–50%
IV	30–70%	5–30%

Reprinted from *Journal of the American College of Cardiology,* 30(7), Uretsky BF, Sheahan RG, Primary prevention of sudden cardiac death in heart failure: will the solution be shocking? 1589–1597, 1997, with permission from American College of Cardiology Foundation.

ly, the patients with HCM who are at highest risk for SCD are those with recurrent syncope, nonsustained VT on Holter monitoring, extreme LV hypertrophy on echocardiogram, and a positive family history of SCD from HCM. It is estimated that up to 60% of patients with HCM and SCD have such a positive family history. An electrophysiology study is indicated in patients with HCM who present with unexplained syncope or documented nonsustained VT. Careful evaluation for HCM is of utmost importance in young persons because HCM is one of the most common causes of SCD in young athletes (Fig. 23-2, top).

Other congenital malformations also represent significant risk for SCD. The congenital malformations that represent the highest risk are aortic stenosis, Ebstein's anomaly, coarctation of the aorta, tetralogy of Fallot, transposition of the great arteries, Eisenmenger's physiology, and congenitally corrected transposition of the great arteries. When surgical correction is possible, the risk of SCD decreases but is not eliminated. A small subset of patients with mitral valve prolapse, that is, patients with a high degree of valve redundancy, thickening, regurgitation, and prolonged corrected QT (QTc) intervals or ST-T wave changes, are at increased risk for SCD.

Arrhythmogenic Right Ventricular Dysplasia

Arrhythmogenic RV dysplasia is an autosomal dominant condition that primarily affects young, otherwise healthy individuals. In arrhythmogenic RV dysplasia, the RV myocardium is replaced by fibrous and fibrofatty tissue, primarily in the apex, in the subtricuspid region, and along the anterior surface of the pulmonary infundibulum. The left

Figure 23-2

Sudden Cardiac Death (SCD)

Structural congenital abnormalities

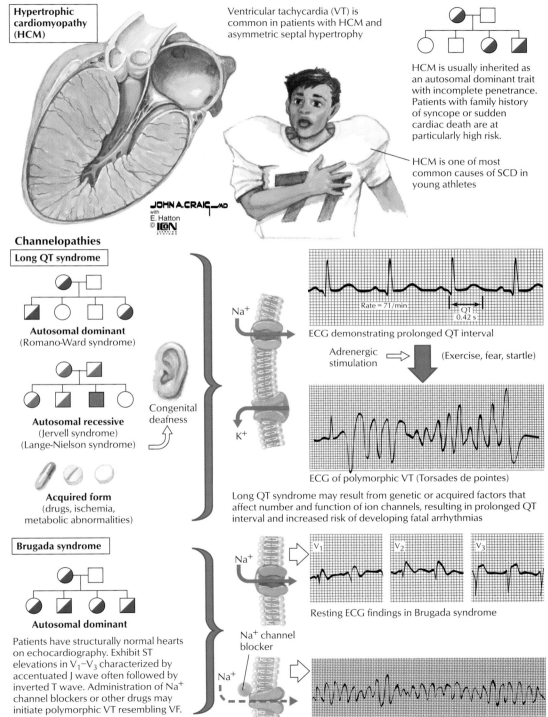

Hypertrophic cardiomyopathy (HCM)

Ventricular tachycardia (VT) is common in patients with HCM and asymmetric septal hypertrophy

HCM is usually inherited as an autosomal dominant trait with incomplete penetrance. Patients with family history of syncope or sudden cardiac death are at particularly high risk.

HCM is one of most common causes of SCD in young athletes

JOHN A. CRAIG—AD
with
E. Hatton
© ICON

Channelopathies

Long QT syndrome

Autosomal dominant
(Romano-Ward syndrome)

Autosomal recessive
(Jervell syndrome)
(Lange-Nielson syndrome)

Congenital deafness

Acquired form
(drugs, ischemia, metabolic abnormalities)

Na^+

K^+

ECG demonstrating prolonged QT interval

Rate = 71/min

QT 0.42 s

Adrenergic stimulation ⟹ (Exercise, fear, startle)

ECG of polymorphic VT (Torsades de pointes)

Long QT syndrome may result from genetic or acquired factors that affect number and function of ion channels, resulting in prolonged QT interval and increased risk of developing fatal arrhythmias

Brugada syndrome

Autosomal dominant

Patients have structurally normal hearts on echocardiography. Exhibit ST elevations in V_1–V_3 characterized by accentuated J wave often followed by inverted T wave. Administration of Na^+ channel blockers or other drugs may initiate polymorphic VT resembling VF.

Na^+

Na^+ channel blocker

Na^+

V_1 V_2 V_3

Resting ECG findings in Brugada syndrome

Polymorphic VT pattern after administration of Na^+ channel blocker

ventricle may be involved in later stages of the disease. A relatively uncommon SCD etiology in the United States, arrhythmogenic RV dysplasia is more common in Italy and, although hereditary, arrhythmogenic RV dysplasia is characterized by variable genetic penetrance.

Patients with arrhythmogenic RV dysplasia often present with presyncope, syncope, or SCD. The ECG may reveal VF or VT with a left bundle branch morphology during syncope or SCD and may demonstrate epsilon waves in leads V_1 through V_3 at baseline. The diagnosis is confirmed by RV wall motion abnormalities, aneurysms, or bulges on echocardiography or right ventriculography, late potentials on signal-averaged ECG, or magnetic resonance imaging. The classic magnetic resonance imaging finding is fatty tissue replacement of the myocardium of the right ventricle. RV biopsy yields relatively little information, because the disease typically spares the septum, the most common biopsy site. The 5-year survival rate after diagnosis is estimated at 95%, but risk assessment and treatment have not been definitively established in the United States.

Coronary Artery Anomalies

Coronary artery anomalies are uncommon (0.17%) but account for a disproportionate percentage of deaths in young athletes (up to 11.8%). The mechanism of SCD is thought to be ischemia from coronary spasm or abnormal tension placed on the ectopic coronary artery by the ascending aorta and the pulmonary trunk. The most consistently fatal anomaly occurs when the left coronary artery originates from the right coronary sinus and courses between the aorta and the pulmonary artery. In patients with coronary artery anomalies who died suddenly, up to 59% had this variant at autopsy. A causal relationship between SCD and anomalous coronary arteries is often not found; that is, irreversible ischemia is not consistently observed. A few anomalies, such as coronary atresia, coronary stenoses, and anomalous origin of the left main coronary artery from the pulmonary artery, show reproducible ischemia analogous to fixed obstructive coronary lesions. Coronary artery bypass surgery is the preferred treatment when appropriate, based on the coronary anatomy (see chapters 11 and 50).

Channelopathies and Sudden Cardiac Death

"Channelopathies" account for up to 5 to 10% of SCDs annually but generate the most interest, because SCD occurs in patients with structurally normal hearts. Abnormalities in a number of ion channels are associated with an increased incidence of ventricular tachyarrhythmias and SCDs. Long QT syndrome (LQTS) encompasses patients with QTc intervals greater than 440 ms (Fig. 23-2, middle). LQTS has an estimated prevalence of 1 in 7000 to 1 in 10,000, with variable penetrance. An estimated 3000 to 4000 patients annually suffer SCD from polymorphic VT (torsades de pointes), the majority from adrenergic stimulation with exercise or when startled or frightened. There are five known genes associated with LQTS, encoding four sodium and potassium channels, with more than 200 characterized mutations (see chapter 62). The most widely described syndromes are the Romano-Ward syndrome (autosomal dominant) and the rare Jervell and Lange-Nielsen syndrome (autosomal recessive), which is associated with congenital deafness. *Acquired LQTS* is LQTS due to secondary causes (medications, electrolyte abnormalities, or ischemia) (Table 23-3). There is interest in determining whether patients with drug-provoked LQTS represent a subset of individuals who have an underlying genetic predisposition.

The Brugada syndrome, an autosomal dominant disease, is another recognized cause of SCD. Patients with this syndrome have structurally normal hearts on echocardiography. The initial diagnosis of the Brugada syndrome is based on 12-lead ECG showing ST elevations in leads V_1 through V_3 characterized by an accentuated J wave (often followed by a negative T wave) (Fig. 23-1, lower). Rapid polymorphic VT that may resemble VF can develop in patients with the Brugada syndrome. The "Brugada" ECG findings may be transient and unmasked by sodium channel blockers such as flecainide, ajmaline, procainamide, disopyramide, and propafenone. ECG changes may also appear during fever or with the use of other drugs, including vagotonics, α-agonists, β-blockers, tricyclic antidepressants, cocaine, and first-generation antihistamines. The risk of SCD in patients with the Brugada syndrome remains controversial, as a wide range of mortality rates have been

Table 23-3
Drugs Implicated in QT Prolongation*

· Antibiotics (erythromycin, clarithromycin, azithromycin, ampicillin, pentamidine, sulfamethoxazole, ketoconazole, itraconazole, chloroquine, mefloquine, fluoroquinolones)

· Antihistamines (terfenadine, astemizole, oxatomide)

· Psychotropic agents (thioridazine, phenothiazines, tricyclic or tetracyclic antidepressants, haloperidol, risperidone)

· Antiarrhythmic agents (quinidine, procainamide, disopyramide, amiodarone, sotalol, dofetilide, ibutilide, mibefradil)

· Motility agents (cisapride)

· Metabolic (hypokalemia, hypomagnesemia, hypocalcemia)

· Bradyarrhythmia (sinus node dysfunction, second- or third-degree atrioventricular block)

· Myocardial ischemia

· Hypothermia

· Intracranial disease

*An updated listing can be found at: http://www.qtdrugs.org/medical-pros/drug-lists/drug-lists.htm.

reported. Patients at highest risk, those who present with resuscitated SCD and a Brugada ECG, have an annual SCD recurrence rate of 69%. Patients who present with syncope and a Brugada ECG have a 19% annual risk of SCD. Asymptomatic patients are further subdivided into patients with a spontaneous Brugada ECG (8% annual recurrence rate) and patients with a provocable Brugada ECG after sodium channel–blocker administration (minimal to no risk). In asymptomatic patients, an electrophysiology study may offer prognostic benefit. The only effective treatment is ICD placement and this is often recommended in first-degree relatives of patients with the Brugada syndrome and SCD.

Commotio cordis is SCD from blunt, nonpenetrating chest blows, occurring in an individual without structural anomalies in the heart and without traumatic injury to the sternum, the ribs, or the heart. It is thought that chest impact occurs during the vulnerable period of repolarization of the monophasic action potential (just before the T-wave peak). In a study of 128 events, it was found that 95% of commotio cordis occurred in males. There were 107 occurrences during sport-

ing events, and 81% were from a precordial blow from a projectile, most often a baseball. The remaining events were caused by precordial contact from body parts (shoulder, fist, knee, etc.). The overall survival rate in these studies is dismal (~25%). In those treated within the first 3 minutes of collapse, survival rates are higher. Of those who did survive, 76% had a normal recovery, with the remainder suffering mild to moderate neurologic impairment. When CPR was initiated after 3 minutes (38 patients), only 3% survived. The majority of the documented arrhythmias were VF and asystole. Prevention with protective sporting equipment, safe work practices, and rapid bystander CPR (including immediate access to automated external defibrillators) represent the best strategies.

DIAGNOSTIC APPROACH

The diagnostic approach should be tailored to the individual. A detailed history must be obtained, including the circumstances of the SCD and the comorbid conditions. Prior events; a family history of SCD; risk factors; other unexplained deaths, such as single-vehicle accidents, drownings, or near-drownings; and medication history, including over-the-counter medications, alternative therapies, or recent additions or dose adjustments, should be documented. A bystander history is useful and should be sought. A thorough physical examination, baseline ECG, blood work, including CBC, glucose, electrolytes (potassium, magnesium, etc.), cardiac enzymes, and drug levels (including a toxicology screen) should be performed. Further diagnostic testing may include any combination of cardiac catheterization, echocardiography, telemetry monitoring, pacemaker placement, provocative testing with an electrophysiology study, T-wave alternans assessment, stress testing (exercise or pharmacologic), myocardial imaging with thallium, magnetic resonance imaging, and transbronchial biopsy. On the basis of these findings, an individualized management strategy should be developed for each patient (Table 23-4).

MANAGEMENT AND THERAPY

Treatment is tailored to the etiology (Table 23-4). The most effective therapies are β-blockers and revascularization in patients with reversible

Table 23-4
Treatment and Prevention of Sudden Cardiac Death

Coronary Artery Disease	
Acute myocardial infarction	ReV, BB, lifestyle modification, smoking cessation, ACE-I
EF <35%	ReV, ICD, BB, ACE-I
EF >35% and <40%	ReV, BB, ACE-I, ICD if nonsustained VT and positive EPS
Nonischemic Cardiomyopathy	
Symptomatic	ICD + BB, RFA (if BBR) for persistent VT
Asymptomatic	BB, ACE-I
EF <35%	ICD, BB, ACE-I
EF >35%	BB, ACE-I
Hypertrophic cardiomyopathy	
Asymptomatic and no family history	BB, CCB, avoidance of competitive sports
Syncope or family history	ICD, BB, avoidance of competitive sports
Long QT syndrome	
Congenital	BB, PM, ICD
Acquired	Avoidance of offending medication, follow-up ETT (BB, ICD, PM if positive.)
Brugada syndrome	ICD
Miscellaneous	
Complete heart block	PM
Valvular heart disease	Surgery if appropriate, BB (if appropriate)
Congenital heart disease	BB, ACE-I, ICD
Right ventricular outflow tract	RFA
Arrhythmogenic right ventricular dysplasia	ICD ± ablation ± surgical isolation
Coronary artery anomalies	Bypass surgery; ICD
Preexcitation/Wolff-Parkinson-White syndrome	RFA
Commotio cordis	Safety equipment, automated external defibrillators
Myocarditis	Supportive initially, later BB, ACE-I, ± ICD
Cardiac sarcoidosis	As for noncardiac sarcoidosis, possible ICD

ACE-I indicates angiotensin-converting enzyme inhibitor; BB, β-blocker; BBR, bundle branch reentry; CB, calcium channel blocker; EF, ejection fraction; EPS, electrophysiology study; ETT, exercise treadmill test; ICD, implantable cardioverter defibrillator; PM, pacemaker; RFA, radiofrequency ablation; ReV, revascularization; VT, ventricular tachycardia.

ischemia or acute MI. Patients with ischemic cardiomyopathy and an EF of less than 35% should receive an ICD after optimization of anti-ischemia therapy (see chapters 12, 17, and 20). For patients with a previous MI, an EF greater than 35% and less than 40%, and nonsustained VT, an electrophysiology study should be performed. If the patient has inducible VT, an ICD should be implanted. Ongoing studies dictate more definitive therapy for these patients and whether to proceed directly to ICD. Aggressive secondary prevention should also be pursued, including the optimal pharmacologic therapy with angiotensin-converting enzyme inhibitors, β-blockers, antiplatelet agents, and lipid-lowering therapy. Aggressive treatment of hypertension, diabetes, hypercholesterolemia, and tobacco abuse should be pursued.

For those patients with dilated cardiomyopathy and an EF less than 35%, an ICD should be placed. Therefore, the clinical picture determines therapy. Electrophysiology studies are predictive of recurrent arrhythmias in most patients in this group. Therefore, in patients with dilated cardiomyopathy and an EF greater than 35%, β-blockers and ACE inhibitors should be initiated. In the case of bundle branch reentry VT, radiofrequency ablation (see chapter 25) may be beneficial, although some patients in this group will still require ICD placement. Other specific diseases require more aggressive approaches. In patients with Wolff-Parkinson-White syndrome and SCD, radiofrequency ablation is necessary; patients with a family history of SCD who have findings of HCM, arrhythmogenic RV dysplasia, LQTS, or Brugada syndrome should undergo ICD placement, and any agent known to precipitate acquired LQTS should be discontinued immediately. Finally, patients without a demonstrable cause for documented VF/VT are still at risk for SCD and should be offered ICD therapy.

β-Blockers have a favorable effect on prevention of SCD and have other benefits in patients with congestive heart failure. The Metoprolol Controlled-release Randomized Intervention Trial in Heart Failure showed a 41% decrease in SCD in heart failure patients with an EF below 40% (mean ~28%) with β-blocker therapy. A β-blocker may be added to amiodarone in most cases without causing worrisome bradycardia. Patients taking amiodarone, shown in a meta-analysis to have a 13% decrease in cardiac death, had a positive interaction when a β-blocker was added. The combined post hoc analysis of the European Myocardial Infarction Amiodarone Trial and the Canadian Amiodarone Myocardial Infarction Arrhythmia Trial revealed a 61% decrease in SCD in post-MI patients treated with both β-blockers and amiodarone.

FUTURE DIRECTIONS

Ongoing research involves finding genetic, electrical, and biochemical markers for increased risk of SCD. Aggressive societal interventions are needed to decrease the incidence of SCD. Genetic research has discovered many links to SCD, including mutations of α-2b-adrenoceptors and cardiac ryanodine receptors. Interestingly, mutations that lead to a prothrombotic state and likely increase the risk of acute MI (e.g., mutations in the prothrombin gene and the factor V Leiden mutation) are not associated with an increased propensity for SCD. Although data are conflicting on serum homocysteine levels, evidence suggests that increased C-reactive peptide, tissue plasminogen activator, B-type natriuretic peptide, autoantibodies against sarcolemmal sodium-potassium adenosine triphosphatase (Na,K-ATPase), and urinary 11-dehydrothromboxane B2 levels predict risk for SCD in patients with coronary artery disease and cardiomyopathies. The role of T-wave alternans assessment in profiling the patients at highest risk also seems promising, but additional prospective evaluations in larger populations are required. Finally, with the epidemic of deaths from SCD occurring outside the hospital and the majority occurring in the context of coronary artery disease, an aggressive primary prevention strategy is needed. Smoking cessation, avoidance of obesity and sedentary lifestyle, and aggressive management of hypertension, hyperlipidemia, and diabetes may provide the greatest decreases in SCD.

SELECTED READING

Al-Khatib SM, Granger CB, Huang Y, et al. Sustained ventricular arrhythmias among patients with acute coronary syndromes with no ST-segment elevation: Incidence, predictors, and outcomes. *Circulation* 2002;106:309–312.

Angelina P, Velasco JA, Flamm S. Coronary anomalies: Incidence, pathophysiology, and clinical relevance. *Circulation* 2002;105:2449–2454.

Bardy G. Sudden Cardiac Death in the Heart Failure Trial (SCD-HeFT). Late Breaking Clinical Trials, American College of Cardiology 2004.

Boutitie F, Boissel JP, Connolly SJ, et al. Amiodarone interaction with beta-blockers: Analysis of the merged EMIAT (European Myocardial Infarct Amiodarone Trial) and CAMIAT (Canadian Amiodarone Myocardial Infarction Trial) databases. The EMIAT and CAMIAT Investigators. *Circulation* 1999;99:2268–2275.

Drugs that cause torsades de pointes: http://www.qtdrugs.org/medical-pros/drug-lists/drug-lists.htm.

Huikuri HV, Castellanos A, Myerburg RJ. Sudden cardiac death due to cardiac arrhythmias. *N Engl J Med* 2001;345:1473–1482.

Maron BJ, Gohman TE, Kyle SB, Estes NAM, Link MS. Clinical profile and spectrum of commotio cordis. *JAMA* 2002;287:1142–1146.

Uretsky BF, Sheahan RG. Primary prevention of sudden cardiac death in heart failure: will the solution be shocking? *J Am Coll Cardiol* 1997;30:1589–1597.

Vincent GM, Timothy K, Zhang L. Congenital long QT syndrome. *Clin Electrophysiol Rev* 2002;6:57–60.

Wilde AAM, Antzelevitch C, Borggrefe M, et al. Proposed diagnostic criteria for the Brugada syndrome. *Circulation* 2002;106:2514–2519.

Chapter 24

Medical Treatment of Tachyarrhythmias

William E. Sanders, Jr and Ali Akbary

Dramatic progress has been made in the treatment of most common tachyarrhythmias. Therapeutic options are widely available that provide symptomatic relief and realistic opportunity for cure. Procedures such as radiofrequency catheter ablation have markedly reduced the necessity for long-term medical therapy in certain populations with paroxysmal supraventricular tachycardias. The mortality risk from sustained ventricular tachycardia and ventricular fibrillation has been virtually eliminated by implantable cardioverter defibrillators (ICDs). The use of medical therapy for tachyarrhythmias has not progressed as rapidly as device therapy, in part because pharmacologic advances have been limited, and in part, because studies have revealed that some antiarrhythmic therapies are detrimental to certain patients with more malignant arrhythmias. However, cardiac arrhythmias and associated symptoms remain a prevalent presentation to primary care physicians and cardiologists. Cardiac arrhythmias are prevalent and because not all are suited for device therapy, medical therapy still plays a major role in the primary treatment of supraventricular arrhythmias and an adjunct role in therapy for ventricular arrhythmias (Table 24-1).

ETIOLOGY AND PATHOGENESIS

Most clinical arrhythmias are reentrant in nature. Automaticity and triggered activity can be a primary cause of tachycardia but represent less than 5% of observed tachycardias. Therefore, medical therapy has focused on preventing tachyarrhythmias due to reentrant mechanisms. Reentry requires alterations in the myocardium, resulting in differing speeds of conduction and recovery in certain regions (Fig. 24-1). These regional electrical discrepancies allow creation of the reentrant loop (Fig. 24-2). Changes in myocardial tissue typically result from myocardial damage secondary to ischemia or dilatation. Drugs that modify repolarization and action potential duration are consequently of therapeutic value in reentrant arrhythmias.

CLINICAL PRESENTATION

Although the pharmacologic treatments of most supraventricular tachycardias are similar, determining the exact mechanism permits drug selection of maximal efficacy. Causes of tachycardia can usually be determined by careful history, physical examination, and 12-lead ECG both in sinus rhythm and during a sustained episode of tachycardia (often such an ECG is not available). A detailed history of syncope, light-headedness, palpitations, chest pain, previous coronary artery disease, and congestive heart failure must be elicited. Information regarding the regularity of palpitations and the abruptness with which they initiate and terminate is essential to accurate identification. Many patients will provide a history of visits to an emergency room where their arrhythmia was stopped by IV medications (adenosine, lidocaine, or calcium channel blockers) and frequently recall the successful drug. When available, this information often will define the type of tachycardia being experienced by the patient. Together, a careful history and an ECG during tachycardia typically permit diagnosis of the specific etiology of the arrhythmia.

DIFFERENTIAL DIAGNOSIS

For several reasons, it can be difficult to give a precise diagnosis for patients presenting with symptoms consistent with tachyarrhythmia. First, if tachycardia is present, discerning the mechanism of the rhythm disturbance can be challenging. Wide-complex tachycardia can be of either supraventricular or ventricular origin. Narrow-complex arrhythmias are, by definition, not ventricular, but further definition is often impossible based solely on the surface ECG and the physical examination. In either case, it

Table 24-1
Antiarrhythmic Agents

	Dose	Major Side Effects
Type IA		
Quinidine (Quinidex)	600–1600 mg qd (divided doses every 6 h)	Gastrointestinal effects, rash, cinchonism, proarrhythmia (↑QT)
Procainamide (Procan)	2000–4000 mg qd (divided doses)	Gastrointestinal effects, lupus, proarrhythmia (↑QT), agranulocytosis
Disopyramide (Norpace)	150–450 mg every 12 h	Anticholinergic effects (urinary retention), proarrhythmia (↑QT)
Type IB		
Lidocaine	IV only (1.5-mg/kg bolus, then 1–4 mg/min IV)	CNS effects (paresthesia, tremor, confusion, seizure)
Mexiletine (Mexitil)	150–300 mg every 8 h	Gastrointestinal effects, CNS effects
Type IC		
Flecainide (Tambocor)	50–200 mg every 12 h	CNS effects, CHF, proarrhythmia
Propafenone (Rythmol)	150–300 mg every 8 h	Gastrointestinal effects, metallic taste, CNS effects, proarrhythmia
Type II		
β-Blockers	Refer to specific agent	Bradycardia, CNS effects (depression), sexual dysfunction
Type III		
Amiodarone (Cordarone)	200–600 mg qd	Bradycardia, pulmonary fibrosis, thyroid, skin effects, CNS effects, liver effects
Sotalol (Betapace)	80–240 mg every 12 h	Bradycardia, fatigue, and torsade de pointes
Type IV		
Diltiazem (Cardizem)	240–360 mg qd	Hypotension, bradycardia
Verapamil (Calan)	240–480 mg qd	Bradycardia, constipation, peripheral edema
Others		
Digoxin (Lanoxin)	0.125–0.35 mg PO qd	Gastrointestinal effects, visual disturbances, proarrhythmia
Adenosine (Adenocard)	IV only (6–18 mg IV)	Facial flushing, chest pain, dyspnea, anxiety (lasting <10 s)
Ibutilide (Corvert)	1 mg IV infusion	Proarrhythmia, headache, chest pain, dizziness
Dofetilide	125–500 mg PO bid	Proarrhythmia, headache, chest pain, dizziness

bid indicates twice daily; CHF, congestive heart failure; CNS, central nervous system; PO, by mouth; qd, once daily.
Adapted with permission from Rakel, Bope: *Conn's Current Therapy*. Elsevier; 2003.

Figure 24-1

Conducting System of Heart
Right side

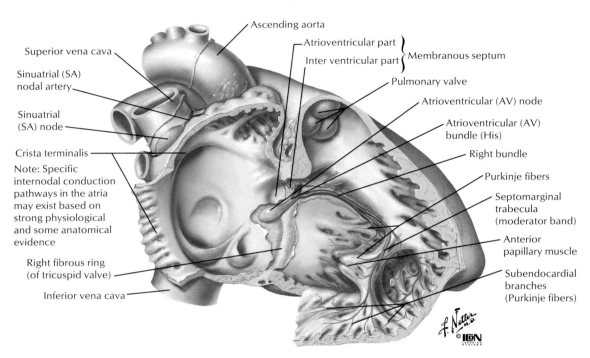

Ascending aorta

Atrioventricular part
Inter ventricular part } Membranous septum

Superior vena cava

Sinuatrial (SA) nodal artery

Pulmonary valve

Atrioventricular (AV) node

Sinuatrial (SA) node

Atrioventricular (AV) bundle (His)

Crista terminalis

Right bundle

Purkinje fibers

Note: Specific internodal conduction pathways in the atria may exist based on strong physiological and some anatomical evidence

Septomarginal trabecula (moderator band)

Anterior papillary muscle

Right fibrous ring (of tricuspid valve)

Subendocardial branches (Purkinje fibers)

Inferior vena cava

should be determined whether the tachycardia is the cause of the symptoms or reflects underlying stresses, such as fever, anemia/blood loss, or hyperthyroidism. In addition, tremors, shivering, and other muscular contractions can mimic arrhythmias on the surface ECG. The tremor of Parkinson's disease is notable for mimicking atrial flutter. Therefore, the differential diagnosis is broad, encompassing any cardiac or metabolic cause of tachycardia and neuromuscular conditions that might alter the ECG.

DIAGNOSTIC APPROACH
AVNRT, SANRT, and AT

Supraventricular tachycardias are best classified based on origin: nodal tissue (sinoatrial [SA] node and atrioventricular [AV] node), atrial tissue, or AV connections (accessory pathway bridging the mitral valve, tricuspid valve, or septum). The most commonly encountered paroxysmal supraventricular tachycardia (SVT) in clinical practice is AV nodal reentrant tachycardia (AVNRT) (Fig. 24-2). However, narrow-complex tachycardias, including sinoatrial nodal reentrant tachycardia (SANRT) and AV reentrant tachycardia (orthodromic reciprocating tachycardia from an accessory retrograde pathway), are approached pharmacologically in a similar fashion. Clues from the surface ECG can enable one to distinguish AVNRT, SANRT, and AT (Fig. 24-2). However, an electrophysiologic study is commonly needed to discern the exact mechanism.

Atrioventricular Reentry

In the healthy heart, the only electrical conduit between the atrium and the ventricle is the AV node. However, congenital abnormalities known as *accessory pathways* bridge the atrium to the ventricular myocardium in some patients, allowing the possibility of a reentrant loop. Paroxysmal tachycardias involving accessory pathways, AV reentrant tachycardia (AVRT), account for up to 30% of supraventricular arrhythmias. Frequently, a narrow-complex tachycardia that is indistinguishable from AVNRT is observed. The accessory pathway

Figure 24-2   **Origin Sites of Supraventricular Tachyarrhythmias**

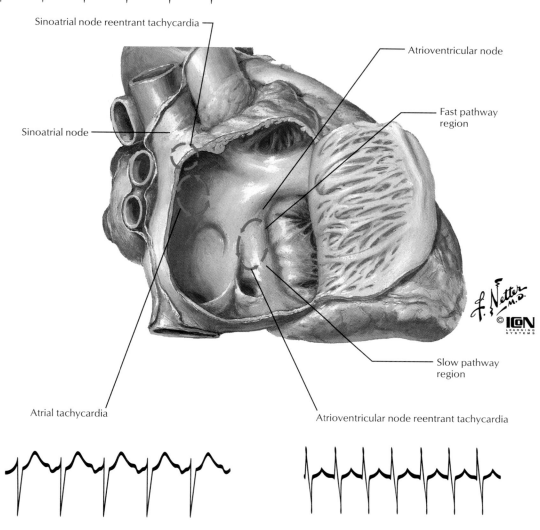

allows the electrical impulse normally transmitted through the AV node to conduct retrogradely and reactivate the atrium.

Pre-excitation Syndrome

A fusion beat results when an accessory pathway functions in an antegrade fashion (atrium to ventricle) in sinus rhythm (Fig. 24-3). The ventricular myocardium is activated through both the accessory pathway and the AV node, which manifests on the ECG as a delta wave. The prototype such entity, the Wolff-Parkinson-White (WPW) syndrome depends on the presence of the electrocardiographic finding of a delta wave for diagnosis.

Figure 24-3

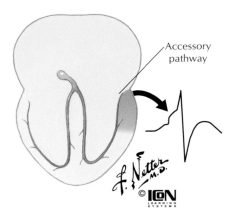

Accessory pathway

Many tachycardias and unusual ECGs can occur when an accessory pathway functions in an antegrade and retrograde fashion. Some of these rhythms can be lethal. The most important therapeutic implications in WPW syndrome are in patients with concomitant atrial fibrillation. Patients with ECG manifestations of WPW syndrome and syncope are at high risk of sudden cardiac death and should be carefully evaluated. Rapid conduction through the accessory pathway during atrial fibrillation results in bizarre ECGs and potentially in ventricular fibrillation. When an irregular ECG is noted with varying degrees of QRS complex width, a diagnosis of atrial fibrillation and WPW syndrome should be considered. It is imperative that AV node–blocking agents not be administered to such patients; instead, IV procainamide is the therapeutic choice. As with all rapid arrhythmias, if a patient is hemodynamically unstable, direct current cardioversion is used.

Wide-complex, rapid, regular arrhythmias can also result from atrial tachycardias and atrial flutter if an accessory pathway is present. Again, AV node–blocking agents should be avoided, and an antiarrhythmic agent should be administered. An unusual type of reentrant tachycardia (<10%) seen in patients with WPW is *antidromic reciprocating tachycardia*. This occurs when an impulse travels through an accessory pathway, activating the entire ventricular myocardium, and returns to the atrium retrogradely through the AV node, resulting in a wide-complex, regular tachycardia that may be difficult to distinguish from ventricular tachycardia.

Atrial Fibrillation

For more information about atrial fibrillation, refer to chapter 19.

Atrial Flutter

Most commonly, the diagnosis of atrial flutter is made based on the presence of flutter waves on the surface ECG (Fig. 24-4). Even in the absence of identifiable flutter waves, atrial flutter should be suspected (1) when a regular, narrow-complex tachycardia is present with a ventricular rate approximating 150 beats/min (suggesting atrial flutter at 300 beats/min with 2:1 atrioventricular block) or (2) when a narrow-complex tachycardia is present with variable ventricular rates, but only at intervals consistent with variable AV block. In the case of a heart rate of 150 beats/min, vagal maneuvers (increasing the AV block to 3:1 or higher) can make flutter waves more apparent. These guidelines do not always apply because with high-grade AV block, tachycardia might not be present, or with aberrant conduction or an underlying bundle branch block, the QRS complex may be prolonged.

Ventricular Tachycardia

Three or more consecutive beats originating from the ventricular myocardium define *ventricular tachycardia*. It is considered sustained when it lasts for more than 30 seconds. Two types of this arrhythmia are recognized: *monomorphic ventricular tachycardia*, in which each complex has uniform morphology in a constant cycle duration (Fig. 24-5), and *polymorphic ventricular tachycardia*, in which different morphologies are present and the cycle duration is not constant. (Fig. 24-6). Some patients present with ventricular tachycardia in a stable hemodynamic state, with normal blood pressure and full cognitive function. Ventricular tachycardia is discussed in more detail in chapter 20.

MANAGEMENT AND THERAPY
AVNRT, SANRT, and AT

In a stable patient with SVT, vagal maneuvers, such as the Valsalva maneuver or carotid sinus massage, can be attempted. If these interventions fail, adenosine is the first-line therapy (Table 25-1). Adenosine can be safely administered in gradually increasing doses (up to 18 mg

Figure 24-4

Atrial Flutter

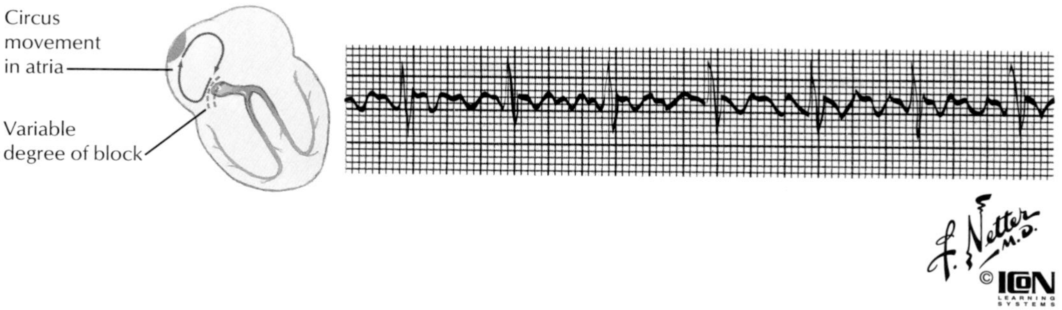

Circus
movement
in atria

Variable
degree of block

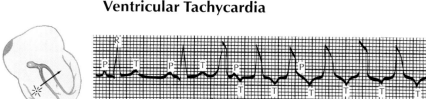

Figure 24-5

Ventricular Tachycardia

Lead II

Onset ventricular tachycardia

IV) to patients presenting with narrow-complex tachycardias that exceed 160 beats/min. It is more than 90% effective in eliminating the most common types of supraventricular arrhythmia. Adenosine is safer and more effective than IV calcium channel blockers. Adenosine consistently terminates reentrant mechanisms that utilize nodal tissue (sinoatrial and AV nodes) as well as accessory pathways, and frequently eliminates reentry within atrial tissue. It also provides diagnostic information for automatic atrial tachycardia. When adenosine is administered during automatic atrial tachycardia, P waves continue uninterrupted at the same tachycardic rate; however, the ventricular response is not observed because of the AV nodal blockade. Tachycardia immediately resumes after the rapid dissipation of the systemic effects of adenosine. On rare occasions, this agent fails to eliminate a narrow-complex SVT, and procainamide should be considered in hemodynamically stable patients. At any time, if hemodynamic status deteriorates or the patient becomes unconscious, immediate direct cur-

rent cardioversion should be used.

When a narrow-complex SVT of any etiology has been diagnosed, options include radiofrequency catheter ablation of the arrhythmia or long-term drug therapy. β-Blockers are the most commonly used pharmacologic agents that reduce incidence of the arrhythmia, limiting symptoms. All β-blockers show similar efficacy in the treatment of paroxysmal supraventricular episodes. Unfortunately, most patients have recurrent symptoms with this therapy. Calcium channel blockers can then be used as the initial agent or as an adjunct to β-blockade. However, strong consideration should be given to a curative approach (radiofrequency ablation) when symptoms recur. Type I antiarrhythmic agents play a small role in long-term therapy of narrow-complex SVTs. Occasionally, flecainide or propafenone is used when radiofrequency catheter ablation has failed to eliminate an accessory pathway, but this approach is reserved for those patients with structurally normal hearts, typically in conjunction with β-blocker therapy. Amiodarone and sotalol, commonly

Figure 24-6

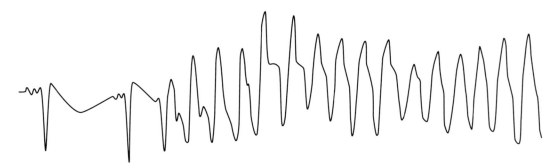

used in the treatment of atrial fibrillation, should rarely be used in SVT therapy, especially in young patients. Radiofrequency ablation is safe and highly efficacious in this setting and avoids any potential problems associated with life-long pharmacologic therapy.

Atrioventricular Reentry

Orthodromic reciprocating tachycardia is treated similarly to AVNRT (β-blockers, calcium channel blockers, and rarely type IC agents). The arrhythmia terminates with IV adenosine administration. Long-term β-blocker therapy allows some modification of symptoms and frequency of tachycardic episodes, but catheter ablation is now the treatment of choice.

Pre-excitation Syndrome

Antidromic tachycardia can be eliminated with the administration of adenosine, but the safest initial approach to a patient with hemodynamically stable wide-complex tachycardia (for which the mechanism is uncertain) is an antiarrhythmic agent, such as procainamide or amiodarone. Long-term medical therapy in patients with WPW syndrome and AVRT has decreased dramatically since the introduction of curative ablative therapy. When patients desire continued drug therapy and no pre-excitation is present on the baseline ECG, therapy is similar to that of AVNRT. AV node–blocking agents are most commonly used. If a delta wave is present, these agents should be avoided. In that circumstance drugs designed to modify conduction through the accessory pathway (type IA and IC agents) are indicated in individuals with structurally normal hearts.

Atrial Flutter

The short-term management of atrial flutter is similar to that of atrial fibrillation and involves initial rate control by drug therapy or cardioversion. Subsequent maintenance of sinus rhythm may necessitate antiarrhythmic therapy, and most patients with atrial flutter should receive appropriate anticoagulation. A combination of AV node–blocking agents, primarily calcium channel blockers, and β-blockers usually produces adequate rate control. If pharmacologic or direct current cardioversion is contemplated and the arrhythmia has persisted for more than 48 hours, transesophageal echocardiography should be performed or the patient should be maintained on anticoagulation for at least 4 weeks before conversion attempts. Chemical cardioversion is associated with similar cerebral vascular accident risks as direct current cardioversion. Ibutilide is recognized as the most effective IV agent for conversion of atrial flutter. Ibutilide must be used in a carefully monitored setting because of the substantial risks of torsades de pointes.

After sinus rhythm has been reestablished, antiarrhythmic agents (dofetilide, amiodarone, or sotalol) are frequently needed to maintain sinus rhythm. The initiation of sotalol should be carefully monitored, with the patient in the hospital. Daily ECGs should assess the QTc interval. The risk of torsades de pointes increases with QTc prolongation and an increasing sotalol dose. Amiodarone therapy should be initiated with a loading dose, while monitoring in a hospital setting, when used in patients with atrial fibrillation/flutter or tachybrady syndrome. In these patients there is a high risk of AV nodal block.

Ventricular Tachycardia

If a patient is hemodynamically stable, without reports of angina at initial evaluation, pharmacologic management is the initial treatment of choice in the acute setting. In all wide-complex tachycardias, procainamide is a safe first-line therapy when the arrhythmia is not believed to be associated with acute ischemia. From an electrophysiologic standpoint, procainamide treatment of wide-complex tachycardia—whether of ventricular or supraventricular origin—can rarely be criticized. The use of calcium channel blockers in the setting of a wide-complex tachycardia of unknown etiology is specifically contraindicated. When treated with calcium channel blockers, ventricular tachycardias frequently deteriorate to ventricular fibrillation. IV amiodarone has been proven effective in emergent situations with patients experiencing wide-complex tachycardia. Amiodarone offers the advantage, when compared with procainamide, of less associated hypotension. However, amiodarone has an extended half-life, and if the arrhythmia diagnosis is uncertain, amiodarone can complicate electrophysiologic evaluation. At any time, if a patient becomes hemodynamically unstable, immediate direct current cardioversion should be performed.

Antiarrhythmic therapy for ventricular arrhythmias is now used only in conjunction with defibrillator placement. Up to 50% of patients with a defibrillator for ventricular arrhythmias are also treated with antiarrhythmic therapy. Amiodarone and sotalol help to reduce the number and frequency of shocks received by patients with a high arrhythmia burden. Obviously, these agents do not reduce the mortality risk and, therefore, cannot be used without an implanted ICD. Low-dose amiodarone therapy (200 mg orally once daily) is the most common adjunct therapy in the ICD population.

Rarely, patients who have undergone ICD placement will present in "storm" with multiple shocks from their device. Careful clinical and laboratory evaluations (electrolyte evaluation, toxicology screens, and other tests) designed to determine possible arrhythmic triggers, including ischemia, must be rapidly pursued. In an emergency, when the device is firing repeatedly, IV amiodarone plus IV β-blocker is the most effective management. Frequently, these patients are discharged from the hospital on oral amiodarone and β-blocker therapy.

FUTURE DIRECTIONS

Pharmacologic management of arrhythmias has diminished with the upsurge of catheter and device therapy. Nonetheless, many agents are used as adjunct treatment for a variety of arrhythmias. β-Blockers and calcium channel blockers still provide adequate, symptomatic relief for certain supraventricular arrhythmias and, for some patients, alleviate the necessity of an invasive procedure. Adenosine has markedly improved the quality of short-term therapy for supraventricular arrhythmias, and ibutilide now offers more effective, rapid chemical cardioversion of atrial fibrillation/flutter. Primary treatment of ventricular arrhythmias is almost entirely device based, but type III antiarrhythmic agents play a prominent role in adjunct therapy. Drugs designed using new methods of molecular, structural, and translational biology might provide more effective pharmacologic therapy in the future.

REFERENCES

Credner SC, Klingenheben T, Mauss O, et al. Electrical storm in patients with transvenous implantable cardioverter-defibrillators: Incidence, management and prognostic implications. *J Am Coll Cardiol* 1998;32:1909–1915.

Epstein AE, Ellenbogen KA, Kirk KA, et al. Clinical characteristics and outcome of patients with high defibrillation thresholds. *Circulation* 1992;86:1206–1216.

Ganz LI, Friedman PL. Supraventricular tachycardia. *N Engl J Med* 1995;332:162–173.

Jackman WM, Beakman KJ, McClelland JH, et al. Treatment of supraventricular tachycardia due to atrioventricular nodal reentry by radiofrequency catheter ablation of slow pathway. *N Engl J Med* 1992;327:313–318.

Masood A. Clinical spectrum of ventricular tachycardia. *Circulation* 1990;82:1561–1572.

Members of the Sicilian Gambit. New approaches to antiarrhythmic therapy: I. Emerging therapeutic applications of the cell biology of cardiac arrhythmias. *Circulation* 2001;104:2865–2873.

Prystowsky EN. Diagnosis and management of the preexcitation syndromes. *Curr Probl Cardiol* 1988;13:225–310.

Saksena S, Poczobutt-Johanos M, Castle LW, et al. Long-term multicenter experience with a second-generation implantable pacemaker-defibrillator in patients with malignant ventricular tachyarrhythmias. *J Am Coll Cardiol* 1992;19:490–499.

Chapter 25

Radiofrequency Catheter Ablation of Supraventricular and Ventricular Arrhythmias

Nitish Badhwar, William E. Sanders, Jr, and Melvin M. Scheinman

The development of radiofrequency catheter ablation (RFCA) as a therapeutic option for the treatment of arrhythmias has dramatically altered the approach to the patient with tachycardia. Since its introduction in 1986, RFCA has provided actual cure for thousands of patients with debilitating symptoms from paroxysmal supraventricular tachycardias and for patients with certain ventricular tachycardias (VTs). This therapy not only improves quality of life, but also reduces risk of mortality in specific populations (Wolff-Parkinson-White syndrome and VT). RFCA is the therapy of choice for a broad range of cardiac arrhythmias.

To appreciate why and how RFCA works, a simple model is required. Most tachycardias can be considered "extra wires" that short-circuit the normal conduction system (Fig. 25-1). The mechanism responsible for the majority of arrhythmias is called "reentry" and requires two distinct pathways ("wires") that have different speeds of conduction ("slow" and "fast") and varying recovery times (refractoriness). Extra, early beats, such as premature atrial or ventricular contractions, may fail to conduct down the normal (fast-conducting but slow-recovering) pathway but can travel down the fast-recovering but slow-conducting extra wire (Fig. 25-1). At the distal junction of the two wires, the arriving slow impulse then returns in a retrograde fashion up the now recovered fast normal pathway. This completes the "short" circuit and activates/depolarizes the myocardial tissue at each end of the wire with every conduction around the circuit. RFCA successfully eliminates the extra wire by the application of thermal energy, typically leaving only normal conduction.

ENERGY SOURCE FOR CATHETER ABLATION

Radiofrequency (RF) energy is alternating current delivered at a frequency of 300 to 1000 kHz when used for catheter ablation. The small lesions created by this method are 5 to 6 mm in diameter and 2 to 3 mm in depth. Usually, RF energy is delivered in unipolar fashion from the tip of the catheter electrode located in the heart to a dispersive (grounded) electrode placed on the patient's skin. Vascular endothelium in the coronary arteries is not damaged by RF application to the endomyocardial surface. It is postulated that the high rate of flow in the epicardial coronary arteries may prevent substantial heating of vascular endothelium during RFCA (a "heat sink" effect). The widespread use of RFCA is attributable not only to remarkable therapeutic success rates, but also to the extremely low occurrence of complications (Table 25-1).

ATRIOVENTRICULAR NODAL REENTRY TACHYCARDIA

Atrioventricular nodal reentry tachycardia (AVNRT) is the most common cause of paroxysmal supraventricular tachycardia, accounting for up to 60% of cases. AVNRT is not typically associated with underlying structural heart disease and can occur at any age. The arrhythmia is most commonly a narrow complex tachycardia that is regular, at rates of 160 to 250 beats/min. The mechanism of AVNRT is reentry involving dual atrioventricular (AV) nodal pathways, a slow pathway (the extra wire) and a fast pathway (the normal conduction wire). The typical form of this arrhythmia uses the slow pathway

Figure 25-1

Models of the Mechanisms of Supraventricular and Ventricular Tachyarrhythmias

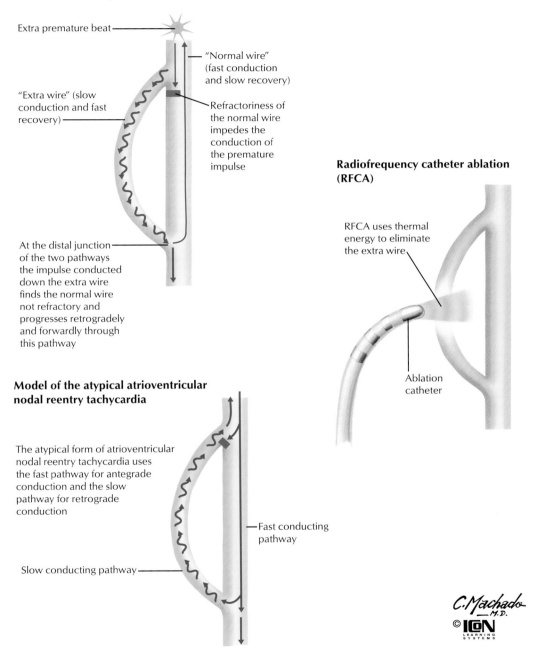

Model of initiation and circuit for a reentrant tachycardia

Extra premature beat

"Normal wire" (fast conduction and slow recovery)

"Extra wire" (slow conduction and fast recovery)

Refractoriness of the normal wire impedes the conduction of the premature impulse

At the distal junction of the two pathways the impulse conducted down the extra wire finds the normal wire not refractory and progresses retrogradely and forwardly through this pathway

Radiofrequency catheter ablation (RFCA)

RFCA uses thermal energy to eliminate the extra wire

Ablation catheter

Model of the atypical atrioventricular nodal reentry tachycardia

The atypical form of atrioventricular nodal reentry tachycardia uses the fast pathway for antegrade conduction and the slow pathway for retrograde conduction

Fast conducting pathway

Slow conducting pathway

C. Machado M.D.

© ICON LEARNING SYSTEMS

Table 25-1
Overview of Catheter Ablation

Type of Arrhythmia/Ablation	Success Rate (%)	Complication
AVNRT	95+	AV block (<1%)
WPW syndrome	85–95 (right-sided) 95+ (left-sided)	AV block, coronary artery occlusion, tamponade
AVJ ablation	98–100	Sudden death (rare)
Atrial flutter	85–95 (typical flutter) 50–60 (atypical flutter)	AV block (rare)
Atrial tachycardia	80 (right-sided) 65 (left-sided)	Stroke (primarily with left-sided lesions)
Focal AF	60–70	Pulmonary stenosis (2–4%), stroke, tamponade
VT associated with CAD	64–81	MI, TIA, arterial complications
Bundle branch reentrant VT	95+	AV block (rare)
Idiopathic VT	85–100	Pericardial tamponade

AF indicates atrial fibrillation; AVNRT, atrioventricular nodal reentry tachycardia; AV, atrioventricular; AVJ, atrioventricular junction; CAD, coronary artery disease; MI, myocardial infarction; TIA, transient ischemic attack; VT, ventricular tachycardia; WPW, Wolff-Parkinson-White.

for antegrade conduction and the fast pathway for retrograde conduction; the atypical form has the opposite sequence. The AV node is located at the apex of the triangle of Koch, formed by the tricuspid annulus, the tendon of Todaro, and the coronary sinus ostium (Fig. 25-2). The atrial insertion of the slow pathway is located around the coronary sinus ostium (the inferior–posterior aspect of the triangle of Koch), and the fast pathway lies in the anterior–superior region of the triangle (close to the AV node). Either form of AVNRT can be cured by RFCA. Elimination of the slow pathway is preferred because ablation of the fast pathway carries a higher risk of destroying the normal conduction—to the extent that a pacemaker may be required. Appropriate targets for RF application to the slow pathway (the extra wire) are selected on the basis of a combined anatomic and electrographic approach (Fig. 25-2, lower). The lesions are placed in the region of the coronary sinus (posterior septum). Success is marked by the noninducibility of AVNRT after ablation. Fast-pathway ablation (cutting the "normal" wire and leaving the extra wire) should be attempted only when slow-pathway ablation has been unsuccessful. Prolongation of the PR interval and noninducibility are the primary markers of successful fast-pathway ablation. Slow-pathway ablation is superior to fast-pathway ablation because of higher success rates (99% vs. 85%) and a very low incidence of high-grade AV block (<1% vs. 10%). RFCA is appropriate first-line therapy for symptomatic patients with AVNRT.

CATHETER ABLATION OF ATRIOVENTRICULAR CONNECTIONS (ACCESSORY PATHWAYS AND THE WOLFF-PARKINSON-WHITE SYNDROME)

In normal cardiac physiology, the only electrical communication between the atrium and the ventricle is via the AV node. However, congenital abnormalities may bridge from the atrium to the ventricle, creating accessory pathways (APs). These tissue connections may cross along the tricuspid or mitral valves and infrequently the septum (Fig. 25-3, upper). Tachycardias resulting from APs are referred to as *AV reentrant tachycardias* and account for 30% of all

Figure 25-2

Atrioventricular Nodal Reentry Tachycardia

Location of the atrioventricular node

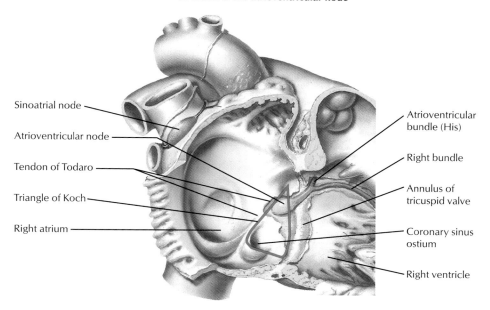

Sinoatrial node

Atrioventricular node

Tendon of Todaro

Triangle of Koch

Right atrium

Atrioventricular bundle (His)

Right bundle

Annulus of tricuspid valve

Coronary sinus ostium

Right ventricle

Catheter ablation of atrioventricular nodal reentry tachycardia (AVNRT)

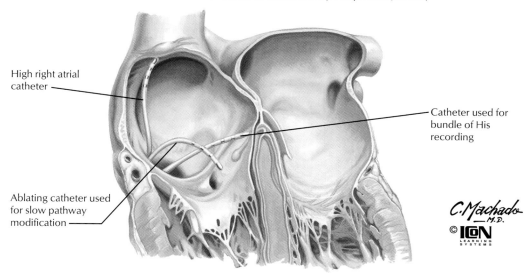

High right atrial catheter

Ablating catheter used for slow pathway modification

Catheter used for bundle of His recording

C. Machado M.D.

© ICON
LEARNING
SYSTEMS

supraventricular tachycardias. **Wolff-Parkinson-White (WPW) syndrome** results from a type of AP that conducts antegrade and is defined electrocardiographically by the presence of a short PR interval and a QRS prolongation (secondary to a delta wave). The abnormality of the QRS morphology is the result of the fusion of normal conduction through the AV node with the ventricular activation via the AP. The AP conduction is faster and "preexcites" the ventricle, causing a delta wave. Therefore, the delta wave represents the early depolarization of a small portion of the ventricular myocardium activated by the AP. ECG findings consistent with WPW syndrome

Figure 25-3

Accessory Pathways and the
Wolff-Parkinson-White Syndrome

Location of atrioventricular accessory pathways and classification

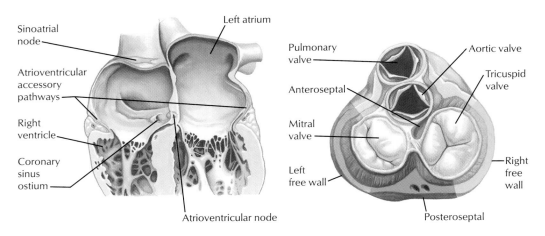

Sinoatrial node

Left atrium

Atrioventricular accessory pathways

Right ventricle

Coronary sinus ostium

Atrioventricular node

Pulmonary valve

Anteroseptal

Mitral valve

Left free wall

Aortic valve

Tricuspid valve

Right free wall

Posteroseptal

Catheter ablation of accessory pathways

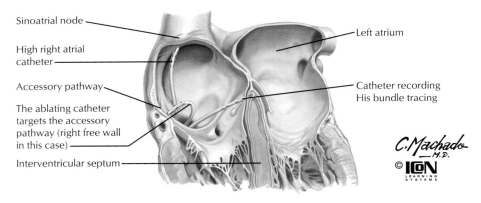

Sinoatrial node

High right atrial catheter

Accessory pathway

The ablating catheter targets the accessory pathway (right free wall in this case)

Interventricular septum

Left atrium

Catheter recording His bundle tracing

C. Machado
M.D.
© ICON
LEARNING SYSTEMS

Radiofrequency ablation

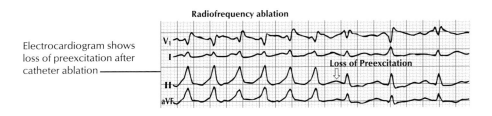

Electrocardiogram shows loss of preexcitation after catheter ablation

V₁

I

Loss of Preexcitation

II

aVF

occur in 1 to 3 individuals per 1000 in the general population. Most of these individuals have structurally normal hearts and no symptoms. No therapy is required for patients without symptoms and with normal physical examinations. APs are best classified as manifest (antegrade conduction producing the WPW ECG) and concealed (retrograde conduction only, usually normal baseline ECG). Many APs can function in both an antegrade and a retrograde fashion. However, most tachycardias result from a macroreentrant circuit that occurs because of conduction through the AV node (normal) with retrograde return to the atrium via the AP. The resultant narrow complex tachycardia is referred to as *orthodromic reciprocating tachycardia*. If this circuit functions in reverse, an unusually wide complex regular tachycardia, called an *antidromic reciprocating tachycardia*, is observed. Orthodromic reciprocating tachycardia is possible with a manifest or a concealed AP, requiring only that the pathway function in a reverse (retrograde) fashion. In reality, a spectrum of arrhythmias may be seen in patients with WPW syndrome, including both narrow complex tachycardias (orthodromic reciprocating tachycardia) and wide complex tachycardias (antidromic reciprocating tachycardia or atrial fibrillation, flutter, or atrial tachycardia conducting down the AP). The risk of sudden cardiac death associated with WPW syndrome (0.05–0.5%) is secondary to atrial fibrillation with subsequent rapid conduction to the ventricle through the AP. Some APs can conduct atrial fibrillation at rates of approximately 300 beats/min. The ventricle cannot indefinitely sustain these extremely fast rates, and ventricular fibrillation ensues. Atrial fibrillation may occur in up to a third of patients with WPW syndrome.

Fortunately, sudden cardiac death is rare and most APs are located on the endomyocardial surface of the AV groove (the mitral and tricuspid valve annuli), making them particularly accessible to RFCA. On the basis of their anatomic location along the AV annulus, APs can be classified as anteroseptal/midseptal (<10%), posteroseptal (20–30%), right free wall (10–20%), and left free wall (50–60%) (Fig. 25-3). In the North American Society for Pacing and Electrophysiology registry, the acute procedure success rate of AP ablations was 84% for anteroseptal sites, 80% for posteroseptal sites, 94% for left free wall sites, and 96% for right free wall sites. In experienced electrophysiology laboratories, the recurrence rates are less than 5%. RFCA is indicated in WPW patients with symptomatic arrhythmias involving APs.

ATRIAL FLUTTER AND ATRIAL TACHYCARDIA

Atrial flutter is characterized electrocardiographically by an atrial rate between 250 to 350 beats/min. Two types of atrial flutter have been described. The most common form, "typical" or type I, occurs in 90% of patients with this arrhythmia. In type I flutter, the ECG shows negative flutter waves in the inferior leads (II, III, aVF) corresponding to the "saw tooth" pattern and positive flutter waves in V1. The circuit of this arrhythmia involves the tissue area (isthmus) between the inferior vena cava and the tricuspid valve (Fig. 25-4). The impulse travels in a counterclockwise fashion in the atrium. By ablating the isthmus region, the circuit is eliminated, and therefore RF catheter techniques are highly effective in treating type I flutter. RF energy is used to produce a lesion line from the ventricular aspect of the tricuspid annulus across the subeustachian isthmus to the inferior vena cava.

In the North American Society for Pacing and Electrophysiology registry, the acute success rate of RFCA in atrial flutter varied from 80 to 90%. The recurrence rate of 10 to 20%, measured by noninducibility of flutter after ablation, is decreased to less than 5% if bidirectional block in the isthmus is documented after RF energy delivery.

Atrial flutter may also develop in areas of the atrium that have been affected by surgical procedures (Mustard/Senning/Fontan, atrial septal defect repair). This unique type of arrhythmia is referred to as *incisional flutter*. Pacing techniques are used to map the circuit, and RFCA can be employed to eliminate the circuit. New mapping systems that provide real-time three-dimensional views of the location of the circuit during tachycardia, greatly facilitating location of the arrhythmic focus and its subsequent treatment by RFCA.

Focal atrial tachycardias, caused by enhanced automaticity or triggered activity, tend to cluster in areas including the crista terminalis, coronary sinus

Figure 25-4

Atrial Flutter, Atrial Tachycardia, and Atrial Fibrillation

Reentry circuit of typical counterclockwise atrial flutter ("Sawtooth" pattern noted on the electrocardiogram)

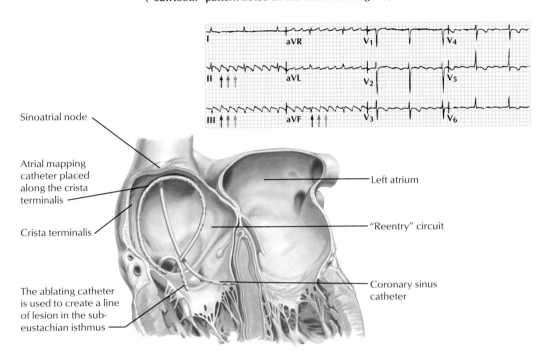

Sinoatrial node

Atrial mapping catheter placed along the crista terminalis

Crista terminalis

The ablating catheter is used to create a line of lesion in the sub-eustachian isthmus

Left atrium

"Reentry" circuit

Coronary sinus catheter

Catheter ablation of focal atrial fibrillation

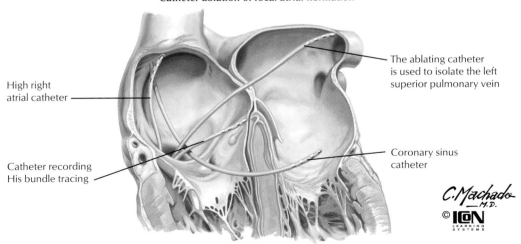

High right atrial catheter

Catheter recording His bundle tracing

The ablating catheter is used to isolate the left superior pulmonary vein

Coronary sinus catheter

ostium, tricuspid annulus, pulmonary veins, and mitral annulus. Mapping systems can identify areas of earliest atrial activation and thereby localize the target for RFCA. RFCA is typically performed during the tachycardia, and termination of the arrhythmia occurs during RF energy application.

Tachycardias may also arise from the sinoatrial node, including sinoatrial node reentrant tachycardia (paroxysmal) and inappropriate sinus tachycardia (usually incessant). Sinoatrial node reentrant tachycardia begins and ends abruptly, with P wave morphology indistinguishable from normal sinus rhythm. It arises from the junction between the atrium and the superior vena cava in the sinus node region. Ablation is performed at the site of earliest atrial activation and has a success rate greater than 95%.

Radiofrequency catheter ablation for inappropriate sinus tachycardia is done in the superior crista terminalis region. Success rates vary from 50 to 60%. Sinus node dysfunction (requiring a pacemaker) and superior vena cava syndrome are significant potential risks associated with inappropriate sinus tachycardia ablation. Hence, RFCA is reserved for symptomatic, drug-refractory cases.

ATRIAL FIBRILLATION

Atrial fibrillation (AF) is the most common sustained arrhythmia, with a prevalence of 5.9% in patients more than 65 years of age (see also chapter 19). The mainstay of managing AF is drug therapy (β-blockers/calcium channel blockers) designed to control rapid ventricular rates. Palliative procedures include AV junction ablation with pacemaker placement and AV node modification. AV junction ablation can be achieved by RFCA in the area of the bundle of His, approached from the right side of the heart. Occasionally, a left ventricular approach is needed. The long-term success is 98 to 100% for AV junction ablation and 70% for AV node modification. These procedures are offered to symptomatic patients with rapid ventricular rates despite optimum drug therapy, particularly when there is evidence of tachycardia-induced cardiomyopathy. The patients are still at risk for thromboembolic events and require warfarin therapy. Long-term improvements in quality of life and ventricular function have been observed.

Multiple catheter-based methods to cure AF have been attempted. Many, such as the catheter maze procedure, were abandoned because of limited success and significant associated complications. Mapping and ablating focal AF originating from pulmonary veins (the majority of the foci) and other sites have been performed in patients with idiopathic paroxysmal AF. Pulmonary veins are known to harbor arrhythmogenic foci that produce premature atrial contractions. Focal ablation within an isolated pulmonary vein has a success rate of 60% for elimination of AF. A repeat procedure is required in 50 to 75% of cases and is associated with symptomatic pulmonary vein stenosis—due to local thermal injury—in 2 to 4% of cases. The most popular curative technique involves segmental isolation of all pulmonary veins by discrete application of RF energy at the ostia (Fig. 25-4). The use of a circular or basket catheter facilitates mapping of the pulmonary vein ostium. These catheters allow accurate anatomic assessment and permit RFCA of the connection between the atrium and the pulmonary vein arrhythmogenic focus. The long-term cure rate is 60 to 70% without antiarrhythmic drugs. The best candidates for this procedure are symptomatic, drug-refractory patients with paroxysmal AF and normal or mildly enlarged left atria.

VENTRICULAR TACHYCARDIA ASSOCIATED WITH STRUCTURAL HEART DISEASE

Reentry within damaged myocardium is the most common mechanism underlying sustained monomorphic VT in patients with coronary artery disease. VT may also present in patients with hypertrophic cardiomyopathy, dilated cardiomyopathy, valvular heart disease, and surgically corrected congenital heart disease (see also Chapter 20). Implantable cardioverter defibrillators are the standard therapy for sustained VT. In patients who experience recurrent shocks from the implantable cardioverter defibrillator , RFCA may be used in an attempt to modify or eliminate the VT circuit and thereby reduce the number of shocks a patient may experience (Table 25-2). The success rates for RFCA of clinical VT (not all VT foci) range from 64 to 81%.

Table 25-2
QRS Polarity in Ventricular Tachycardia

VT Location	Negative QRS Leads	Positive QRS Leads
Basal	VR, inferior leads	Precordial leads
Apical	Precordial leads	
Anterior	Precordial leads	Inferior leads
Septal		I/a, VL
Lateral	I/a, VL	

VT indicates ventricular tachycardia.

Bundle branch reentrant ventricular tachycardia is commonly seen in patients with idiopathic dilated cardiomyopathy and is usually associated with a significant conduction delay in the His-Purkinje system. Bundle branch reentrant ventricular tachycardia usually shows a left bundle branch block QRS morphology, a leftward axis and a reentrant tachycardia using the right bundle as the antegrade limb and the left bundle as the retrograde limb. RFCA is performed to terminate conduction through the right bundle and consequently disrupt the abnormal circuit. Most patients require an implantable cardioverter defibrillator implantation because other forms of VT commonly coexist with Bundle branch reentrant ventricular tachycardia.

IDIOPATHIC VENTRICULAR TACHYCARDIA

Patients with normal hearts can have monomorphic ventricular tachycardia from several right and left ventricular sites. The most common is the right ventricular outflow tract VT, which has left bundle branch block and an inferior axis. The mechanism of tachycardia is thought to be catecholamine-dependent triggered activity, usually responsive to adenosine. Right ventricular outflow tract VT is easily treated with RFCA. It typically originates just below the pulmonary valve, in an anteroseptal or septal location.

Idiopathic fascicular left ventricular VT has a narrow, right bundle branch block superior axis morphology and is responsive to verapamil. This form of VT is a reentrant tachycardia that uses the Purkinje network and that usually arises in the inferoapical septum of the left ventricle. RFCA at the ideal site results in characteristic tachycardia acceleration and termination of the tachycardia. High success rates (85–100%) make RFCA a good alternative to drug therapy for this arrhythmia.

COMPLICATIONS

There is a 2 to 4% incidence of significant complications associated with RFCA. The risk of life-threatening complications including pericardial tamponade, pulmonary embolism, complete heart block, myocardial infarction, valvular injury, stroke, and death is less than 1% (Table 25-1).

FUTURE DIRECTIONS

Catheter ablation of supraventricular and ventricular arrhythmias is progressing rapidly. Advances in mapping techniques (basket catheters, noncontact mapping) and catheter design (delivery of deeper lesions) have made RFCA the first-line therapy for most symptomatic arrhythmias. Improved techniques for curative ablation of AF and RFCA for scar-related VT are potential developments in this field.

REFERENCES

Jackman WM, Beckman KJ, McClelland JH, et al. Treatment of supraventricular tachycardia due to atrioventricular nodal reentry, by radiofrequency catheter ablation of slow-pathway conduction. N Engl J Med 1992;327:313–318.

Jackman WM, Wang XZ, Friday KJ, et al. Catheter ablation of accessory atrioventricular pathways (Wolff-Parkinson-White syndrome) by radiofrequency current. N Engl J Med 1991;324:1605–1611.

Jais P, Haisseguerre M, Shah DC, et al. A focal source of atrial fibrillation treated by discrete radiofrequency ablation. Circulation 1997;95:572–576.

Klein LS, Shih HT, Hackett FK, Zipes DP, Wiles WM. Radiofrequency catheter ablation of ventricular tachycardia in patients without structural heart disease. Circulation 1992;85:1666–1674.

Morady F, Harvey M, Kalbfleisch SJ, el-Atassi R, Calkins H, Langberg JJ. Radiofrequency catheter ablation of ventricular tachycardia in patients with coronary artery disease. Circulation 1993;87:363–372.

Sanders WE Jr, Sorrentino RA, Greenfield RA, Shenasa H, Hamer ME, Wharton JM. Catheter ablation of sinoatrial nodal reentrant tachycardia. J Am Coll Cardiol 1994;23:926–934.

Scheinman MM, Huang S. The 1998 NASPE prospective catheter ablation registry. Pacing Clin Electrophysiol 2000;23:1020–1028.

Scheinman MM, Morady F, Hess DS, Gonzalez R. Catheter-induced ablation of the atrioventricular junction to control refractory supraventricular arrhythmias. JAMA 1982;248:851–855.

Chapter 26

Cardiac Pacemakers and Defibrillators

Margaret C. Herbst and William E. Sanders, Jr

Technological advances have improved the versatility and function of implantable devices used to treat arrhythmias, resulted in marked reduction of device size, and fostered the development of facile implant techniques. Surgical placement of pacemakers and implantable cardioverter defibrillators (ICDs) can be performed as outpatient procedures, and patients are encouraged to return to functional capacity shortly after the procedure.

The American College of Cardiology, in collaboration with the American Heart Association, has published guidelines for ICD and pacemaker implantation and antiarrhythmia devices. The recommendations are divided into three classes: Class I indications include conditions for which there is evidence or general agreement that device therapy is beneficial. Class IIa encompasses conditions for which there is a divergence of opinion but for which the weight of evidence favors device therapy, while Class IIb delineates the conditions for which efficacy is less well established. In Class III conditions, device therapy is considered not useful or possibly harmful. Table 26-1 outlines the American College of Cardiology/American Heart Association indications for Class I and IIa pacemaker and ICD implantation. Typical circumstances for device implantation are the focus of this chapter.

ETIOLOGY AND PATHOGENESIS

The pathologic states that necessitate pacemaker implantation are remarkably diverse. The most common indications involve defects in electrical impulse initiation or conduction through the specialized conduction system of the heart. Sinus node dysfunction, frequently referred to as sick sinus syndrome, is a major cause of bradycardia and an indication for pacemaker placement (see chapter 21). Damage to the sinoatrial node can result from infiltration (fibrosis, sarcoidosis, amyloidosis, etc.), infection, or infarction. This complex tissue is influenced significantly by parasympathetic and sympathetic tone and by many pharmacologic agents, electrolyte imbalance,

hypothermia, hyperthyroidism, and increased intracranial pressure. Elucidation of the precise etiology is imperative in determining whether device therapy is indicated.

The atrioventricular conduction system (including the atrioventricular node and bundle of His) is subject to disruption by the same conditions that affect the sinoatrial node; however, focal injury from infarction, infection, and catheter trauma is more common. Autonomic input plays a major role in the manifestation of most conduction system abnormalities.

An ICD is typically placed in patients with structural heart disease who are at risk for malignant tachyarrhythmias. Damage to the ventricular myocardium fosters the development of abnormal circuits. Usually, tissue damage is the result of myocardial infarction (MI), but can also be seen in infection (primarily viral), infiltration, and dysplasia.

CLINICAL SETTINGS

The strength of the recommendations for device therapy in conditions that result in Class I indications is primarily based on mortality data. Symptoms of bradycardia or tachycardia may be subtle (palpitations, dizziness) or dramatic (syncope or cardiac arrest). The correlation of symptoms to a specific arrhythmia helps establish the diagnosis and the indication for therapy (Table 26-1). Natural history studies of bradyarrhythmias suggest significant mortality in untreated acquired heart block and congenital heart block. Improved survival has also been demonstrated with pacing for high-degree heart

Table 26-1
Class I and Class IIa Indications for Permanent Pacing in Adults

Pacing for Acquired Atrioventricular Block in Adults

Class I
1. Third-degree and advanced second-degree atrioventricular (AV) block at any anatomic level, associated with any one of the following conditions:
   a. Bradycardia with symptoms (including heart failure) presumed to be due to AV block.
   b. Arrhythmia and other medical conditions that require drugs that result in symptomatic bradycardia.
   c. Documented periods of asystole greater than or equal to 3.0 seconds or any escape rate less than 40 beats/min in awake, symptom-free patients.
   d. After catheter ablation of the AV junction. There are no trials to assess outcome without pacing, and pacing is virtually always planned in this situation unless the operative procedure is AV junction modification.
   e. Postoperative AV block that is not expected to resolve after cardiac surgery.
   f. Neuromuscular diseases with AV block, such as myotonic muscular dystrophy, Kearns-Sayre syndrome, Erb's dystrophy (limb-girdle), and peroneal muscular atrophy, with or without symptoms, because there may be unpredictable progression of AV conduction disease.

Class IIa
1. Asymptomatic third-degree AV block at any anatomic site with average awake ventricular rates of 40 beats/min or faster, especially if cardiomegaly or left ventricular (LV) dysfunction is present.
2. Asymptomatic type II second-degree AV block with a narrow QRS. When type II second-degree AV block occurs with a wide QRS, pacing becomes a Class I recommendation (see section "Pacing for Chronic Bifascicular and Trifascicular Block," below).
3. Asymptomatic type I second-degree AV block at intra- or infra-His levels found at electrophysiology study performed for other indications.
4. First- or second-degree AV block with symptoms similar to those of pacemaker syndrome.

Pacing for Chronic Bifascicular and Trifascicular Block

Class I
1. Intermittent third-degree AV block.
2. Type II second-degree AV block.
3. Alternating bundle branch block.

Class IIa
1. Syncope not demonstrated to be due to AV block when other likely causes have been excluded, specifically ventricular tachycardia (VT).
2. Incidental finding at electrophysiology study of markedly prolonged HV interval ($\geq$100 ms) in asymptomatic patients.
3. Incidental finding at electrophysiology study of pacing-induced infra-His block that is not physiological.

Pacing for Atrioventricular Block Associated With Acute Myocardial Infarction

Class I
1. Persistent second-degree AV block in the His-Purkinje system with bilateral bundle branch block or third-degree AV block within or below the His-Purkinje system after acute myocardial infarction (MI).
2. Transient (second- or third-degree) infranodal AV block and associated bundle branch block. If the site of block is uncertain, an electrophysiology study may be necessary.
3. Persistent and symptomatic second- or third-degree AV block.

Pacing in Sinus Node Dysfunction

Class I
1. Sinus node dysfunction with documented symptomatic bradycardia, including frequent sinus pauses that produce symptoms. In some patients, bradycardia is iatrogenic and will occur as a consequence of essential long-term drug therapy of a type and dose for which there are no acceptable alternatives.
2. Symptomatic chronotropic incompetence.

Table 26-1
Class I and Class IIa Indications for Permanent Pacing in Adults (continued)

Class IIa

1. Sinus node dysfunction occurring spontaneously or as a result of necessary drug therapy with heart rates less than 40 beats/min when a clear association between significant symptoms consistent with bradycardia and the actual presence of bradycardia has not been documented.
2. Syncope of unexplained origin when major abnormalities of sinus node function are discovered or provoked in electrophysiological studies.

Pacing in Hypersensitive Carotid Sinus and Neurocardiogenic Syncope

Class I

1. Recurrent syncope caused by carotid sinus stimulation; minimal carotid sinus pressure induces ventricular asystole of more than 3-second duration in the absence of any medication that depresses the sinus node or AV conduction.

Class IIa

1. Recurrent syncope without clear, provocative events and with a hypersensitive cardioinhibitory response.
2. Syncope of unexplained origin when major abnormalities of sinus node function or AV conduction are discovered or provoked in electrophysiological studies.
3. Significantly symptomatic and recurrent neurocardiogenic syncope associated with bradycardia documented spontaneously or at the time of tilt-table testing.

Pacing in Idiopathic Dilated Cardiomyopathy

Class I

1. Class I indications for sinus node dysfunction or AV block as previously described.
2. Biventricular pacing in medically refractory, symptomatic New York Heart Association class III or IV patients with idiopathic dilated or ischemic cardiomyopathy, prolonged QRS interval (≥130 ms), LV end-diastolic diameter greater than or equal to 55 mm, and ejection fraction less than or equal to 35%.

Class I and Class IIa Indications for Implantable Cardioverter Defibrillator Therapy in Adults

Indications for Implantable Cardioverter-Defibrillator Therapy

Class I

1. Cardiac arrest due to ventricular fibrillation (VF) or VT not due to a transient or reversible cause.
2. Spontaneous sustained VT in association with structural heart disease.
3. Syncope of undetermined origin with clinically relevant, hemodynamically significant sustained VT or VF induced at electrophysiological study when drug therapy is ineffective, not tolerated, or not preferred.
4. Nonsustained VT in patients with coronary disease, prior MI, LV dysfunction, and inducible VF or sustained VT at electrophysiological study that is not suppressible by a Class I antiarrhythmic drug.
5. Spontaneous sustained VT in patients who do not have structural heart disease that is not amenable to other treatments.

Class IIa

Patients with LV ejection fraction of less than or equal to 30%, at least 1 month post-MI and 3 months post–coronary artery revascularization surgery.

block and for second-degree atrioventricular block (type II). Patients with acute MI, especially inferior infarction, have a high incidence of heart block that may be associated with excess mortality. Patients with acute MI and persistent high-degree heart block (>48 hours after MI) or transient advanced atrioventricular block associated with bundle branch block are candidates for temporary, and ultimately permanent, pacing. Patients with a symptomatic vasovagal syncope (history of syncope, positive tilt-table test demonstrating induced syncope or presyncope, and bradycardia) are known to have a reduced likelihood of syncope after implantation of a dual-chamber pacemaker. Individuals with a hypersensitive response (asystole of >3 seconds) during carotid sinus massage frequently experience presyncope and syncope, which are eliminated by pacemaker implant. It should be noted that pacing may only partially resolve symptoms because not all complaints are related to heart rate variations but may be the manifestation of vasodilatation.

Biventricular pacing is approved for treatment of patients with moderate to severe congestive heart failure (New York Heart Association class III or IV), reduced left ventricular ejection fraction, a widened QRS on the baseline ECG, and symptoms despite optimal medical therapy. Biventricular resynchronization is achieved by positioning pacemaker leads in the right ventricle and in a distal left-sided branch of the coronary sinus. This allows simultaneous pacing of both ventricles and corrects asynchronous ventricular contraction. Biventricular pacing improves exercise tolerance and quality of life in individuals with congestive heart failure.

Sudden cardiac death (SCD) from cardiac arrest not associated with MI or a reversible cause, and sustained ventricular tachycardia (clinical or induced during electrophysiology study), remain the traditional Class I indications for ICD implant. Although ischemic heart disease may produce the substrate for the development of tachyarrhythmia, there is increasing recognition of the high risk of SCD in cardiomyopathies from different etiologies (viral, infiltrative, hypertrophic, and hypertensive) and of the therapeutic benefits of ICD placement. In addition, indications for ICD placement are expand-

ing to include primary prevention of SCD in certain populations with congestive heart failure. In patients with structurally normal hearts (normal ejection fraction), but electrical genetic abnormalities, such as long QT syndrome, Brugada syndrome, and right ventricular dysplasia, ICD placement is also frequently warranted.

MANAGEMENT AND THERAPY
Pacemaker Technology and Application

Pacemaker technology offers many device choices: single versus dual chamber, fixed rate versus rate responsive, and various sensors and lead options (Fig. 26-1). To clarify pacemaker characteristics, the North American Society for Pacing and Electrophysiology and the British Pacing and Electrophysiology Group published a four-letter code that describes features specific to each pacemaker. The first letter or category of the code indicates the chamber(s) paced and the second describes the chamber(s) sensed. Options for these positions include O (none), A (atrium), V (ventricle), and D (dual = A+V). The code's third position indicates the response of the device to sensing; options include O (none), T (triggered), I (inhibited), and D (dual triggered and inhibited). The fourth position indicates programmability of rate modulation. The letter R in this position indicates that the device has an active rate responsive sensor. The North American Society for Pacing and Electrophysiology/British Pacing and Electrophysiology Group generic pacemaker code allows the programmed functions and pacemaker settings of a particular device to be easily described and communicated. A pacemaker programmed to the DDDR mode, for example, paces both chambers (D), senses both chambers (D), employs a dual response (D) for sensing (inhibits with a sensed beat and triggers ventricular activation after atrial sensing or pacing), and utilizes a rate responsive sensor (R).

Implantable Cardioverter Defibrillator Technology and Application

Although the first devices used clinically in the 1980s required open chest procedures, the development of intravascular lead systems has made it possible for ICD implantation to be performed on an outpatient basis for most patients,

Figure 26-1

Implantable Cardiac Pacemaker
(Dual-Chamber Cardiac Pacing)

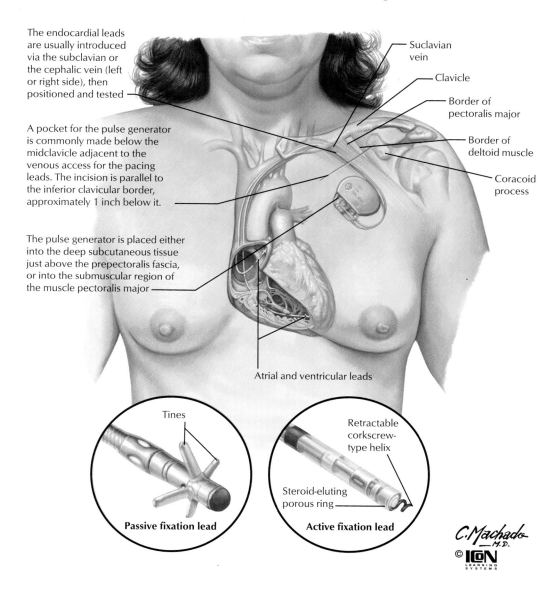

The endocardial leads are usually introduced via the subclavian or the cephalic vein (left or right side), then positioned and tested

Suclavian vein

Clavicle

Border of pectoralis major

A pocket for the pulse generator is commonly made below the midclavicle adjacent to the venous access for the pacing leads. The incision is parallel to the inferior clavicular border, approximately 1 inch below it.

Border of deltoid muscle

Coracoid process

The pulse generator is placed either into the deep subcutaneous tissue just above the prepectoralis fascia, or into the submuscular region of the muscle pectoralis major

Atrial and ventricular leads

Tines

Passive fixation lead

Retractable corkscrew-type helix

Steroid-eluting porous ring

Active fixation lead

C. Machado
—M.D.
© ICON
LEARNING
SYSTEMS

The leads connecting the pulse generator to the endocardium can be different types: unipolar or bipolar and of active fixation or passive fixation. The unipolar system has a single electrode (cathode, negative pole) in contact with the endocardium, and the anode is the pulse generator itself. The bipolar system lead has both a cathode and an anode at the tip of the same lead. Passive fixation leads have tines, barbs that anchor the lead to the endocardial trabecular muscle of the chamber in which it is implanted. Active fixation leads have a corkscrew-type device or helix that is placed into the myocardium. Both types irritate the myocardium, causing inflammatory reaction and cellular growth around the lead. To minimize the inflammatory reaction, most leads have steroid-eluting tips.

Figure 26-2

Implantable Cardiac Defibrillator
(Dual-Chamber Leads)

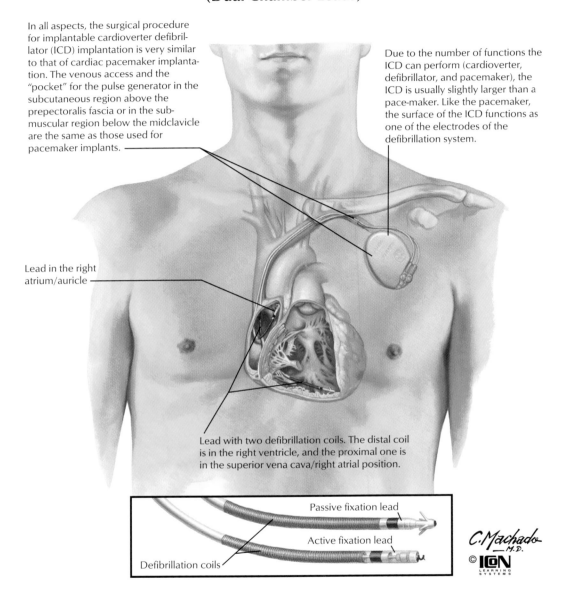

In all aspects, the surgical procedure for implantable cardioverter defibrillator (ICD) implantation is very similar to that of cardiac pacemaker implantation. The venous access and the "pocket" for the pulse generator in the subcutaneous region above the prepectoralis fascia or in the submuscular region below the midclavicle are the same as those used for pacemaker implants.

Due to the number of functions the ICD can perform (cardioverter, defibrillator, and pacemaker), the ICD is usually slightly larger than a pace-maker. Like the pacemaker, the surface of the ICD functions as one of the electrodes of the defibrillation system.

Lead in the right atrium/auricle

Lead with two defibrillation coils. The distal coil is in the right ventricle, and the proximal one is in the superior vena cava/right atrial position.

Passive fixation lead

Active fixation lead

Defibrillation coils

C. Machado
—M.D.
© **ICON**
LEARNING SYSTEMS

ICD leads have a tip electrode that can sense the heart rate and deliver an electrical stimulus to pace the heart. The defibrillation coils that are part of ICD leads are not found on standard pacemaker leads. At least one coil (in the right ventricle) is necessary for defibrillation. Some models have a second defibrillation coil, which is positioned in the superior vena cava/right atrium.

as is the case with pacemaker placement. The therapeutic capabilities have expanded with concomitant reduction in device size. ICDs provide defibrillation, lower energy cardioversion, antiarrhythmic pacing, and dual chamber cardiac pacing (Fig. 26-2). ICD therapy is superior to therapy with antiarrhythmic drugs for treatment of life-threatening ventricular arrhythmias.

Serial electrophysiologic testing and Holter-guided drug studies have no role in the treatment of patients with documented sustained ventricular arrhythmias. Indeed, the indications for ICD implantation have continued to expand as ongoing trials demonstrate mortality reduction in different patient populations. The recent demonstration that patients with left ventricular dysfunction following MI benefit from ICD implantation has drastically changed the way in which cardiologists practice.

Device Implant and Function

Pacemaker and ICD systems consist of a pulse generator and endocardial leads placed in the atrium, ventricle, or both, positioned using fluoroscopy. Endocardial system leads are introduced via access through the subclavian or cephalic vein; rarely used epicardial leads require a more invasive surgical approach. After the endocardial lead system is positioned and tested, the pulse generator is implanted into the subcutaneous or submuscular region below the mid-clavicle. Leads are secured to the endocardial surface of the right ventricle, the right atrium and, in the case of biventricular pacing devices, the coronary sinus. A pacemaker lead typically has two electrodes (bipolar) in contact with the ventricular or atrial myocardium. Impulses delivered by the pulse generator through these electrodes pace the heart (Fig. 26-1). An ICD lead has a similar distal structure, but it has an additional coil in the right ventricle and usually in the atrium (see Fig. 26-2). These coils act as shock electrodes in conjunction with the ICD (pulse generator) itself. Hence, the ICD works as a pacemaker (when necessary) and a defibrillator.

Postoperative Care

Postoperatively, patients are instructed to keep the surgical incision clean and dry for approximately 10 days and to notify their provider of any evidence of infection. They are asked to limit ipsilateral arm use to below shoulder level and to avoid heavy lifting for a few weeks to prevent lead dislodgment. Driving restrictions are typically imposed for approximately 6 months in patients who have had an ICD placed for documented sustained ventricular tachycardia or ventricular fibrillation. Occa-sionally, it may be reasonable to shorten the driving restrictions. Patients who undergo ICD implant for primary prevention are generally not restricted from driving. It is recommended that commercial driving be permanently prohibited.

Pacemaker patients are followed transtelephonically every 3 months, with clinic evaluations for complete battery voltage and lead testing every 6 to 12 months. Although some ICD patients can be evaluated transtelephonically, the general follow-up entails clinic evaluation approximately every 4 months for device testing and evaluations of electrogram recorded by the device during a tachyarrhythmia.

Electromagnetic Interference

Electromagnetic interference occurs when a source emits electromagnetic waves that interfere with the proper function of the device. There is no restriction on the use of household items such as microwaves, televisions, radios, or electric blankets as these are not sources of electromagnetic interference. Although passage through a metal detector will not harm ICD or pacemaker function, it is recommended that patients with these devices not be in close contact with hand-held metal detectors or scanning "wands" containing magnets. Instead, patients are advised to present their device identification card to security personnel and request a hand search. Cellular telephone use is not prohibited, although patients are advised to use the phone on the contralateral ear (≥10 cm from the device) and to not carry the phone in the breast pocket on top of the implanted device. Electronic article surveillance systems are not likely to cause a negative interaction with an implanted device as long as the patient is not standing close to the scanning system for a prolonged period of time. Patients are instructed to walk normally through such devices.

Medical sources of potential electromagnetic interference include magnetic resonance imaging scanners, radiation therapy, transthoracic cardioversion, and electrocautery. The effect of a strong magnetic field differs for pacemakers and ICDs: pacemaker exposure to an electromagnetic field usually results in asynchronous pacing; exposure of an ICD can result in "blinding" of the device, potentially causing therapy for tachyarrhythmias to be inappropriately withheld. Magnetic resonance imaging scans are generally contraindicated in patients with implanted devices. Direct radiation of an implanted pacemaker or ICD is not recommended; if necessary, the device should be moved to the opposite side and shielded from the direct beam. Implanted ICDs and pacemakers should be evaluated before and after electrical cardioversion, and the external electrodes used for cardioversion (anterior–posterior position) should be positioned as far as possible (≥5 cm) from the implanted device. Surgical electrocautery presents unique concerns for the ICD patient because electrical output from the cautery can be mistakenly detected by the ICD, resulting in inappropriate delivery of therapy during a normal rhythm. Hence, the detection function of the ICD should be inactivated before any surgery or procedure during which electrocautery may be used. Electrocautery may also interfere with pacemaker sensing and inhibit output. In the pacemaker-dependent patient, the anesthesiologist may need to apply a magnet to the pacemaker to provide asynchronous pacing in this event. Electrocautery in close proximity to an older pacemaker may render it nonoperational. It is recommended that postoperative electrocardiograms, with and without magnet application, be performed after the use of electrocautery to confirm proper pacemaker function.

FUTURE DIRECTIONS

Advances in pacemaker and ICD technology have substantially improved survival and quality of life for patients with cardiac arrhythmias. In addition to patients with recognized bradycardic and tachycardic arrhythmias for whom established indications exist for pacemaker and ICD implant, future studies will evaluate these devices in the treatment of atrial fibrillation, congestive heart failure, and primary prevention of SCD. Implantable devices are considered the most effective way to prevent SCD mortality in high-risk groups and may also provide hope for improved quality of life in this population.

REFERENCES

Abraham WT, Fisher WG, Smith AL, et al. Cardiac resynchronization in chronic heart failure. N Engl J Med 2002;346:1845–1853.

AVID Investigators. A comparison of antiarrhythmic-drug therapy with implantable defibrillators in patients resuscitated from near-fatal ventricular arrhythmias. N Engl J Med 1997;337:1576–1583.

Bernstein AD, Camm AJ, Fletcher RD, et al. The NASPE/BPEG generic pacemaker code for antibradyarrhythmia and adaptive-rate pacing and antitachyarrhythmia devices. PACE 1987;10(pt 1):794.

Buxton AE, Lee KL, Fisher JD, et al. A randomized study of the prevention of sudden death in patients with coronary artery disease. N Engl J Med 1999;341:1882–1890.

Glikson M, Hayes DL. Cardiac pacing: A review. Med Clin North Am 2001;85:369–421.

Mangrum JM, DiMarco JP. The evaluation and management of bradycardia. N Engl J Med 2000;342:703–709.

Moss AJ, Hall WJ, Cannom DS, et al. Improved survival with an implanted defibrillator in patients with coronary disease at high risk for ventricular arrhythmia. N Engl J Med 1996;335:1933–1940.

Moss AJ, Zareba W, Hall WJ, et al. Prophylactic implantation of a defibrillator in patients with myocardial infarction and reduced ejection fraction. N Engl J Med 2002;346:877–883.

Section V

VALVULAR HEART DISEASE

Chapter 27
Aortic Stenosis

Timothy A. Mixon and Gregory J. Dehmer

The leaflets of the aortic valve form three pocketlike cusps of approximately equal size that separate the left ventricle from the aorta. The normal aortic valve opens completely during systole, allowing unimpaired ejection of blood from the left ventricle. Closure of the aortic valve prevents retrograde blood flow from the aorta into the left ventricle and allows the left ventricle to fill solely from the left atrium in preparation for the next beat. The outflow of blood from the left ventricle can become obstructed at several levels. The most common cause of aortic stenosis is an abnormality within the valve apparatus that obstructs flow by impairing valve mobility and opening.

Nonvalvular obstruction of left ventricular (LV) outflow usually results from a congenital narrowing and may occur above or below the valve. Hypertrophic cardiomyopathy, which produces a dynamic subaortic obstruction is also an important cause and is the focus of chapter 13.

ETIOLOGY AND PATHOGENESIS

The etiology of valvular aortic stenosis varies with the patient's age at presentation. In childhood, valvular **congenital abnormalities** are the usual cause of stenosis. The aortic valve may be unicuspid, bicuspid, tricuspid, or, rarely, even quadricuspid (Fig. 27-1). Unicuspid valves usually are severely narrowed at birth and produce symptoms in infancy. Bicuspid and malformed tricuspid valves rarely cause symptoms during childhood. More frequently, the abnormal architecture of bicuspid and malformed tricuspid valves alters flow patterns across the valve, slowly traumatizing the leaflets, leading to progressive fibrosis, calcification, and stenosis between age 50 and 70 years. **Acquired abnormalities** from senile, calcific degeneration of a previously normal valve predominate in patients diagnosed after age 70 years (Fig. 27-2).

Rheumatic involvement of the aortic valve, less prevalent now than a generation ago, usually results in a combination of stenosis and regurgitation, often with mitral valve disease. Less common causes of aortic valve stenosis include obstructive vegetations from endocarditis, prior radiation therapy, and rheumatoid involvement with severe nodular thickening of the valve leaflets. Aortic stenosis may also be associated with systemic diseases including Paget's, Fabry's, ochronosis, and end-stage renal disease.

Aortic stenosis is more common in older patients (>70 years) and men, but there is no apparent racial predilection. An association has been noted between aortic stenosis and some risk factors for coronary artery disease, including diabetes and hypercholesterolemia, supporting a concept that degenerative, calcific aortic stenosis is a proliferative, inflammatory disease.

CLINICAL PRESENTATION

Aortic stenosis is often asymptomatic for years. Prolonged, severe pressure overload imposed by outflow tract obstruction results in concentric LV hypertrophy (LVH), a compensatory adaptation that lowers wall stress and maintains forward flow but also has detrimental effects, including an abnormal diastolic filling pattern and subendocardial ischemia.

The principal symptoms of aortic stenosis are angina, syncope, and overt congestive heart failure. The average survival period without valve replacement is 5 and 3 years in patients who present with angina or syncope, respectively. The most concerning symptom is CHF. In patients with aortic stenosis presenting with CHF, the average survival without valve replacement is 2 years. Angina occurs in two thirds of patients with severe aortic stenosis, and approximately half of these have concomitant coronary artery disease. In the absence of coronary artery disease, angina is caused by subendocardial ischemia induced by increased wall thickness

Figure 27-1 ## Anomalies of the Left Ventricular Outflow Tract

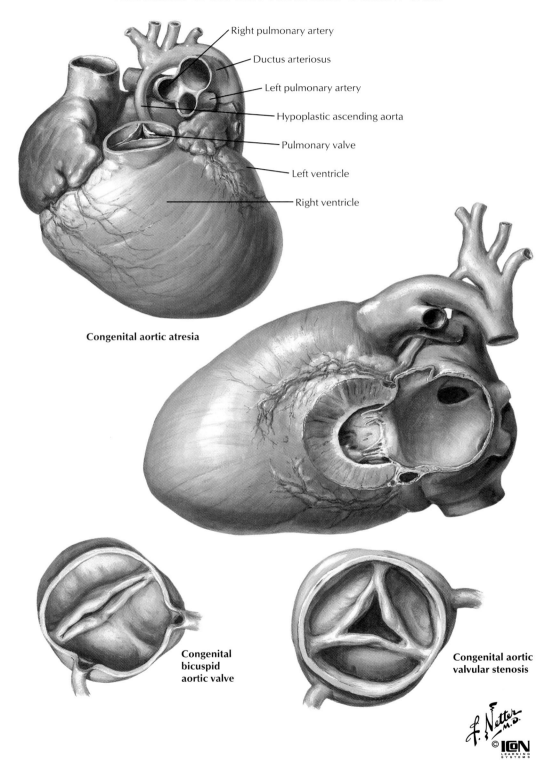

Right pulmonary artery

Ductus arteriosus

Left pulmonary artery

Hypoplastic ascending aorta

Pulmonary valve

Left ventricle

Right ventricle

Congenital aortic atresia

Congenital bicuspid aortic valve

Congenital aortic valvular stenosis

Figure 27-2

Rheumatic and Nonrheumatic
Causes of Aortic Stenosis

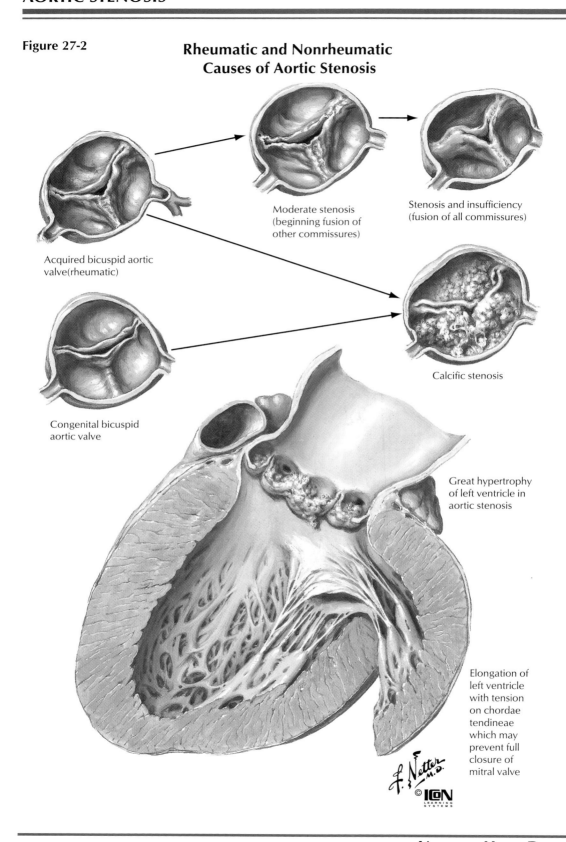

Moderate stenosis
(beginning fusion of
other commissures)

Stenosis and insufficiency
(fusion of all commissures)

Acquired bicuspid aortic
valve(rheumatic)

Calcific stenosis

Congenital bicuspid
aortic valve

Great hypertrophy
of left ventricle in
aortic stenosis

Elongation of
left ventricle
with tension
on chordae
tendineae
which may
prevent full
closure of
mitral valve

with relatively decreased capillary density, prolonged ejection time, and increased LV end-diastolic pressure, which reduces the diastolic transmyocardial perfusion gradient.

The causes of syncope include exertion, LVH, and arrhythmias. Exertion lowers the systemic vascular resistance while an increase in cardiac output is limited by the fixed outflow tract obstruction; this combination leads to cerebral and cardiac hypoperfusion. LVH from the development of aortic stenosis may cause an exaggerated vasodepressor response when activity increases the already elevated LV systolic pressure. Arrhythmias, including atrial fibrillation, ventricular tachycardia, ventricular fibrillation, and atrioventricular conduction abnormalities, may cause syncope at rest or on exertion.

Congestive heart failure is often caused by diastolic dysfunction, related to the development of LVH-related abnormal ventricular relaxation and decreased compliance. Systolic dysfunction with progressive ventricular dilation may occur late in the disease course. To compensate for the LV pressure load, the left atrium hypertrophies and develops vigorous contractions that allow adequate filling of the left ventricle despite increased LV end-diastolic pressure. However, as the disease progresses or with physical activity, left atrial pressure increases further, leading to higher pulmonary venous pressures and eventually to pulmonary congestion and edema. Pulmonary edema may develop abruptly during activity or with the loss of atrial function, as in atrial fibrillation.

Other manifestations of aortic stenosis may include gastrointestinal bleeding from angiodysplasia, the development of infective endocarditis, embolic phenomenon from an infective vegetation or detachment of small calcium deposits, and sudden cardiac death from serious ventricular arrhythmias.

Physical Examination

One of the most reliable findings in severe aortic stenosis is decreased pulsation of the carotid arteries, slowed arterial upstroke (pulsus parvus et tardus), with the maximum carotid upstroke noticeably delayed after the apical impulse (Fig. 27-3). A marked vibration may be felt in the carotid artery. The jugular venous pressure is not elevated

unless heart failure is present. In mild aortic stenosis, the jugular venous pulsation may show a prominent *a* wave, whereas late in the disease a prominent *v* wave may occur from tricuspid insufficiency caused by pulmonary hypertension and bulging of the hypertrophied septum into the right ventricle. The LV apical impulse is usually displaced inferiorly and laterally, with a palpable presystolic pulsation ("palpable S_4"). If the apical impulse is hyperdynamic, concomitant aortic or mitral insufficiency should be considered. The first heart sound is usually normal; the second heart sound may be single because of the absence of the aortic component from immobile aortic leaflets, or it may be paradoxically split from a marked delay of LV ejection. The murmur may be preceded by an early systolic ejection click, heard more frequently with a bicuspid valve or a congenital aortic stenosis in which the leaflets have preserved pliability. The murmur is characteristically described as crescendo-decrescendo and harsh in quality, most prominent at the right upper sternal border, with transmission to the carotids. High-frequency resonations may be heard at the apex ("Gallavardin murmur") and can be misinterpreted as mitral regurgitation. As aortic stenosis worsens, the murmur can continue into mid systole and late systole with progressively later peaking.

The murmur of aortic sclerosis is similar to that heard in aortic stenosis, but tends to be an early-peaking murmur, and carotid pulsations are normal. The murmur of mitral regurgitation is usually easily distinguished from aortic stenosis. It is pansystolic, with a more musical quality and constant intensity despite variable cardiac cycle length. The murmur of aortic stenosis is accentuated after pauses such as those associated with post-extrasystolic beats or long cycles in atrial fibrillation. The LV outflow tract murmur associated with hypertrophic obstructive cardiomyopathy can be similar in character, but responds to provocative maneuvers in a very characteristic manner (see chapters 1 and 13). The murmur of valvular aortic stenosis increases with increased flow across the valve resulting from squatting or maneuvers to increase preload and decreases in intensity with a Valsalva maneuver. The murmur of hypertrophic cardiomyopathy with obstruction becomes more

Figure 27-3

Aortic Stenosis

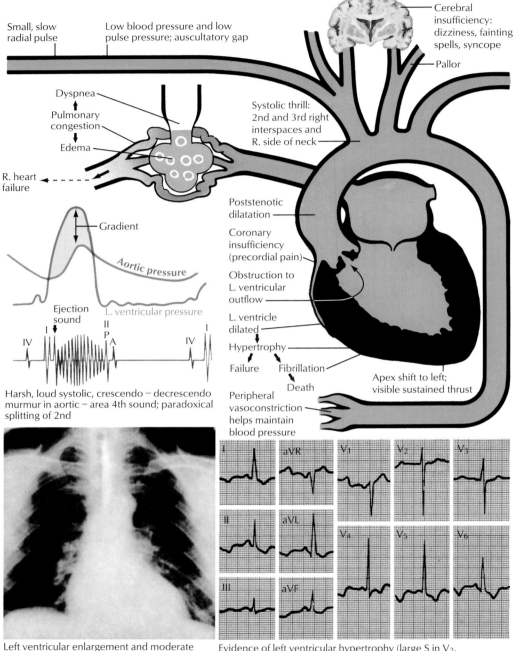

Small, slow radial pulse

Low blood pressure and low pulse pressure; auscultatory gap

Cerebral insufficiency: dizziness, fainting spells, syncope

Pallor

Dyspnea

Pulmonary congestion

Edema

R. heart failure

Systolic thrill: 2nd and 3rd right interspaces and R. side of neck

Gradient

Aortic pressure

L. ventricular pressure

Ejection sound

II
P
A

IV
I
IV
I

Harsh, loud systolic, crescendo – decrescendo murmur in aortic – area 4th sound; paradoxical splitting of 2nd

Poststenotic dilatation

Coronary insufficiency (precordial pain)

Obstruction to L. ventricular outflow

L. ventricle dilated

Hypertrophy

Failure Fibrillation

Death

Peripheral vasoconstriction helps maintain blood pressure

Apex shift to left; visible sustained thrust

Left ventricular enlargement and moderate dilatation of ascending aorta (poststenotic)

I aVR V_1 V_2 V_3

II aVL V_4 V_5 V_6

III aVF

Evidence of left ventricular hypertrophy (large S in V_2, large R in V_5) and "strain" (inverted T and depressed S–T in I, II, aVL, V_5, V_6)

prominent with decreasing preload, such as the straining phase of the Valsalva maneuver or standing upright. Further, the carotid upstroke in hypertrophic cardiomyopathy with obstruction is rapid and has a bisferious quality.

DIFFERENTIAL DIAGNOSIS

Differentiation of valvular aortic stenosis from other causes of LV outflow tract obstruction is important because the treatment and prognosis differs depending on the precise disease etiology. **Subvalvular** outflow tract obstruction may be due to a discrete subaortic membrane, a fibromuscular deformity (tunnel defect), or disproportionate muscular hypertrophy of the intraventricular septum with dynamic obstruction of the outflow tract (previously called idiopathic hypertrophic subaortic stenosis). **Supravalvular** outflow tract obstruction is much less common than the other varieties. It occurs in three forms: a circumferential hourglass narrowing of the aorta above the valve, a discrete fibromembranous ring, or a hypoplastic variety with diffuse narrowing of the ascending aorta.

DIAGNOSTIC APPROACH

In patients with an aortic stenosis, the ECG most commonly shows sinus rhythm until late in the disease course. The most common findings are LVH (>80%) (Fig. 27-4) and left atrial abnormality manifested by a negative terminal deflection of P waves in lead V_1 corresponding to left atrial hypertrophy. Less common findings include ST-segment depression in leads V_4 through V_6 (the left ventricular "strain pattern") and conduction system disease from calcification of the specialized conduction tissue, manifested as atrioventricular block, left anterior fascicular block, or a nonspecific intraventricular conduction delay.

A chest x-ray usually shows a normal-sized cardiac silhouette, as the ventricles may be hypertrophied but usually not grossly dilated. Left atrial enlargement and signs of pulmonary venous congestion may be present. It is uncommon to see calcification of the aortic valve leaflets on standard chest x-ray examination, but some calcium near the aortic and mitral valve annuli is common and poststenotic dilatation of the ascending aorta may be present. Calcified aortic valve leaflets can often be visualized by careful cardiac fluoroscopy.

Two-dimensional echocardiography with Doppler is useful for evaluating suspected aortic stenosis. A complete echocardiogram can reveal the location of the aortic outflow obstruction, estimate the severity of valvular obstruction, and provide supplemental information such as the function of the left ventricle, the degree of LVH, the size of the left atrium, and the presence or absence of associated valvular abnormalities (most notably, mitral regurgitation or aortic insufficiency) (Fig. 27-5). Doppler interrogation of the flow across the aortic valve can be used to estimate the transvalvular aortic pressure gradient, using a modification of the Bernoulli equation. The measured pressure decrease across the valve depends on the severity of the stenosis and the flow volume across the valve. With valvular aortic stenosis, the valve area is fixed, but flow across the valve, and hence the pressure gradient, varies depending on a number of factors, including exercise, anxiety, anemia, or concomitant aortic insufficiency and LV systolic dysfunction, sedation, or hypovolemia. Transvalvular gradients are reported as a mean value or as a peak instantaneous gradient. Although these measures are linearly related, neither corresponds exactly to the peak-to-peak gradient frequently reported from simultaneous measurements made with catheters. In general, a peak transvalvular gradient of greater than 100 mm Hg or a mean transvalvular gradient of greater than 50 mm Hg is consistent with severe aortic stenosis. Aortic valve areas can be calculated via the continuity equation or estimated directly by planimetry. Because the pressure gradient can vary considerably under different conditions, the calculated aortic valve area is generally thought to be a more reliable measure of severity. A calculated aortic valve area of less than 1.0 cm^2 or 0.5 cm^2/m^2 is consistent with severe aortic stenosis.

Because of the relationship of flow and pressure across the valve, some patients with low cardiac output secondary to left-sided heart failure have a low transvalvular pressure gradient (<30 mm Hg) despite the presence of significant aortic stenosis. Valve area calculations in this circumstance may be misleading; it is often helpful to increase the cardiac output with intravenous inotropic drugs and to use the new data to recalculate the valve area. If the increase in cardiac output causes a sub-

Figure 27-4

Left Ventricular Hypertrophy

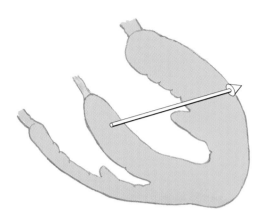

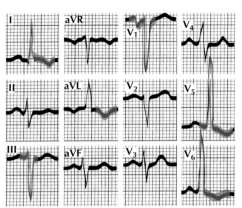

High voltage in limb leads (R I + S III ≥25 mm) or precordial leads (S V_1 + R V_5 or R V_6 ≥35mm). Often, left atrial enlargement. ST–T abnormalities.

Causes

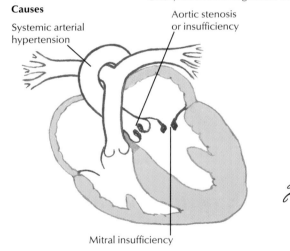

Systemic arterial hypertension

Aortic stenosis or insufficiency

Mitral insufficiency

stantial increase in the calculated valve area, the primary problem is likely to be a primary cardiomyopathy, rather than aortic stenosis. If the increase in cardiac output results in a substantial increase in the gradient (and decrease in the calculated valve area), the primary problem is likely to be a stenotic valve. Patients with severe aortic stenosis and impaired LV systolic function generally benefit from aortic valve replacement, although the immediate risk of surgery is higher than that in individuals with aortic stenosis and normal LV systolic function before surgery. After valve replacement, LV systolic function returns to normal in many patients with impaired LV systolic function as a result of aortic stenosis.

In the past, the degree of stenosis was commonly confirmed with invasive hemodynamic measurements; it is now acceptable to forgo invasive hemodynamic evaluation unless the historic, physical, and echocardiographic findings are discordant. In this circumstance, right- and left-sided heart catheterization is indicated to directly obtain pressure gradients and measure of cardiac output. Valve resistance can also be calculated and is less dependent on flow across the stenotic valve orifice. Before replacement of the aortic valve, coronary angiography is indicated for all patients who are older than 35 years or who have two or more risk factors for coronary artery disease.

Figure 27-5 Two-Dimentional Echocardiography and Doppler Analysis in a Patient With Aortic Stenosis

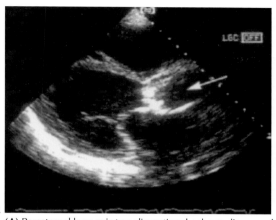
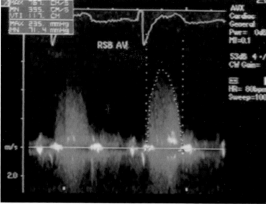

A   B

(A) Parasternal long axis two-dimentional echocardiogram showing an immobile, heavily calcified aortic valve (arrow). (B) continuous wave Doppler echocardiography shows the velocity profile across the aortic valve. Standard on-line software assists in determining the peak velocity and time + velocity integral, which are used to determine the valve area based on the continuity equation. It is essential to intergrate the jet from multiple transducer positions to obtain the true maximal jet, which is found when the transducer is parallel to the direction of flow.

MANAGEMENT AND THERAPY

Medical therapy for valvular aortic stenosis is usually limited to the treatment of complications, such as heart failure, rhythm disturbances, and infective endocarditis. Heart failure is treated with digoxin and the judicious use of diuretics. Volume depletion must be avoided, because aggressive diuresis may lead to severe hypotension. Elevated blood pressure may be controlled with medications, but excessive afterload reduction is not helpful and should be avoided. Because the ability of cardiac output to increase is limited in severe aortic stenosis, lowering the systemic pressure can increase the transvalvular gradient and worsen symptoms. Atrial fibrillation may occur late in the disease course of patients with aortic stenosis, raising the question of concomitant mitral valve disease. Atrial fibrillation is treated in the usual manner, with emphasis on the maintenance of sinus rhythm and appropriate anticoagulation. In patients with aortic stenosis, loss of atrial contraction can result in a marked decrease in cardiac output. Rarely, the onset of atrial fibrillation may be catastrophic in terms of hemodynamic decompensation due to loss of effective ventricular filling; urgent electrical cardioversion may be necessary in this circumstance. Infective endocarditis occurs more frequently with congenital valvular abnormalities

and is less common with senile, calcific aortic stenosis. Patients with moderate to severe degrees of outflow tract obstruction should not engage in vigorous, unsupervised exercise.

Aortic valve replacement is indicated for the treatment of symptomatic aortic stenosis. In fact, replacement is frequently delayed until symptoms develop. Prosthetic, bioprosthetic, and homograft valves all provide excellent symptom relief and improve the mortality rate, with the expected survival rate approaching that of the unaffected population. Asymptomatic patients with a severe aortic stenosis generally have an excellent prognosis without valve replacement, but 1 to 2% die suddenly or have rapid progression, with syncope and sudden cardiac death. Nevertheless, valve replacement is not recommended for most asymptomatic individuals because the rate of mortality for the operation is similar to the rate without the operation and placement of a prosthetic valve exposes the patient to associated risks (valve dysfunction, prosthetic valve endocarditis, bleeding from anticoagulant therapy). Surgery may be considered for asymptomatic patients who have LV dysfunction, exercise-induced hypotension, ventricular tachycardia, very severe valvular aortic stenosis, or extreme LVH.

Balloon valvotomy is useful in the palliation of congenital aortic stenosis (in young patients) but late restenosis and a need for valve replacement often occur. In older patients with calcific aortic stenosis, balloon valvotomy is indicated only as a bridge to surgery in critically ill patients, in patients who require urgent noncardiac surgery, or as palliation for terminal patients with a limited life expectancy.

FUTURE DIRECTIONS

Minimally invasive aortic valve replacement surgery via a right parasternal incision is gradually replacing the traditional approach of a median sternotomy. Percutaneous alternatives to surgical valve replacement are also being developed and tested in patients. Although valve replacement surgery has been considered the only treatment option, there is now preliminary evidence that therapy with statin drugs reduces the rate of progression of aortic stenosis by about half compared to the rate in patients not receiving statin drugs.

REFERENCES

Carabello BA. Aortic stenosis. *N Engl J Med* 2002;346: 677–682.

Ford LE, Feldman T, Chiu C, Carroll JD. Hemodynamic resistance as a measure of functional impairment in aortic valvular stenosis. *Circ Res* 1990;66:1–7.

Lester SJ, Heilbron B, Gin K, Dodek A, Jue J. The natural history and rate of progression of aortic stenosis. *Chest* 1998;113:1109–1114.

Lombard JT, Selzer A. Valvular aortic stenosis: A clinical and hemodynamic profile of patients *Ann Intern Med* 1987;106:292–298.

Marcus ML, Doty DB, Hiratzka LF, Wright CB, Eastman CL. Decreased coronary reserve: A mechanism for angina pectoris in patients with aortic stenosis and normal coronary arteries. *N Engl J Med* 1982;307:1362–1367.

Perloff JK. Clinical recognition of aortic stenosis: The physical signs and differential diagnosis of the various forms of obstruction to left ventricular outflow. *Prog Cardiovasc Dis* 1968;10:323.

Roberts WC. Valvular, subvalvular, and supravalvular aortic stenosis: Morphological features. *Cardiovasc Clin* 1973;5:97–126.

Chapter 28

Aortic Insufficiency

Timothy A. Mixon and Gregory J. Dehmer

Incompetence of the aortic valve results in volume overload of the left ventricle. The distinction between acute and chronic forms of aortic regurgitation is important in terms of etiologies, associated diseases, prognosis, and treatment.

ETIOLOGY AND PATHOGENESIS

Common causes of acute aortic regurgitation include ascending aortic dissection with distortion of the normal valve architecture, infective endocarditis with destruction of a valve leaflet, traumatic disruption, and spontaneous rupture or prolapse of a valve cusp secondary to degenerative diseases of the valve. Acute aortic regurgitation also may occur with sudden dehiscence of the sewing ring of a prosthetic valve and after operative or balloon valvuloplasty.

The many causes of chronic aortic regurgitation are fundamentally related to two structural defects: those involving the valve leaflets and cusp or those involving the aortic root. Causes of valve leaflet disease include rheumatic heart disease, congenital abnormalities of the aortic valve (especially bicuspid valves), calcific degenerative valve disease, myxomatous degeneration, or infective endocarditis. Rheumatic disease is characterized by shortening and scarring of the cusps and is frequently accompanied by mitral valve involvement (Fig. 28-1). Congenitally bicuspid valves occur in up to 2% of the population, with a marked male predominance. This abnormality often presents as aortic stenosis or a mixed stenosis–regurgitation lesion, but 10% have pure regurgitation. Infective endocarditis may cause aortic regurgitation by several mechanisms, including perforation of a single leaflet or a flail leaflet or by weakening of the cusp and valve annulus as a result of an expanding aortic root abscess.

Aortic root disease is responsible for approximately half of all clinically significant regurgitation cases. Common aortic root problems causing aortic regurgitation include Marfan's syndrome with annuloaortic ectasia and ascending aortic dissection that may distort valve structure and undermine support of the leaflets. In systemic hypertension, aortic regurgitation may occur because the presence of long-standing hypertension can result in dilation of the ascending aorta with distortion of the valve and chronic damage to the valve leaflets. Less common causes of aortic regurgitation include syphilitic aortitis, ankylosing spondylitis, osteogenesis imperfecta, systemic lupus erythematosus, rheumatoid arthritis, psoriatic arthritis, Behçet's syndrome, ulcerative colitis, discrete subaortic stenosis, and ventricular septal defect with prolapse of an aortic cusp (Fig. 28-2).

Natural History

The natural history of chronic aortic regurgitation is incompletely known. Data from the presurgical era indicate that patients with chronic, severe aortic insufficiency who have angina or heart failure have a prognosis similar to those with severe aortic stenosis, with mortality rates of at least 10 to 20% per year. Asymptomatic patients with normal left ventricular (LV) function develop symptoms or LV dysfunction at a rate of about 4% annually, but the occurence of sudden death is rare (<0.2% per year). It is important to note, however, that 25% of patients die or progress to LV dysfunction before manifesting symptoms, emphasizing the importance of serial quantitative assessments of LV function. The subset of asymptomatic patients who have LV dysfunction predictably has higher event rates, with more than 25% developing symptoms annually.

CLINICAL PRESENTATION

The presentation of aortic insufficiency varies with the onset (acute or chronic) and the degree of compensatory changes to volume overload (Table 28-1). In acute aortic regurgitation, the

Figure 28-1

Rheumatic Heart Disease XI
Aortic Insufficiency

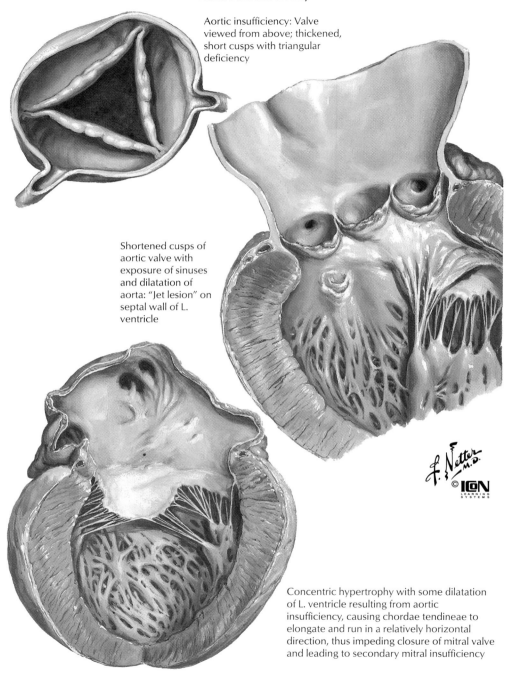

Aortic insufficiency: Valve viewed from above; thickened, short cusps with triangular deficiency

Shortened cusps of aortic valve with exposure of sinuses and dilatation of aorta: "Jet lesion" on septal wall of L. ventricle

Concentric hypertrophy with some dilatation of L. ventricle resulting from aortic insufficiency, causing chordae tendineae to elongate and run in a relatively horizontal direction, thus impeding closure of mitral valve and leading to secondary mitral insufficiency

Figure 28-2

Syphilitic Heart Disease

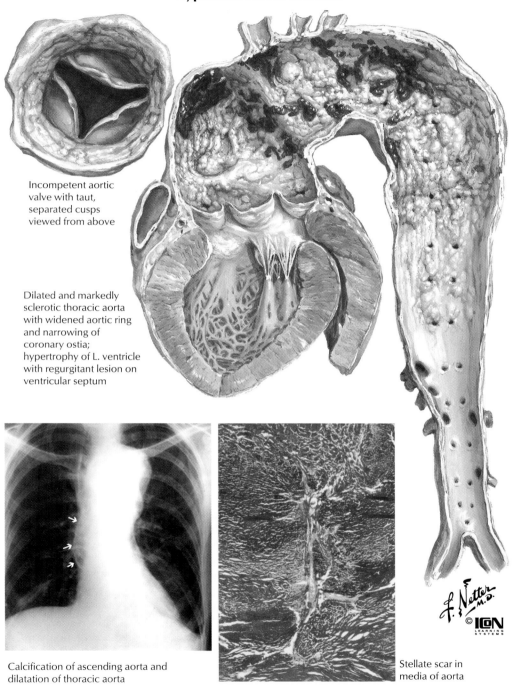

Incompetent aortic valve with taut, separated cusps viewed from above

Dilated and markedly sclerotic thoracic aorta with widened aortic ring and narrowing of coronary ostia; hypertrophy of L. ventricle with regurgitant lesion on ventricular septum

Calcification of ascending aorta and dilatation of thoracic aorta

Stellate scar in media of aorta

Table 28-1
Hemodynamic Features of the Stages of Severe Aortic Regurgitation

	Acute Severe Regurgitation	Chronic, Severe Regurgitation (Compensated)	Chronic, Severe Regurgitation (Late Decompensation)
LV compliance	Not increased	Increased	No longer increased
LVEDP	↑↑↑	Normal	↑↑↑
LV dimensions	Normal	↑↑	↑↑
Aortic SBP	Normal or low	↑	Normal or low
Aortic DBP	Normal	↓↓	Normal
Pulse pressure	Normal / ↑	↑↑↑	Normal
LVEF	Normal	Normal / ↑	↓
Total stroke volume	↑	↑↑↑	↑
Heart rate	↑↑↑	Normal	↑↑
Regurgitant volume	Large	Very large	Large
Effective cardiac output	↓↓	Normal	↓
Arterial pulse volume	Normal / ↑	↑↑↑	Normal

↑ indicates slight increase; ↑↑, moderate increase; ↑↑↑, severe increase; ↓, slight decrease; ↓↓, moderate decrease; ↓↓↓, severe decrease; LV, left ventricular; LVEDP, left ventricular end-diastolic pressure; LVEF, left ventricular ejection fraction.
Arrows are not used in the first row because the changes in LV compliance are complex. In acute severe regurgitation, compliance is not really normal, but not increased. In last column, compliance is not really normal, but is reduced compared with the state described in the middle column.

presentation is often dramatic. LV hypertrophy has not developed, so ventricular compliance is normal and remains so despite the sudden regurgitation. The acute volume overload is poorly tolerated because the left ventricle is abruptly and dramatically distended, resulting in impaired systolic function (based on the diastolic pressure–volume curve). The left ventricle is unable to acutely compensate for the large regurgitant volume. Forward cardiac output is reduced and LV end-diastolic pressure is greatly increased. Tachycardia occurs in a futile attempt to increase cardiac output. The regurgitation results in premature mitral valve closure with occasional diastolic mitral regurgitation. As a result, the patient with acute regurgitation usually appears severely ill, manifesting tachycardia, hypotension, peripheral vasoconstriction, and pulmonary congestion and edema, but lacks many physical signs of chronic regurgitation. Fatigue, apathy, agitation, or a decline in mental function may develop as a manifestation of the abrupt decrease in forward cardiac output.

Chronic aortic regurgitation may be asymptomatic for years. When symptoms develop, they are usually indolent, reflecting the slow, progressive nature of the disease. Frequent complaints include exertional dyspnea, orthopnea, and paroxysmal nocturnal dyspnea, all reflecting congestive heart failure (CHF), and palpitations. Angina pectoris may be produced by concurrent coronary artery disease or low diastolic perfusion pressure and a reduction in coronary blood flow during diastole because of the aortic regurgitation–induced LV hypertrophy. As aortic regurgitation develops, the left ventricle slowly enlarges primarily with eccentric hypertrophy, although concentric hypertrophy also occurs from increased afterload (Fig. 28-3). LV end-diastolic volume increases in response to the regurgitation with an increase in chamber compliance; accordingly the increased end-diastolic volume is not associated with major increases in end-diastolic pressure. Increased stroke volume maintains normal forward cardiac output, usually without significant increases in heart rate. Greatly augmented stroke volume leads to many of the classic findings of chronic aortic regurgitation (Table 28-2 and Fig. 28-3); the patient sometimes experiences an unpleasant

Figure 28-3

Manifestations of Aortic Insufficiency

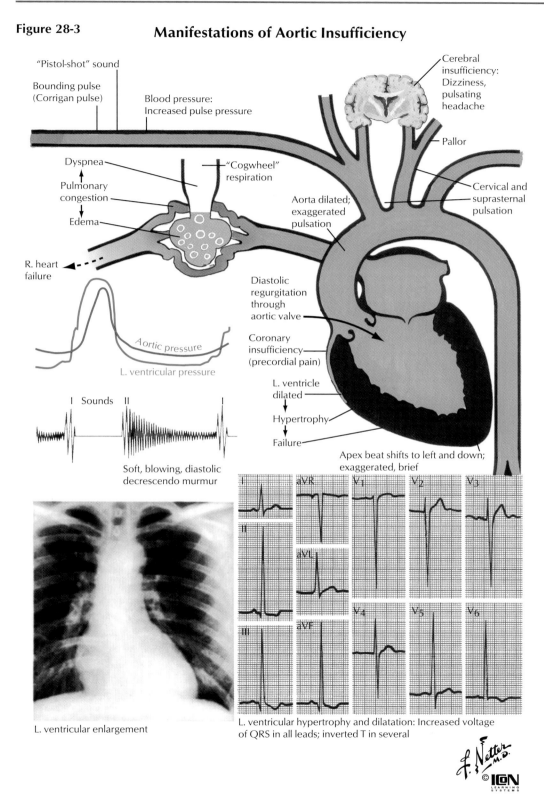

"Pistol-shot" sound

Bounding pulse (Corrigan pulse)

Blood pressure: Increased pulse pressure

Cerebral insufficiency: Dizziness, pulsating headache

Pallor

Dyspnea

Pulmonary congestion

Edema

R. heart failure

"Cogwheel" respiration

Aorta dilated; exaggerated pulsation

Cervical and suprasternal pulsation

Aortic pressure

L. ventricular pressure

Diastolic regurgitation through aortic valve

Coronary insufficiency (precordial pain)

L. ventricle dilated

Hypertrophy

Failure

I Sounds II I

Soft, blowing, diastolic decrescendo murmur

Apex beat shifts to left and down; exaggerated, brief

L. ventricular enlargement

I aVR V₁ V₂ V₃

II aVL V₄ V₅ V₆

III aVF

L. ventricular hypertrophy and dilatation: Increased voltage of QRS in all leads; inverted T in several

Table 28-2
Physical Examination Findings With Severe Aortic Regurgitation

Finding	Description
de Musset's sign	Head bob with each systolic pulsation
Corrigan's pulse	Bounding pulse, alternatively named "water-hammer pulse"
Traube's sign	Booming systolic and diastolic sounds ("pistol shots") over the femoral arteries
Muller's sign	Systolic pulsation of the uvula
Duroziez's sign	Systolic murmur over the femoral artery when compressed proximally, diastolic murmur when compressed distally
Quincke's sign	Capillary pulsations noted in the nail beds or fingertips with each cardiac cycle
Hill's sign	Popliteal systolic pressure exceeding brachial pressure by 30–60 mm Hg

awareness of each contraction, especially if irregular beats lead to a pause with a further increase in preload. Low aortic diastolic pressure from the regurgitation of the incompetent valve into the left ventricle usually results in a wide pulse pressure. During exercise, systemic vascular resistance and diastolic filling period decrease, resulting in less regurgitation per cardiac cycle. This increases forward cardiac output without substantial increases in LV end-diastolic pressure. In some patients, the ability of the left ventricle to compensate for the chronic volume overload eventually is exceeded and LV failure develops. As the LV ejection fraction (EF) decreases, the ventricle dilates further, initiating a vicious cycle. Throughout this process, fibrosis of the myocardium slowly contributes to the development of irreversible LV dysfunction. Typical symptoms of CHF may become evident at this stage.

Physical Examination

In acute severe aortic regurgitation, systolic BP is normal or decreased and diastolic BP is slightly elevated, resulting in a pulse pressure that is usually normal. Although tachycardia is usually present, the precordium is relatively quiet. The first heart sound is soft because of premature closure of the mitral valve and may be absent in severe acute regurgitation. The second heart sound is also soft, and a third heart sound is frequently present due to the rapid early diastolic filling of the ventricle. A fourth heart sound is uncommon. In contrast to chronic aortic regurgitation, the diastolic murmur of acute regurgitation is often short, ending well before the end of diastole, and soft in intensity. A systolic murmur is also present, but not particularly loud due to the reduced forward output. A second diastolic murmur, the Austin Flint murmur, is a mid diastolic rumble similar to mitral stenosis best heard at the apex. Possible mechanisms of this murmur include relative mitral stenosis from the regurgitant jet displacing the anterior mitral leaflet, impedance of left atrial outflow, or vibrations induced by the regurgitant jet. An Austin Flint murmur indicates that aortic regurgitation is severe.

In chronic, compensated aortic regurgitation, increased carotid pulse volumes may be accompanied by a bruit or transmitted systolic murmur. Peripheral pulses are bounding due to the wide pulse pressure, with systolic hypertension and a low diastolic BP. The LV apical impulse is enlarged and displaced inferiorly and laterally. The first heart sound is normal or soft and the second heart sound may be normal, single, or paradoxically split. Ejection clicks may be heard, especially in patients with a dilated aortic root. A fourth heart sound can be detected as LV hypertrophy develops and a third heart sound occurs when the left ventricle decompensates. The diastolic murmur of chronic aortic regurgitation is best heard at the base of the heart along the left sternal edge or in the second right intercostal space. It is best detected with the diaphragm of the stethoscope while the patient is leaning forward during held expiration. The etiology of the regurgitation is more likely to be valvular if the murmur is louder to the left of the sternum, whereas aortic root disease is often the cause if the murmur is louder to the right of the sternum.

The diastolic murmur begins at the second heart sound and continues for a variable portion of diastole. Severity of the regurgitation is better correlated with the length rather than the intensity of the murmur. However, when the left ventricle begins to fail and end-diastolic pressure increases, the murmur shortens again. A systolic murmur may be present from increased forward flow across the aortic valve or concomitant aortic stenosis. An Austin Flint murmur, if present, indicates severe aortic regurgitation.

DIFFERENTIAL DIAGNOSIS

The hallmarks of chronic aortic regurgitation are an increased pulse pressure and diastolic decrescendo murmur heard at the upper sternal border. Several other conditions can mimic aortic regurgitation and should be considered in the differential diagnosis. First, patients with pulmonic regurgitation have a blowing diastolic decrescendo murmur, but would not usually have a wide pulse pressure or bounding carotid pulse. The murmur of pulmonic regurgitation should increase with inspiration; the pulmonic valve closure sound is often increased in intensity and a right ventricular (RV) heave may be present. ECG would show signs of RV strain or hypertrophy rather than left-sided abnormalities and chest radiography would show signs of RV enlargement. In adults, there is usually a comorbid condition causing pulmonary hypertension and therefore the pulmonary regurgitation. Second, in those presenting at a younger age the diagnosis of a patent ductus arteriosus should be considered. It causes a wide pulse pressure, as seen in aortic regurgitation, but the murmur is continuous with a low-pitched diastolic component. ECG in this condition would be normal or show signs of LV hypertrophy and chest radiography would show increased flow in the pulmonary vasculature. Third, if symptoms of dyspnea and chest pain begin suddenly, a ruptured sinus of Valsalva aneurysm should be considered. The pulse pressure is usually increased, but the murmur would be continuous rather than diastolic only. Chest radiography would show signs of increased flow in the pulmonary vasculature. Finally, a coronary arteriovenous fistula may present with a murmur that can be confused with aortic regurgitation. The murmur should be continuous, but occasionally the diastolic component can dominate, mimicking aortic regurgitation. Echocardiography and, if necessary, cardiac catheterization can be performed to distinguish all of these conditions from aortic regurgitation.

DIAGNOSTIC APPROACH

With chronic aortic regurgitation, the ECG frequently shows left-axis deviation and LV hypertrophy. The findings are nonspecific and may include interventricular conduction defects, nonspecific ST-segment and T-wave changes, and PR-interval prolongation, especially if the etiology is inflammatory. These findings are not accurate predictors of the severity of regurgitation.

Chest radiography in chronic aortic insufficiency shows LV dilatation that may be massive (so called "cor bovinum"). Enlarged aortic root size suggests the etiology of the regurgitation. The pulmonary vasculature may be engorged with fluid during a decompensated state. With acute aortic insufficiency, there is minimal cardiac enlargement, with florid pulmonary edema the only finding.

Echocardiography is valuable for the initial assessment of acute and chronic aortic regurgitation and for serial follow-up examinations (Fig. 28-4). Complete echocardiography provides information about the etiology and severity of aortic regurgitation, the presence of concomitant valve disorders, and the state of LV compensation assessed by chamber size, function, and wall thickness. The severity of regurgitation can be estimated semiquantitatively by measuring the width or cross-sectional area of the regurgitant jet in relation to the LV outflow tract cross-sectional area by the finding of holodiastolic flow reversal in the descending aorta or by measuring the pressure half-time of the regurgitant jet. Severity can be determined quantitatively by the pressure half-time method or by the continuity equation that yields the regurgitant volume and fraction. Additionally, information from echocardiography, notably LVEF and chamber dimensions, can be followed serially to determine the timing of surgical intervention.

Aortic regurgitation can also be evaluated by cardiac catheterization. Hemodynamic tracings in severe aortic regurgitation show a wide pulse pressure and an elevated LV end-diastolic pressure (Fig. 28-3). Aortic root angiography provides

Figure 28-4 **Hemodynamics and Heart Sounds in Patients With Acute and Chronic Severe Aortic Regurgitation**

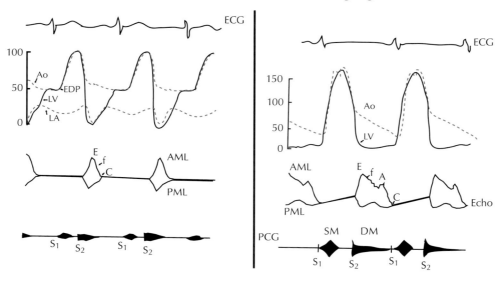

ECG, pressure tracings, M-mode echocardiogram (Echo), and phonocardiograms (PCG) from a patient with acute severe (**left**) and chronic severe (**right**) aortic regurgitation.

A indicates A point corresponding to the peak upward motion of the mitral valve leaflet after atrial systole; AML, anterior mitral valve leaflet; Ao, aorta; C, C point where the two mitral leaflets come together; DM, diastolic murmur; E, E point corresponding to the maximal excursion of the anterior mitral valve leaflet after early diastolic opening; EDP, end-diastolic pressure; f, flutter of anterior mitral valve leaflet; LA, left atrium; LV, left ventricle; PML, posterior mitral valve leaflet; S_1, first heart sound; S_2, second heart sound; SM, systolic murmur.

With permission from Morganroth J, Perloff JK, Zeldis SM, Dunkman WB. Acute severe regurgitation: Pathophysiology, clinical recognition, and management. *Ann Intern Med* 1977;87:223–232.

a semiquantitative assessment of severity, based on the speed and completeness of LV opacification. Quantitatively, regurgitant volume and regurgitant fraction are calculated using the stroke volume from LV angiography and forward cardiac output obtained by the thermodilution or Fick methods.

MANAGEMENT AND THERAPY
Acute Aortic Regurgitation

Whatever the etiology, acute aortic insufficiency necessitates rapid diagnosis, with aggressive medical and surgical therapy, if feasible. Medical stabilization includes afterload-reducing agents to augment forward cardiac output, but worsening hypotension may preclude implementation of afterload-reducing therapy. Intraaortic balloon counterpulsation is contraindicated because it increases regurgitation. Slowing the heart rate is not recommended because it prolongs the diastolic filling period and thus lengthens the time during which regurgitation can occur. However, if acute aortic dissection is the etiology of the regurgitation, β-blockers may reduce the force of LV ejection. Long-term administration of β-blockers is important in patients with Marfan's syndrome because it slows the rate of aortic dilatation and progression to aortic complications, a favorable effect while awaiting definitive surgical intervention.

With acute aortic dissection, the clinical picture may be dominated by other sequelae, including myocardial infarction (MI) from compromise of a coronary artery (most commonly the right coronary artery), hemopericardium with tamponade, hemorrhagic shock, or stroke due to involvement of a great vessel. When aortic regurgitation occurs as a result of infective endocarditis, surgery occasionally can be delayed a few days, allowing further antibiotic therapy, but should not be postponed if there is significant hemodynamic instability or CHF. Despite concerns about placing a prosthetic valve during an infection, the risk of recurrence of infection is fairly low.

Chronic Aortic Regurgitation

Valve replacement should be considered for most patients with symptomatic severe aortic regurgitation, unless comorbid conditions preclude surgery. Preoperative LV systolic performance is the major determinant of postoperative prognosis in terms of LV function, symptoms of heart failure, and survival rate. In general, symptomatic patients with reduced LV function who undergo valve replacement have reduced postoperative survival rates, whereas those with preserved LV function have an excellent prognosis. However, there is a subgroup of patients with reduced LV function who show substantial improvement in LV function after valve replacement. In this subgroup, improvement in LV function resulted from the elimination of valve regurgitation and left ventricle volume overload and reversal of the imbalance between excessive afterload and the combination of preload reserve and compensatory hypertrophy (so called "afterload mismatch"). Key factors for improvement in LV function and prognosis after surgery are early identification of patients with minimal or no symptoms yet early signs of LV dysfunction and potential valve replacement, before severe symptoms develop.

There is controversy, however, regarding the timing of surgery in asymptomatic patients with severe regurgitation. Vasodilator therapy can reduce the degree of regurgitation, increase forward cardiac output, and delay the necessity of valve replacement. Accordingly, vasodilator therapy is recommended for asymptomatic patients with severe aortic regurgitation who have hypertension or a normal EF with enlarged LV volumes. Vasodilators are not recommended in patients with lesser degrees of regurgitation or if the EF and cardiac volumes are normal. Surgery is recommended in asymptomatic patients with severe aortic regurgitation who have a depressed LVEF (<0.50), severe ventricular dilatation (LV end-systolic dimension >55 mm or end-diastolic dimen-

sion >75 mm) or are undergoing surgery on a different valve, the aorta, or coronary arteries. Data that suggest that an exercised-induced decrease in LVEF has independent prognostic value in patients undergoing surgery are inconsistent. The most common surgical procedure is valve replacement, but alternative approaches include use of the patient's pulmonary valve (Ross procedure) or valve repair (see chapter 34). Valve repair is most feasible in patients with perforation of a leaflet due to endocarditis or when redundancy of the free edge of one of the leaflets results in leaflet prolapse. Concomitant aortic root reconstruction is often necessary in aortic dissection and Marfan's syndrome.

FUTURE DIRECTIONS

Minimally invasive aortic valve replacement surgery is becoming more common as surgical techniques are perfected. The entire surgical procedure is performed through a small incision to the right of the sternum rather than the traditional median sternotomy. This approach appears to shorten length of stay and recovery periods before returning to work, but it is unclear whether there are any long-term advantages or hazards. Percutaneous alternatives to surgical valve replacement are also being developed.

REFERENCES

al Jubair K, al Fagih MR, Ashmeg A, Belhaj M, Sawyer W. Cardiac operations during active endocarditis. *J Thorac Cardiovasc Surg* 1992;104:487–490.

Bonow RO, Carabello B, deLeon AC Jr, et al. ACC/AHA guidelines for the management of patients with valvular heart disease: a report of the American College of Cardiology/American Heart Association Task Force on Practice Guidelines (Committee on Management of Patients with Valvular Heart Disease). *J Am Coll Cardiol* 1998;32:1504–1514.

Cosgrove DM, Rosenkranz ER, Hendren WG, et al. Valvuloplasty for aortic insufficiency. *J Thorac Cardiovasc Surg* 1991;102:571–576.

Scognamiglio R, Rahimtoola SH, Fasoli G, Nistri S, Dalla Volta S. Nifedipine in asymptomatic patients with severe aortic regurgitation and normal left ventricular function. *N Engl J Med* 1994;331:689–694.

Shores J, Berger KR, Murphy EA, Pyeritz RE. Progression of aortic dilatation and the benefit of long term beta-adrenergic blockade in Marfan's syndrome. *N Engl J Med* 1994;330:1335–1341.

Tribouilloy C, Shen WF, Leborgne F, Trojette F, Rey JL, Lesbre JP. Comparative value of Doppler echocardiography and cardiac catheterization for management decision-making in patients with left-sided valvular regurgitation. *Eur Heart J* 1996;17:272–280.

Chapter 29

Mitral Valve Disease

Thomas R. Griggs

Mitral valve leaflets consist of thin, pliable, fibrous material. The two leaflets—anterior and posterior—open by unfolding against the ventricular wall and close by apposition when the pressure in the left ventricle becomes greater than that in the left atrium. *Mitral stenosis* occurs when the mitral valve leaflets become stiffened, calcified, and unable to fully open during diastole. This process often involves the chordae tendineae, in addition to the mitral valve leaflets. *Mitral valve regurgitation* (MR) occurs when the leaflets are unable to fully close in systole. In the United States, more than 20,000 patients annually require surgery for manifestations of mitral stenosis and MR, and thousands more require monitoring and treatment.

ETIOLOGY AND PATHOGENESIS

Rheumatic fever is responsible for a majority of cases of mitral stenosis. The initial infection and its sequelae result in thickened valve leaflets and fusion of the commissure between the leaflets. Chordae tendineae are also affected and become thickened and shortened. Most valves that are affected by rheumatic fever show abnormalities of all these structures. Few patients with rheumatic mitral valve disease have pure mitral stenosis; most patients have a combination of stenosis and regurgitation. Approximately two thirds of the cases of mitral stenosis in the United States occur in women.

The normal mitral valve cross-sectional area in diastole is 4 to 6 cm^2. Blood flow is impaired when the valve orifice is narrowed to less than 2 cm^2, creating a pressure gradient with exertion. A valve area smaller than 1 cm^2 is considered critical mitral stenosis and causes a gradient across the valve at rest with chronically increased left atrial pressures (Fig. 29-1).

Chronically increased pressures in the left atrium associated with mitral stenosis result in left atrial enlargement and a predisposition for atrial fibrillation. Valves affected by mitral stenosis are also vulnerable to recurrent thrombosis and implantation of bacteria that lead to infective endocarditis.

The hemodynamic effects of chronic mitral stenosis include pulmonary venous and arterial hypertension, right ventricular (RV) hypertrophy and failure, peripheral edema, ascites, and hepatic injury with cirrhosis (Fig. 29-2).

Numerous etiologies contribute to MR. These include mitral valve prolapse, rheumatic heart disease, cardiomyopathy with ventricular dilation, ischemic heart disease involving the papillary muscles, ischemic cardiomyopathy, bacterial or fungal endocarditis, and certain collagen–vascular diseases. Disease of any component of the mitral apparatus can cause a functional failure of the valve.

With moderate or severe MR, with left ventricular contraction in systole, blood is discharged into the left atrium, in addition to traveling its usual route through the aortic valve and into the aorta. If the regurgitant volume is large, the left ventricle dilates to accommodate increased volumes (Fig. 29-3).

Infectious endocarditis, spontaneous rupture of chordae tendineae, or ischemic injury of a papillary muscle may cause acute loss of integrity of the mitral valve and acute MR. In these cases, there is no adaptation of the left atrium or pulmonary vasculature to the increased regurgitant volumes; sudden onset of acute pulmonary edema may result. Aggressive use of afterload-reducing agents is the emergent treatment, but survival usually depends on emergency repair or replacement of the valve.

CLINICAL PRESENTATION
Mitral Stenosis

Patients notice the effects of moderate (1–2 cm^2) mitral stenosis with activity. With severe stenosis, dyspnea with minimal exertion and paroxysmal nocturnal dyspnea may occur. In

Figure 29-1

Mitral Stenosis

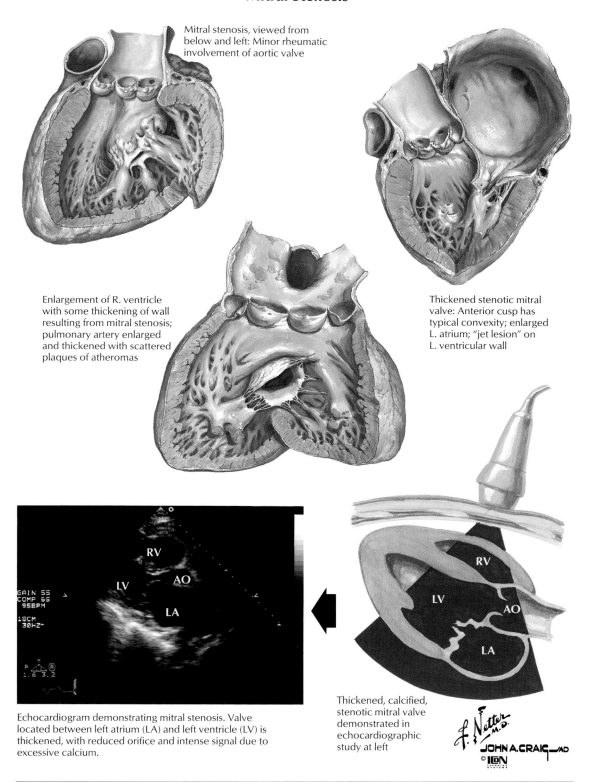

Mitral stenosis, viewed from below and left: Minor rheumatic involvement of aortic valve

Enlargement of R. ventricle with some thickening of wall resulting from mitral stenosis; pulmonary artery enlarged and thickened with scattered plaques of atheromas

Thickened stenotic mitral valve: Anterior cusp has typical convexity; enlarged L. atrium; "jet lesion" on L. ventricular wall

GAIN 55
COMP 65
95BPM

18CM
30HZ

P
1.6 3.2

Echocardiogram demonstrating mitral stenosis. Valve located between left atrium (LA) and left ventricle (LV) is thickened, with reduced orifice and intense signal due to excessive calcium.

Thickened, calcified, stenotic mitral valve demonstrated in echocardiographic study at left

Figure 29-2 **Pathophysiology and Clinical Aspects of Mitral Stenosis**

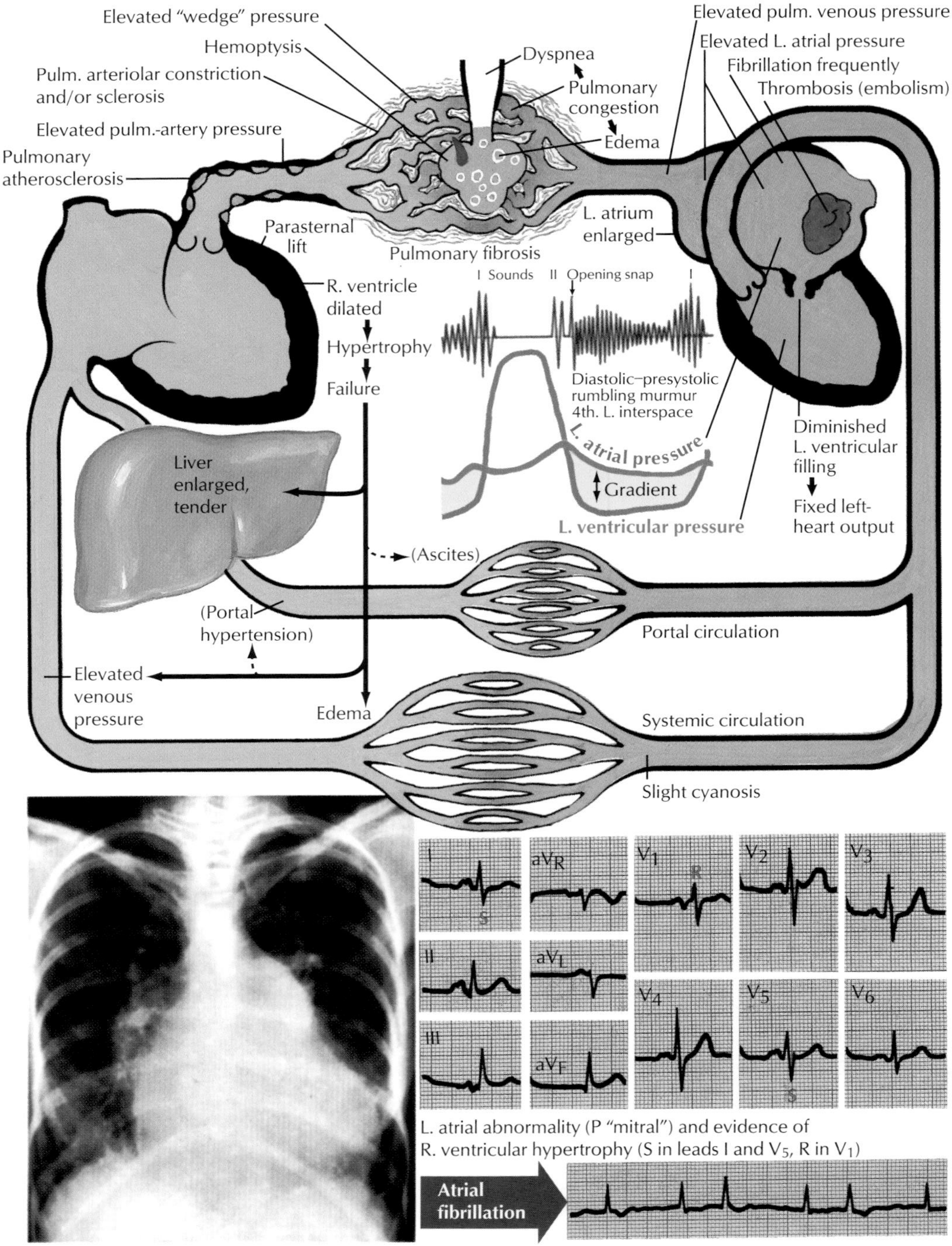
Elevated "wedge" pressure
Hemoptysis
Pulm. arteriolar constriction and/or sclerosis
Elevated pulm.-artery pressure
Pulmonary atherosclerosis
Dyspnea
Pulmonary congestion
Edema
Elevated pulm. venous pressure
Elevated L. atrial pressure
Fibrillation frequently
Thrombosis (embolism)
L. atrium enlarged
Parasternal lift
Pulmonary fibrosis
R. ventricle dilated
Hypertrophy
Failure
I Sounds II Opening snap I
Diastolic–presystolic rumbling murmur 4th. L. interspace
L. atrial pressure
Gradient
L. ventricular pressure
Diminished L. ventricular filling
Fixed left-heart output
Liver enlarged, tender
(Ascites)
(Portal hypertension)
Portal circulation
Elevated venous pressure
Edema
Systemic circulation
Slight cyanosis
I
aVR
V1
V2
V3
S
R
II
aVL
III
aVF
V4
V5
V6
S
L. atrial abnormality (P "mitral") and evidence of R. ventricular hypertrophy (S in leads I and V5, R in V1)
Atrial fibrillation

Figure 29-3

Mitral Regurgitation

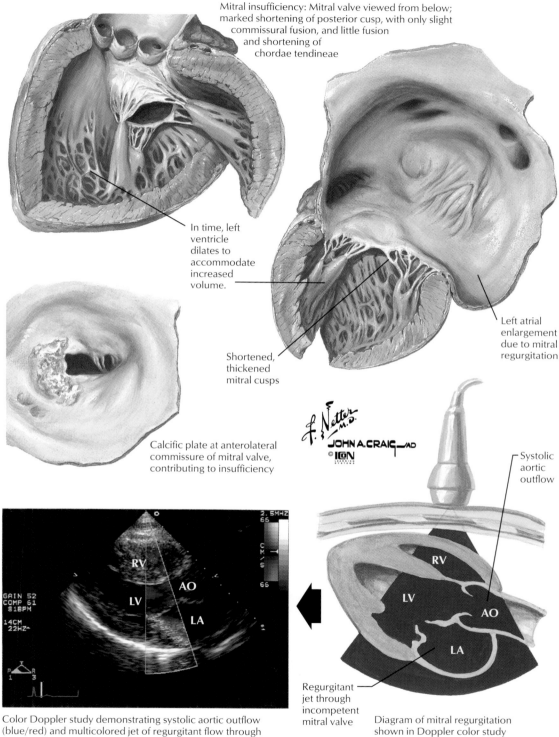

Mitral insufficiency: Mitral valve viewed from below; marked shortening of posterior cusp, with only slight commissural fusion, and little fusion and shortening of chordae tendineae

In time, left ventricle dilates to accommodate increased volume.

Left atrial enlargement due to mitral regurgitation

Shortened, thickened mitral cusps

Calcific plate at anterolateral commissure of mitral valve, contributing to insufficiency

Systolic aortic outflow

Regurgitant jet through incompetent mitral valve

Color Doppler study demonstrating systolic aortic outflow (blue/red) and multicolored jet of regurgitant flow through incompetent mitral valve into left atrium (LA)

Diagram of mitral regurgitation shown in Doppler color study at left

Figure 29-4

Pathophysiology and Clinical Aspects
of Mitral Regurgitation

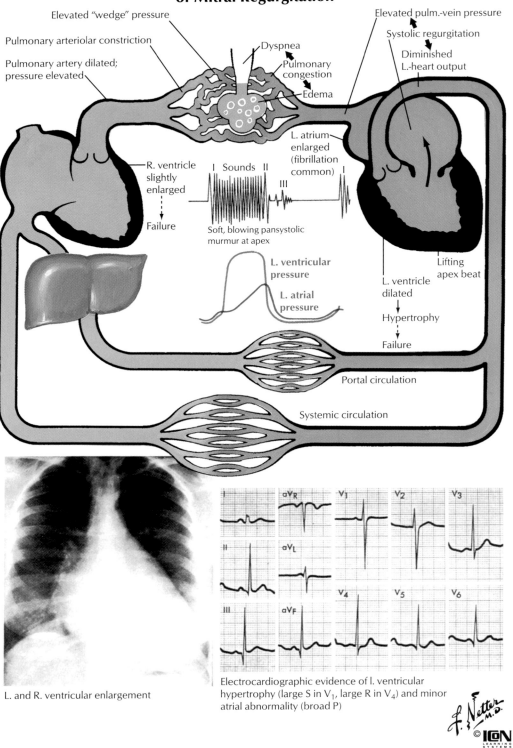

Elevated "wedge" pressure

Pulmonary arteriolar constriction

Pulmonary artery dilated; pressure elevated

Dyspnea

Pulmonary congestion

Edema

Elevated pulm.-vein pressure

Systolic regurgitation

Diminished L.-heart output

L. atrium enlarged (fibrillation common)

R. ventricle slightly enlarged

Failure

Sounds

Soft, blowing pansystolic murmur at apex

L. ventricular pressure

L. atrial pressure

Lifting apex beat

L. ventricle dilated

Hypertrophy

Failure

Portal circulation

Systemic circulation

L. and R. ventricular enlargement

Electrocardiographic evidence of l. ventricular hypertrophy (large S in V_1, large R in V_4) and minor atrial abnormality (broad P)

some cases, a sudden, dramatic onset of atrial fibrillation produces the first symptoms, occasionally resulting in fatal pulmonary edema. When the development of atrial fibrillation is clinically silent, the initial event may be a stroke or other thromboembolic event. The classic presentation of severe cor pulmonale with ascites and edema is rarely seen today except in medically underserved populations. Mitral valve disease increases the risk for bacterial endocarditis, which should always be considered when symptoms worsen in a previously stable patient with mitral valve disease.

Auscultation of symptomatic mitral stenosis is characterized by a loud first heart sound, an opening snap after the second heart sound, and a low-pitched diastolic murmur with presystolic accentuation if the patient is in sinus rhythm. The *opening snap* is the sound generated by sudden full opening of the mitral valve. It can reflect the severity of the pressure gradient across the mitral valve because greater left atrial pressures generate earlier opening than do lesser ones. Therefore, the shorter the interval from A2 to opening snap, the greater the pressure gradient, and the more severe the stenosis.

The characteristic diastolic, low-frequency "rumble" or murmur associated with mitral stenosis is best heard at the apex, with the patient in the left lateral decubitus position and the bell over the point of maximal ventricular intensity. The rumble occurs throughout diastole, with accentuation in late diastole (presystole) in patients who have preserved normal sinus rhythm. This murmur can be difficult to hear and is soft and brief when the mitral stenosis is minor. Therefore, heightened awareness of possible mitral stenosis is necessary. If the murmur is inaudible during this maneuver, it can be accentuated by having the patient exercise before auscultation. This murmur sequence—loud first sound, opening snap, and diastolic rumble—is quite specific for mitral stenosis. Murmurs that mimic mitral stenosis include the Austin Flint murmur with aortic regurgitation, mitral diastolic murmurs in patients with large intracardiac shunts, and occasionally murmurs that are caused by a left atrial myxoma. However, none have all three components of classic mitral stenosis.

Electrocardiographic changes in mitral stenosis may range from minor ST-segment and T-wave abnormalities to electrocardiographic evidence of severe pulmonary hypertension and RV enlargement. The ECG pattern of left atrial and RV enlargement is a classic indicator. Atrial fibrillation is common.

Mitral Regurgitation

Even severe MR may be clinically silent. Many cases are discovered during routine examinations when the characteristic murmur is noticed. Symptoms usually begin as dyspnea on exertion. Patients may also present with acute pulmonary edema or evidence of RV failure. Sudden decompensation can occur with the onset of atrial fibrillation or the development of bacterial endocarditis.

With MR, palpation may be normal or may show a displaced, sustained left ventricular (LV) impulse with a rapid filling wave. On auscultation, the most prominent feature is a high-pitched holosystolic murmur that usually radiates to the axilla. The intensity may not correlate with the severity of the MR; even highly severe MR can be associated with virtually no murmur. ECG changes in MR are nonspecific and are primarily changes of LV hypertrophy and strain; atrial fibrillation is common.

DIFFERENTIAL DIAGNOSIS

Primary pulmonary diseases (pneumonia, tuberculosis, chronic obstructive lung disease, and pulmonary thromboembolism) have presentations similar to that of mitral valve disease: dyspnea on exertion or pulmonary edema. Dyspnea may also be present in chronic interstitial pulmonary diseases, pulmonary hypertension, and malignancies that involve the chest. Heart diseases to consider are ischemic heart disease, congenital heart disease, dilated cardiomyopathy, and hypertrophic cardiomyopathy. Chronic pericardial disease with restriction can cause RV failure that mimics the pulmonary hypertension associated with mitral valve disease.

DIAGNOSTIC APPROACH

Many pulmonary diseases can be differentiated from mitral valve disease by means of chest imaging, including both radiography and computerized tomographic scanning. When an initial evaluation has focused the differential diagnosis on mitral valve disease, the most helpful clinical tool is echocardiography (see also chapter 4). In rheumatic mitral valve disease, echocardiography can demonstrate thickening, calcification, poor mobility of the valve, and thickening of subvalvular structures. The degree of valvular stenosis or regurgitation can be estimated using Doppler ultrasonography. When necessary, the anatomy of the valve and subvalvular apparatus can be further defined by transesophageal echocardiography. The goals of echocardiography are to evaluate the severity of the stenosis or regurgitation, the mobility of the valve, the involvement of subvalvular structures, and the degree of calcification and to detect intracardiac thrombi. Echocardiography provides information about LV contractile function and an accurate estimation of pulmonary artery pressure and RV function. It can also identify bacterial and fungal vegetations, intracardiac masses (especially left atrial myxoma), and intraventricular septal defects, all conditions that can complicate the diagnosis of mitral valve disease.

Cardiac catheterization is indicated in the few patients with a questionable diagnosis and in those patients for whom surgical treatment is contemplated. Catheterization is performed to quantify the mitral valve area; document key elements of hemodynamics, such as cardiac output and systemic resistance; define the degree of pulmonary hypertension; and to determine whether coexistent coronary artery disease is present.

MANAGEMENT AND THERAPY

Asymptomatic patients with mild, uncomplicated mitral valve disease may require only prophylaxis for endocarditis. In symptomatic patients, diuretics can help to reduce pulmonary congestion. With mitral stenosis, the time for ventricular filling is critically important; HR should be maintained as low as is practical with a β-blocker or a calcium channel blocker, such as verapamil or diltiazem. Patients with atrial fibrillation must be treated with warfarin anticoagulation unless it is contraindicated.

Symptomatic mitral stenosis can be improved by means of percutaneous balloon mitral valvotomy, surgical valvotomy, or surgical replacement of the mitral valve. Various criteria are used to determine the timing of surgery, ranging from the development of symptoms in a patient with known severe mitral stenosis to the new diagnosis of severe mitral stenosis in a young person. In selected patients, in whom there is little valvular calcification, little involvement of the subvalvular apparatus, and minimal or no mitral valve regurgitation, percutaneous balloon valvotomy is the treatment of choice. Longitudinal studies have documented event-free survival to be greater than 70% at 7 years.

Open valvotomy is a repair procedure that involves direct visualization by the surgeon, allowing for débridement of the valve structure and reconstruction of subvalvular apparatus. Because the approach used also allows for valve replacement, in patients who are questionable candidates for valvotomy, the decision can be made during surgery whether repair or replacement is the most appropriate choice. Mitral valve replacement continues to be an alternative for patients with severe mitral stenosis and is especially appropriate for patients with significant MR (see chapter 34).

The timing of surgical intervention for patients with MR is critical. In most cases, MR is well tolerated, and the patient is asymptomatic for many years. Delaying surgery as long as possible avoids the trauma, expense, and risk of surgery. However, every effort must be made to proceed with surgery before ventricular function has degenerated. Assessments of LV systolic function involve measurement of the ejection fraction. The reduced wall tension and afterload of MR allow the ejection fraction to be preserved late into the course of the disease; therefore, any decrement in ejection fraction may represent a considerable decrease in myocardial functional reserve. In general, mitral valve surgery should be considered in a patient with known moderate to severe MR when the patient is symptomatic or there is objective evidence of decreased LV function.

Valve repair for severe MR improves mortality and decreases the frequency of complications. Valves must be relatively free of calcification and have pliable leaflets with chordae tendineae that can be separated, reinforced, or reattached as needed. Placement of a reinforcing mitral ring

Figure 29-5

Bacterial Endocarditis in Mitral Valvular Disease

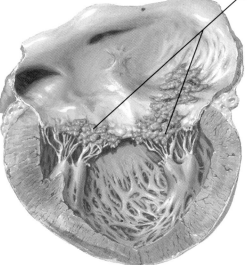

Bacterial vegetations first appear along "contact line" of mitral valve but spread to involve atria and chordae tendineae with subsequent rupture and shrinkage of the latter.

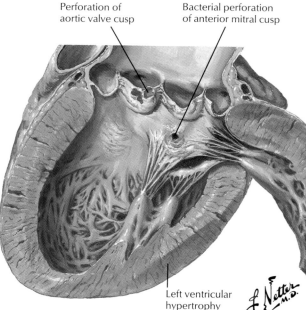

Perforation of aortic valve cusp

Bacterial perforation of anterior mitral cusp

Left ventricular hypertrophy

Late sequelae of bacterial endocarditis may result in mitral regurgitation via destruction of mitral valve cusps or by widening of annular valve ring due to left ventricular enlargement due to aortic insufficiency.

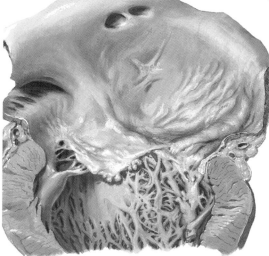

Thickening and erosion of mitral valve with stumps of ruptured chordae tendineae resulting in valvular incompetence, regurgitation, and atrial enlargement

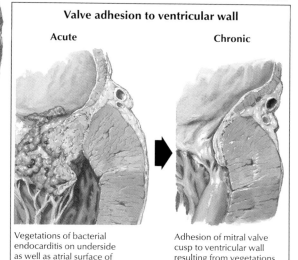

Valve adhesion to ventricular wall

Acute

Chronic

Vegetations of bacterial endocarditis on underside as well as atrial surface of mitral valve

Adhesion of mitral valve cusp to ventricular wall resulting from vegetations on undersurface of valve

is frequently included in the repair. Advantages of valve repair over replacement are that it provides patients with functional subvalvular components, including the papillary muscles, and that the natural tissues in the valve are much more resistant to thrombogenicity than any artificial surface, obviating the use of warfarin anticoagulant.

Mitral regurgitation resulting from dilated cardiomyopathy is an especially troublesome problem that is caused by dilation of the mitral ring and ventricles and results in anatomic deformity of the relation of the papillary muscles and chordae tendineae to the mitral valve leaflets. The resulting MR increases the need for ejection volume and decreases forward blood flow. In this situation, repair or replacement of the mitral valve may fail to improve symptoms and is associated with an extremely high risk of operative death. New percutaneous approaches for mitral valve repair in this circumstance are currently in clinical trials to determine safety and efficacy.

Coronary heart disease can cause MR by means of several mechanisms. The mitral valve is tethered to papillary muscles that are dependent on myocardial blood flow. Acute ischemia to the area providing blood flow to the papillary muscles can cause temporary MR. Infarction of the papillary muscle will cause permanent failure of the subvalvular apparatus. Acute myocardial infarction that involves a papillary muscle causes severe, acute, life-threatening MR, with mortality rates of nearly 30% if not surgically and emergently corrected. In some circumstances, an infarction results in rupture of the tip of the papillary muscle with acute MR. This is almost always fatal unless surgically corrected. Finally, patients with extensive myocardial scarring caused by previous infarction and associated dilation of the ventricle, ischemic cardiomyopathy, can have severe MR because of dilation of the mitral ring and abnormal alignment of the papillary muscles, chordae tendineae, and valve leaflets.

Any structural abnormality of the valve can result in flow aberrations that promote deposition of microthrombi. These can be the nidus for a bacterial or fungal infection with simultaneous septicemia, resulting in further damage associated with endocarditis (Fig. 29-5). Endocarditis can affect valve competency because of interference in valve function by vegetations or by destruction or fenestration of the valve leaflets. Although endocarditis is usually managed with antibiotics, the damage effected by the bacteria is permanent, as is the resultant MR. Indications for surgery after cured bacterial endocarditis are identical to those for other causes for MR. In addition, acute surgical care is indicated for extremely large vegetations, when heart failure is otherwise unmanageable, when a myocardial abscess is documented, and for patients with persistent bacteremia.

FUTURE DIRECTIONS

Improving worldwide morbidity and mortality associated with rheumatic heart disease necessitates better systems of hygiene and improved prophylactic treatment of streptococcal infection, especially the current drug-resistant strains. The prevalence of MR will increase as the population ages, spurring improvements in several areas: imaging with more accurate estimates of ventricular reserve, surgical technology with early repair of severely regurgitant valves, balloon valvotomy with improved patient selection and equipment, and minimally invasive surgical techniques with reduced recovery time and morbidity. Better treatment for atrial fibrillation and improved therapies for prevention of thrombosis will greatly improve the quality of life for patients with mitral valve disease and valve prostheses.

REFERENCES

Bonow RO, Carabello B, de Leon AC Jr, et al. ACC/AHA guidelines for the management of patients with valvular heart disease: A report of the American College of Cardiology/American Heart Association Task Force on Practice Guidelines (Committee on Management of Patients With Valvular Heart Disease). J Am Coll Cardiol 1998;32:1486–1588.

Enriquez-Sarano M. Timing of mitral valve surgery. Heart 2002;87:79–85.

Marcus RH, Sareli P, Pocock WA, et al. The spectrum of severe rheumatic mitral valve disease in a developing country: Correlations among clinical presentation, surgical pathologic findings, and hemodynamic sequelae. Ann Intern Med 1994;120:177–183.

Chapter 30
Mitral Valve Prolapse

Lee R. Goldberg and Park W. Willis IV

Mitral valve prolapse (MVP) is the most common form of congenital heart disease in adults, affecting 4 to 5% of the US population. MVP refers to the superior and posterior displacement of one or both mitral leaflets into the left atrium during systole. Although MVP is usually benign, important complications, including infective endocarditis and severe mitral regurgitation (MR), can occur.

Mitral valve prolapse can be classified as primary, secondary, or functional. Primary MVP occurs in the absence of connective tissue disease. Myxomatous degeneration of the tricuspid valve may be present; the aortic and pulmonic valves are sometimes involved. Primary MVP can be associated with skeletal abnormalities, von Willebrand's disease, and hypomastia. Secondary MVP occurs in the presence of a known connective tissue disorder, such as Marfan's syndrome, Ehlers-Danlos syndrome, adult polycystic kidney disease, osteogenesis imperfecta, and pseudoxanthoma elasticum. The pathologic changes of the mitral valve apparatus are identical to those found in primary MVP. In functional MVP, the mitral valve is anatomically normal, but both superior and posterior displacement of the valve can occur secondary to other cardiac conditions. Causes of functional MVP include a dilated mitral annulus and ischemic papillary muscle dysfunction. In hypertrophic cardiomyopathy, the left ventricular (LV) cavity may be too small to accommodate the mitral valve, causing functional MVP. In atrial septal defect, left-to-right shunting and right ventricular chamber dilation secondary to volume overload can cause a small left ventricle and functional MVP.

ETIOLOGY AND PATHOGENESIS

The etiology of MVP is unknown. In families with MVP, the abnormal gene is inherited in an autosomal dominant fashion, with variable penetrance. Pathologic findings in primary and secondary MVP often involve the mitral leaflets and the chordae tendineae. Typical gross pathologic findings include thickened, redundant mitral leaflets and elongated chordae tendineae.

Although both the anterior and posterior mitral leaflets may be affected, the middle scallop of the posterior leaflet is most commonly involved in the myxomatous process. Histologic examination of the mitral valve leaflets reveals interruption of collagen bundles and an accumulation of acid mucopolysaccharides within the spongiosa layer.

CLINICAL PRESENTATION

The clinical presentation of MVP is highly variable. Most patients with MVP are asymptomatic. The most common complaint is atypical chest pain. Other nonspecific symptoms associated with MVP include palpitations, dizziness, dyspnea, anxiety, numbness, and tingling. There is ongoing controversy about whether these complaints are caused by MVP or are a coincidental finding. The original descriptions of MVP were probably influenced by selection bias. Several subsequent studies have not shown truly increased frequency of symptoms such as chest pain, dyspnea, or dizziness.

Mitral valve prolapse is usually discovered incidentally on routine physical examination, and cardiac auscultation is the key to making the clinical diagnosis. One or more nonejection systolic clicks in midsystole or late systole with or without a late systolic murmur are characteristic of MVP. The systolic click, or clicks, heard in MVP are thought to originate from the chordae tendineae snapping as the mitral leaflets bow into the left atrium. Multiple systolic clicks can cause a scratching sound occasionally likened to a pericardial friction rub. Mitral regurgitation at the time of leaflet prolapse results in the late systolic murmur. This murmur typically has a crescendo contour and envelops the second heart sound (S_2); it is commonly preceded by a nonejection click but may occur alone. A late systolic murmur usually indicates mild MR; with more significant MR, the murmur can be pansystolic and a click may not be audible. Although late systolic accentuation is often preserved, the murmur can become indistinguishable from the murmur related to MR from other causes. In the case of posterior leaflet prolapse, the mitral regurgitant flow is commonly directed anteriorly toward the aortic root and the murmur may be transmitted along the left sternal border and to the aortic area. With anterior leaflet prolapse, the murmur radiates to the left axilla and back.

Mitral valve prolapse is a dynamic, load-dependent phenomenon, and the most sensitive and specific physical diagnostic criteria are based on characteristic postural changes in auscultatory findings. A complete examination with the patient in the supine, standing, and sitting positions is required to alter hemodynamics and ventricular loading conditions and detect the characteristic findings with the highest degree of accuracy (see also chapter 1). The postural auscultatory changes are related primarily to changes in LV volume, augmented by alterations in heart rate and myocardial contractility. Generally, measures that decrease LV volume produce earlier and more prominent systolic prolapse of the mitral leaflets, causing the systolic click and murmur to move closer to the first heart sound (S_1) (Fig. 30-1).

DIFFERENTIAL DIAGNOSIS

The differential diagnosis of a nonejection systolic click includes semilunar ejection sounds arising from the aortic and pulmonic valves, splitting of S_1 or S_2, and clicks arising from nonvalvular structures such as an atrial septal aneurysm, pericardial sounds, and clicks heard in patients with a pneumothorax. Aortic and pulmonic ejection sounds are high-frequency sounds that occur in early systole. An aortic ejection sound is best heard with the diaphragm and simulates wide splitting of S_1. Although audible over the entire precordium, these sounds are usually loudest at the mitral area, where the S_1–ejection click sequence is commonly mistaken for a fourth heart sound

followed by S_1. Pulmonary ejection sounds can be difficult to differentiate from the splitting of S_1, but the characteristic loud and "clicky" quality of these sounds, exaggerated in the expiratory phase of respiration and disappearing on inspiration, is a reliable diagnostic feature. Ejection clicks are not perceptibly affected by altering preload with postural changes. Because the ejection clicks occur as the semilunar valve opens, they precede the carotid upstroke, whereas the nonejection clicks of MVP occur afterward. A midsystolic click can occur with an atrial septal aneurysm, and then there is no associated late systolic murmur. Clicking pneumothorax can mimic MVP, but extra sounds do not show a consistent relationship to the cardiac cycle and can also occur in diastole. A prolonged period of continuous cardiac auscultation is useful in diagnosis.

DIAGNOSTIC APPROACH

When the diagnosis of MVP is made by cardiac auscultation, transthoracic echocardiography can be useful to confirm the physical findings. Both two-dimensional and M-mode techniques are sensitive in detecting MVP. Echocardiography provides additional information, including the degree of leaflet prolapse, the severity of the MR, and the thickness of the mitral leaflets (Fig. 30-2). The improvement in echocardiographic methods and technology and changing diagnostic criteria have resulted in a degree of variability in the clinical interpretation of the information generated. Today, far fewer patients are diagnosed as having MVP than were diagnosed 20 years ago. However, the load-dependent nature of MVP does make its diagnosis more difficult since patients routinely are studied in a supine position.

The originally described M-mode criteria for MVP required displacement of the mitral leaflet echo beyond the CD segment in systole. Either 3 mm of holosystolic displacement or 2 mm of late systolic displacement were sufficient to meet M-mode criteria for MVP. Because of the saddle shape of the mitral annulus, the diagnosis of MVP by two-dimensional echo is limited to parasternal long-axis views. Prolapse in the parasternal long axis is defined by the bowing of mitral leaflets beyond an imaginary line that connects the anterior and posterior annular

Figure 30-1

Auscultation in Mitral Valve Prolapse

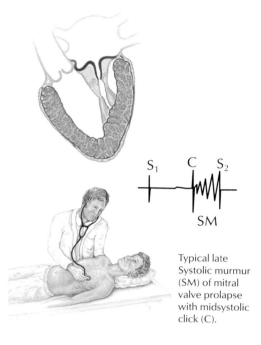

S_1 C S_2

SM

Typical late
Systolic murmur
(SM) of mitral
valve prolapse
with midsystolic
click (C).

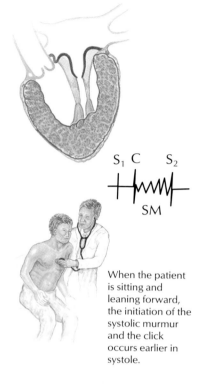

S_1 C S_2

SM

When the patient
is sitting and
leaning forward,
the initiation of the
systolic murmur
and the click
occurs earlier in
systole.

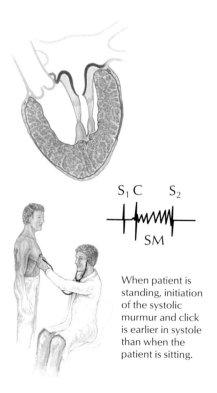

S_1 C S_2

SM

When patient is
standing, initiation
of the systolic
murmur and click
is earlier in systole
than when the
patient is sitting.

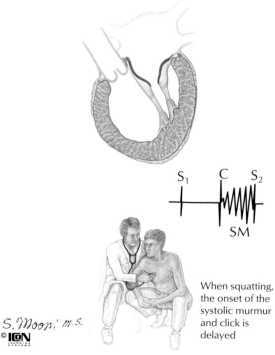

S_1 C S_2

SM

When squatting,
the onset of the
systolic murmur
and click is
delayed

S. Moon, M.S.
© ICON

Figure 30-2

Mitral Valve Prolapse

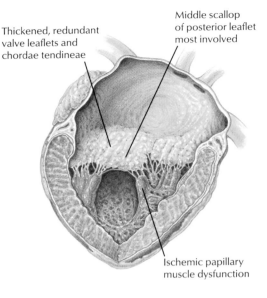

Thickened, redundant valve leaflets and chordae tendineae

Middle scallop of posterior leaflet most involved

Ischemic papillary muscle dysfunction

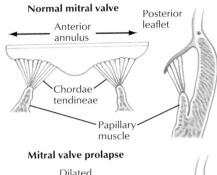

Normal mitral valve

Anterior annulus

Posterior leaflet

Chordae tendineae

Papillary muscle

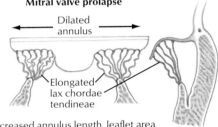

Mitral valve prolapse

Dilated annulus

Elongated lax chordae tendineae

Increased annulus length, leaflet area and elongated chordae tendineae allow "buckling" or prolapse of valve leaflets into left atrium during systole.

Findings in mitral valve prolapse

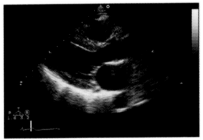

2-D echocardiogram showing normal configuration of mitral valve leaflets in systole

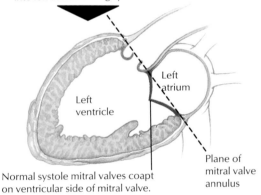

Left atrium

Left ventricle

Plane of mitral valve annulus

Normal systole mitral valves coapt on ventricular side of mitral valve.

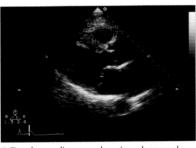

2-D echocardiogram showing abnormal configuration of mitral valve leaflets in systole

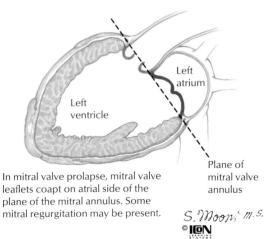

Left atrium

Left ventricle

Plane of mitral valve annulus

In mitral valve prolapse, mitral valve leaflets coapt on atrial side of the plane of the mitral annulus. Some mitral regurgitation may be present.

S. Moon, M.S.

© ICN

Figure 31-1

Tricuspid Stenosis and/or Insufficiency

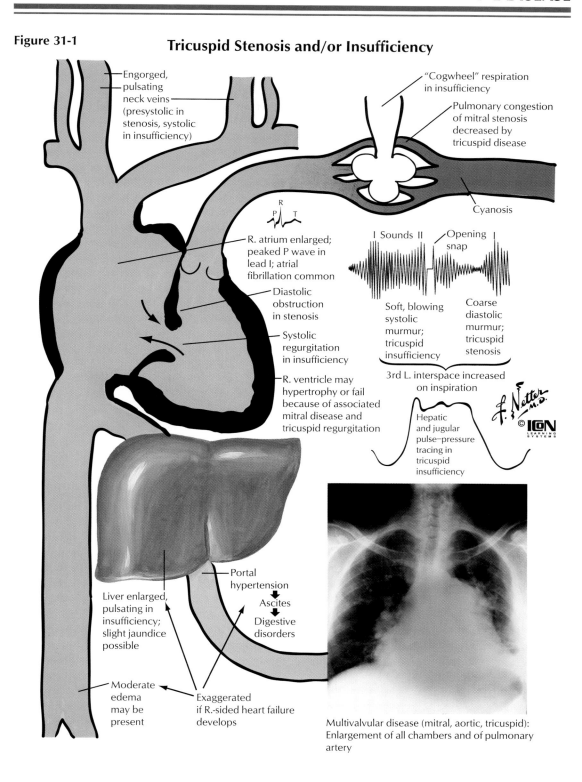

Engorged, pulsating neck veins (presystolic in stenosis, systolic in insufficiency)

"Cogwheel" respiration in insufficiency

Pulmonary congestion of mitral stenosis decreased by tricuspid disease

Cyanosis

R. atrium enlarged; peaked P wave in lead I; atrial fibrillation common

I Sounds II — Opening snap

Diastolic obstruction in stenosis

Systolic regurgitation in insufficiency

Soft, blowing systolic murmur; tricuspid insufficiency

Coarse diastolic murmur; tricuspid stenosis

R. ventricle may hypertrophy or fail because of associated mitral disease and tricuspid regurgitation

3rd L. interspace increased on inspiration

Hepatic and jugular pulse–pressure tracing in tricuspid insufficiency

Portal hypertension
↓
Ascites
↓
Digestive disorders

Liver enlarged, pulsating in insufficiency; slight jaundice possible

Moderate edema may be present

Exaggerated if R.-sided heart failure develops

Multivalvular disease (mitral, aortic, tricuspid): Enlargement of all chambers and of pulmonary artery

Figure 31-2

Right Atrial Enlargement

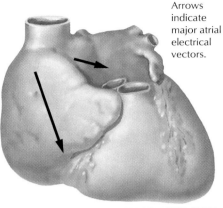

Arrows indicate major atrial electrical vectors.

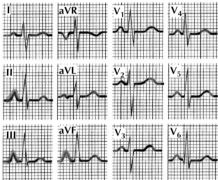

Tall P waves in leads II, III, and aVF ≥2.5 mm
(P pulmonale)

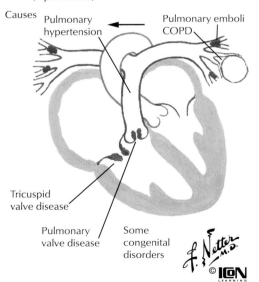

Causes

Pulmonary hypertension

Pulmonary emboli
COPD

Tricuspid valve disease

Pulmonary valve disease

Some congenital disorders

TRICUSPID REGURGITATION

Tricuspid regurgitation may be due to primary disease of the valve apparatus or diseases causing pulmonary hypertension with secondary annular dilatation. Secondary tricuspid regurgitation is seen in any condition associated with increased pulmonary artery pressures, and is the predominant cause of tricuspid regurgitation. The most common secondary causes are LV failure, mitral regurgitation, mitral stenosis, primary pulmonary disease, and primary pulmonary hypertension. The rare causes of primary tricuspid regurgitation include rheumatic heart disease, myxomatous disease (prolapse), infective endocarditis, carcinoid heart disease, and trauma.

Symptoms are often due to associated left-sided heart disease or pulmonary disease. Prominent signs and symptoms of right-sided heart failure suggest tricuspid regurgitation as a component. Endocarditis or carcinoid syndrome may be associated with characteristic systemic symptoms.

Jugular venous pressure is usually increased, and there is a prominent cv wave produced by regurgitant flow into the right atrium. The typical murmur is holosystolic and located at the left sternal edge. Augmentation of the murmur with inspiration helps distinguish tricuspid from mitral regurgitation.

Chest radiography often reveals RV enlargement manifested as filling of the retrosternal space. Dilation of the right ventricle often causes incomplete or complete right bundle branch block, seen on the ECG.

Doppler echocardiography is helpful in evaluating tricuspid regurgitation. Two-dimensional echocardiography evaluates the structure of the valvular apparatus and size of the right atrium and ventricle. Pulse-wave or color flow Doppler reveals the presence, direction, and magnitude of the regurgitant jet. Finally, continuous wave Doppler and the modified Bernoulli equation can be used to estimate the RV and pulmonary artery systolic pressures. In tricuspid regurgitation, the gradient between the right ventricle and the right atrium during systole equals four times the square of the velocity. This gradient is then added to the estimated right atrial pressure (the jugular venous pressure) to estimate RV systolic pressure. In the absence of pulmonic stenosis, this also equals pulmonary systolic pressure. Note that the calculation estimates the severity of the pulmonary hypertension, not the severity of the tricuspid regurgitation.

The mainstay of therapy for tricuspid regurgitation is treatment of the condition causing pulmonary hypertension. Diuretics may be useful for refractory fluid retention. Tricuspid valve replacement or repair is appropriate for patients refractory to medical therapy or sometimes at the time of surgery for coexistent mitral valve disease. Often a prosthetic ring is used for annuloplasty. If valve replacement is necessary, bioprostheses are favored because the tricuspid valve may be relatively prone to thrombosis.

PULMONIC STENOSIS

Right ventricular outflow obstruction may be subvalvular, valvular, or supravalvular. Both the subvalvular and the supravalvular forms are usually associated with other congenital heart disease, as discussed in section VIII. True valvular pulmonic stenosis, however, usually occurs as an isolated congenital defect. Rarely, pulmonic stenosis is due to rheumatic disease, endocarditis, or carcinoid syndrome (Fig. 31-3).

Patients with pulmonic stenosis are often asymptomatic. Patients may reach the fourth through sixth decades of life with significant pressure gradients across the pulmonic valve, but with no symptoms and no evidence of right-sided heart failure. If right-sided heart failure does develop, abdominal swelling, peripheral edema, abdominal discomfort, and fatigue may be present. Patients seldom present with chest pain or exertional syncope.

The physical examination typically reveals a mid systolic crescendo–decrescendo murmur at the left sternal edge. Often, an associated ejection click, which usually decreases with inspiration, is present. P_2 is soft and delayed, producing a widely split S_2, but one that does narrow with appropriate physiologic changes (unlike the fixed, widely split S_2 present in patients with an atrial septal defect). An RV lift may also be present. If RV failure is present, there may be peripheral edema, hepatomegaly, abdominal swelling, and jugular venous distention with a prominent a wave.

Electrocardiography usually reveals RV hypertrophy, right axis deviation, and right atrial enlargement. A complete or incomplete right bundle branch block is sometimes present. Chest radiography reveals poststenotic dilatation of the pulmonary artery but diminished peripheral pulmonary vascular markings. RV hypertrophy and enlargement are highly variable.

Echocardiography with Doppler evaluation is useful for establishing the diagnosis and assessing therapy. Morphologic assessment is best performed with the parasternal short axis view and the subcostal view. Transesophageal echocardiography is not usually necessary but can be performed if a transthoracic study fails to provide an adequate assessment. The right ventricle may be normal, particularly in childhood, but stenosis of long duration, greater severity, or both may be associated with RV hypertrophy and enlargement. Paradoxical motion of the interventricular septum is often apparent. Continuous wave Doppler evaluation is highly reliable in establishing the gradient across the pulmonic valve. Cardiac catheterization is usually not necessary but may be performed if Doppler studies are suboptimal or if balloon valvuloplasty will be performed.

Adult patients with mild-to-moderate pulmonic stenosis generally do well and require no intervention. When symptoms develop, it is often in the fourth decade of life. Balloon valvuloplasty is highly effective and indicated in symptomatic patients and possibly in patients with severe stenosis even in the absence of symptoms (see chapter 33). The most recent ACC/AHA task force has recommended balloon valvuloplasty as a class I indication in asymptomatic adolescents and young adults with transvalvular gradients greater than 50 mm Hg. A gradient of 40 to 49 mm Hg was considered a class IIa indication (meaning that this consideration should be based on individual patient circumstances) based on these recent guidelines.

PULMONIC REGURGITATION

Pulmonic valve regurgitation is usually secondary to severe pulmonary hypertension, pulmonary artery dilatation, or both. Rarely, it is secondary to endocarditis, carcinoid syndrome, rheumatic heart disease, trauma, or congenital valvular abnormalities. Accordingly, the dominant symptoms in pulmonic regurgitation are

Figure 31-3   **Pulmonary Valvular Stenosis and Atresia**

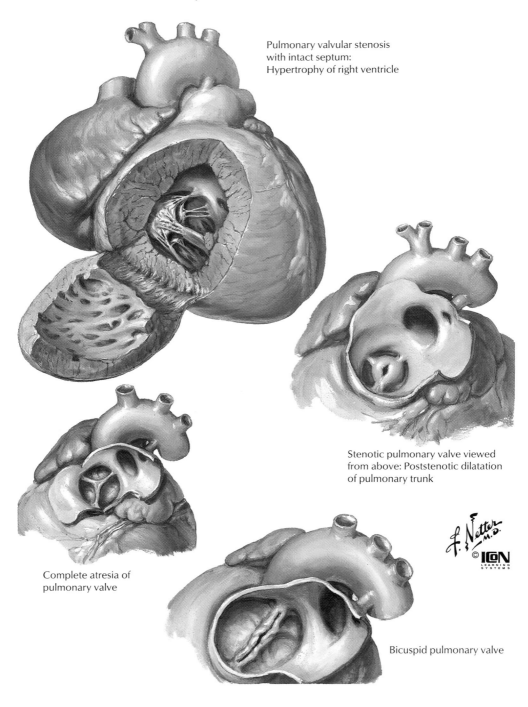

Pulmonary valvular stenosis
with intact septum:
Hypertrophy of right ventricle

Stenotic pulmonary valve viewed
from above: Poststenotic dilatation
of pulmonary trunk

Complete atresia of
pulmonary valve

Bicuspid pulmonary valve

usually those of the underlying disease process. Patients without severe underlying disease are often asymptomatic. However, patients with severe pulmonic regurgitation may ultimately have typical symptoms and signs of right-sided heart failure.

The characteristic physical finding is a decrescendo diastolic murmur, loudest at the left third and fourth intercostal spaces, which increases with inspiration. S_2 is usually widely split with an accentuated pulmonic component. There is often an associated systolic murmur from increased flow across the valve. Jugular venous distention and signs of right-sided heart failure may be apparent.

Right ventricular hypertrophy and dilatation may be evident by chest radiography and ECG. Echocardiography with Doppler can identify and grossly quantitate pulmonic regurgitation and assess the size and contractility of the right ventricle.

Treatment is generally directed at the underlying disease. If regurgitation is severe, valve surgery may be necessary. Patients should receive endocarditis prophylaxis for dental or other nonsterile procedures.

FUTURE DIRECTIONS

The treatment of pulmonic and tricuspid valve disease will continue to benefit from the steady evolution of percutaneous techniques. Pulmonic valvuloplasty was introduced in the early 1980s. Follow-up studies confirm the continued long-term effectiveness of a percutaneous approach. It is clear that most patients have a subsequent further decrease in the RV outflow gradient due in part to resolution of infundibular hypertrophy. This success has led to a generally lower threshold for intervention, as reflected in the most recent ACC/AHA guidelines discussed previously and in chapter 33. With respect to tricuspid stenosis, valvuloplasty techniques that use multiple balloons or the newer Inoue balloon appear promising.

REFERENCES

ACC/AHA Guidelines for the Management of Patients With Valvular Heart Disease. A Report of the American College of Cardiology/American Heart Association Task Force on Practice Guidelines. *J Am Coll Cardiol* 1998;32:1486.

Daniels SJ, Mintz GS, Kotler MN. Rheumatic tricuspid valve disease: Two-dimensional echocardiographic, hemodynamic, and angiographic correlations. *Am J Cardiol* 1983; 51:492–496.

DePace NL, Ross J, Iskandrian AS, et al. Tricuspid regurgitation: noninvasive techniques for determining causes and severity. *J Am Coll Cardiol* 1984;3:1540–1550.

Rao PS, Patnana M, Buck SH, et al. Results of three to ten year follow-up of balloon dilatation of the pulmonic valve. *Heart* 1998;80:591.

Yock PG, Popp RL. Noninvasive estimation of right ventricular systolic pressure by Doppler ultrasound in patients with tricuspid regurgitation. *Circulation* 1984;70:657–662.

Yousof AM, Shafei MZ, Endrys G, Khan N, Simo M, Cherian G. Tricuspid stenosis and regurgitation in rheumatic heart disease: A prospective cardiac catheterization study in 525 patients. *Am Heart J* 1985;110:60–64.

Chapter 32
Infective Endocarditis

Lisa B. Hightow and Meera Kelley

The term *infective endocarditis* (IE) refers to infection of the endocardial surface of the heart and implies a physical presence of microorganisms in the lesion. Despite many advances, IE continues to be associated with high morbidity and mortality rates. Early diagnosis, prompt and appropriate antimicrobial therapy, and timely surgical intervention are paramount to successful management.

The incidence of IE infection is difficult to determine because the criteria for diagnosis vary among the numerous series that have been reported. Estimates from the American Heart Association place the annual incidence of IE at 10,000 to 20,000 new cases per year. The mean age of patients has increased—from younger than 30 years in 1926 to older than 50 years currently. This change is likely due to dramatic decreases in the incidence of rheumatic fever because of the development of antimicrobial therapy. Degenerative valvular heart disease is now the major predisposing factor for endocarditis (see also chapters 27–31). The mitral valve is most commonly affected, followed by the aortic valve. The tricuspid and pulmonic valves are only rarely involved, usually in association with injection drug use.

ETIOLOGY AND PATHOGENESIS

The development of IE requires two events. First, the surface of the heart valve must be damaged, creating a suitable site for platelet and fibrin deposition. Subsequently, bacteria must reach the site and adhere to the lesion (Fig. 32-1).

Transient bacteremia occurs when an area heavily colonized with bacteria (and usually distant to the heart) is traumatized. The most common of such areas includes the oropharynx, the gastrointestinal tract, and the genitourinary tract. Bacteremia can occur in areas where skin breakdown accompanies bacterial colonization or after manipulation of the area (for instance, after dental cleaning, cystoscopy or endoscopy, or colonoscopy with biopsy). After colonization of the valve, bacteria replicate to a critical mass, and the vegetation enlarges by deposition of platelets and fibrin and continued bacterial replication (Fig. 32-2).

Patient Population

Approximately 60 to 80% of patients with endocarditis have an identifiable predisposing cardiac lesion such as degenerative or congenital heart disease, mitral valve prolapse, or rheumatic heart disease. The exception to this is patients with infective endocarditis associated with intravenous drug abuse. These individuals typically present with IE of the right heart valves, involving the tricuspid or pulmonic valves that were probably structurally normal before infection. Although the typical patient with IE secondary to intravenous drug abuse is young and male, intravenous drug abuse should be considered in any individual with tricuspid valve endocarditis. In addition to these causes, bacteremia from intravenous catheters, TPN indwelling catheters, arteriovenous shunts (used for hemodialysis), pacemakers, postoperative wound infections, and genitourinary manipulation have become an important cause of IE in chronically ill patients.

CLINICAL PRESENTATION

Four processes contribute to the clinical picture of IE: the infectious process on the heart valve, including local intracardiac complications; bland or septic embolization to virtually any organ; persistent bacteremia, possibly with metastatic foci of infection; and circulating immune complexes and other immunopathologic factors (Fig. 32-3).

Fever is present in approximately 95% of patients, but may be absent in those with congestive heart failure (CHF), renal failure, liver disease, and history of antibiotic usage, as well as in elderly individuals. Fever lasting longer than 2 weeks despite adequate antimicrobial therapy is

Figure 32-1

Bacterial Endocarditis I

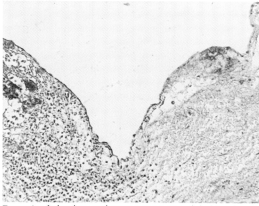

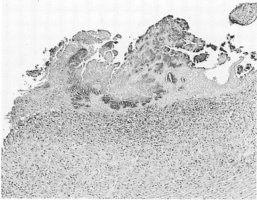

Deposit of platelets and organisms (stained dark), edema, and leukocytic infiltration in very early bacterial endocarditis of aortic valve

Development of vegetations containing clumps of bacteria on tricuspid valve

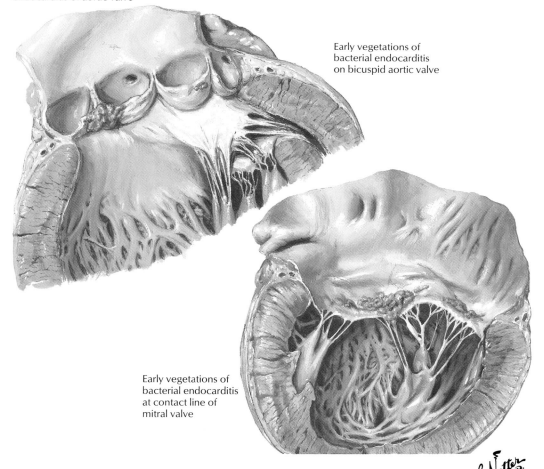

Early vegetations of bacterial endocarditis on bicuspid aortic valve

Early vegetations of bacterial endocarditis at contact line of mitral valve

Figure 32-2 ## Common Portals of Bacterial Entry in Bacterial Endocarditis

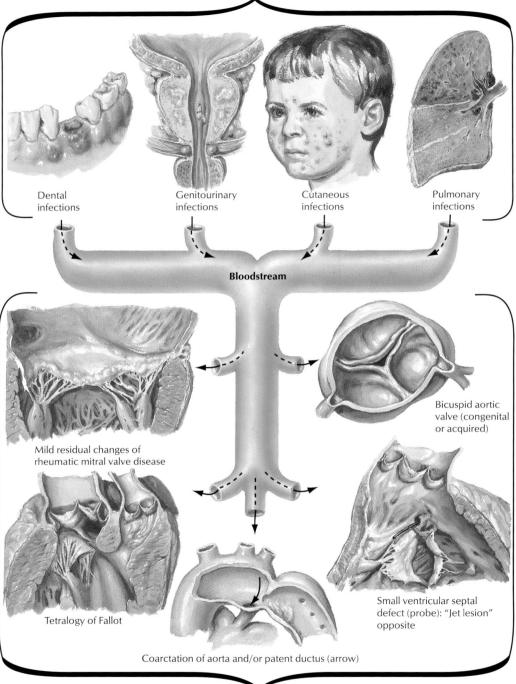

Dental infections

Genitourinary infections

Cutaneous infections

Pulmonary infections

Bloodstream

Mild residual changes of rheumatic mitral valve disease

Bicuspid aortic valve (congenital or acquired)

Tetralogy of Fallot

Small ventricular septal defect (probe): "Jet lesion" opposite

Coarctation of aorta and/or patent ductus (arrow)

Common Predisposing Lesions

Figure 32-3

Bacterial Endocarditis II

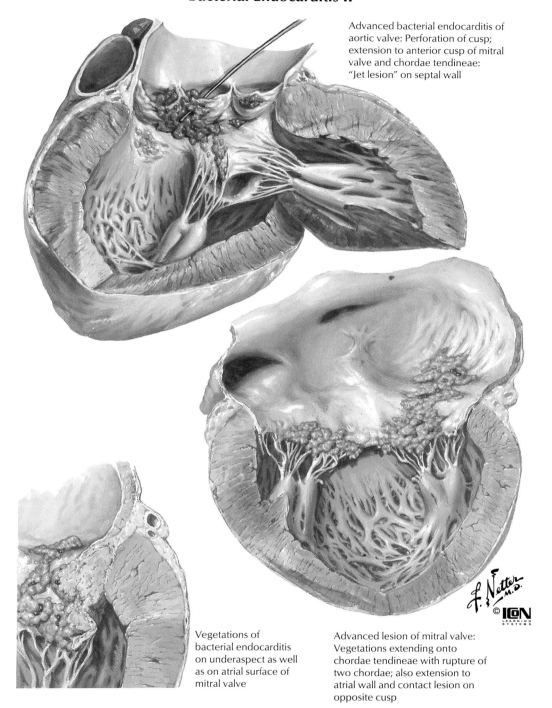

Advanced bacterial endocarditis of aortic valve: Perforation of cusp; extension to anterior cusp of mitral valve and chordae tendineae: "Jet lesion" on septal wall

Vegetations of bacterial endocarditis on underaspect as well as on atrial surface of mitral valve

Advanced lesion of mitral valve: Vegetations extending onto chordae tendineae with rupture of two chordae; also extension to atrial wall and contact lesion on opposite cusp

associated with specific etiologic agents, such as *Staphylococcus aureus*, gram-negative rods, fungi, culture-negative IE, embolization, myocardial abscess, tissue infarction, the need for cardiac surgery, and a higher mortality rate.

Heart murmurs can be detected in more than 85% of cases because of the predisposing valvular or congenital abnormality. In patients with IE diagnosed at an early stage, a documented change in their murmur or the appearance of a new murmur is uncommon and predicts an adverse outcome. CHF results primarily from progressive valvular insufficiency, and CHF develops in more than 90% of patients who demonstrate a new regurgitant murmur. Heart block, arrhythmias, pericarditis, abscesses, fistulas, and perforations can also occur (Fig. 32-4).

Peripheral manifestations are found in up to half of the cases and often reflect serious systemic consequences of IE. These include splinter hemorrhages, petechiae, Osler nodes, Janeway lesions, Roth spots, and clubbing (Fig. 32-5). Splenomegaly and musculoskeletal symptoms are also common.

Embolic episodes occur in at least one third of cases, and the clinical findings are unique to the organ involved. Neurologic manifestations (20–40% of cases) are associated with increased mortality. Embolic stroke is more commonly observed than other systemic emboli, due to the sensitivity of the brain to ischemic damage. Neuroemboli may result in hemiplegia, sensory loss, ataxia, aphasia, or an alteration in mental status (Fig. 32-5).

Many patients have symptoms for weeks to months before diagnosis because symptoms and signs can be nonspecific. The diagnosis of IE should be considered in any patient with persistent fever, weight loss, or unexplained failure to thrive.

DIFFERENTIAL DIAGNOSIS

An initial set of criteria published in 1981 to help diagnose IE did not use echocardiographic findings in the case definitions. With improved methods and recognition of the central diagnostic role of echocardiography in suspected IE, new case definitions and diagnostic criteria (Duke criteria) were proposed in 1994 and are now widely used (Table 32-1).

Microbiology
Streptococci

Streptococci are the pathogens in 55% of cases of native valve IE (if IE is excluded due to intravenous drug abuse). Approximately 35% of all cases are due to *Streptococcus viridans*, a normal inhabitant of the oropharynx.

Streptococcus bovis is a normal inhabitant of the human gastrointestinal tract. *S. bovis* endocarditis is more likely to develop in elderly individuals, and more than one third of those infected have a predisposing malignant or premalignant gastrointestinal tract lesion. To screen for underlying colon cancer, colonoscopy is indicated when *S. bovis* is recovered from the bloodstream.

Streptococcus pneumoniae is a rare cause of IE seen more commonly with alcohol abuse; its course is usually fulminant. Presentation may be associated with perivalvular abscess formation, pericarditis, or concurrent meningitis. Left-sided involvement is the rule, with a predilection for the aortic valve. The overall mortality rate remains high, with death resulting from rapid valvular destruction and hemodynamic compromise.

Enterococcal endocarditis usually has a subacute course, similar to the viridans streptococci. It is more common in older men after genitourinary manipulation and in younger women after obstetric procedures. More than 40% of the patients have no underlying heart disease, although a heart murmur develops in more than 95% during the illness. Classic peripheral manifestations are uncommon. Resistance of enterococci to conventional antimicrobial therapy makes the infection more difficult to treat.

Staphylococci

Staphylococci are responsible for at least 20 to 30% of the cases of IE, and 80 to 90% of these are due to the coagulase-positive *S. aureus*. Endocarditis resulting from this organism may involve previously normal heart valves. *S. aureus* endocarditis progresses rapidly and carries with it a high risk. Rapid valve destruction, widespread metastatic infections, myocardial abscesses, purulent pericarditis, and valve ring abscesses—and hemodynamic compromise—are more common with this agent than with more common

Figure 32-4

Bacterial Endocarditis III: Cardiac Sequelae

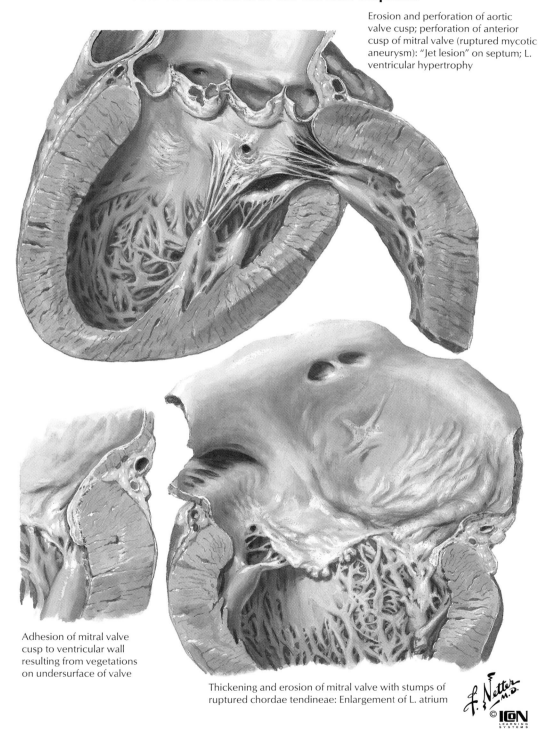

Erosion and perforation of aortic valve cusp; perforation of anterior cusp of mitral valve (ruptured mycotic aneurysm): "Jet lesion" on septum; L. ventricular hypertrophy

Adhesion of mitral valve cusp to ventricular wall resulting from vegetations on undersurface of valve

Thickening and erosion of mitral valve with stumps of ruptured chordae tendineae: Enlargement of L. atrium

Figure 32-5   ## Bacterial Endocarditis IV: Remote Embolic Effects

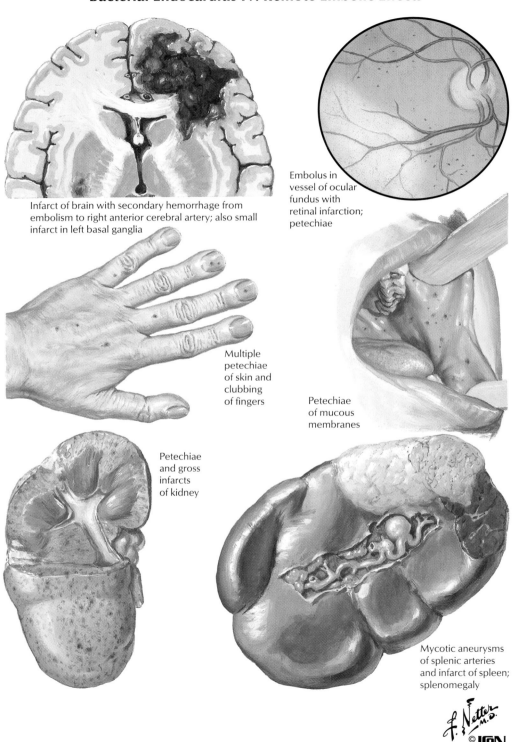

Infarct of brain with secondary hemorrhage from embolism to right anterior cerebral artery; also small infarct in left basal ganglia

Embolus in vessel of ocular fundus with retinal infarction; petechiae

Multiple petechiae of skin and clubbing of fingers

Petechiae of mucous membranes

Petechiae and gross infarcts of kidney

Mycotic aneurysms of splenic arteries and infarct of spleen; splenomegaly

Table 32-1
Duke Criteria

Definite IE

Pathologic criteria

- Microorganism: demonstrated by culture or histology in a vegetation, in a vegetation that has embolized, or in an intracardiac abscess **or**
- Pathologic lesions: vegetation or intracardiac abscess, confirmed by histology showing active endocarditis

Clinical criteria

- Two major criteria **or**
- One major and three minor criteria **or**
- Five minor criteria

Possible IE

Findings consistent with IE that fall short of "definite" but not rejected

Rejected IE

Firm alternate diagnosis for manifestations of endocarditis **or**

Resolution of manifestations of endocarditis, with antibiotic therapy for 4 days or less **or**

No pathologic evidence of IE at surgery or autopsy after antibiotic therapy for 4 days or less

Major criteria

1. Positive blood cultures for IE
   a. Typical microorganism for IE from two separate blood cultures in absence of a primary focus
      - Viridans streptococci
      - *Streptococcus bovis*, including nutritional variant strains
      - HACEK group
      - Community-acquired *Staphylococcus aureus* or enterococci
   b. Persistently positive blood culture, defined as recovery of a microorganism consistent with IE from:
      - Blood cultures drawn more than 12 hours apart **or**
      - All of three or a majority of four or more separate blood cultures, with first and last drawn at least 1 hour apart

2. Evidence of endocardial involvement
   a. Positive echocardiogram for IE
      - Oscillating intracardiac mass, on valve or supporting structures, or in the path of regurgitant jets, or on implanted material, in the absence of an alternate anatomic explanation **or**
      - Abscess **or**
      - New partial dehiscence or prosthetic valve **or**
   b. New valvular regurgitation (increase or change in preexisting murmur not sufficient)

Minor criteria

1. Predisposition: predisposing heart condition or intravenous drug use

2. Fever 38.0°C or higher (100.4°F)

3. Vascular phenomena: major arterial emboli, septic pulmonary infarcts, mycotic aneurysm, intracranial hemorrhage, conjunctival hemorrhages, Janeway lesions

4. Immunologic phenomena: glomerulonephritis, Osler nodes, Roth spots, rheumatoid factor

5. Microbiologic evidence: positive blood culture but not meeting major criterion as noted previously or serologic evidence of active infection with organism c/w IE

6. Echocardiogram consistent with IE but not meeting major criterion

---

IE indicates infective endocarditis.

Reprinted from *Am J Med*, Vol 96, Durack et al. New criteria for diagnosis of infective endocarditis: Utilization of specific echocardiographic findings, 200–209, 1994, with permission from Excerpta Medica.

---

causes of endocarditis. In many cases, urgent or emergent surgery is needed to remove the infected valve and surrounding area. *S. aureus*, including methicillin-resistant *S. aureus,* is the most common pathogen in conjunction with intravenous drug abuse. Coagulase-negative staphylococci, generally less virulent, are important pathogens in prosthetic valve IE.

Gram-Negative Bacilli

Persons who inject drugs or have prosthetic valves or cirrhosis are at increased risk for gram-negative bacillary IE. *Salmonella* species have an affinity for abnormal heart valves and may cause valvular perforation or destruction, atrial thrombi, myocarditis, and pericarditis. *Pseudomonas* IE is seen mainly in patients who inject drugs and tends to affect normal valves. Common complications include major embolic phenomena, inability to sterilize valves, neurologic complications, ring and annular abscesses, splenic abscesses, bacteremic relapse, and heart failure. Early surgery is recommended for left-sided disease.

HACEK Organisms

Bacteria in the HACEK group include *Haemophilus* species, *Actinobacillus actinomycetemcomitans, Cardiobacterium hominis, Eikenella corrodens,* and *Kingella kingae.* All of these organisms are fastidious and may require 2 to 3 weeks of incubation for isolation from blood. The typical clinical syndrome produced includes large friable vegetations, frequent emboli, and the development of heart failure.

Fungi

Most patients with fungal endocarditis have predisposing factors, such as intravenous drug abuse, reconstructive cardiovascular surgery, or prolonged intravenous therapy. *Candida parapsilosis* and *Candida tropicalis* predominate in those persons injecting drugs, whereas *Candida albicans* and *Aspergillus* species predominate in others. Fungal endocarditis carries a poor prognosis secondary to large bulky vegetations, a tendency for myocardial invasion, widespread systemic septic emboli, and inadequate antifungal therapy due to poor penetration and lack of fungicidal activity. Surgical intervention is usually necessary.

Culture-Negative Infective Endocarditis

The most common causes of culture-negative IE include recent administration of antibiotics, slow growth of fastidious organisms or organisms that are difficult to culture (HACEK organisms, *Brucella, Coxiella, Mycoplasma, Chlamydia, Bartonella, Legionella*), fungal endocarditis, and noninfective endocarditis or alternative diagnoses.

DIAGNOSTIC APPROACH

Blood cultures remain the single most important laboratory test in the diagnosis of IE. Bacteremia is usually continuous and low grade; blood cultures are positive for growth in 85 to 95% of cases. At least three sets of blood cultures should be drawn in the first 24 hours. More cultures may be necessary if the patient has received antibiotics in the preceding 2 weeks. Negative blood culture results are usually secondary to previous antibiotic usage, but some organisms, such as those in the HACEK group and *Brucella*, grow slowly and may require up to 4 weeks' incubation. Blood cultures are more likely to be negative when fungi are the pathogens. If embolization to a major vessel occurs, embolectomy should be performed and material should be sent for routine bacterial and fungal stains and culture. Serologic studies may be necessary for the diagnosis of Q fever, brucellosis, legionellosis, and psittacosis.

Echocardiography should be performed in all patients. Transthoracic echocardiography (TTE) is a rapid, noninvasive test with excellent specificity for vegetations (98%). However, the sensitivity of TTE is variable (from <50% to >90% positive). Transesophageal echocardiography (TEE) is substantially more sensitive (76–100%) and is particularly useful in patients with suboptimal TTE due to pulmonary disease, obesity, or chest wall deformities and for evaluating tricuspid, pulmonic, and prosthetic valves. TEE is also superior for evaluating complications of IE, such as extravalvular extension of infection and abscess. Negative TEE and TTE confer a 95% negative predictive value. However, when clinical suspicion of IE is high and the result of initial echocardiography is negative, a repeat examination in 7 to 10 days is warranted.

Laboratory abnormalities are common but nonspecific in IE. Hematologic parameters are often abnormal, but none are diagnostic. Normochromic, normocytic anemia is usually present, characteristic of an anemia of chronic disease. The erythrocyte sedimentation rate is elevated in most patients (90–100%), and positive rheumatoid factor is found in 40 to 50% of cases, particularly when illness duration is more than 6 weeks. Other findings include thrombocytopenia, leukocytosis or leukopenia, hypergammaglobulinemia, and abnormal urinalysis results.

MANAGEMENT AND THERAPY

Antimicrobial Therapy

Empiric, broad-spectrum antibiotic therapy—directed against the most likely causative agents—should be initiated after blood cultures have been obtained. Subsequent selection of antimicrobial agents is based on susceptibility testing of the causative microbe. Treatment requires prolonged use of bactericidal antibiotics; the parenteral route is usually indicated (Table 32-2).

Indications for Cardiac Surgery

Indications for surgical therapy of infective endocarditis are shown in Table 32-3. Deciding whether and when to proceed to surgery can be difficult. Most often, complications occur suddenly and the first embolic event can be devastating (one significant embolic episode is an indication for surgery). Ideally, surgical therapy proceeds when a serious complication is imminent but has not yet occurred. Predicting which patients are at highest risk is as much art as it is science. The size and mobility of vegetations imaged by echocardiography can be helpful, but is not absolute. Thus, the decision to proceed with surgery must be made carefully, with early discussion among cardiologists, infectious disease physicians, and cardiac surgeons, after well-informed input from patients and families.

Course of Endocarditis

Symptomatic improvement, a decrease in fever, and clearance of bacteremia are usually prompt with appropriate antibiotic therapy. Anemia usually persists through therapy, and it may take weeks or months to resolve. Recurrent or persistent fever may be secondary to failure to control infection, metastatic abscess formation, recurrent emboli, IV-related phlebitis,

superimposed infections, or medication (most likely antibiotic) related. The most frequent causes of death in IE are neurologic and septic complications, CHF, embolic phenomena, rupture of mycotic aneurysm, and complications from cardiac surgery.

Special Considerations

Prosthetic Valve Endocarditis

Prosthetic valve endocarditis (PVE) accounts for 10 to 15% of all cases of IE. It is classified as early when the infection occurs within the first 2 months after surgery and as late thereafter. Early PVE infection is believed to result from organisms acquired at the time of surgery or in the early postoperative period. Coagulase-negative staphylococci such as *Staphylococcus epidermidis* are the most common organisms, with occasional infections caused by *S. aureus*, diptheroids, Gram-negative rods, and fungi. Late PVE is presumably caused by bacteremia unrelated to the initial surgical procedure. Although the pathogens overlap with those of early PVE, the more usual agents of endocarditis, such as *S. viridans* and enterococci, also are found.

The clinical signs and symptoms of PVE are similar to those encountered in patients with native valve endocarditis. Because TTE typically fails to adequately visualize prosthetic valves, TEE is generally necessary.

Treatment of infective endocarditis is much more challenging when it involves the foreign material of a prosthetic valve. Empiric treatment usually includes a combination of vancomycin, gentamicin, and rifampin, but effective therapy frequently also necessitates removal and replacement of the prosthesis.

Prophylaxis

Antimicrobial prophylaxis is recommended for patients with increased risk of endocarditis from underlying cardiac conditions who undergo invasive procedures likely to generate bacteremia. For dental procedures, the recommendation for adults is a single 2.0-g dose of amoxicillin to be administered 1 hour before the anticipated procedure. For details regarding prophylaxis for other procedures, see the American Heart Association Web site: http://www.americanheart.org.

Table 32-2
Antimicrobial Therapy for Infective Endocarditis

Etiology	Antimicrobial Therapy
Viridans streptococci and *Streptococcus bovis* susceptible to penicillin (MIC ≤0.1 µg/mL)	Penicillin G 12–18 million U/24 h IV in six doses* for 4 weeks or ceftriaxone 2 g IV once daily for 4 weeks **or** Penicillin G 12–18 million U/24 h IV in six doses* for 2 weeks **WITH** gentamicin 1 mg/kg IV every 8 h[†] for 2 weeks **or** Vancomycin 30 mg · kg[-1] · 24 h[-1] IV in two divided doses for 4 weeks (only recommended for patients allergic to β-lactams)
Viridans streptococci and Streptococcus bovis relatively resistant to penicillin (MIC >0.01 to <0.5 µg/mL)	Penicillin G 18 million U/24 h IV continuously or six doses for 4 weeks **WITH** gentamicin 1 mg/kg IV every 8 h for 2 weeks (First-generation cephalosporins may be substituted for penicillin in patients with penicillin hypersensitivity not of the immediate type.) **or** Vancomycin 30 mg · kg[-1] · 24 h[-1] IV in two divided doses for 4 weeks (only recommended for patients allergic to β-lactams)
Enterococci (and viridans streptococci with penicillin MIC >0.5 µg/mL, nutrient variant viridans streptococci)	Penicillin G 18–30 million U/24 h IV in six doses **WITH** gentamicin 1 mg/kg IV every 8 h for 4–6 weeks **or** Ampicillin 12 g/24 h in six doses **WITH** gentamicin 1 mg/kg IV every 8 h for 4–6 weeks **or** Vancomycin 30 mg · kg[-1] · 24 h[-1] IV in two divided doses for 4–6 weeks **WITH** gentamicin 1 mg/kg IV every 8 h[†] for 4–6 week (Only recommended for patients allergic to β-lactams; cephalosporins are not acceptable alternatives for patients allergic to penicillin.)[‡]
Staphylococci (penicillin susceptible)	Penicillin G 20 million U/24 h IV in six doses for 4–6 weeks*
Staphylococci (methicillin susceptible, penicillin resistant)	Nafcillin (or oxacillin) 2 g IV every 4 h* for 4–6 weeks **WITH** gentamicin 1 mg/kg IV[†] every 8 h for 3–5 days* **or** Cefazolin (or other first-generation cephalosporin) 2 g IV every 8 h for 4–6 weeks with gentamicin 1 mg/kg IV every 8 h[†] for 3–5 days
Staphylococci (methicillin resistant)	Vancomycin 30 mg · kg[-1] · 24 h[-1] IV in two divided doses for 4–6 weeks
HACEK microorganisms	Ceftriaxone 2 g IV once daily for 4 weeks **or** Ampicillin 2 g every 4 h or 12 g/24 h IV continuously **WITH** gentamicin 1 mg/kg IV every 8 h[†] for 4 weeks

*Dosing of penicillin, nafcillin, and oxacillin is quite frequent and often considered problematic for patients stable enough for home therapy. However, because these drugs are stable for 24 h at room temperature, they may be given via a pump that remains continuously at the patient's side, requiring adjustment by a nurse or other caregiver only once every 24 h.

†Aminoglycosides are used in endocarditis for synergy for gram-positive infections. Therefore, doses are lower than those used to treat gram-negative infections but require a continuous therapeutic level such that once-daily therapy is not an option.

‡The infecting strain of *Enterococcus* bacteria must be tested for resistance to aminoglycosides. High-level resistance means loss of synergy, and thus, aminoglycosides should not be used in these instances. Therapy should be prolonged to 8–12 weeks.

With permission from Wilson WR, Sande MA. *Current Diagnosis and Treatment in Infectious Diseases.* New York, NY: McGraw Hill; 2001:155–163.

Table 32-3
Indications for Surgical Therapy for Infective Endocarditis

· CHF refractory to medical therapy

· At least one significant embolic episode

· Persistent bacteremia despite appropriate antibiotic therapy

· Physiologically significant valve dysfunction, as demonstrated by echocardiography

· Inadequate antimicrobial therapy (as in fungal IE)

· Mycotic aneurysm

· Early prosthetic valve endocarditis and some cases of late PVE, especially with resistant organisms

· Evidence of extension of infection (development of persistent heart block or bundle branch block, perivalvular or myocardial abscess)

CHF indicates congestive heart failure; IE, infective endocarditis; PVE, prosthetic valve endocarditis.

FUTURE DIRECTIONS

The increase of antimicrobial resistance is likely to continue and will complicate treatment decisions in patients with IE. Future studies will be needed to evaluate treatment effectiveness for resistant species of streptococci, staphylococci, and enterococci. Some clinicians believe that the size of the vegetation and other echocardiographic characteristics may predict which patients are at risk for poor outcome and will need early surgery. Advances in imaging methods may make predictions based on characteristics of the vegetations more feasible. In addition, future studies will help to determine whether echocardiographic findings other than perivalvular or myocardial abscess should be added to the list of surgical indications.

REFERENCES

American Heart Association. Prevention of bacterial endocarditis: Recommendations by the American Heart Association. *Circulation* 1997;96:358–366.

Bayer AS. Infectious endocarditis. *Clin Infect Dis* 1993;17:313–322.

Durack DT, Lukes AS, Bright DK. New criteria for diagnosis of infective endocarditis: Utilization of specific echocardiographic findings. *Am J Med* 1994;96:200–209.

Ellis M. Fungal endocarditis. *J Infect* 1997;35:99–103.

Mandell GL, Bennett JE, Dolin R. *Principles and Practice of Infectious Diseases.* 5th ed. New York: Churchill Livingstone; 2000.

Wilson WR, Sande MA. *Current Diagnosis and Treatment in Infectious Diseases.* New York: McGraw Hill; 2001:155–163.

Chapter 33

Percutaneous Balloon Valvuloplasty

Thomas M. Bashore

Charles Dotter is credited with noting that the stenotic severity of a high-grade iliac lesion was lessened when a diagnostic catheter was passed through it. Early vascular efforts used progressively larger catheters to open the lesions by blunt dilatation. Eventually, this approach using progressively larger bougies was replaced by the use of elastic balloon-tipped catheters, first for peripheral vascular disease, then for coronary angioplasty. Reports from the National Heart, Lung, and Blood Institute (NHLBI) registry, the Mansfield balloon catheter registry, and large institutional experiences subsequently shaped the development of percutaneous balloon procedures for stenotic valvular lesions.

As technology advances resulted in more effective percutaneous approaches to the treatment of valvular stenosis, the terminology used to describe these procedures evolved as well. The term "commissurotomy" originated from the surgical procedure developed for commissural mitral valve stenosis (see chapter 34), and some thought valvuloplasty should be reserved for surgical procedures that more directly altered the valvular structure. As an initial compromise, the NHLBI registry suggested that the term "valvotomy" be used for aortic and pulmonic procedures and commissurotomy for mitral procedures. These terms are often used in the older literature. In recent years, "valvuloplasty" has become the term of choice to describe procedures in which stenotic valves are opened by balloon dilatation. This term, analogous to balloon angioplasty, is established in the cardiology community and is used in this chapter.

PULMONARY VALVE STENOSIS
Pathophysiology

Pulmonary valve stenosis results from fusion of the valve cusps during mid to late fetal development. The most common form of isolated right ventricular (RV) obstruction, pulmonary valvular stenosis occurs in approximately 7% of individuals with congenital heart disease (see also chapters 44 and 45). Pulmonary valve stenosis may be associated with significant RV hypertrophy and infundibular narrowing. The fusion of the valvular cusps produces a classic systolic "doming" appearance angiographically (Fig. 33-1). Tissue pads within the valve sinuses

may exist and result in a thickened, rigid valve that is considered dysplastic. Excessive thickening in dysplastic valves usually renders the valve unsuitable for percutaneous valvuloplasty, although attempts have occasionally been successful. The dysplastic form is common in Noonan's syndrome. The greater the severity of congenital pulmonary valvular stenosis, the more likely the RV outflow tract will also be narrowed and the lesion will resemble pulmonary valve atresia. Balloon valvuloplasty is contraindicated in individuals with annular hypoplasia. Fortunately, in adults, the most common form of pulmonary valve stenosis results from commissural fusion, making this lesion amenable to percutaneous balloon methods.

Figure 33-2 demonstrates the gradient between the right ventricle and the pulmonary artery before and after successful percutaneous balloon valvuloplasty. The RV outflow track may have considerable subpulmonic stenosis, which may be masked when valvular obstruction is present. The sudden removal of the valvular stenosis after valvuloplasty may result in acute decompensation from marked RV infundibular obstruction, sometimes called the "suicide RV." Fluid loading, calcium channel blockers, and β-blockers can be used for emergent treatment. After pulmonary valvuloplasty, the subpulmonic hypertrophy may regress considerably over the next several months.

Indications

Valvular regurgitation is generally graded from 1+ (mild) to 4+ (severe). In patients with less

Figure 33-1

Pulmonary Stenosis

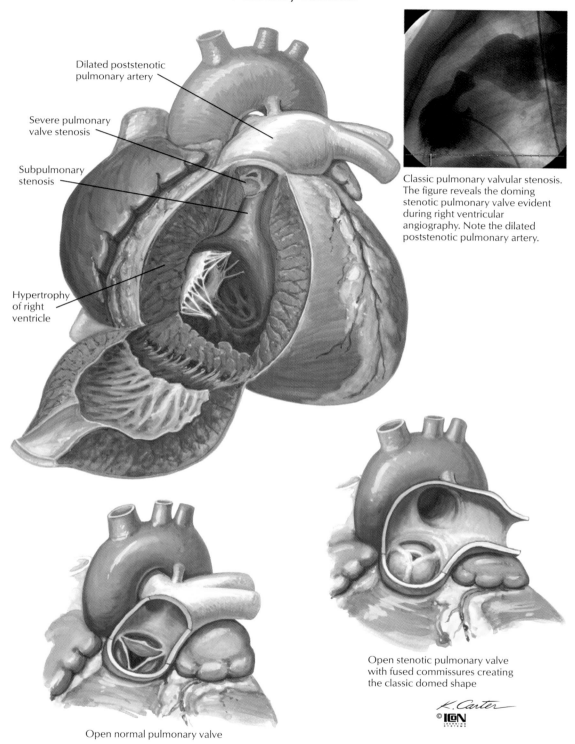

Dilated poststenotic
pulmonary artery

Severe pulmonary
valve stenosis

Subpulmonary
stenosis

Hypertrophy
of right
ventricle

Classic pulmonary valvular stenosis.
The figure reveals the doming
stenotic pulmonary valve evident
during right ventricular
angiography. Note the dilated
poststenotic pulmonary artery.

Open stenotic pulmonary valve
with fused commissures creating
the classic domed shape

K. Carter
©ICN

Open normal pulmonary valve

Figure 33-2

Pulmonary Balloon Valvuloplasty

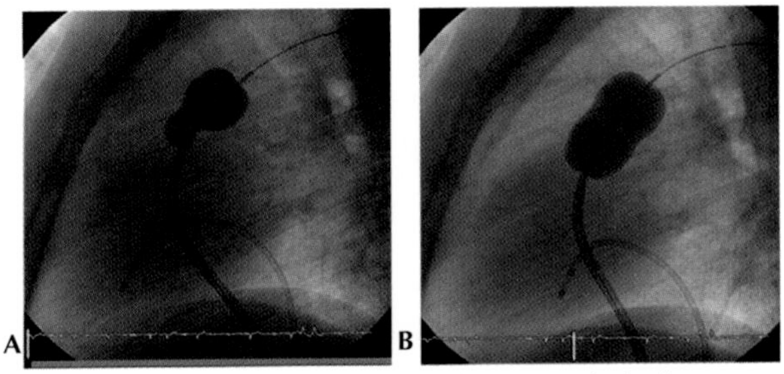

The Inoue balloon used for pulmonary valvuloplasty; partially inflated inoue balloon (**A**) and completed inflated Inoue balloon (**B**)

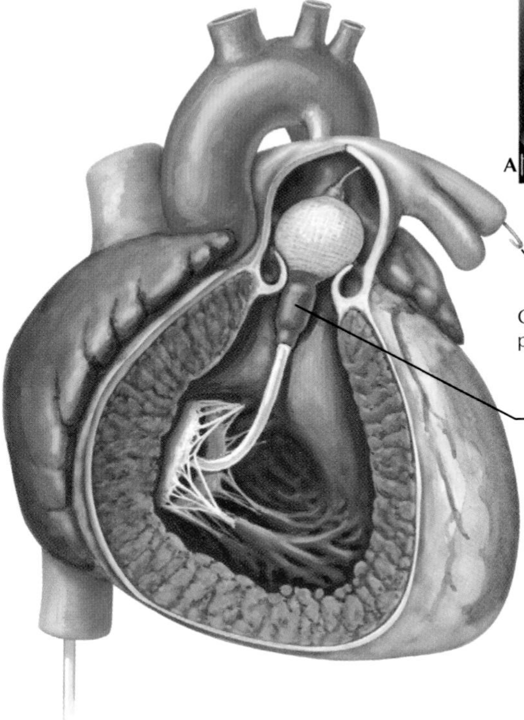

Guide wire in left pulmonary artery

Inoue valvuloplasty balloon in place across stenotic pulmonary valve

Percutaneous catheter from femoral vein

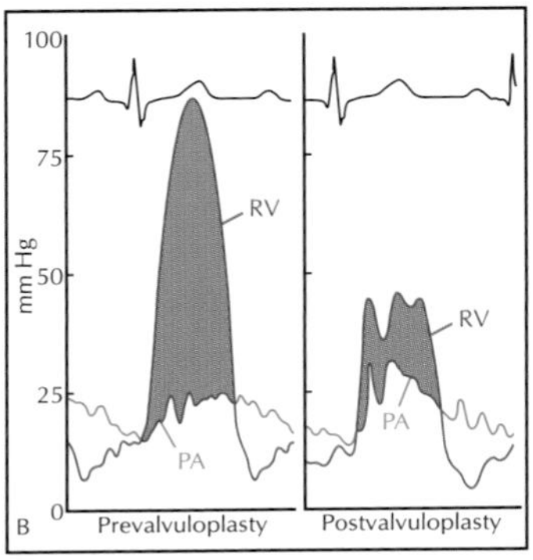

The pulmonary artery–RV gradient before and after pulmonary valvuloplasty

With permission from Bashore TM, Davidson CJ. Acute hemodynamic effects of percutaneous balloon aortic valvuloplasty. In: Bashore TM, Davidson CJ, eds. *Percutaneous Balloon Valvulopasty and Related Techniques*. Baltimore: Williams & Wilkins; 1991:99–111.

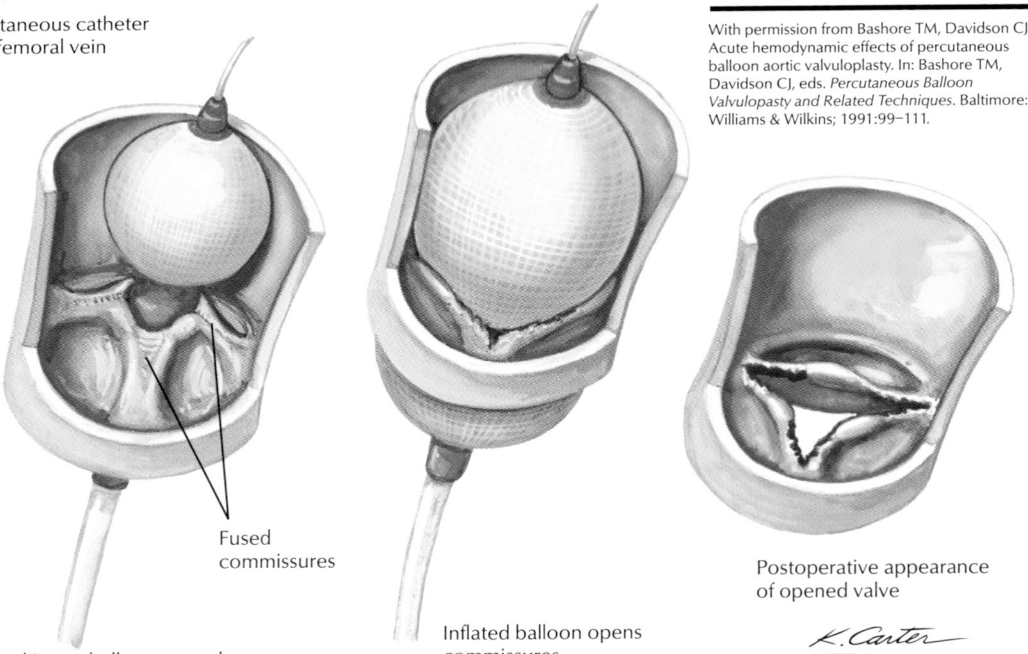

Fused commissures

Deflated Inoue balloon passed across stenotic valve, inflated distally and positioned

Inflated balloon opens commissures

Postoperative appearance of opened valve

K. Carter

© ICN

Inoue Balloon Catheter, Toray Industries, Inc., Tokyo, Japan.

than 2+ pulmonic insufficiency and a doming pulmonic valve, a peak pulmonary valve gradient of 50 mm Hg at cardiac catheterization is sufficient to warrant balloon valvuloplasty even without symptoms. Any evidence of RV dysfunction or associated RV failure and tricuspid regurgitation should prompt intervention. For the reasons described previously, procedural success is much lower in patients with pulmonary valve dysplasia. Percutaneous balloon valvuloplasty of the pulmonary valve has also been reported to be of some limited success in patients with carcinoid involvement of the pulmonic valve.

Technique

Before the procedure, RV angiography in the cranial right anterior oblique and straight lateral views is performed. Pulmonary angiography assesses preprocedural pulmonic insufficiency. Severe pulmonic insufficiency is a contraindication to valvuloplasty; severe insufficiency as a result of the procedure represents an adverse outcome. Baseline annular size is determined by echocardiography, magnetic resonance imaging, or contrast angiography. In the cardiac catheterization laboratory, a catheter (with radioopaque markers a known distance apart) may be used for angiography at the valve level to determine appropriate balloon size. Quantitative angiographic methods may be similarly applied.

The dilating balloon or balloons are percutaneously inserted into the femoral vein without a sheath. The maximum inflation of the balloon(s) should be equal to 1.2 to 1.4 times the estimated annular size (Fig. 33-2). In contrast to the aortic valve (see Aortic Valve Stenosis section), the pulmonary artery is elastic and often requires oversizing for adequate results. The goal of the procedure is a final peak valvular gradient less than 30 mm Hg. Recurrence rates are much lower if that threshold is reached. A single balloon, often 23 mm in diameter in adults, may be used, although two balloons side by side may be necessary in patients with a large annulus. In some laboratories, trefoil or bifoil balloon catheters are available and preferred. The Inoue mitral valvuloplasty balloon has increasingly been used for pulmonary valvuloplasty because of its stability during inflation.

Careful measurement of postprocedural gradients allows differentiation of infundibular stenosis from residual valvular stenosis. Postprocedural RV and pulmonary artery angiography help assess the severity of pulmonic insufficiency that has developed as a result of the procedure and also can address the presence and significance of infundibular stenosis.

Short-Term Results and Complications

Numerous groups have reported excellent short-term results in children and adults, as exemplified by a report of 66 infants and children in whom the peak gradient across the pulmonic valve fell from 92 ± 43 mm Hg to 29 ± 20 mm Hg with no change in cardiac output. The NHLBI adult registry included 37 adult patients, the procedure was completed in 97%, and the average peak gradient decreased from 46 to 18 mm Hg. Larger balloon sizes, up to 30 to 50% larger than the annulus, resulted in greater reductions in the valvular gradient without increasing complications.

Minimal complications in the acute setting include vagal symptoms and ventricular ectopy from catheters in the right ventricle. Pulmonary edema, presumably from increasing pulmonary flow to previously underperfused lungs, perforation of a cardiac chamber, high-grade atrioventricular nodal block, and transient RV outflow obstruction have also been reported. Pulmonary valve insufficiency occurs in about two thirds of the patients after the procedure, but it is rarely clinically significant.

Long-Term Results

Long-term data are available for up to 10 years after percutaneous balloon valvuloplasty of the pulmonary valve. In one representative study, 62 children undergoing this procedure, with an average balloon-to-pulmonary annulus ratio of 1.4, were followed up for a mean of 6.4 ± 3.4 years. Persistent pulmonary valve insufficiency was found in 39% of the patients, there was evidence of a progressive resolution of infundibular hypertrophy, and the restenosis (>35 mm Hg gradient) rate was only 4.8%. Restenosis was more common in patients with dysplastic valves. If restenosis occurred, repeat valvuloplasty appeared to be effective in patients without dysplastic pulmonary valves.

These data compare quite favorably with the outcomes of surgical valvotomy. One large study of surgical valvotomy in children reported a surgical mortality rate of 3%, with poor surgical results (residual gradient >50 mm Hg) in 4%. Restenosis rates after surgery were 14 to 33% at up to 34 months of follow-up. Thus, percutaneous balloon valvuloplasty for valvular pulmonic stenosis appears to be the treatment of choice and provides excellent short- and long-term relief from pulmonary valvular obstruction.

AORTIC VALVE STENOSIS
Pathophysiology

The normal aortic valve has thin, flexible cusps composed of three tissue layers sandwiched between layers of endothelium on both sides of the valve. The layers include a fibrosa with collagen fibers oriented parallel to the leaflet that support the major leaflet, a ventricularis layer composed of elastic fibers oriented perpendicularly to the leaflet edge that provide flexibility, and a spongiosa layer of loose connective tissue in the basal third of each leaflet.

Congenitally deformed aortic valves can generally be described as either unicuspid or bicuspid. Unicuspid valves are inherently stenotic at birth and cause symptoms early in life. Unicuspid aortic valves account for about 10% of all cases of isolated aortic valve stenosis in adulthood, whereas bicuspid aortic valves account for about 60% of isolated aortic valve stenosis in patients aged 15 to 65 years of age. Bicuspid aortic valves generally have two cusps of nearly equal size with little commissural fusion, but with a false commissure (raphe) present in one cusp. Over time, progressive valvular fibrosis and calcium deposition occurs, worsening the functional stenosis. Some commissural fusion may occur, but the major limitation is usually valvular rigidity from calcium buildup and scarring.

Aortic valve stenosis in elderly persons generally involves a trileaflet valve and likely represents a continuum, from benign aortic valvular sclerosis to severe aortic valvular stenosis. The prevalence of aortic valve sclerosis has been reported to be 25% in individuals older than 65 years of age, with severe aortic valve stenosis evident in 1 to 2% of the population. There is evidence that the mechanism of calcific aortic valve stenosis in the elderly is related to atherosclerosis. Little commissural fusion exists; large accretions of calcium can be present in the sinuses of Valsalva. The leaflets gradually lose their flexibility due to these calcium deposits. In calcific aortic valve stenosis, the minimal reduction in the gradient that can be obtained by balloon procedures has generally been attributed to cracks in the calcific nodules, cuspal tears, and aortic wall expansion (Fig. 33-3).

When left ventricular (LV) outflow is obstructed at the valvular level, a gradient develops between the left ventricle and the aorta (Fig. 33-4). The relationship between the gradient and the aortic valve area (AVA) is complex, however, and depends on the severity of the lesion as measured by the AVA and on the cardiac output or the aortic flow. After aortic valvuloplasty, aortic flow may increase because of an improvement in the cardiac output or the development of aortic insufficiency. Either result could increase the gradient, even if the actual AVA increases. Alternatively, the cardiac output may fall and the gradient may appear lower even if the AVA has increased. Thus, the short-term postprocedural valvular gradient change may not always reflect the actual change in the AVA.

Using just the change in the AVA can be problematic for other reasons. For instance, if the baseline AVA is severe, an improvement in the AVA of 0.3 cm^2 from baseline has a dramatic effect on the peak LV systolic pressure (e.g., when the AVA increases from 0.5 to 0.8 cm^2), but if the baseline AVA is less severe, the same incremental change may have much less consequence (e.g., when the AVA increases from 0.8 to 1.1 cm^2). Hence, either an improvement in the gradient, or an improvement in both the gradient and the final valve area can be used to define a successful result (i.e., a final valve gradient of <50 mm Hg and/or a 50% improvement in the AVA).

Indications

The decision whether to intervene in aortic valve stenosis usually depends on the presence of symptoms of congestion, angina, or exertional syncope, and an assessment of the likelihood of successful improvement in AVA. Serial measurements of transvalvular pressure gradients, by Doppler echocardiography, can be helpful to

Figure 33-3

Effect of Valvuloplasty on Aortic Valve Area

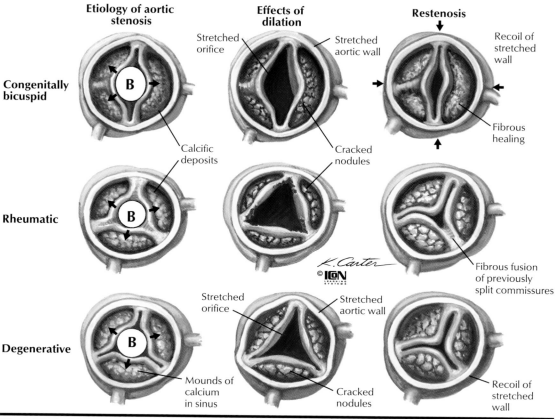

With permission from Waller BF, van Tassel JW, McKay C. Anatomic basis for and morphologic changes produced by catheter balloon valvuloplasty. In: Bashore TM, Davidson CJ, eds. *Percutaneous Balloon Valvuloplasty and Related Techniques*. Baltimore: Williams & Wilkins; 1991:34.

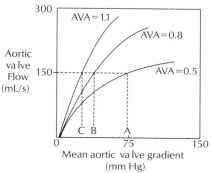

The relation between the aortic valve area and aortic flow (cardiac output). Note the curvilinear relation. The more flat the curves at the smaller aortic valve areas, the greater the gradient at any particular aortic flow. Because of this relation, a change in the aortic valve of 0.3 cm² has a much greater impact on the gradient going from 0.5 cm² to 0.8 cm² (A to B) than the same incremental change going from 0.8 cm² to 1.1 cm² (B to C).

With permission from Bashore TM, David CJ. *Acute Hemodynamics Effects of Percutaneous Balloon Aortic Valvuloplasty and Related Techniques.* Baltimore: Williams & Wilkins; 1991:105.

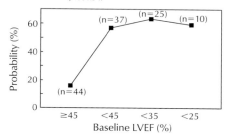

The relation between the baseline ejection fraction (EF) and the probability of recurrent symptoms at the 1-year outcome in elderly patients undergoing percutaneous balloon aortic valvuloplasty. Only those with an EF >45% experienced acceptable results.

With permission from Davidson CJ, Harrison JK, Pieper KS, et al. Determinants of one-year outcome from balloon aortic vavuloplasty. *Am J Cardiol* 1991;68:79.

Figure 33-4

Aortic Balloon Valvuloplasty

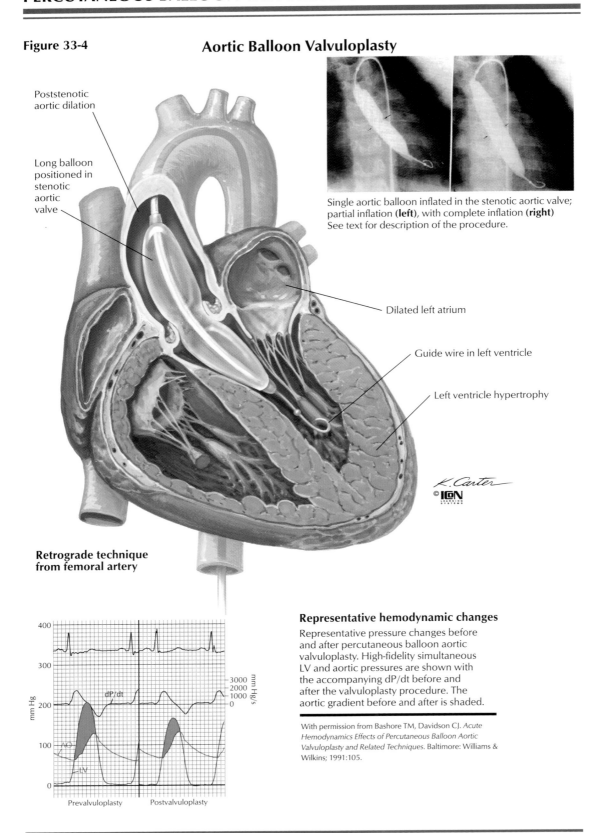

Poststenotic aortic dilation

Long balloon positioned in stenotic aortic valve

Single aortic balloon inflated in the stenotic aortic valve; partial inflation (**left**), with complete inflation (**right**) See text for description of the procedure.

Dilated left atrium

Guide wire in left ventricle

Left ventricle hypertrophy

Retrograde technique from femoral artery

Representative hemodynamic changes

Representative pressure changes before and after percutaneous balloon aortic valvuloplasty. High-fidelity simultaneous LV and aortic pressures are shown with the accompanying dP/dt before and after the valvuloplasty procedure. The aortic gradient before and after is shaded.

With permission from Bashore TM, Davidson CJ. *Acute Hemodynamics Effects of Percutaneous Balloon Aortic Valvuloplasty and Related Techniques.* Baltimore: Williams & Wilkins; 1991:105.

Prevalvuloplasty   Postvalvuloplasty

the physician who follows up on the patient. When the maximum velocity exceeds 4 m/sec (estimated gradient of 64 mm Hg), symptoms emerge relatively quickly. A change in the Doppler gradient of more than 0.3 m/sec within 1 year also portends symptoms. Because of the variable means for measuring valvular gradients and the dependence of the valve gradient on the aortic valvular flow and the effective orifice area, the use of a specific AVA to make a decision on operability is tenuous. In symptomatic patients with reduced LV systolic function and poor forward cardiac output, the use of an inotropic agent or nitroprusside to augment aortic flow may help determine whether the low output (and the subsequently low gradient) is a consequence of the valvular stenosis or is attributable to poor ventricular function. Most physicians use an AVA of below 0.8 cm^2 and a mean aortic gradient of at least a 50 mm Hg in symptomatic patients as indications for aortic valve intervention.

Whether to use percutaneous intervention depends on the clinical situation and the type of valvular disease responsible for the aortic valve stenosis. In the rare case of rheumatic aortic valve stenosis without significant aortic insufficiency, commissural fusion is present. Percutaneous balloon valvuloplasty would be expected to be beneficial in this situation, but very few patients have isolated aortic valve stenosis due to rheumatic disease.

In neonates and very young children, the initial success rates for percutaneous intervention are not encouraging, although older children may benefit and should be considered for the procedure. In adults, surgical intervention has consistently proven superior to percutaneous balloon valvuloplasty. The use of percutaneous balloon valvuloplasty in adults should be restricted to situations in which the risk of surgical intervention is very high (e.g., in a pregnant patient or in an elderly patient with cardiogenic shock). In these circumstances, percutaneous balloon valvuloplasty may serve as a bridge to eventual aortic valve replacement. Also, in the rare elderly adult with preserved LV systolic function and severe aortic valve stenosis who is not a candidate for surgical aortic valve replacement because of comorbid conditions, valvuloplasty can provide short-term symptomatic benefit, but long term outcomes are poor.

Technique

The balloon catheter used for aortic valvuloplasty should have a maximum inflated diameter slightly smaller than the measured size of the aortic annulus. In adults, a 20-mm diameter balloon is usually used, although a 23-mm balloon may be required for larger patients. Smaller sizes are used in children or in very small adults. Longer balloons (i.e., 5.5 cm vs. 3 cm in length) are advantageous to help prevent slippage in the stenotic valve orifice during balloon inflation.

Hemodynamics are measured at baseline and after the completion of the procedure to determine the efficacy of the procedure. The balloon catheter is placed in the middle of the valve plane and inflated, using dilute (25%) radiographic contrast in saline (Fig. 33-4). Inflation pressures do not seem to significantly influence the outcome, and these pressures are no longer measured. Usually one to three separate 15- to 20-second inflations are adequate.

Whether the approach is percutaneous (via the femoral artery, with or without a sheath), cutdown (using the brachial artery), or transseptal (using an antegrade approach to the aortic valve via the right femoral artery), similar results are obtained. The transseptal approach is particularly useful in patients with significant aortoiliac atherosclerosis, which is common in elderly individuals. Following the transseptal puncture, an 0.038-inch wire is navigated through the left atrium and the left ventricle, across the aortic valve, and down the descending aorta for stability. The intraatrial septum is expanded using an 8-mm balloon catheter before insertion of the aortic valvuloplasty balloon catheter. The remainder of the procedure is similar to the retrograde approach.

Acute Results and Complications

A review of 18 studies of balloon valvuloplasty in elderly patients showed that the mean aortic gradient can be expected to fall from about 55 to 29 mm Hg acutely, with the AVA increasing from 0.5 to 0.8 cm^2. Patients in these studies generally had no measurable increase in cardiac output.

In those patients for whom pressure–volume data were derived before and immediately after the procedure, systolic function was largely unchanged, with the ejection fraction rising only slightly, the peak positive dP/dt falling slightly, and stroke volume and peak and end-systolic wall stress all modestly reduced. A greater impact was noted on diastolic measures of ventricular function, including a significant decrease in peak negative dP/dt and a prolongation of tau (a measure of active diastolic relaxation). Transient mild ischemia during the procedure was considered responsible for some of the acute changes.

Results in children and neonates vary broadly depending on the patient's clinical status and associated cardiac anomalies. Many neonates with critical aortic valve stenosis have severe LV hypoplasia or endocardial fibroelastosis and do poorly with either percutaneous aortic valvuloplasty or surgery. After the neonatal period, the results from valvuloplasty improve. Data from 232 patients with a mean age of about 9 years showed the aortic gradients decreased approximately 60% from about 75 mm Hg to 30 mm Hg after percutaneous balloon valvuloplasty. Thus, the procedure appears to work reasonably well in the adolescent age group, importantly offering an opportunity to delay surgery until the individual has reached their full adult size. It should be noted that, even with an excellent outcome, restenosis will occur over time. This may be a good trade-off because surgical replacement of the aortic valve before adulthood may be followed by a need for subsequent surgery due to relative valvular stenosis (for instance a prosthetic valve that was appropriate in an adolescent may be undersized for the adult heart).

The rate of serious life-threatening complications from aortic valvuloplasty is remarkably low given the elderly population in whom it was initially applied. Almost all protocols require patients to be noncandidates for surgical intervention. In a review of 791 such patients, in-hospital mortality rates of 5.4% with a risk of serious morbidity (cerebrovascular accident, cardiac perforation, myocardial infarction, or serious aortic insufficiency) of up to 1.5%. Vascular complications were overwhelmingly the greatest complicating feature, with a 10.6% incidence.

In the NHLBI registry of 671 patients, complications were significant. At least one complication was reported in 25% of the patients within 24 hours, and 31% had some complication before hospital discharge. The most common complication was the need for transfusion (23%), followed by the need for vascular surgery (7%) or the occurrence of a cerebrovascular accident (3%), a systemic embolization (2%), or a myocardial infarction (2%). All cause mortality was 3%, with death usually related to multiorgan failure and poor preprocedural LV function. In patients who survived to 30 days, 75% had improved at least one New York Heart Association (NYHA) functional class.

Long-Term Results

Short-term studies after aortic valvuloplasty have revealed that an increase in the aortic gradient can occur as early as 2 days after the procedure, undoubtedly related to aortic recoil. There may also be progressive early improvement in cardiac output over this initial period that, while beneficial, adds to the increased gradient observed. By 6 months, most patients have evidence of restenosis. In a study of 41 patients undergoing recatheterization at 6 months, essentially all of the patients demonstrated hemodynamic restenosis. Of interest, symptoms at follow-up appear more related to diastolic dysfunction than to the measured AVA or gradient.

In one study, at 1-year follow-up, the probability of recurrent symptoms was predicted by a baseline ejection fraction below 45. This implies that patients with poor LV systolic function are not good candidates for percutaneous balloon aortic valvuloplasty. Because most patients with preserved LV systolic function would clearly be candidates for aortic valve replacement surgery, only a small population of adult patients would be expected to benefit from the resultant short-term improvement in symptoms. This situation is most likely to occur in those aortic valve stenosis patients at an extreme age (over 90 years), in whom the risk of surgery is usually prohibitive.

MITRAL VALVE STENOSIS
Pathophysiology

Obstruction to LV inflow through the mitral valve is usually attributed to rheumatic heart disease. Congenital mitral valve stenosis (MS) may also occur, generally from chordal fusion, often to each other, or abnormal papillary muscle positioning. The papillary muscles may be so close that a single papillary muscle is evident (parachute mitral valve). Rarely, a mitral web on the atrial side of the mitral leaflet can obstruct flow. In the elderly, mitral valve annular calcification may result in leaflet stiffening and MS, in which calcium invades from the annulus toward the center of the valve; mitral regurgitation (MR) is frequently associated. Other causes of MS are rare: carcinoid (usually associated with a patent foramen ovale or an atrial septal defect), systemic lupus erythematosus, rheumatoid arthritis, Fabry's disease, and amyloidosis. Rheumatic involvement predominates as a cause for MS, however, and other valves are often involved as well.

The interval between an episode of acute rheumatic fever and symptomatic MS averages about 16 years. Most patients do not recall the acute event when they ultimately present with MS. Fusion of the commissures between the anterior and posterior leaflets is the most characteristic feature of rheumatic MS. Fusion, thickening, and retraction of the chordae; thickening of the valvular leaflets; and calcium deposition contribute to the obstructive process. The severity of these features has led to an echocardiographic qualitative scoring system in which numbers are assigned to each characteristic. The mobility of the anterior mitral valve leaflet, the presence of valvular thickening or submitral scarring, and evidence of calcification are weighted into a score to help define the suitability of the valve for percutaneous valvuloplasty (discussed under Indications). Figure 33-5 represents the spectrum of involvement from chest wall two-dimensional echocardiography.

The location of the commissural fusion may help predict success of balloon dilation. Because the procedure works by tearing the commissural fibrosis that causes leaflet fusion, the presence of minimal commissural fusion suggests that the procedure will be ineffective. If there is eccentric commissural fusion on only one side of the leaflet, the inflated balloon(s) might be forced to the nonfused side of the leaflet, increasing the risk of valvular or ventricular trauma. If the fusion is only on the septal side of the mitral valve, for instance, the risk that the inflated balloons will tear into the mitral annulus increases.

The area of the mitral valve measured by planimetry usually correlates well with the Doppler-derived valve area. When the planimetric area seems much larger than the Doppler-derived area, this dichotomy may signal the presence of a significant submitral gradient. Such a valve may not respond to balloon valvuloplasty.

Indications

Mitral valve stenosis results in obstruction to LV inflow and an elevated left atrial (LA) pressure. Any activity that increases flow (e.g., exercise) or shortens diastolic time (e.g., the onset of a rapid tachycardia, such as atrial flutter or fibrillation) increases the mitral gradient. When the pressure gradient across the mitral valve is increased, symptoms of dyspnea and pulmonary congestion emerge. The decision to intervene in MS is based primarily on exertional symptoms.

Pulmonary hypertension that is greater than would be expected from the magnitude of the left atrial pressure alone may be present. Pulmonary hypertension is also an indication for correcting the valvular stenosis; significant improvement can be expected after the procedure. Pulmonary vascular resistance only roughly correlates with the MVA. Pulmonary vascular resistance can be disproportionately elevated compared with the pulmonary capillary wedge pressure. Although the trigger for the excessive elevation in the pressure of the pulmonary artery is unknown, endothelin and adrenomedullin, both potent pulmonary vasoconstrictors, may be involved. Because pulmonary hypertension in this situation may regress following balloon valvuloplasty, pulmonary hypertension or right-sided heart failure even without congestive symptoms is an indication for intervention in MS.

Whether to proceed with valve replacement or valvuloplasty depends on the morphology of the stenosed mitral valve. Several echocardiographic scoring systems have been suggested, the most popular being the Massachusetts General Hospital system, in which each of four characteristics is graded 0 to 4, with 0 being normal (Table 33-1). The higher the score, the less likely it is that a satisfactory result will be by percutaneous balloon dilation. The scoring system has successfully predicted acute results in many studies; a score greater than 8 is more likely to be associated with a suboptimal result. When treated as a continuous

Figure 33-5

Mitral Balloon Valvuloplasty

Echocardiographic scoring of mitral valve stenosis severity

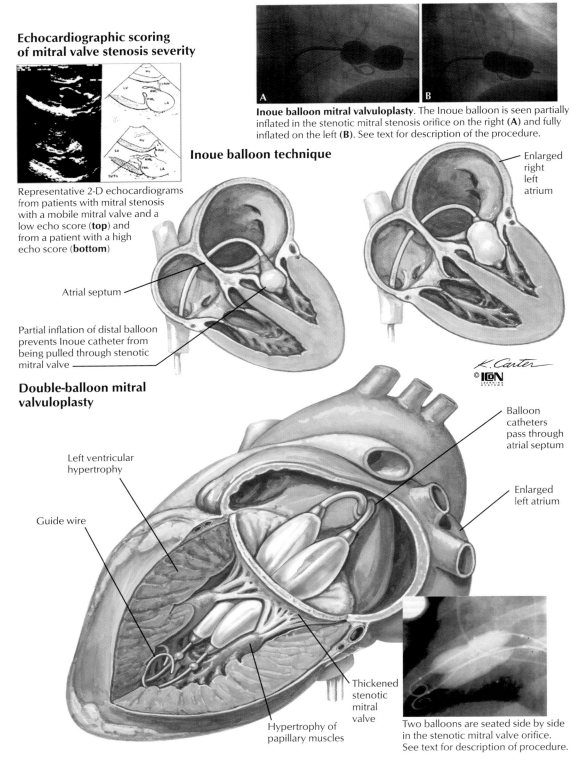

Representative 2-D echocardiograms from patients with mitral stenosis with a mobile mitral valve and a low echo score (**top**) and from a patient with a high echo score (**bottom**)

Inoue balloon mitral valvuloplasty. The Inoue balloon is seen partially inflated in the stenotic mitral stenosis orifice on the right (**A**) and fully inflated on the left (**B**). See text for description of the procedure.

Inoue balloon technique

Enlarged right left atrium

Atrial septum

Partial inflation of distal balloon prevents Inoue catheter from being pulled through stenotic mitral valve

Double-balloon mitral valvuloplasty

Left ventricular hypertrophy

Guide wire

Balloon catheters pass through atrial septum

Enlarged left atrium

Thickened stenotic mitral valve

Hypertrophy of papillary muscles

Two balloons are seated side by side in the stenotic mitral valve orifice. See text for description of procedure.

Table 33-1
Anatomic Classification of the Stenotic Mitral Valve: The Massachusetts General Hospital Scoring System

Measurement	Valve Score
A. Leaflet mobility	1. Highly mobile valve with only leaflet tip restriction 2. Midportion and base of leaflets with reduced mobility 3. Valve leaflets move forward in diastole mainly at the base 4. No or minimal forward movement of the leaflets in diastole
B. Valvular thickening	1. Leaflets minimally thickened (4–5 mm) 2. Midleaflet thickening, pronounced thickening of the margins 3. Thickening extends through the entire leaflets (5–6 mm) 4. Pronounced thickening of all leaflet tissue (>8 mm)
C. Subvalvular thickening	1. Minimal thickening of chordal structures just below the valve 2. Thickening of the chordae extending up to one third of the chordal length 3. Thickening extending to the distal third of the chordae 4. Extensive thickening and shortening of all chordae extending down to the papillary muscles
D. Valvular calcification	1. A single area of increased echo brightness 2. Scattered areas of brightness confined to the leaflet margins 3. Brightness extending to the midportion of the leaflets 4. Extensive brightness through most of the leaflet tissue
Assessment	A "0" score implies normal valve morphology. A total valve score of ≤8 implies a mobile valve amenable to percutaneous valvuloplasty. Progressively higher total valve scores result in less favorable outcomes, both acutely and long term.

With permission from Wilkins GT, Weyman AE, Abascal VM, Block PC, Palacios IF. Percutaneous balloon dilatation of the mitral valve: An analysis of echocardiographic variables related to outcome and the mechanism of dilatation. *Br Heart J* 1988;60:299–308.

variable, however, the relationship between the morphology score and either the increase in MVA or the final MVA after the procedure is relatively poor. The scoring system weighs each factor equally, even though certain factors may weigh more heavily toward a negative result than others. For instance, commissural calcium may be a stronger predictor of outcome than the total score.

Before the procedure, patients should undergo transesophageal echocardiography to ensure that no atrial thrombus is present and to provide an additional assessment of the valvular morphology. If an atrial thrombus is present, patients are placed on warfarin for 4 to 6 weeks and the transesophageal echocardiography is repeated. The procedure can be done when an atrial thrombus is deep inside the appendage, but resolution of any atrial clot before proceeding is advisable.

Patient age or a history of surgical commissurotomy does not significantly influence the acute results of the procedure, provided the valvular morphology is favorable. In general, a symptomatic patient with a reasonably low morphology score and less than 2+ MR is a candidate for percutaneous mitral valvuloplasty. Essentially all patients with symptoms related to MS have a calculated MVA of less than 1.5 cm^2.

Technique

Early experience and suboptimal results with single-balloon techniques initially prompted the development of double-balloon techniques. Since then, a unique single-balloon technique using the Inoue balloon has become popular.

Most laboratories use an antegrade method that requires transseptal catheterization. Right-sided heart catheterization and ventriculography initially determine the degree of MR, cardiac output, pulmonary pressure, the valve gradient, and the MVA. Some interventionalists use a right atrial angiogram with LA levophase filling to guide transseptal needle placement.

Transseptal catheterization uses a hollow Brockenbrough needle within an 8F Mullins sheath. Continuous pressure monitoring alerts the operator if the needle punctures the aorta or enters the pericardium. Once the sheath has been advanced into the left atrium, the needle is removed, the mitral gradient remeasured, and the MVA obtained.

Double-balloon techniques are complex. Some operators favor using double balloons that are positioned side by side using two guidewires. Other systems are available that use two balloons on a single catheter (the bifoil system) or two balloons on a single guidewire (the Multi-Track System). In any approach, the dilating balloons are then positioned side by side across the mitral valve and simultaneously inflated one to four times with dilute contrast (Fig. 33-5). When the procedure is completed, the mitral gradient is remeasured and the left ventriculogram repeated to assess any residual MR.

The Inoue balloon method simplifies the procedure. The 12F balloon catheter is designed so the distal end of the balloon inflates before the proximal end, allowing balloon positioning across the mitral valve, inflation of the distal end, and pulling of the remaining balloon into the mitral orifice before inflation of the entire balloon. With double balloons, the maximum diameter is predetermined and dependent on the inflated maximum balloon diameter(s). With the Inoue system, the diameter depends on the amount of contrast used to inflate the balloon. This feature allows for graded increases in the diameter of the balloon during the procedure without replacing the entire balloon catheter. The balloon size can be determined from echocardiographic measurements of the mitral annulus or by the patient's height. The most commonly used sizes are maximum diameters of 26 mm and 28 mm.

Once in the left ventricle, the balloon is sequentially inflated in the mitral valve orifice in increments of 1 to 2 mm. The LA pressure and the mitral gradient are reevaluated following each balloon inflation. Echocardiography of the chest wall between each inflation allows observation of any change in the mitral valve and any Doppler evidence of MR. If MR is present or if the valvular gradient has been satisfactorily reduced, the procedure is completed. Repeat cardiac output measures, a shunt run to evaluate evidence of any atrial septal defect created by the transseptal puncture, and repeat right-sided heart pressures are then performed before the postprocedural ventriculogram. A final valve area greater than 1.5 cm^2 with no more than 2+ MR is the goal.

Acute Results and Complications

Immediate improvement in the hemodynamic and clinical outcomes was found in all 19 studies that addressed the immediate results of mitral valvuloplasty. A 50 to 70% decrease in the transmitral gradient with an accompanying 50 to 100% increase in the MVA is a reasonable expectation based on these studies. A representative example would be a preprocedural MVA of 0.9 cm^2 improving to a postprocedural MVA of 1.9 cm^2. Similarly, a representative preprocedural mitral gradient would be about 14 mm Hg before and 6 mm Hg following valvuloplasty. Cardiac output tends to remain unchanged. The postprocedural valve areas are similar with the double-balloon method and the Inoue system. About 8 to 10% of valve areas will not improve to a final valve area of greater than 1.0 cm^2.

Pulmonary pressures fall immediately, consistent with the change in LA pressure. In patients with severe pulmonary hypertension, the pulmonary pressures drop further by 24 hours and continue to decline during the ensuing months.

The issues involved in the relationship between the valve area and valve flow discussed in the assessment of the results of aortic valvuloplasty also pertain mitral valvuloplasty. A successful procedure is generally defined as a 50% improvement in the MVA or a final MVA of more than 1.5 cm^2 plus no more than 2+ MR. An acute success rate of about 90% can be expected, depending on the valvular morphology. The major factors identified as predictive of success are a low valvular score by whatever method and the absence of significant baseline MR.

Complications from percutaneous mitral valvuloplasty have declined as the learning curve of the procedure has improved, and the procedure has largely been restricted to the relatively few centers that perform the procedure frequently. Table 33-2 summarizes figures for acute complications from several reviews. With the routine use of transesophageal echocardiography before the procedure, the risk of embolic events has virtually disappeared. Major complications are related to the transseptal technique and the development of significant MR from injury to the mitral valve apparatus. The use of serial echocardiography following each balloon dilation has increased awareness of any developing MR, allowing the procedure to be aborted before serious MR develops. Careful attention to the change in the LA *v* wave during the procedure is also important, with an increase predictive of acutely worsening MR.

Long-Term Results

Survival and Event-Free Survival Data

Ten-year survival rates have been reported at 85 to 97%, with event-free survival rates of 61 to 72%. Event-free survival appears to be dependent on optimal valve morphology, the presence of sinus rhythm, lower MVA pressures, and no more than 2+ MR following the procedure. A review of the Massachusetts General Hospital experience showed that although incidence of adverse events (death, mitral valve surgery, and redo-valvuloplasty) were low within the first 5 years of follow-up, a progressive increase in adverse events occurred beyond this period, probably related more to the disease process more than to complications of the procedure. Survival (82% vs. 57%) and event-free survival (38% vs. 22%) rates at 12-year follow-up were better in patients with an echocardiography score of 8 or below than in those with scores above 8. Cox regression analysis identified independent predictors of combined events at long-term follow-up: postvalvuloplasty MR of 3+ or more, an echocardiography score above 8, older age, prior surgical commissurotomy, NYHA functional class 4, prevalvuloplasty MR of 2+ or more, and higher postvalvuloplasty pulmonary artery pressure. Atrial fibrillation has a negative effect on event-free survival, and some reports have

Table 33-2
Contemporary Complications Associated With Percutaneous Mitral Valvuloplasty

Complication	Estimates (%)
Emergency cardiac surgery	1–4
Cardiac perforation/tamponade	0.5–4
Significant mitral regurgitation	2–3
Cerebrovascular accident/ embolic events	0.5–1.5
Death	0–1

also noted the negative effect of valvular calcium and baseline MR. As expected, patients with suboptimal initial results do less well clinically.

Symptomatic Improvement and Restenosis

Essentially all studies emphasize the impressive improvement in patients' symptoms after percutaneous balloon mitral valvuloplasty. Symptoms are more likely to occur in patients with suboptimal results and in those with poorer valve morphology. Postprocedural restenosis is difficult to define because of issues related to the definition of an initial hemodynamic success. Initial studies defined restenosis as at least 50% loss of the initial MVA gain, whereas other studies have advocated including an MVA of less than 1.5 cm^2 in the definition.

Serial hemodynamic studies suggest that clinical restenosis may not correlate well with anatomic restenosis. One report of serial echocardiographic restenosis data in 310 patients with high baseline echocardiography scores assessed restenosis, defined as an MVA of less than 1.5 cm^2 and/or at least 50% loss of the initial MVA increase. Acute procedural success (a final valve area >1.5 cm^2) occurred in 66% of patients. The cumulative restenosis rate was about 40% at 6 years after successful valvuloplasty. The only independent predictor of restenosis was the echocardiographic score (the probability of restenosis at 5 years was 20% for scores <8 vs. 61% for scores ≥8). The decline in MVA and the occurrence of restenosis were gradual and progressive during follow-up. Echocardiographic restenosis was related to adverse events or to

NYHA functional class 3 or 4 symptoms, but it was not an independent predictor of clinical outcome by multivariate analysis.

Clinical restenosis data are more impressive. Mitral valve anatomy always appears to predict the symptomatic outcome. Clinically, the restenosis rate has been reported at 20 to 39% at 7 years after valvuloplasty. A 10-year clinical restenosis rate of 23% was found for those with an echocardiography score of 8 or lower, 55% for those with an echocardiography score of 9 to 11, and 50% for those with a score of 12 or higher.

Comparative Data With Surgical Commissurotomy

Studies comparing surgery and balloon valvuloplasty have shown similar initial results. In 60 patients with favorable anatomy randomized to valvuloplasty (using the double-balloon technique) or open surgical commissurotomy, excellent early results were reported with both techniques. However, at 3 years, the MVAs of the balloon valvuloplasty patients were actually better than those of the surgical group (2.4 cm^2 vs. 1.8 cm^2) and 72% of the valvuloplasty patients were in NYHA functional class 1 compared with 57% of the surgical group.

In another study, 90 patients were randomized to valvuloplasty, open commissurotomy or closed commissurotomy and were followed for 7 years. Little difference existed between the valvuloplasty patients and the open commissurotomy patients at the conclusion of the study. The valvuloplasty and open surgical procedure groups had less clinical restenosis than the closed commissurotomy group (0% for the valvuloplasty and open commissurotomy groups, 27% for the closed surgical group). At 7 years, 87% of the valvuloplasty patients and 90% of the open commissurotomy patients were in NYHA functional class 1 compared with 33% of the closed surgical commissurotomy patients.

It appears that balloon valvuloplasty is equivalent or superior to surgical commissurotomy for symptomatic MS, at least through the first 7 years after the procedure, as long as the preprocedural valve score falls within an acceptable range. Hence, the percutaneous approach is advocated in those with appropriate valve morphology.

TRICUSPID VALVE STENOSIS
Pathophysiology

Tricuspid valve anatomy is more variable than mitral anatomy. The three leaflets of the tricuspid valve are of unequal size; the septal leaflet is the smallest, the anterior leaflet the largest. Although some chordae attach to distinct papillary muscles in the right ventricle, they also attach directly to the right ventricular endocardium. Therefore, tricuspid regurgitation is a frequent occurrence when the right ventricle dilates from any cause. The orifice of the tricuspid valve is considerably larger than the mitral orifice, the normal tricuspid valve area being about 10 cm^2. Considerable valve stenosis must be present to obstruct the RV inflow. Although a mean gradient of 2 mm Hg establishes the diagnosis, most consider a mean gradient of at least 5 mm Hg or a calculated valve area of less than 2.0 cm^2 to indicate significant tricuspid valve stenosis (TS).

Tricuspid valve stenosis is decidedly uncommon and never an isolated lesion. Rheumatic disease accounts for 90% of cases of TS. Of patients with rheumatic mitral valve disease, about 3 to 5% have associated TS. Commissural fusion is present, but the fibrosis and/or the fusion of the chordae is seen less often than is observed in rheumatic MS. Leaflet calcium is also uncommon.

In the United States, the second most common cause of TS is carcinoid syndrome, in which tricuspid regurgitation is also usually present. Carcinoid plaque thickens the leaflets and the chordae, and commissural fusion is unusual. Congenital forms of TS exist and are generally due to abnormalities in the leaflets (absent or decreased number), the chordae (absent, reduced number, or shortened) and the papillary muscles (reduced number). Percutaneous balloon techniques have been attempted in congenital TS, but the role of these techniques is limited in the treatment of this condition.

Open surgical commissurotomy on the tricuspid valve is also rarely performed because of the high risk of tricuspid regurgitation. It is inadvisable to open the commissure between the anterior and posterior leaflets, although surgical commissurotomy may succeed if fusion is relieved between the anterior and septal or the posterior and septal leaflets. On the basis of surgical experience, the use of balloon valvuloplasty seems anatomically limited.

Indications

Patients with TS usually present with low cardiac output, fatigue, anasarca, and abdominal swelling from hepatomegaly and ascites. Giant *a* waves may be visible in the neck and even felt by the patient. Symptomatic TS is an acceptable reason to consider intervention. The limiting factor is usually associated tricuspid regurgitation. The procedure could be considered in the unlikely circumstance that a patient was not a surgical candidate and had limited tricuspid regurgitation or would clinically benefit from conversion from TS to tricuspid regurgitation.

Procedure and Results

There are few data on the use of percutaneous balloon tricuspid valvuloplasty. The technical aspects are similar to percutaneous mitral valvuloplasty except that no transseptal procedure is required. In the NHLBI Balloon Valvuloplasty Registry, only three patients underwent the procedure on a native valve.

Most tricuspid valvuloplasty procedures have been performed in patients who had both mitral and tricuspid valvuloplasty at the same setting. Results of these procedures have been mixed in the treatment of TS from carcinoid syndrome. No long-term reports exist about the efficacy of tricuspid valvuloplasty in any setting.

BIOPROSTHETIC VALVE STENOSIS

Pathophysiology

Porcine or bovine pericardial prosthetic valves may be implanted in any valvular position. All of these valves have a limited lifespan because of eventual mineralization and collagen degeneration. Cuspal tears, fibrin deposition, disruption of the fibrocollagenous structure, perforation, fibrosis, and calcium infiltration appear after a few years; by 10 years, tissue valve failure occurs in about 30% of patients. By 15 years, more than 50% of the valves have failed. The degenerative structural changes occur earlier in valves in the mitral compared with the aortic position, because of greater hemodynamic stress on the mitral valve. Patients on dialysis appear to be particular-

ly susceptible to early valve failure. Other identified factors associated with valve failure include younger age, pregnancy, and hypercalcemia.

Commissural fusion is uncommon in these valves, the major problem being leaflet immobility. At times, these valves become relatively stenotic from undersizing (patient-prosthetic mismatch). From an anatomic standpoint, the use of percutaneous balloon valvuloplasty procedures appears problematic given the lack of commissural fusion.

Prosthetic Valvuloplasty

Limited data exist about the use of balloon procedures in prosthetic valve stenosis. Success in two patients with porcine TS has been described, although limited follow-up data were available and "restenosis" quickly occurred in one patient. The NHLBI Balloon Valvuloplasty Registry reported four successful procedures with no follow-up. In every instance of our investigations of explanted porcine valves, considerable trauma occurred to the explanted valve and balloon techniques did not appear to be a viable option. No prospective studies have addressed the safety and efficacy of this procedure, and on the basis of the evidence available, it is not recommended.

REFERENCES

al Zaibag M, Ribeiro P, Al Kasab S. Percutaneous balloon valvotomy in tricuspid stenosis. *Br Heart J* 1987;57:51–53.

Ben Farhat M, Ayari M, Maatouk F, et al. Percutaneous balloon versus surgical closed and open mitral commissurotomy: Seven-year follow-up results of a randomized trial. *Circulation* 1998;97:245–250.

Dotter CT, Judkins MP. Transluminal treatment of atherosclerotic obstruction: Description of a new technique and a preliminary report of its application. *Circulation* 1964;30:654–670.

Harrison JK, Wilson JS, Hearne SE, Bashore TM. Complications related to percutaneous transvenous mitral commissurotomy. *Cathet Cardiovasc Diagn* 1994; (suppl 2):52–60.

Multicenter experience with balloon mitral commissurotomy. NHLBI Balloon Valvuloplasty Registry Report on immediate and 30-day follow-up results. The National Heart, Lung, and Blood Institute Balloon Valvuloplasty Registry Participants. *Circulation* 1992;85:448–461.

Percutaneous balloon aortic valvuloplasty: Acute and 30-day follow-up results in 674 patients from the NHLBI Balloon Valvuloplasty Registry. *Circulation* 1991;84:2383–2397.

Rao PS, Fawzy ME, Solymar L, Mardini MK. Long-term results of balloon pulmonary valvuloplasty of valvular pulmonic stenosis. *Am Heart J* 1988;115:1291–1296.

Reyes VP, Raju BS, Wynne J, et al. Percutaneous balloon valvuloplasty compared with open surgical commissurotomy for mitral stenosis. *N Engl J Med* 1994;331:961–967.

Chapter 34

Surgical Treatment for Valvular Heart Disease

Peter J. K. Starek

Competency of the atrioventricular valves allows blood to enter the ventricles, where pressure is generated. When adequate systolic blood pressure (SBP) is generated, the aortic and pulmonary valves open, allowing the blood to enter the arterial system. The atrioventricular valves close, preventing the flow of blood into the atria. During diastole, the aortic and pulmonary valves close, the atrioventricular valves open, the ventricles fill and ultimately begin the cycle of pulsatile blood flow through the systemic and pulmonary vascular tree.

Malfunction of any of the cardiac valves results in a less efficient circulatory system. Valvular dysfunction causes work overload in one or both ventricles. In extreme cases, resultant congestive heart failure can cause death. More information about etiology, pathogenesis, differential diagnoses, and diagnostic approaches used for evaluation of valvular diseases can be found in chapters 27–33.

BACKGROUND

Before the discovery of penicillin, rheumatic heart disease was widespread. Physicians recognized that mitral valve stenosis frequently followed rheumatic fever. This obstruction to blood flow through the mitral valve was not medically treatable however. For "stenosed" mitral valves, physicians described the need to relieve the obstruction surgically. The first successful attempt at surgical treatment involved incising the left atrial appendage, placing a finger through the incision into the left atrium, feeling the stenotic mitral valve, and relieving the obstruction by simple finger pressure. Soon after these initial therapeutic approaches, special knives and dilators were developed to relieve mitral valve stenosis. In the early days of cardiovascular surgery, these procedures were all performed on the beating heart.

The notion of using anticoagulant heparin to allow blood to circulate outside a patient's vasculature without clotting led to the development of cardiac and pulmonary bypass machines in the 1950s. It was then possible to keep the patient alive while stopping the heart for surgical repair. The ability to stop the heart, examine valve pathology, and try to repair it stimulated surgeons' collaboration with mechanical engineers in developing prosthetic valves to replace those that were too diseased to repair. Initial attempts to duplicate valve leaflets with flexible, nonbiologic materials failed. The leaflets of these valves were too stiff in comparison with normal valve leaflets.

FIRST-GENERATION PROSTHETIC VALVES

Attempts at using nonflexible leaflets by constructing hinged valve leaflets resulted in hinge thrombosis and malfunction. Design engineers then focused on free-floating occluders, such as discs or balls retained in a cage-like housing. This general valve design produced the first clinically useful valves, including the Hufnagel, Starr-Edwards, Smeloff-Cutter, and Beall valves (Fig. 34-1). In 1958, the Starr-Edwards valve was used in the first clinically successful valve replacement.

Although these early designs functioned as intended, the first caged-ball valves had major shortcomings: (1) they were bulky in design and did not fit well into a small ventricle or aorta; (2) they had a small internal orifice, making them relatively stenotic; and (3) they stimulated thrombus formation, which precipitated thromboembolic events, necessitating long-term anticoagulation therapy.

Figure 34-1   ## First Generation of Synthetic Prosthetic Valves

The first generation of clinically useful synthetic valves had a free-floating ball or disc occluder retained in a cage-like house.

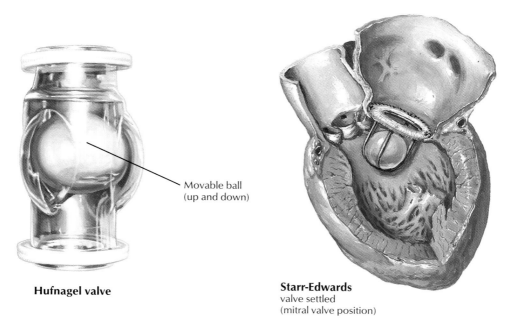

Hufnagel valve

Movable ball
(up and down)

Starr-Edwards
valve settled
(mitral valve position)

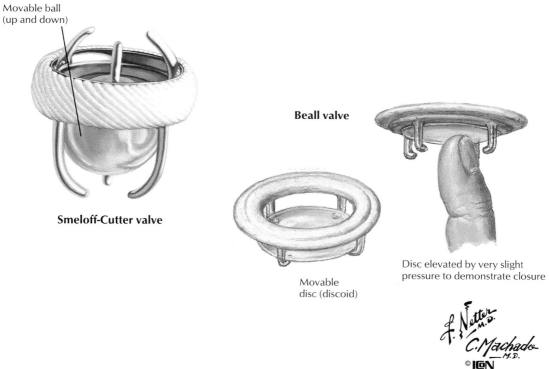

Movable ball
(up and down)

Smeloff-Cutter valve

Beall valve

Movable
disc (discoid)

Disc elevated by very slight
pressure to demonstrate closure

SECOND-GENERATION PROSTHETIC VALVES

The disadvantages of early prosthetic valves led to the development of two divergent lines of valve design using synthetic materials or biologic tissue. The caged-ball valves were modified, and pivoting hingeless disc valves, such as the Lillehei-Kaster, Medtronic-Hall, and Björk-Shiley valves, were developed. The St. Jude and Carbomedic valves were the first successful hinged leaflet valves (Fig. 34-2).

Homograft valves harvested at autopsy and preserved in antibiotic solution or frozen were the first nonsynthetic valves to be implanted successfully. Their limited availability prompted the use of porcine valves procured from slaughterhouses. Porcine valves were preserved with glutaraldehyde and mounted on a modified nylon–covered plastic or metal stents. Valves made of pericardium were also developed and used successfully (Fig. 34-3, lower). Many of these valve designs are still in use today.

ETIOLOGY AND PATHOGENESIS

Cardiac valve pathology comprises two broad categories, congenital valve deformity and acquired valvular dysfunction. Congenital deformity can occur in one or more cardiac valves (see section VIII). Patients with severe congenital valvular dysfunction can die if prompt surgical intervention is not undertaken. In patients with normally developed hearts, infection can cause valvular dysfunction at any age. Rheumatic heart disease secondary to untreated streptococcal infection and bacterial endocarditis can destroy a normal heart valve. Generalized inflammatory illnesses, such as lupus erythematosus, rheumatoid arthritis, and eosinophilic endocarditis, as well as carcinoid disease, similarly can cause valvular dysfunction. Connective tissue diseases, such as Ehlers-Danlos syndrome and myxomatous degeneration, can cause valve deformity and dysfunction. Severe myocardial ischemia and injury can cause papillary muscle dysfunction, which can result in mitral valve insufficiency. Finally, just as aging often results in atherosclerotic changes and calcium deposition in arterial walls, so can it affect the aortic valves, sometimes with severe calcification of the leaflets.

The mitral valve annulus can also be severely calcified, with or without valvular dysfunction.

CLINICAL PRESENTATION

The presenting symptoms in patients with dysfunctional valves vary considerably, depending on the type and severity of dysfunction and the location of the affected valves. Diseased valves can become incompetent, stenotic, or both. Young patients with moderate aortic valve stenosis are often asymptomatic. Likewise, many patients with moderate mitral valve stenosis or insufficiency may be asymptomatic. In general, patients whose valve dysfunction progresses eventually experience dyspnea on exertion. Syncope or angina pectoris, alone or in association with dyspnea, can develop in patients with aortic stenosis.

DIFFERENTIAL DIAGNOSIS

In patients presenting with dyspnea and fatigue, noncardiac causes, such as anemia, hypertension, pulmonary pathology, and hypothyroidism, should be excluded. Primary cardiac myopathy (see chapters 12–16) should be considered. Coronary artery disease must be ruled out if angina pectoris is a symptom.

DIAGNOSTIC APPROACH

Physical findings such as cardiac murmurs, wide pulse pressure, cardiomegaly, hepatomegaly, ascites, or pedal edema help to confirm abnormal circulatory conditions. Chest radiography and ECG offer supportive evidence of cardiac pathology. The most descriptive and definitive tests pinpointing cardiac valve anomalies are echocardiography in association with hemodynamic data from cardiac catheterization.

MANAGEMENT AND THERAPY
Surgical Therapy

A variety of procedures are available to treat cardiac valvular disease. Replacing diseased valves with prosthetic valves has become a routine procedure and valve repair—particularly mitral and tricuspid valve repair—has evolved dramatically. Techniques routinely used in the repair of mitral and tricuspid insufficiencies include ring annuloplasty, resection of prolapsing portions of leaflets not supported by chor-

Figure 34-2

Second Generation of Synthetic Prosthetic Valves and Biologic Valves

Second-generation synthetic prosthetic valves were hingeless pivoting disk valves and hinged bileaflet valves.

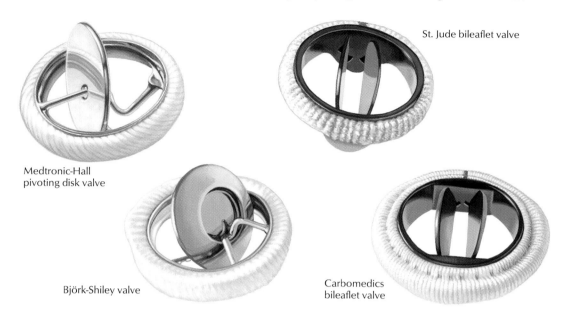

St. Jude bileaflet valve

Medtronic-Hall
pivoting disk valve

Björk-Shiley valve

Carbomedics
bileaflet valve

Tissue valves made of porcine aortic valves, pericardium, or cadaver homografts are also important in valve replacement surgical therapy.

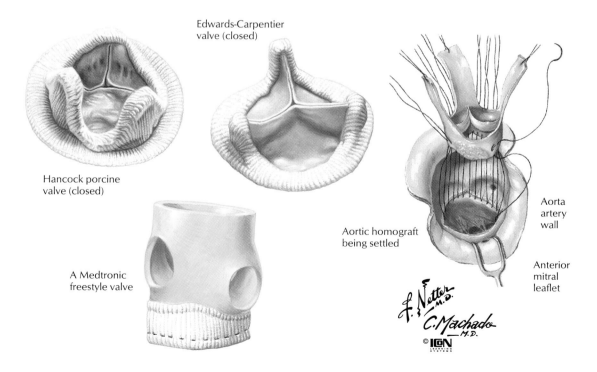

Edwards-Carpentier
valve (closed)

Hancock porcine
valve (closed)

Aorta
artery
wall

Aortic homograft
being settled

Anterior
mitral
leaflet

A Medtronic
freestyle valve

Figure 34-3

Chordal Transfer, Sliding Annuloplasty, and Ring Annuloplasty

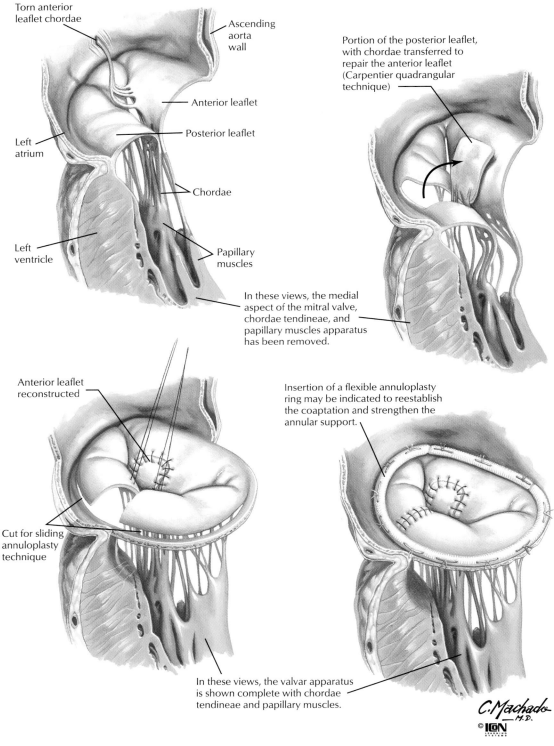

Torn anterior leaflet chordae

Ascending aorta wall

Anterior leaflet

Posterior leaflet

Left atrium

Chordae

Left ventricle

Papillary muscles

Portion of the posterior leaflet, with chordae transferred to repair the anterior leaflet (Carpentier quadrangular technique)

In these views, the medial aspect of the mitral valve, chordae tendineae, and papillary muscles apparatus has been removed.

Anterior leaflet reconstructed

Cut for sliding annuloplasty technique

Insertion of a flexible annuloplasty ring may be indicated to reestablish the coaptation and strengthen the annular support.

In these views, the valvar apparatus is shown complete with chordae tendineae and papillary muscles.

C. Machado
—M.D.
© ICON
LEARNING SYSTEMS

dae, shortening or using artificial chordae, and increasing or decreasing the leaflet area by sliding annuloplasty (Fig. 34-4). In patients who need aortic valve replacement, some surgeons advocate the Ross procedure, which entails transplanting a patient's pulmonary valve into the aortic position. This provides the patient with a living, durable, nonthrombogenic, and hemodynamically superior valve. The pulmonary valve is then reconstructed using a tissue homograft valve. The choice of procedure depends on many factors, including the patient's valve pathology, age, and ability to tolerate and comply with long-term anticoagulation.

Mitral and Tricuspid Valves

Patients with mitral and tricuspid valve pathology should be considered for valve repair rather than replacement because the operative mortality associated with repair of these valves is lower than that associated with their replacement. After surgery for either valve repair or replacement, patients need to receive anticoagulants for 3 to 6 months until the surgical site is endothelialized. Patients with repaired valves or valves replaced with biologic tissue can then discontinue anticoagulation if they remain in sinus rhythm. The long-term incidence of thromboembolic events is generally lower in patients with repaired valves in comparison with patients with replaced valves. This is one of the reasons that valve repair is preferable to valve replacement, when the repair is technically feasible.

Conditions precluding satisfactory repair of the mitral and tricuspid valves include severe scarring and deformation by a disease process such as advanced rheumatic heart disease, advanced lupus, or another inflammatory process involving the valve leaflets and destruction of valve leaflets and annuli by endocarditis. Under these circumstances, the valve should be replaced. Mitral valve replacement should include preservation of a portion of the subvalvular chordae and papillary muscles to aid in preserving normal ventricular contractility.

Aortic Valves

Adult patients with aortic valve pathology are seldom candidates for valve repair; valve replacement is usually necessary for significant aortic stenosis or regurgitation. The patient's age, the patient's lifestyle, and the preferences of the surgeon and the patient dictate the type of prosthetic valve replacement.

Patients with prosthetic valves made of biologic tissue have a lower incidence of bleeding because long-term anticoagulation is not required in patients in sinus rhythm. Unfortunately, all tissue valves eventually deteriorate and become insufficient. Deterioration of tissue valves occurs at an accelerated rate in younger patients and in patients with end-stage renal disease on hemodialysis. For older patients, particularly those with a risk of falling, a tissue valve may be the most appropriate choice. Younger patients, with a natural life expectancy exceeding 15 to 20 years, should have prosthetic valves made of durable synthetic materials, such as pyrolytic carbon, titanium, stainless steel, or a combination of these.

Postoperatively, all patients with prosthetic heart valves must be anticoagulated until endothelialization of the sewing ring is complete, as discussed previously herein. Use of non-tissue valves necessitates indefinite anticoagulation.

Issues With Prosthetic Valve Replacement

Nontissue valves must have an appropriate sewing ring sutured to the annulus of the patient's valve after the leaflets are excised. Sewing rings are usually circular and rigid and vary in thickness. The rigid sewing rings change the natural shape of the valve annulus and, depending on thickness, decrease the size of the internal orifice of the prosthetic valve. Implanting a valve with a circular sewing ring into a noncircular annulus can generate unnatural tension between the valve annulus and sewing ring, which can lead to paravalvular leaks; the surgical approach in these instances must take this possibility into account.

The use of rigid circular sewing rings is unnecessary in biologic tissue valves implanted in the aortic position. Freehand suturing is used to insert autograft pulmonary valves into the aortic position (the Ross procedure). It is also used in homograft cadaver valve implantation and with nonstented freestyle porcine valves.

Figure 34-4 Approaching the Mitral Valve Through the Interatrial Septum
(sometimes extending the incision onto the roof of the left atrium)

Exposing the mitral valve through the interatrial septum and an extension of the incision through the roof of the left atrium is common. This surgical exposure allows excellent visualization of the mitral and tricuspid valves and can be performed through a standard sternotomy, as well as through a variety of partial sternotomy and right thoracotomy incisions.

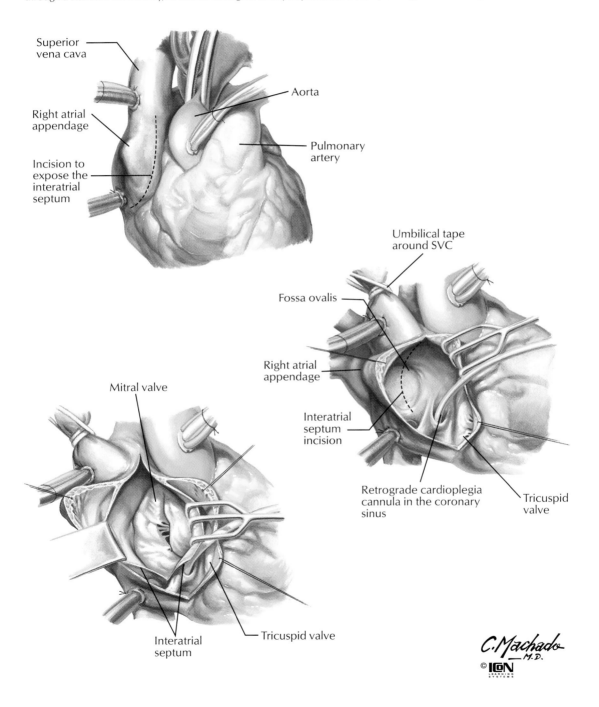

Superior vena cava

Aorta

Right atrial appendage

Pulmonary artery

Incision to expose the interatrial septum

Umbilical tape around SVC

Fossa ovalis

Right atrial appendage

Mitral valve

Interatrial septum incision

Retrograde cardioplegia cannula in the coronary sinus

Tricuspid valve

Interatrial septum

Tricuspid valve

C. Machado
—M.D.
©ICN
LEARNING
SYSTEMS

Minimally Invasive Techniques

Minimally invasive coronary artery revascularization surgery uses small incisions and therefore is performed on a beating heart, obviating the use of cardiopulmonary bypass (CPB). In valve repair and replacement procedures, the use of smaller incisions is possible, but eliminating CPB is not feasible with current techniques and prosthetic valves.

Good visualization of the operative field is a prerequisite for proper valve repair or replacement. Smaller incisions limit visualization, although the use of miniature video cameras improves the view of the operative field. The mitral valve is generally the most difficult to visualize, so many surgeons approach it through the intra-atrial septum, sometimes extending the incision to the roof of the left atrium (see Fig. 34-4).

FUTURE DIRECTIONS

Refinements in manufacturing synthetic prosthetic valves and their sewing rings will continue to decrease thromboembolic complications while improving their hemodynamic characteristics. Better chemical preservation of tissue valves will improve their longevity and resistance to deterioration and make tissue valves a more attractive choice for younger patients.

The teaching of valve repair techniques to surgical trainees is already becoming more standardized. The appropriate surgical repair technique will be more predictable from the preoperative, noninvasive echocardiographic examination and hemodynamic evaluation. Freehand valve implantation techniques will find increased use in selected patients, particularly for patients in whom the annulus is small and the valve sewing rings make the prosthetic valves too stenotic. Finally, with clinical acceptance of genetic engineering, farms of genetically altered pigs and baboons might provide viable biologic leaflets, valves, and entire hearts for implantation.

REFERENCES

Carpentier A. Cardiac valve surgery: The "French connection." *J Thorac Cardiovasc Surg* 1983;86:323–337.

Duran CG, Pomar JL, Revuelta JM, et al. Conservative operation for mitral insufficiency: Critical analysis supported by postoperative hemodynamic studies in 72 patients. *J Thorac Cardiovasc Surg* 1980;79:326–337.

Katholi RE, Nolan SP, McGuire LB. Living with prosthetic heart valves: Subsequent noncardiac operations and the risk of thromboembolism or hemorrhage. *Am Heart J* 1976;92:162–167.

Khan SS, Trento A, DeRobertis M, et al. Twenty-year comparison of tissue and mechanical valve replacement. *J Thorac Cardiovasc Surg* 2001;122:257–269.

Ross DN. Replacement of aortic and mitral valves with a pulmonary autograft. *Lancet* 1967;2:956–958.

Rozich JD, Carabello BA, Usher BW, et al. Mitral valve replacement with and without chordal preservation in patients with chronic mitral regurgitation: Mechanisms for differences in postoperative ejection performance. *Circulation* 1992; 86:1718–1726.

Shumacker HB Jr. *The Evolution of Cardiac Surgery.* Bloomington: Indiana University Press; 1992:39.

Section VI

PERICARDIAL DISEASES

Chapter 35

Pericardial Disease: Clinical Features and Treatment

Christopher D. Chiles and George A. Stouffer

The *pericardium* is a two-layered sac that encircles the heart (Fig. 35-1). The *visceral pericardium* is a mesothelial monolayer that adheres to the epicardium. It is reflected back on itself at the level of the great vessels, where it joins the parietal pericardium, the tough fibrous outer layer. Under normal conditions, a small amount of fluid (approximately 5–50 mL) separates the two layers and decreases friction between them.

The normal pericardium serves three primary functions: fixing the heart within the mediastinum, limiting cardiac distension during sudden increases in intracardiac volume, and limiting the spread of infection from the adjacent lungs. However, the importance of these functions has been questioned because of the benign prognosis associated with congenital absence of the pericardium. This chapter discusses the clinical features and treatment of four pathologic conditions involving the pericardium: acute pericarditis, chronic pericarditis, constrictive pericarditis, and pericardial effusions. The complex hemodynamic effects of pericardial pathology are discussed in chapter 36.

ACUTE PERICARDITIS

The most common presentation of a pericardial abnormality is *acute pericarditis*, inflammation of the pericardium (Fig. 35-2). In general, this is a self-limited disease that is responsive to oral anti-inflammatory medication; acute pericarditis infrequently necessitates hospital admission. It is more common in men than in women and more common in adults than in children. The two most common causes of acute pericarditis in the United States are viral and idiopathic. Other causes include uremia, pericardiectomy associated with cardiac surgery, pulmonary embolism, collagen–vascular diseases, Dressler's syndrome, malignancy, tuberculosis, fungus (e.g., histoplasmosis), parasites (e.g., amoeba), myxedema, radiation, acute rheumatic fever, and trauma (Fig. 35-3).

Clinical Presentation

The clinical presentation of pericarditis most often is dominated by chest pain, which is generally sharp, pleuritic, and positional in nature. Classically, the pain is increased by lying supine and improved by leaning forward. Symptoms may include dyspnea, palpitations, coughing, and subjective fever, and the patient may have a history of a viral prodrome. On physical examination, a pericardial friction rub is generally the most remarkable finding. The classic description is of a scratchy sound heard best along the lower left sternal border. It typically has three components (when the patient is in sinus rhythm), which correspond to atrial systole, ventricular systole, and rapid ventricular filling during early diastole. The component corresponding to rapid ventricular filling (atrial systole) may be absent, resulting in a two-component friction rub. In one series of 100 patients with acute pericarditis, a three-component friction rub was detected in approximately 50% of the patients, whereas any friction rub (one component, two components, or three components) was present in almost all cases.

Laboratory and Imaging Studies

There are four stages of ECG changes associated with the evolution of acute pericarditis (Figs. 35-2, ECG, and 35-4). Stage I changes accompany the onset of chest pain and include the classic ECG changes associated with acute pericarditis: diffuse concave ST elevation with PR depression (see chapter 3). Stage II occurs several days later and is represented by the return of ST segments to baseline and T-wave flattening. In stage III, T-wave inversion is seen in

Figure 35-1

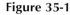

Pericardial Sac

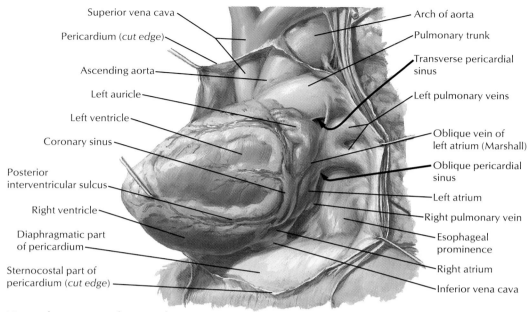

Superior vena cava

Pericardium (*cut edge*)

Ascending aorta

Left auricle

Left ventricle

Coronary sinus

Posterior
interventricular sulcus

Right ventricle

Diaphragmatic part
of pericardium

Sternocostal part of
pericardium (*cut edge*)

Arch of aorta

Pulmonary trunk

Transverse pericardial
sinus

Left pulmonary veins

Oblique vein of
left atrium (Marshall)

Oblique pericardial
sinus

Left atrium

Right pulmonary vein

Esophageal
prominence

Right atrium

Inferior vena cava

**Heart drawn out of opened
pericardial sac: Left lateral view**

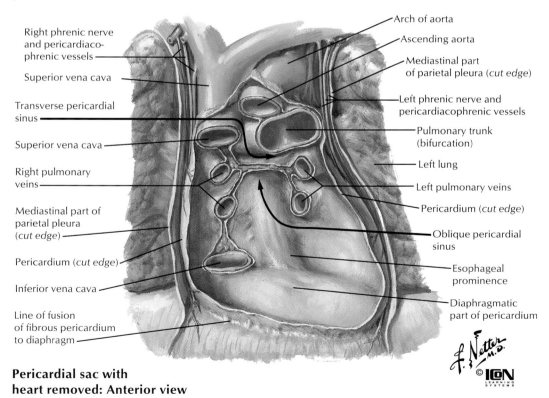

Right phrenic nerve
and pericardiaco-
phrenic vessels

Superior vena cava

Transverse pericardial
sinus

Superior vena cava

Right pulmonary
veins

Mediastinal part of
parietal pleura
(*cut edge*)

Pericardium (*cut edge*)

Inferior vena cava

Line of fusion
of fibrous pericardium
to diaphragm

Arch of aorta

Ascending aorta

Mediastinal part
of parietal pleura (*cut edge*)

Left phrenic nerve and
pericardiacophrenic vessels

Pulmonary trunk
(bifurcation)

Left lung

Left pulmonary veins

Pericardium (*cut edge*)

Oblique pericardial
sinus

Esophageal
prominence

Diaphragmatic
part of pericardium

**Pericardial sac with
heart removed: Anterior view**

Figure 35-2

Diseases of Pericardium

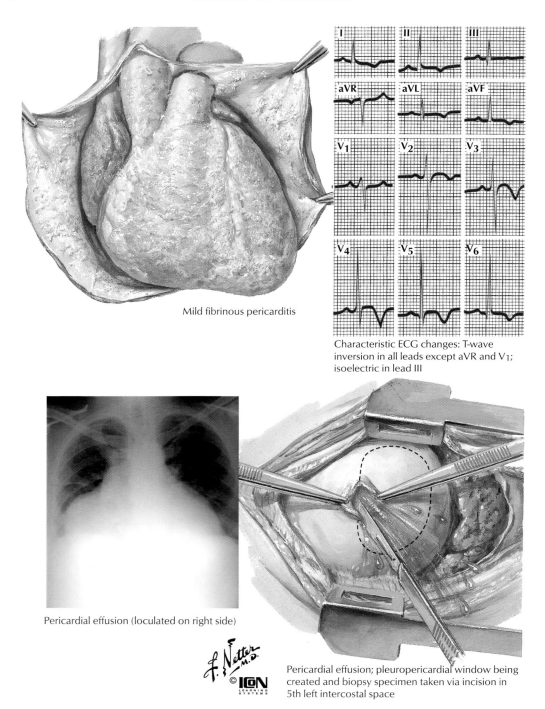

Mild fibrinous pericarditis

Characteristic ECG changes: T-wave inversion in all leads except aVR and V_1; isoelectric in lead III

Pericardial effusion (loculated on right side)

Pericardial effusion; pleuropericardial window being created and biopsy specimen taken via incision in 5th left intercostal space

Figure 35-3

Diseases of Pericardium

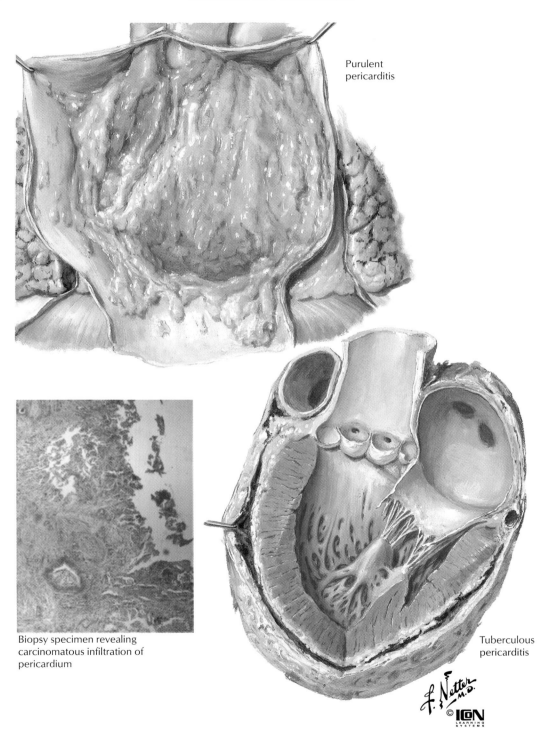

Purulent
pericarditis

Biopsy specimen revealing
carcinomatous infiltration of
pericardium

Tuberculous
pericarditis

most leads. The ECG in stage IV shows the return of T waves to an upright position. The approximate time frame for passage through all four stages of ECG changes in most cases of acute pericarditis is 2 weeks.

Electrocardiographic abnormalities are present in approximately 90% of patients with acute pericarditis, but only approximately 50% of patients show all four stages. Other ECG presentations include isolated PR depression, absence of one or more stages, and persistence of T-wave inversion. Atrial arrhythmias are seen in 5 to 10% of cases.

Laboratory studies are nondiagnostic in acute pericarditis. Nonspecific markers of inflammation may be present, including an elevated white blood cell count. If concurrent myocarditis is present, serum levels of cardiac biomarkers (creatine kinase and troponin) may be elevated.

Management and Therapy

Most cases of acute pericarditis are self-limited, although symptoms can persist for weeks. The goals of acute pericarditis management include pain relief, identification and treatment of the underlying cause, and observation to detect the development of tamponade. Nonsteroidal anti-inflammatory agents are generally first-line therapy for pain relief, but steroids may be used if pain does not improve within 48 hours. Tamponade has been reported in up to 15% of patients with acute pericarditis. Transient constrictive physiology within the first 30 days after an acute episode of pericarditis was found in 9% of the patients in one study but abated by 3 months. Constrictive pericarditis develops in a small group of patients with acute pericarditis but generally is not clinically evident for many years (discussed in more detail below).

CHRONIC OR RECURRENT PERICARDITIS

Recurrent or chronic symptoms develop in approximately one quarter of patients with acute pericarditis. Most of these patients are treated with reinstitution of nonsteroidal anti-inflammatory agents or steroids. Some investigators have advocated the use of colchicine or even pericardiectomy if symptoms are severe.

CONSTRICTIVE PERICARDITIS

Constrictive pericarditis is characterized by a dense, fibrous thickening of the pericardium that adheres to and encases the myocardium, resulting in impaired diastolic ventricular filling (Fig. 35-5). The general paradigm is that constrictive pericarditis occurs over a period of years as a result of an acute injury (e.g., a viral infection) that elicits a chronic fibrosing reaction or as a result of a chronic injury that stimulates a persistent reaction (e.g., renal failure). Clinically, constrictive pericarditis generally is a chronic disease with symptom progression over a period of years. The presentation is that of right-sided heart failure and may resemble restrictive cardiomyopathy, cirrhosis, cor pulmonale, or other conditions. Because pericardial constriction is uncommon, patients occasionally have an incorrect diagnosis (left- or right-sided heart failure, hepatic failure, or others) for years. Indeed, patients with pericardial constriction often have been admitted to the hospital for symptoms attributed to other causes before a definitive diagnosis of constriction is made. Newer diagnostic technologies and a change in the predominant etiologies of constriction have increased the recognition of subacute presentations occurring over a period of months.

Etiology

The causes of constriction that are most common in industrialized countries are cardiac surgery, mediastinal radiation, pericarditis, and idiopathic etiologies (Table 35-1). Other causes include infection (e.g., fungal or tuberculosis), malignancies such as breast cancer or lymphoma, connective tissue disease (e.g., systemic lupus erythematosus or rheumatoid arthritis), trauma, and drugs.

Clinical Presentation
History

The symptoms and signs of constrictive pericarditis result from reduced cardiac output (CO), elevated systemic venous pressure, and pulmonary venous congestion. The typical history is progressively worsening dyspnea, edema, or other volume overload symptoms. Patients generally have features of right-sided heart failure with ascites and edema, but other features may

Figure 35-4

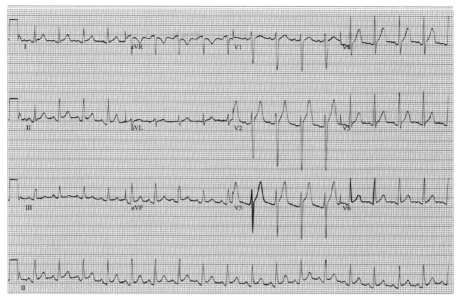

include anorexia, nausea, fatigue, orthopnea, and, sometimes, cardiac tamponade, atrial arrhythmia, and frank liver disease. Chest pain typical of angina may be related to underperfusion of the coronary arteries or compression of an epicardial coronary artery by the thickened pericardium.

Physical Examination

Physical examination generally reveals increased jugular venous pressure (JVP), prominent y descent in the jugular pulse, and an increase of JVP on inspiration (Kussmaul's sign), resulting from the thickened pericardium's impairment of venous return to the right side of the heart. The pulse pressure may be reduced, and a pulsus paradoxus may be present in up to one third of patients. Tachycardia may develop to compensate for the diminished stroke volume. The apical impulse is reduced and rarely displaced because the heart size is generally normal. The heart sounds may be distant, and the first heart sound is typically soft because the mitral and tricuspid valves are nearly closed at end diastole (because almost all ventricular filling occurs early in diastole). A pericardial knock (heard best along the left sternal border) often occurs shortly after the second heart sound as a result of a sudden deceleration of ventricular filling. A pericardial knock may be confused with an S3 gallop, but knocks usually occur earlier in the cardiac cycle and have a higher acoustic frequency. Pericardial knocks can also be confused with the opening snap of mitral stenosis. Murmurs found at diagnosis are generally unrelated to pericarditis. Ascites, pleural effusions, and peripheral edema may be found. Additionally, hepatosplenomegaly and its clinical sequelae, such as protein-losing enteropathy from impaired lymphatic drainage from the gut, may occur. Because the most impressive physical findings are often the insidious development of hepatomegaly and ascites, patients with constrictive pericarditis may initially be mistakenly thought to have hepatic cirrhosis or an intra-abdominal tumor.

Laboratory and Imaging Studies

Laboratory evaluation might show the result of congestive hepatopathy with an elevated bilirubin concentration, mild elevation of hepatic transaminase concentrations, a low albumin concentration, and an elevated prothrombin time.

Electrocardiographic results are rarely normal in constriction. They may reveal low-voltage QRS and diffuse flattening of the T waves. Low voltage

Figure 35-5

Diseases of Pericardium

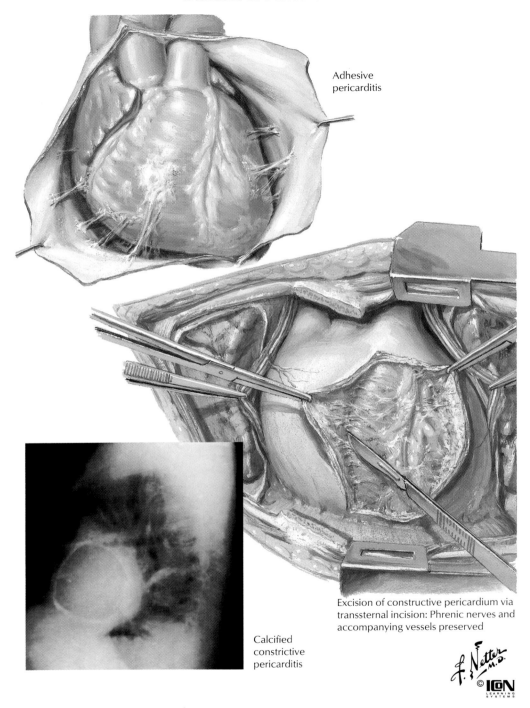

Adhesive pericarditis

Excision of constructive pericardium via transsternal incision: Phrenic nerves and accompanying vessels preserved

Calcified constrictive pericarditis

Table 35-1

Mayo Clinic Experience: Causes of Constrictive Pericarditis and Pericardial Effusions Requiring Pericardiocentesis in Different Cohorts

	CP		PE		
	1936–1982 (n = 231) %	1985–1995 (n = 135) %	1979–1986 (n = 182) %	1986–1993 (n = 354) %	1993–2000 (n = 441) %
Idiopathic	73	33	9	8	8
Infectious	6	3	7	4	7
After cardiac surgery	2	18	21	22	28
Connective tissue disease	2	7	6	3	4
Exposure to radiation	5	13	—	—	—
Acute pericarditis	10	16	—	—	—
Invasive procedure	—	—	4	9	14
Neoplastic	—	—	41	39	25

CP indicates constrictive pericarditis; PE, pericardial effusion requiring pericardiocentesis.

Adapted from Ling LH, Oh JK, Schaff HV, et al. Constrictive pericarditis in the modern era: Evolving clinical spectrum and impact on outcome after pericardiectomy. *Circulation* 1999;100:1380–1386; and Tsang TS, Enriquez-Sarano M, Freeman WK, et al. Consecutive 1127 therapeutic echocardiographically guided pericardiocenteses: Clinical profile, practice patterns, and outcomes spanning 21 years. *Mayo Clin Proc* 2002;77:429–436.

can result from effusive constrictive disease or myocardial atrophy. Conduction abnormalities and other nonspecific abnormalities may be present. Atrial fibrillation occurs in approximately one third of patients.

When tuberculous pericarditis was common, chest radiography showed classic pericardial calcification in up to one third of chronic cases, but this finding is less common today (Fig. 35-5). Indeed, the lack of pericardial calcification in constrictive pericarditis is the rule rather than the exception today. Alveolar edema and radiographic evidence of congestive heart failure are rarely present and should suggest consideration of alternative diagnoses. Cardiac size is generally normal.

The two-dimensional echocardiographic features of constriction include a thickened pericardium, abnormal ventricular septal motion, flattening of the left ventricular (LV) posterior wall during diastole, respiratory variation in ventricular size, and a dilated inferior vena cava.

Doppler echocardiographic features include impaired diastolic filling and dissociation of intracardiac and intrathoracic pressures. The thickened pericardium acts as a buffer to the transmission of the usual intrathoracic pressure changes on the intrapericardial structures. This dissociation between the respiratory (intrathoracic) pressure variations is one feature of constriction but may also occur in tamponade. This may be seen as a decrease in the mitral inflow velocity greater than 25%. A decrease in LV filling allows more room for right ventricular (RV) filling as the interventricular septum moves to the left and hepatic diastolic flow velocities increase during inspiration. During expiration, LV filling increases, with a concomitant decrease in right-sided heart filling and a decrease in hepatic diastolic forward-flow velocity. In constriction, diastolic forward flow is usually greater than systolic forward flow. Additionally, hepatic diastolic flow reversal is increased because the inflow across the tricuspid valve is interrupted by the pericardium and movement of the septum toward the right ventricle with expiration.

CT and magnetic resonance imaging (MRI) of the heart can be important in determining pericardial thickness. These modalities directly visualize the pericardium and can detect thickness greater than 2 mm. The finding of normal pericardial thickness does not exclude constrictive pericarditis because up to 20% of patients with surgically confirmed disease have normal pericardial thickness on these imaging modalities. Similarly, not all patients with a thickened pericardium have constrictive pericarditis; however a thickness of greater than 6 mm adds considerable specificity to the diagnosis.

Left- and right-sided heart catheterization provides important information in evaluating potential constrictive pericarditis. There are three key features: elevation and equalization of the diastolic pressures in each of the cardiac chambers, an early diastolic "dip-and-plateau" configuration in the RV and LV tracings, and a prominent y descent on right atrial (RA) pressure tracings. (For a more detailed discussion of hemodynamics, see chapter 36.) Cardiac catheterization can also be used to evaluate for concomitant disease, such as coronary artery disease (CAD), before pericardiectomy.

Management and Therapy

Chronic constrictive pericarditis is a progressive disease without spontaneous reversal of pericardial abnormalities, symptoms, or hemodynamics. A minority of patients survive for years with modest jugular venous distension and peripheral edema controlled by the judicious use of diet and diuretics. Drugs that slow the HR, such as β-blockers and calcium channel blockers, should be avoided because mild sinus tachycardia is a compensatory mechanism. The majority of patients become progressively more disabled and experience the complications of severe cardiac cachexia.

The mainstay of therapy is surgical removal of the pericardium. In cases with a firmly adherent pericardium, scoring of the pericardium may "loosen" the pericardium, but results are less optimal. Pericardiectomy is associated with significant risk for morbidity and mortality, especially in elderly patients or those with significant

preoperative symptoms, organ dysfunction, or coexisting CAD. Mortality with pericardiectomy has also been reported to range from 5.6 to 19% and to correlate with RA pressure. In one series, survivals at 5 and 10 years were 78 ± 5 and 57 ± 8%, respectively, and were inferior to those of an age- and sex-matched US population.

Of those patients who survive the pericardiectomy, 90% report symptomatic improvement, and approximately 50% become asymptomatic. Symptom resolution may be immediate but can take weeks to months. However, symptoms may recur.

PERICARDIAL EFFUSION

Pericardial effusions are a response to injury of the pericardium. Transudative effusions result from obstructed fluid drainage, which occurs through lymphatic channels. Exudative effusions occur secondary to inflammatory, infectious, malignant, or autoimmune processes within the pericardium.

Etiology

There are few data regarding etiologies of pericardial effusions in a community setting or in patients who do not require drainage. The most common etiologies requiring pericardiocentesis include malignancy, postoperative causes, cardiac perforation during a percutaneous procedure (e.g., pacemaker lead placement), idiopathic etiologies, connective tissue disorder, and infection (Table 35-1). Other causes include acute pericarditis, renal failure, coagulopathy, hypothyroidism, trauma, postradiation, HIV, and myocardial infarction. Transudative effusions are rarely seen in congestive heart failure, cirrhosis, nephrosis, and pregnancy.

Pericardial effusions are common after cardiac surgery, occurring in more than 80% of cases. The maximal size is apparent by 10 days, and the effusions usually resolve spontaneously within 1 month after surgery.

Malignancy is one of the most common causes of pericardial effusions, reported in up to 20% of patients with cancer in autopsy series. The primary tumors most often associated with pericardial effusions are lung (40%), breast (23%), lymphoma (11%), and leukemia (5%). Pericardial effusions in patients with cancer are malignant approximately 50% of the time. Nonmalignant causes of pericardial effusions in patients with cancer include radiation-induced pericarditis and infections.

Clinical Presentation

Clinical manifestations of pericardial effusion depend on the intrapericardial pressure, which, in turn, depends on the amount and rate of fluid accumulation in the pericardial sac. As intrapericardial pressure increases, ventricular diastolic pressure increases. Atrial pressures increase to maintain forward flow across the tricuspid and mitral valves. Further increases in intrapericardial pressure cause ventricular filling to decrease, leading to impaired CO and hypotension. Rapid accumulation of pericardial fluid may elevate intrapericardial pressures with as little as 80 mL of fluid, whereas slowly progressing effusions can grow to 2 L without symptoms. When pericardial fluid accumulation is rapid or sustained, pericardial tamponade may result, the hemodynamics of which are discussed in detail in chapter 36.

History and Physical Examination

Most pericardial effusions are asymptomatic. Once symptoms occur, the most common complaints include dyspnea (85%), coughing (30%), orthopnea (25%), and chest pain (20%). The common signs of pericardial effusion are a paradoxic pulse (45%), tachypnea (45%), tachycardia (40%), hypotension (25%), and peripheral edema (20%), all of which raise the possibility that pericardial tamponade is present.

Small pericardial effusions are generally not detectable by means of physical examination. Large effusions result in muffled heart sounds and occasionally in Ewart's sign, dullness to percussion beneath the angle of the left scapula from compression of the left lung by pericardial fluid.

Patients with pericardial tamponade generally are tachycardic and tachypneic and appear ill (Fig. 35-6). Pericardial tamponade is an emergent condition that necessitates hospital admission and intervention to relieve the associated hemodynamic abnormalities. Beck's description of pericardial tamponade included the classic triad of hypotension, muffled heart sounds, and jugular venous distension. Tamponade is generally associated with a *pulsus paradoxus*, a decrease in SBP of more than 10 mm Hg with inspiration. SBP normally decreases during inspiration, but cardiac tamponade causes an exaggeration of physiologic respiratory variation in systemic blood pressure from decreasing CO during inspiration. However, pulsus paradoxus is neither sensitive nor specific for cardiac tamponade. It can also occur in constrictive pericarditis, obstructive lung disease, RV infarction, pulmonary embolus, or large pleural effusions.

Electrocardiography

Typical findings include sinus tachycardia and low voltage. If associated pericarditis is present, PR segment depression, diffuse ST elevation, and possibly atrial tachyarrhythmias may be apparent. *Electrical alternans*, in which R wave voltage varies from beat to beat, is the most specific ECG finding but is rarely found and only in association with large pericardial effusions.

Chest Radiography

An enlarged cardiac silhouette is seen after the accumulation of at least 200 mL of fluid. A large pericardial effusion results in a so-called water bottle appearance. One third to one half of patients have a coexisting pleural effusion, with left being more common than right. Separation of the epicardial fat pad from the outer border of the cardiac silhouette can occasionally be observed, especially in the lateral view.

Echocardiography

Echocardiography is the gold standard test for evaluating pericardial effusions. Pericardial fluid appears as an echo-free space between the visceral and parietal pericardia. Effusions can be circumferential (completely surrounding the heart) or loculated. In pericardial tamponade, echocardiographic findings include diastolic collapse of the right atrium and ventricle. Doppler interrogation demonstrates marked respiratory variation in flow across the tricuspid and mitral valves. Echocardiography is a sensitive and specific test for pericardial effusions; however, false-positive results can occur in pleural effusions, pericardial thickening, increased pericardial fat (especially the anterior epicardial fat pad), atelectasis, and mediastinal lesions. Transthoracic echocardiography is generally diagnostic, and transesophageal echocardiography is rarely needed for the diagnosis of pericardial tamponade.

Figure 35-6

Cardiac Tamponade

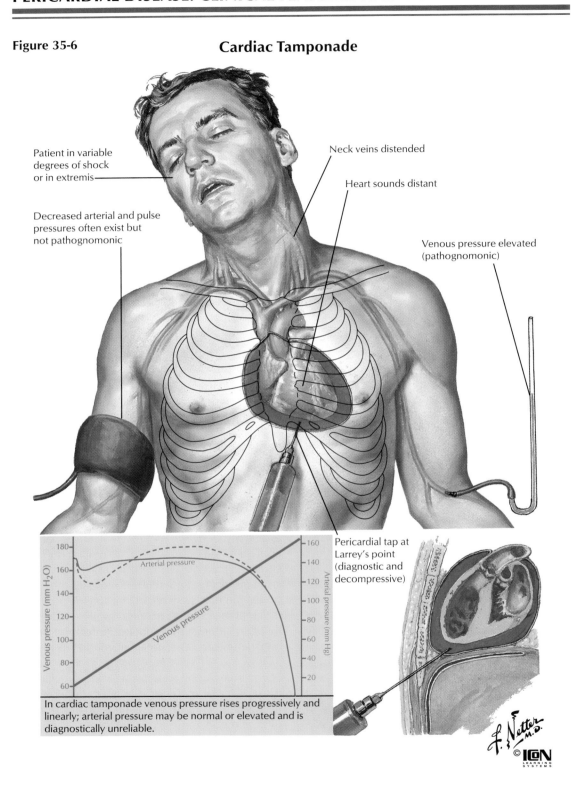

Patient in variable degrees of shock or in extremis

Decreased arterial and pulse pressures often exist but not pathognomonic

Neck veins distended

Heart sounds distant

Venous pressure elevated (pathognomonic)

Pericardial tap at Larrey's point (diagnostic and decompressive)

In cardiac tamponade venous pressure rises progressively and linearly; arterial pressure may be normal or elevated and is diagnostically unreliable.

Computed Tomography

A CT scan may detect as little as 50 mL of fluid. This modality is rarely used to evaluate patients with suspected effusions; more commonly, effusions are incidentally found in patients undergoing chest CT evaluation for other indications (e.g., lung cancer, unexplained dyspnea).

Magnetic Resonance Imaging

An MRI can detect as little as 30 mL of pericardial fluid and may be used to distinguish hemorrhagic and nonhemorrhagic effusions based on T1 and T2 signal intensities.

Management and Therapy

Most pericardial effusions resolve without drainage. In some patients, however, pericardiocentesis is needed as emergent treatment for tamponade (Fig. 35-6) or for diagnostic purposes. Pericardiocentesis can be performed percutaneously or surgically. Surgical procedures have several advantages, including complete drainage of loculated effusions and access to pericardial tissue for biopsy. However, percutaneous pericardiocentesis is simpler, is more rapid, and necessitates less time for recovery.

A subxyphoid approach is generally used for percutaneous pericardiocentesis, although echocardiographically guided approaches via the chest wall are widely used. Needle insertion can be performed under electrocardiographic, echocardiographic, or radiographic guidance. Although pericardiocentesis usually leads to clinical improvement, pulmonary edema, hypotension, and acute ventricular dysfunction have been reported after the procedure. The safety and efficacy of this procedure is dependent on the skill of the operator and the size of the effusion. Recurrence rates of 12 to 40% have been reported after successful drainage.

Malignant pericardial effusions tend to recur, and several approaches have been advocated to prevent the need for recurrent pericardiocentesis. The literature consists primarily of small prospective or larger retrospective studies, and no consensus on the best approach has formed. Balloon pericardotomy involves tearing a hole in the pericardium with a balloon placed in the pericardial space under fluoroscopy. This hole enables pericardial fluid to drain into the pleural space. Pericardial sclerosis involves application of a sclerosing agent (e.g., tetracycline, doxycycline, cisplatin, 5-fluorouracil, bleomycin) into the pericardial space to scar the visceral and parietal pericardia with elimination of the pericardial space. Success rates of as high as 91% are reported at 30 days, but potential complications include intense pain, atrial dysrhythmias, fever, and infection. Another viable approach, surgical creation of a subxyphoid pericardial window, is associated with low morbidity, mortality, and recurrence rates and can be performed under local anesthesia. However, this approach is not effective with loculated pericardial effusion. In some cases, a pleuropericardial window can be created by means of thoracotomy under general anesthesia.

FUTURE DIRECTIONS

The diagnosis of pericardial diseases continues to become more accurate, resulting in improved therapies. Challenges for the future include the development of more effective therapies for the more serious pericardial diseases, including refractory pericarditis, pericardial constriction, and pericardial tamponade. In this area, little improvement has occurred in the past decade, perhaps because of the inaccuracies of diagnosis. The subtleties of diagnosis are the focus of chapter 36, and advances that are likely to occur offer hope for improved therapy.

REFERENCES

Bilchick KC, Wise RA. Paradoxical physical findings described by Kussmaul: Pulsus paradoxus and Kussmaul's sign. *Lancet* 2002;359:1940–1942.

Hoit BD. Management of effusive and constrictive pericardial heart disease. *Circulation* 2002;105:2939–2942.

Hoit BD. Pericardial heart disease. *Curr Probl Cardiol* 1997; 22:357–400.

Laham RJ, Cohen DJ, Kuntz RE, et al. Pericardial effusion in patients with cancer: Outcome with contemporary management strategies. *Heart* 1996;75:67–71.

Nishimura RA. Constrictive pericarditis in the modern era: A diagnostic dilemma. *Heart* 2001;86:619–623.

Spodick DH. Diagnostic electrocardiographic sequences in acute pericarditis: Significance of PR segment and PR vector changes. *Circulation* 1973;48:575.

Spodick DH. Pericardial rub: Prospective, multiple observer investigation of pericardial friction rub in 100 patients. *Am J Cardiol* 1975;35:357.

Wilkes JD, Fidias P, Vaickus L, et al. Malignancy-related pericardial effusion: 127 cases from the Roswell Park Cancer Institute. *Cancer* 1995;76:1377–1387.

Chapter 36

Pericardial Disease: Diagnosis and Hemodynamics

Thomas M. Bashore

Pericardial pathology can present as an outpatient disease, in a setting requiring invasive diagnostic testing and surgery, or anywhere in between (see chapter 35). This chapter focuses on the more serious presentations that result in hemodynamic abnormalities. In these cases, pericardial diseases inhibit diastolic filling of the heart. Clinically, constrictive pericarditis presents with evidence for right-sided heart failure, whereas pericardial tamponade presents with distinctive hypotension. Diagnosis of these conditions is not always simple, as combinations of the disease processes can exist (effusive-constrictive pericarditis) and milder forms require fluid loading to bring out characteristic hemodynamic findings (occult constrictive pericarditis). In addition, localized and transient forms of constrictive pericarditis have been described. The differential diagnosis between constrictive pericarditis and restrictive cardiomyopathy, addressed primarily in chapter 14, can also be a challenge.

ETIOLOGY AND PATHOGENESIS
Normal Physiology

To understand the hemodynamics of pericardial diseases, it is important to understand that the pericardial cavity (the space between the visceral and parietal layers that holds a usually small collection of fluid), is a space in which large volumes of fluid may accumulate.

The fluid within the pericardial space is in dynamic equilibrium with the blood serum. A normal amount of pericardial fluid is less than 50 cc and normally pericardial fluid is transudative with low protein. Because there are many smaller sinuses and recesses in the pericardial space (around the atria, the superior vena cava, the great vessels, the pulmonary veins, and the inferior vena cava), a minimum of about 250 cc of fluid forms the normal pericardial reserve volume.

The pericardium provides a thin tissue barrier between the heart and the surrounding structures and exerts constant pressure on the heart, affecting thin structures (the atria and the right ventricle) more than the thicker-walled left ventricle. Resting diastolic pressures within the heart are directly affected by this pericardial constraint (pericardial removal results in right ventricular [RV] dilatation rather than left ventricular [LV] dilatation, for instance).

Normal intrapericardial pressures range from −6 to −3 mm Hg, directly reflecting intrapleural pressures. The pressure differential between the pericardium and the cardiac chambers (transmural pressure) is about 3 mm Hg. The pericardium is much stiffer than cardiac muscle, and once the pericardial reserve volume is exceeded, the pressure–volume curve of the normal pericardium rises steeply. The pericardium has little effect on ventricular systole; however, interactions between the right- and left-sided cardiac chambers are enhanced by the pericardium because atrial and ventricular septal movement are independent of pericardial constraint.

Intracardiac pressures are a reflection of the contraction and relaxation of individual cardiac structures and the changes imparted to them by the pleural and pericardial pressures (Fig. 36-1). Thus, changes in pleural or pericardial pressure affect the measured intracardiac pressure. With inspiration, the intrapleural pressures drop and the abdominal cavity pressure increases. Blood flow to the right side of the heart increases, whereas blood return to the left side of the heart decreases slightly. The fall in the intrapleural pressures also causes an increase in the transmural aortic root pressure, effectively increasing impedance to LV ejection. The reverse occurs during expiration. In the normal setting, the respiratory changes are reflected in the intrapericardial and intracardiac pressures, with inspiration lowering the measured right atrial pressures

Figure 36-1

Normal Cardiac Blood Flow During Inspiration and Expiration

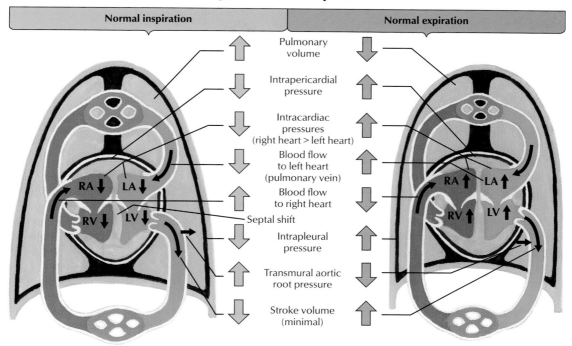

Normal inspiration	Normal expiration

Pulmonary volume

Intrapericardial pressure

Intracardiac pressures (right heart > left heart)

Blood flow to left heart (pulmonary vein)

Blood flow to right heart

Septal shift

Intrapleural pressure

Transmural aortic root pressure

Stroke volume (minimal)

On inspiration, intrapleural pressure drops and abdominal pressure increases with increased blood flow to right heart and slight decrease in flow to left heart. Increased aortic root transmural pressure adds a minor amount of increased LV afterload.

On expiration, intrapleural pressure increases and abdominal pressure decreases with decreased blood flow to right heart and increase in flow to left heart

JOHN A.CRAIG—AD
© ICON

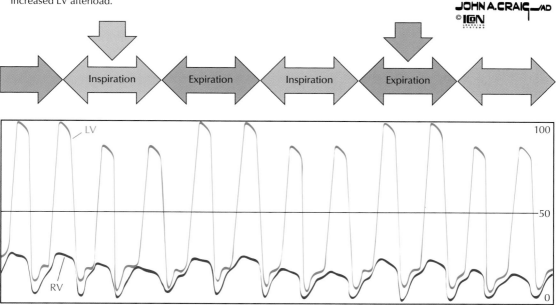

Inspiration — Expiration — Inspiration — Expiration

Simultaneous measurement of RV and LV systolic pressure reveals a concordant decrease in pressure in both chambers during inspiration, with a similar concordant increase in pressure in both ventricles during expiration and the systolic RV pressure more than the left-sided heart pressures.

The trivially reduced LV filling and increased impedance to ejection with inspiration produce a modest decline in the LV stroke volume and a slightly lower aortic pulse pressure with inspiration. Marked swings in the intrapleural pressure from very negative during inspiration to very positive during expiration (as occur in asthma or severe COPD) exaggerate the changes in LV filling and may produce a paradoxical pulse (>10 mm Hg decline in the aortic systolic pressure) purely from the pleural pressure swings. This phenomenon of a paradoxical pulse must be differentiated from the same phenomenon due to cardiac tamponade.

The normal atrial and ventricular waveforms are shown in Figure 36-2. With atrial contraction, the atrial pressures rise (a wave). With the onset of ventricular contraction, the atrioventricular (AV) valves bulge toward the atria and a small c wave results (the c wave is evident on hemodynamic tracings but often is not visible to the examiner observing the jugular venous pulsations). As ventricular contraction continues, the AV annular ring is pulled into the ventricular cavity and the atria enter diastole, enlarging the atria and decreasing the atrial pressure (represented by the x descent). Passive filling of the atria during ventricular systole produces a slow rise in the atrial pressure (the v wave) until the AV valves reopen at the peak of the v wave, and the pressure then falls rapidly as the ventricles actively relax. Passive filling of the ventricles continues while the AV valves are open until atrial contraction again occurs, and the cycle repeats. For this discussion, following ventricular systole, ventricular diastole can be divided into an initial active phase (a brief period when the ventricle fills about halfway) and a passive filling phase. The nadir, or lowest, diastolic pressure during ventricular diastole occurs during the early active relaxation phase (suction effect).

Hemodynamics of Pericardial Constriction and Pericardial Tamponade

Constrictive pericarditis and cardiac tamponade alter the normal intracardiac pressures in a number of ways. Some of the hemodynamic abnormalities seen are present in both entities,

whereas others are unique to either pericardial constriction or tamponade (Fig. 36-2).

Constrictive Pericarditis

Constrictive pericarditis was recognized at autopsy in the 19th century and described as a "chronic fibrous callous thickening of the wall of the pericardial sac that is so contracted that the normal diastolic filling of the heart is prevented" (Fig. 36-3). The variable severity of the constrictive process results in a spectrum of hemodynamic change. Table 36-1 outlines the major features of the subacute (elastic) and the more chronic (rigid shell) forms of pericardial constriction.

The difference between the subacute and the more chronic forms relates to whether only the visceral pericardium is fused to the epicardium of the heart (subacute) or both the visceral and the parietal pericardial layers are fused together (chronic). In both instances, the diastolic pressures in the atria are elevated, due to the restriction of ventricular diastolic relaxation. The elevated atrial pressures result in a high driving pressure across the AV valves as they open with an immediate, rapid decrease in atrial pressure that is responsible for the rapid y descent seen in pericardial constriction (Fig. 36-2). However, the constraint imposed by the constricted pericardium results in the sudden halting of this rapid early filling. The consequence is a rapid rise in the ventricular diastolic pressures to levels exceeding those in the atria, with the result that atrial filling suddenly ceases. This produces the "square root sign" or the "dip and plateau" in the AV tracings seen during ventricular diastole in patients with pericardial constriction. The x descent is generally unaffected; thus, the y descent is usually greater than the x descent in constrictive pericardial disease. The high right atrial pressure coupled with the normal or only mildly elevated RV systolic pressures causes the RVEDP to usually be greater than one third the RV systolic pressure. Transmitral Doppler patterns (Fig. 36-3) reflect the initial high driving pressure (high initial E velocity), the abrupt change in flow with the rapid rise in the LV pressure (short deceleration of initial flow) and a reduced velocity observed with atrial contraction (reduced A velocity).

The normal respiratory changes in cardiac flow are altered in constriction. The right atrial

Table 36-1

Comparison of Features Characteristic of Subacute (Elastic) and Chronic (Rigid Shell) Constrictive Pericarditis

Subacute (Elastic)	Chronic (Rigid Shell)
Paradoxical pulse usually present. Signs of ventricular interdependence prominent.	Paradoxical pulse usually minimal or absent. Ventricular interdependence less prominent.
Prominent x and y descents ("M" or "W" waveform in the JVP)	Prominent y descent; x descent sometimes minimal
Dip and plateau pattern less obvious	Conspicuous dip and plateau pattern
Early diastolic nadir may not approach zero	Early diastolic nadir approaches zero
Calcification of pericardium rare	Calcification of pericardium more likely
Pericardial effusion may be present	Pericardial effusion absent
Constriction primarily due to visceral pericardium	Constriction due to fusion of visceral and parietal pericardium and with epicardium of the heart
ECG "P" waves usually normal	ECG "P" waves wide, notched, and low amplitude
Atrial fibrillation or flutter uncommon	Atrial fibrillation or flutter common

With permission from Hancock EW. Differential diagnosis of restrictive cardiomyopathy and constrictive pericarditis. *Heart* 2001;86:343–349.

pressure normally falls with inspiration, however, it may fail to fall (Kussmaul's sign) in constrictive pericarditis or it may even rise. Also reflecting the loss of normal RV filling with respiration, the inferior vena cava diameter, as seen by echocardiography, may be reduced less than the expected 50% with inspiration. The precise mechanisms responsible for the loss of respiratory effects on cardiac flow are the subject of some debate. It seems most likely that the rigid pericardium in constrictive pericarditis acts to disassociate the usually related intrathoracic and intracardiac pressures. Conceptually, the increased flow to the right side of the heart is mandated by the negative intrathoracic pressures. In constriction, the right side of the heart is forced to fill to more than its capacity (which is limited by pericardial constriction) and pressure rises rather than falls. In addition with inspiration, the falling diaphragm may actually reduce the overall cardiac volumes during pericardial constriction. Kussmaul's sign is not specific for pericardial constriction. Other conditions that result in high right atrial pressures can

produce Kussmaul's sign; it can be seen in acute or chronic RV failure, RV infarction, or restrictive cardiomyopathy. In most of these conditions, the constrictive physiology is due more to RV volume overload (reaching the limit of RV capacity) rather than to pericardial capacity.

Normally, with inspiration, the LV minimal pressure and the left atrial (LA) pressures fall equally and no change is noted in the Doppler mitral inflow velocities. In constriction, the high LA pressures inhibit filling from the pulmonary venous bed. The reduced initial flow into the left ventricle during inspiration can be observed in the transmitral Doppler flow pattern by noting a greater than 25% decrease in the previously described high initial driving force across the mitral valve (decreased E velocity) during inspiration (Fig. 36-3).

Because the atrial and ventricular septa are unaffected by the pericardial process, changes in atrial and ventricular filling on the right side of the heart can affect left-sided filling (chamber interdependence). In constriction when the ventricular pressures are simultaneously assessed, the normal inspiratory decrease in both ventric-

Figure 36-2 Comparison of Normal and Pathologic Intracardiac Pressures

Normal

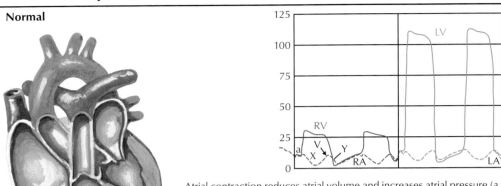

Atrial contraction reduces atrial volume and increases atrial pressure (*a* wave). Ventricular contraction causes initial small *c* wave and as AV ring pulled into atria and atrial relaxation ensues, atrial enlargement occurs with pressure decrease (*x* descent). Passive atrial filling causes *v* wave until AV valves open and pressure rapidly drops (*y* descent) as ventricles relax. Following ventricular systole, an active and passive filling phase follows—pressure lowest in active phase.

Constrictive pericarditis

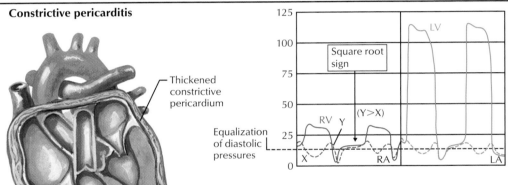

Thickened constrictive pericardium

Equalization of diastolic pressures

High atrial pressures when the AV valves open result in rapid early filling (rapid *y* descent) until filling abruptly stops (square root sign). There is equalization of late diastolic pressures. The RV diastolic is usually $> 1/3$ RV systolic pressure.

Cardiac tamponade

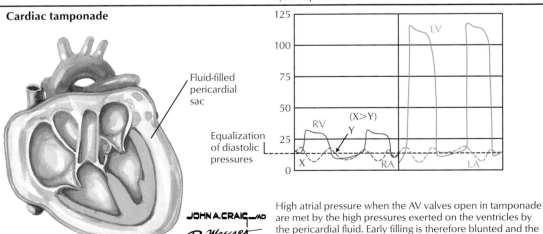

Fluid-filled pericardial sac

Equalization of diastolic pressures

JOHN A. CRAIG—AD
D. Mascaro
© ICON

High atrial pressure when the AV valves open in tamponade are met by the high pressures exerted on the ventricles by the pericardial fluid. Early filling is therefore blunted and the *y* descent less than the *x* descent. There is equalization of late diastolic pressures, and the pulmonary pressure is usually normal.

Figure 36-3

Pericarditis

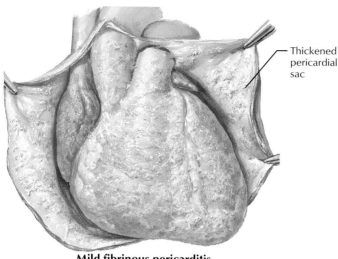

Thickened pericardial sac

Mild fibrinous pericarditis

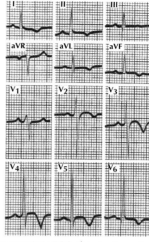

Characteristic ECG changes in pericarditis T-wave inversion in all leads except AVR and V$_1$, isoelectric in lead III

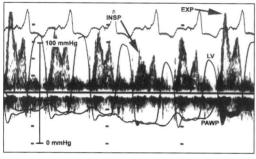

Doppler flow in constrictive pericarditis during peak inspiration and expiration. There is a decrease in initial gradient between LV diastolic pressure and pulmonary wedge pressure (PAWP). This results in initial decrease in E velocity. The transmittal gradient is re-established in expira-tion with an ↑ in E velocity and transmitted flow velocity.

With permission from Nishimura RA. Constrictive pericarditis in the modern era: A diagnostic dilemma. *Heart* 2001;86:619–623.

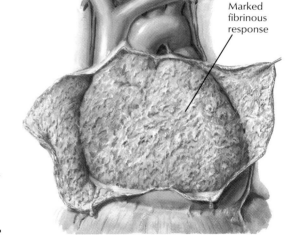

Marked fibrinous response

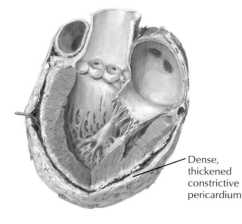

Dense, thickened constrictive pericardium

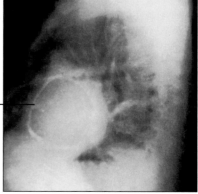

Calcification of pericardium in chronic pericarditis

Figure 36-4

Comparison of Blood Flow in Constrictive Pericarditis and Cardiac Tamponade

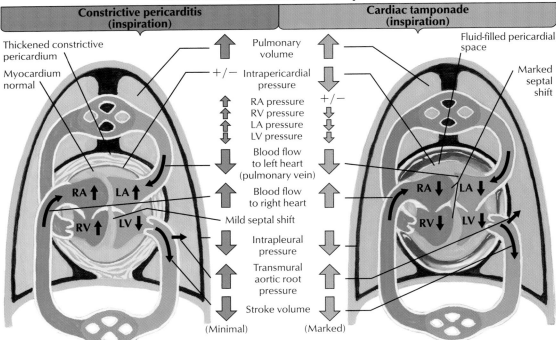

Constrictive pericarditis (inspiration)		Cardiac tamponade (inspiration)
Thickened constrictive pericardium	Pulmonary volume	Fluid-filled pericardial space
Myocardium normal	+/− Intrapericardial pressure	Marked septal shift
	RA pressure / RV pressure / LA pressure / LV pressure	+/−
	Blood flow to left heart (pulmonary vein)	
RA↑ LA↑ / RV↑ LV↓	Blood flow to right heart	RA↓ LA↓ / RV↓ LV↓
	Mild septal shift	
	Intrapleural pressure	
	Transmural aortic root pressure	
(Minimal)	Stroke volume	(Marked)

Reduced intrapleural pressure not transmitted to RA and RV due to tethering of pericardium to descending diaphragm. The negative intrapleural pressure and expanding lung bring blood into lungs, and pressures may actually rise in heart. (Kussmaul's) ↑ in RV systolic pressure contrasts with ↓ in LV systolic pressure since ↑ LA pressure further reduces the normal modest ↓ in pulmonary venous flow. (This reduction is generally inadequate to cause paradoxical pulse.)

In cardiac tamponade, ↓ intrapleural pressure in inspiration is usually transmitted to right heart structures, so no Kussmaul's is noted. ↑ flow to right heart expands RA and RV at the expense of LA and LV. The normal ↓ in pulmonary venous flow is further reduced by smaller left heart chamber sizes and ↑ filling pressures. A substantial ↓ in stroke volume occurs, creating paradoxical pulse.

JOHN A. CRAIG—AD
©ICON LEARNING SYSTEMS

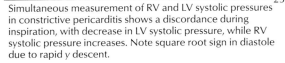

Inspiration

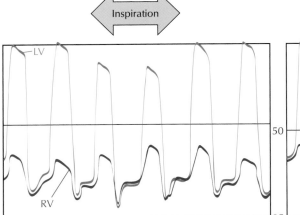

Simultaneous measurement of RV and LV systolic pressures in constrictive pericarditis shows a discordance during inspiration, with decrease in LV systolic pressure, while RV systolic pressure increases. Note square root sign in diastole due to rapid y descent.

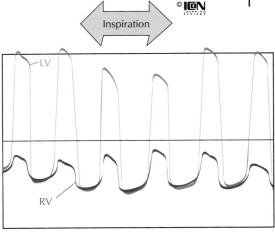

Inspiration

50
25

Simultaneous measurement of RV and LV pressures in cardiac tamponade. There is loss of rapid early filling of ventricles. Inspiration results in blood being drawn into RV, with RV systolic pressure rising. Increased RV volumes result in marked septal shifting and LV volumes decline (ventricular interdependence). Subsequent decrease in LV stroke volume results in paradoxical pulse.

Figure 36-5

Pressure–Volume Relationship of Pericardium

Acute pericardial effusion

hours/days

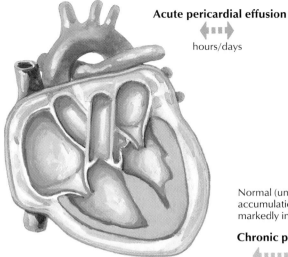

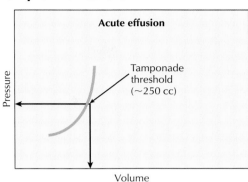

Acute effusion

Pressure

Tamponade
threshold
(~250 cc)

Volume

Normal (unstretched) pericardium is able to accommodate acute fluid accumulation up to ~250 cc, beyond which additional volume markedly increases intrapericardial pressure.

Chronic pericardial effusion

weeks/months

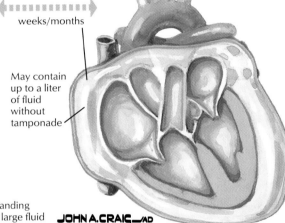

Chronic effusion

Pressure

Tamponade
threshold

Volume

May contain
up to a liter
of fluid
without
tamponade

Pericardium that has been stretched over time by long-standing effusion is more distensible and is able to accommodate large fluid volume without critical increase in intrapericardial pressure.

JOHN A. CRAIG—MD
© ICON

Echocardiographic findings in cardiac tamponade

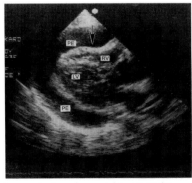

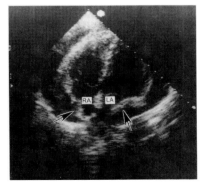

Long-axis view shows right ventricular (RV) collapse due to large pericardial effusion (PE).

Four-chamber view demonstrates collapse of both right (RA) and left (LA) atria due to tamponade.

ular systolic pressures is altered, as the increase in RV filling results in a rise in the RV systolic pressure while there occurs the normal fall (Fig. 36-4) in the LV systolic pressure. This finding is particularly useful in differentiating constrictive pericarditis from restrictive cardiomyopathy, in which there is a concordant fall in both ventricular systolic pressures with inspiration.

Pericardial Tamponade

Cardiac tamponade occurs when pericardial fluid exceeds pericardial reserve volume. The result is cardiac compression and restricted diastolic filling of all the cardiac chambers (see Fig. 36-5). The amount of pericardial fluid required for tamponade depends on the parietal pericardial compliance and the fluid accumulation rate. Acute tamponade can result with even a small increase in pericardial fluid because of the normally steep pericardial pressure–volume relationship. When fluid accumulates slowly, as in patients with metastatic cancer or chronic uremia, the parietal pericardium adapts and stretches and tamponade occurs only after the accumulation of a large amount (sometimes >1 L) of fluid. Therefore, the rate of fluid accumulation determines the clinical presentation.

As fluid accumulates in the pericardium, the thinnest-walled chambers (the right atrium and the right ventricle) are affected first. Right-sided diastolic pressures are normally lower than left-sided diastolic pressures, and collapse of the right atrium and the right ventricle are observed early in tamponade (often before a paradoxical pulse, for instance). The high intrapericardial pressures are transmitted to the early diastolic atrial and ventricular pressures. When the AV valves open, the diastolic pressure is already elevated, as reflected in the reduced *y* descent (following the opening of AV valve) from the loss of rapid ventricular filling (Fig. 36-2). These high diastolic pressures also cause premature closure of the AV valves. However, as the ventricles contract to eject blood, the pericardial space is actually increased and the atria can fill in atrial diastole (preserving the *x* descent). The *x* descent is therefore greater than the *y* descent in cardiac tamponade. Increasing intrapericardial pressures progressively affect the right atrial diastolic pressure, then the RV diastolic pressure

(especially in the thinner RV outflow tract), and eventually the left-sided heart diastolic pressure, finally resulting in the equalization of diastolic pressures throughout the heart.

As in constriction, the increased filling of the right side of the heart, mandated by the negative intrathoracic pressure during inspiration, increases the early filling of the right side structures. However, because there is a fixed space for the heart chambers, a leftward shift in the atrial and ventricular septa occurs as the right side of the heart fills. This reduces LV chamber compliance and impairs LV filling. Atrial reservoir function increases in importance during cardiac tamponade; the left atrium may fill only during expiration, with subsequent LV filling only during atrial systole. The reduced LV filling also reduces LV preload and contractile function, further lowering the stroke volume. The paradoxical pulse in cardiac tamponade results from this inspiratory reduction in LV filling. In the most extreme cases of tamponade, the aortic valve may open only during expiration. A paradoxical pulse may not occur in extreme hypotension; in patients with pericardial tamponade and severe aortic insufficiency, an atrial septal defect, a single ventricle; or in some cases of acute LV infarction. Table 36-2 outlines the major hemodynamic differences between constrictive pericarditis and cardiac tamponade.

DIAGNOSTIC APPROACH
History and Physical Examination

The classic findings of pericardial constriction and tamponade are presented in chapter 35. This chapter reviews the key findings with an emphasis on understanding the underlying hemodynamics that they represent and how these findings are helpful in some cases (and not in others) for distinguishing pericardial constriction from pericardial tamponade.

Pericardial Constriction

Pericardial constriction may be subtle, but significant constriction presents as primarily right-sided heart failure with normal LV systolic function. A history of antecedent pericarditis, pericarditis-inducing drug use, uremia, cardiac surgery, or thoracic radiation may be a clue. There is usually evidence for venous congestion,

Table 36-2
Major Hemodynamic Differences Between Constrictive Pericarditis and Cardiac Tamponade

Constrictive Pericarditis	Cardiac Tamponade
Atrial pressures elevated with rapid y descent	Atrial pressures elevated with blunted y descent
y descent greater than x descent	x descent greater than y descent
Kussmaul's sign often present	Kussmaul's sign occasionally present
Square-root sign in diastole	Blunted early filling in diastole
Nadir of early ventricular pressure near zero	Elevated early ventricular diastolic pressure
Paradoxical pulse uncommon	Paradoxical pulse common
Normal heart size on chest radiograph	Water-bottle cardiac enlargement
Calcification of the pericardium occasionally present	Calcification rarely seen
Atria normal in size and shape on echo	Right atrial, right ventricular, and occasional left atrial collapse on echo
No or trivial pericardial effusion on echo, CT, or MRI	Pericardial effusion present
Often, thickened pericardium seen on CT or MRI	Normal or minimally thickened pericardium seen on CT or MRI

MRI indicates magnetic resonance imaging.

pedal edema, ascites (often out of proportion to peripheral edema), fatigue, dyspnea, and low cardiac output. Most patients compensate with tachycardia. Atrial arrhythmias are common. The retinal veins are often engorged. Jugular venous distention is universal, and a positive Kussmaul's response is expected. The sharp, rapid x and y descents are often seen in the jugular venous pulsations at bedside. Because the jugular veins may be so distended, patients need to be examined in an upright position. To time the pulse waveforms, one should feel the opposite carotid pulse: the x descent occurs during ventricular systole. Precordial palpation may be normal, or the apex may even retract with systole. The rapid filling of the ventricles may produce a loud filling sound (pericardial knock) on auscultation. The liver is often enlarged, and ascites is often the prominent examination feature. A paradoxical pulse is not usually demonstrated unless associated lung disease or concurrent pericardial tamponade exists.

Cardiac Tamponade

Cardiac tamponade symptoms are generally more related to low output than to right-sided heart failure. The setting for acute tamponade often includes chest trauma, recent cardiac surgery, recent (but generally not acute) myocardial infarction, or evidence of aortic dissection. Chronic tamponade is generally related to malignancy, uremia, or other causes of inflammatory pericarditis. Tachypnea and dyspnea are common. Orthopnea from pulmonary interstitial edema, which increases lung stiffness, is also common. Cough, dysphagia, and presyncope or frank syncope are often seen, along with fatigue, weakness, and anorexia. Anemia, common in uremia and malignancies, exacerbates the symptoms. Eventually, shock, with accompanying renal and hepatic failure and mesenteric ischemia, may be seen.

The physical examination may be deceptive, with hypotension and shock predominating. Tachycardia is the rule (although the heart rate

Table 36-3
Differences in the Physical Examination of Patients With Constrictive Pericarditis Versus Patients With Cardiac Tamponade

Constrictive Pericarditis	Cardiac Tamponade
Clear lung fields	Clear lung fields, with occasional Ewart's sign in large pericardial effusions
Ascites often present. Peripheral edema occasionally present.	Ascites and peripheral edema rare
Evidence of pleural effusions common	Pleural effusions uncommon
JVP markedly elevated. Rapid x and y descents	JVP moderately elevated. Loss of y descent evident.
Pericardial rub rare	Pericardial rub common
Apical pulse localized and may retract with systole	Apical pulse large and diffuse
Loud filling sound ("knock") occasionally present with normal S_1 and S_2	Heart sounds often diminished

JVP indicates jugular venous pressure.

may be lower in patients with hypothyroidism or in some patients with uremia). The JVP is usually elevated (often dependent on the absence of hypovolemia), and a Kussmaul's sign is usually not evident unless there is associated constrictive physiology. At times, the JVP elevation may be striking and may result in venous distention of the scalp, the forehead, and the ocular veins. The jugular venous waveforms reveal a normal or even diminished y descent (as opposed to the rapid y descent seen in constriction) and preservation of the x descent during ventricular systole (as assessed by palpation of the opposite carotid). A paradoxical pulse is usually present unless there is marked hypotension, and the presence of a paradoxical pulse should be aggressively sought. Pericardial rubs are variable and may exist even in the presence of large pericardial effusions. At times, very large pericardial effusions produce dullness and bronchial breathing between the left scapula and the spine (Bamberger-Pins-Ewart's sign). The cardiac impulse may not be palpable. Evidence for chronic right-sided heart failure, such as ascites, is usually absent. Table 36-3 outlines the differences in the physical examination of patients with pericardial constriction and patients with pericardial tamponade.

ECG and Chest X-ray

As discussed in chapter 35, while often helpful, the ECG and chest radiograph should not be relied on to make the diagnosis of either pericardial constriction or pericardial tamponade, or to distinguish the two. In pericardial constriction, the ECG is frequently abnormal, with low voltage being common. Interatrial block demonstrated by a wide P wave is common. An RV strain pattern may present with right-axis deviation. In chronic constriction, myocardial calcification and fibrosis can affect coronary perfusion and the conduction system. Stress tests in patients with pericardial constriction can produce a "false-positive" result, with ECG changes due to myocardial calcification and fibrosis rather than to typical coronary artery disease. Atrial arrhythmias, especially fibrillation, are common. In pericardial tamponade, nonspecific findings such as P-R depression, S-T elevation, and low voltage may be seen. When the pericardial effusion is large, the heart may swing within the pericardium, producing an electrical alternans that primarily affects the QRS and not the T waves. Atrial arrhythmias are common.

In pericardial constriction, chest x-ray findings may reveal a normal or only modestly enlarged cardiac silhouette. However, in pericardial tamponade (particularly when a large effusion is present) the chest radiography can be very useful, demonstrating clear lung fields with evidence of a markedly enlarged cardiac silhouette (water-bottle heart). Identification of the cardiac fat pad may reveal that the cardiac enlargement is from an increase in the extracardiac space. The superior vena cava and the azygous veins may be dilated also.

Doppler Echocardiography
Constrictive Pericarditis

Doppler echocardiography studies can help confirm or refute the diagnosis of constrictive pericarditis. Before considering constrictive pericarditis as the definitive diagnosis, other causes of right-sided heart failure, such as LV dysfunction, pulmonary hypertension, mitral valve disease, or congenital heart disease must be ruled out. The three major echocardiographic findings seen in constrictive pericarditis are the septal bounce, the ventricular septal shift with respiration, and the lack of significant atrial enlargement (a hallmark of restrictive cardiomyopathy) (Table 36-4). The rapid filling that occurs in early diastole does not occur at the same time in both the right and left ventricles and can result in an abrupt bounce or notch in the interventricular septal motion. Inspiration also causes a shift of the interventricular septum toward the left ventricle because of ventricular interdependence. Expiration results in a septal shift back toward the right ventricle. It is important to note that echocardiography is an insensitive method for measuring pericardial thickness and the absence of a thickened pericardium by echocardiography does not rule out the diagnosis of pericardial constriction.

The mitral inflow Doppler can be particularly valuable for distinguishing pericardial constriction from other entities. In healthy patients, there is a concurrent drop in the LA and LV pressures with inspiration and, thus, no change in the mitral inflow velocities with inspiration is seen. In most patients with constrictive pericarditis, inspiration results in a greater reduction in LA pressure than in the LV minimal pressure and the mitral flow gradient is reduced. In patients with severe constrictive pericarditis, this reduction in mitral flow velocity is often lost

because there is little change in either the LV minimal pressure or the LA pressure. This lack of an effect of inspiration on mitral flow velocity is due to the fact that diastolic pressures are operative on the steeper portion of the pericardial pressure–volume curve, which is already compromised in severe constriction. In severe instances of constriction, the respiratory variation is thus preload-dependent and the inspiratory changes can be reinstituted by having the patient assume the upright posture or by means of diuresis.

In constrictive pericarditis, there is also an exaggerated variation in the velocity of the early diastolic filling between the two ventricles with respiration. With inspiration, the tricuspid valve velocity E increases as the right ventricle fills and the mitral valve E velocity decreases. The same changes can be seen in the pulmonary venous flow pattern, with reciprocal changes in the hepatic venous flow. As described earlier, one also expects mitral flow velocities to demonstrate a high initial E velocity, a short deceleration of the initial flow, and a reduced atrial contraction velocity. In addition, if a tricuspid regurgitation jet is present (and can be evaluated by Doppler as a surrogate for RV pressures) the RV systolic pressure can be observed to increase in late inspiration in constrictive pericarditis rather than decrease, as would be expected normally. These findings are summarized in Table 36-4 and compared to those expected in cardiac tamponade.

Cardiac Tamponade

Two-dimensional echocardiography is critical to the diagnosis of pericardial tamponade, because it confirms the presence of a pericardial effusion. An echo-free space must be demonstrated and differentiated from epicardial fat. In large effusions, the heart may swing within the pericardial fluid, correlating with electrical alternans on the ECG. Systolic function is preserved. During inspiration, the aortic valve may demonstrate early closure and the LV ejection time may decrease from the inspiratory reduction in the LV stroke volume. With tamponade, there is evidence of a reduced RV diameter (usually <7 mm) and early diastolic RV collapse. RV collapse is most marked in expiration, during which time RV

Table 36-4
Comparison of the Doppler Echocardiography Findings in Constrictive Pericarditis Versus Cardiac Tamponade

Constrictive Pericarditis	Cardiac Tamponade
Pericardial effusion small or not present	Pericardial effusion evident and often large
Atria normal in size	Atria demonstrate free wall collapse
Right ventricle normal in size. Septal shift occasionally noted with inspiration.	Right ventricle (especially outflow) may demonstrate free wall collapse. Septal shift with inspiration common.
Distinct interventricular septal bounce in early ventricular diastole	No interventricular septal bounce
Mitral valve motion usually normal	Delayed mitral valve opening and reduced E-F slope of mitral opening. Aortic valve may close prematurely.
With inspiration, LVET normal or slightly shortened and RVET prolonged	With inspiration, LVET shortened and RVET prolonged
Mitral valve E wave initially high with short deceleration and reduced "A" wave	Mitral valve E wave height usually blunted
With inspiration or sniff, IVC does not decrease >50% in diameter	Similarly, with inspiration or sniff, IVC does not decrease >50% in diameter
With inspiration, >25% decline in mitral valve E wave height	Similarly, with inspiration, >25% decline in mitral valve E wave height
With inspiration, RV pressure may rise (as noted on tricuspid regurgitation jet, if present)	With inspiration, RV systolic pressure may fall normally or rise modestly
With inspiration, tricuspid valve E wave increases >40% and mitral valve E wave decreases	Similarly, with inspiration, tricuspid valve E wave increases >40% and mitral valve E wave decreases
With inspiration, hepatic vein flow increases and pulmonary vein flow decreases	Similarly, with inspiration, hepatic vein flow increases and pulmonary vein flow decreases

IVC indicates inferior vena cava; LVET, left ventricular ejection time; RV, right ventricular; RVET, right ventricular ejection time.

volume is reduced. The duration of RV collapse is directly related to the pericardial pressure. RV collapse is a more sensitive and specific marker of tamponade physiology than right atrial collapse. The right atrial free wall often shows late diastolic collapse lasting at least one third of the cardiac cycle. Occasionally, the LA free wall is also indented. The superior and inferior vena cava diameters are usually greater than 2.2 cm, and these diameters collapse less than 50% with inspiration or during a brief sniff (the patient is asked to sniff to increase negative inspiratory pressure). The inspiratory increase in the RV size, the septal shift, the reduced LV size, the delayed mitral valve opening, and the decreased mitral E-F slope reflect the hemodynamic changes that characterize pericardial tamponade.

Doppler studies similarly reflect the flow variation that occurs with respiration. Many of these changes in flow are similar to those seen in constrictive pericarditis, including a greater than 25% variation in the peak E wave with inspiration (decreased mitral inflow and increased tricuspid inflow). These reciprocal changes with respiration are also seen in the respective pulmonary venous flow or mitral annular movements (tissue Doppler) and in the hepatic venous flows. The hepatic venous flow may also demonstrate marked atrial reversal of flow with expiration. The LV ejection time may decrease and the RV ejection time may increase during inspiration, again documenting the expected respiratory changes between the ventricles.

Computed Tomography and Magnetic Resonance Imaging

Constrictive Pericarditis

Thickening of the pericardium may help confirm pericardial disease and constriction, but constrictive physiology can clearly be present with minimal changes on CT or magnetic resonance imaging. When detected by CT or MRI, pericardial thickness is usually greater than 3 mm. Focal areas of thickening can also be identified by CT and/or MRI. A significant number of patients with surgically-documented pericardial constriction do not have pericardial thickening by CT or MRI. Thus, the absence of observed thickening by CT or MRI should not rule out constriction if other compelling findings are present. Magnetic resonance imaging has the advantage of not requiring contrast media or x-ray radiation. Neither modality can yet identify respiratory differences because of the need for temporal averaging of the images and breath holding. Calcification, present in about 25% of cases, is useful, but it is not a sensitive measure. Electron beam and multislice CT may be more sensitive to pericardial calcium than chest radiography or standard CT methods are, although the specificity of these newer methods is not resolved.

Cardiac Tamponade

Neither chest CT nor cardiac magnetic resonance imaging provides additional information that is not available from Doppler echocardiography for the diagnosis of cardiac tamponade. Both studies can confirm the presence of an effusion. From an etiologic standpoint, both studies provide additional data about the involvement of contiguous structures, enlarged lymph nodes, lung lesions, evidence for pleural involvement, and so forth, that may help determine the cause of the pericardial effusion.

Cardiac Catheterization

Constrictive Pericarditis

The hemodynamics of constrictive pericarditis were described earlier in this chapter (see Table 36-2; Fig. 36-4). It is important to track all right-sided heart pressures versus the left-sided heart pressures and to note any respiratory changes in systolic and diastolic pressures. Right-sided heart catheterization by itself is inadequate for diagnosing pericardial disease. Observations to be made at cardiac catheterization include nearly equal levels of end-diastolic pressure in all chambers, relatively normal or only slightly elevated pulmonary pressures with a normal pulmonary vascular resistance, a discrepancy of less than 5 mm Hg between the LVEDP and the RVEDP, a positive Kussmaul's sign in the right atrium, the classic square-root (dip and plateau) pattern in the atrial and diastolic ventricular waveforms, and discordant peak systolic RV and LV pressures with inspiration (the RV pressure rising and the LV pressure falling with inspiration). The RVEDP is usually greater than one third the RV systolic pressure. A paradoxical pulse is unusual. In significant constriction, the nadir of the ventricular pressures usually approaches zero. At times, rapid fluid loading is required to reveal the constrictive physiology in patients with hypovolemia. In addition, a right atrial angiogram in the anteroposterior view may reveal a cardiac "peel" or thickening at the interface of the right atrial free wall and the lung fields. Similarly, contrast angiography of the coronary arteries may reveal a "peel" or a radiographic shadow between the coronary arteries and the lung fields. Portions of the coronaries may appear frozen in the pericardium during cardiac motion.

Cardiac Tamponade

In cardiac tamponade, the expected findings include marked elevation in the atrial and ventricular diastolic pressures, loss of the y descent in the atrial tracings, no Kussmaul's sign (in general), blunting of the early diastolic filling pressures in the ventricles, normal pulmonary pressure and pulmonary resistance, equalization of the diastolic pressures, and a paradoxical pulse. On fluoroscopy, the heart may be observed to swing within the pericardial sac. When the issue of mixed disease (i.e., effusive-constrictive disease) is present, pericardiocentesis may remove the tamponade component and reveal the underlying constrictive physiology.

FUTURE DIRECTIONS

Advances in the diagnosis of pericardial diseases range from the use of magnetic resonance imaging and CT to diagnose pericardial thickness to the development of sensitive Doppler echocardiographic approaches to diagnose hemodynamic compromise in pericardial pathology. However, the diagnosis of more subtle presentations, whether differentiation of recurrent pericarditis from chronic pain syndromes or differentiating constrictive pericarditis from restrictive cardiomyopathy, is still challenging. It is estimated that more than 10% of patients with presumed constrictive pericarditis who undergo surgery are found to have a normal pericardium. As cardiovascular imaging techniques advance and noninvasive assessment of cardiovascular hemodynamics improves, it is hoped that the diagnosis of pericardial diseases and their sequelae will become more accurate.

REFERENCES

Breen JF. Imaging of the pericardium. *J Thorac Imaging* 2001;16:47–54.

Hancock EW. Differential diagnosis of restrictive cardiomyopathy and constrictive pericarditis. *Heart* 2001;86: 343–349.

Klodas E, Nishimura RA, Appleton CP, Redfield MM, Oh JK. Doppler evaluation of patients with constrictive pericarditis: Use of tricuspid regurgitation velocity curves to determine enhanced ventricular interaction. *J Am Coll Cardiol* 1996;28:652–657.

Myers RBH, Spodick DH. Constrictive pericarditis: Clinical and pathophysiologic characteristics. *Am Heart J* 1999;138:219–232.

Nishimura RA. Constrictive pericarditis in the modern era: A diagnostic dilemma. *Heart* 2001;86:619–623.

Oh JK, Tajik AJ, Appleton CP, Hatle LK, Nishimura RA, Seward JB. Preload reduction to unmask the characteristic Doppler features of constrictive pericarditis: A new observation. *Circulation* 1997;95:796–799.

Schutzman JJ, Obarski TP, Pearce GL, Klein AL. Comparison of Doppler and two-dimensional echocardiography for assessment of pericardial effusion. *Am J Cardiol* 1992;70:1353–1357.

Spodick DH. Pericardial diseases. In: Braunwald E, Zipes DP, Libby P, eds. *Heart Disease.* 6th ed. Philadelphia: WB Saunders; 2001:1823–1876.

Section VII

VASCULAR DISEASES

Chapter 37

Angiogenesis and Atherosclerosis

Cam Patterson

Revascularization via coronary artery bypass surgery and percutaneous coronary interventions (PCIs) remains the definitive therapy for patients with refractory ischemic heart disease, particularly when accompanied by left ventricular (LV) dysfunction. Bypass surgery in particular improves mortality in patients with multivessel coronary artery disease and LV dysfunction. However, it is invasive and is associated with significant mortality and morbidity. In addition, many patients are poor candidates for bypass based on their coronary anatomy, coexisting conditions, or the severity of their heart failure. Likewise, anatomic complications may make PCIs such as balloon angioplasty and stent implantation a poor choice for many of these patients. An alternative means of revascularization is needed. The identification of endogenous pathways that regulate angiogenesis—the growth of new blood vessels from existing vessels—would mean that these same pathways could be used to augment blood vessel formation to revascularize tissues in myocardial ischemic zones.

MECHANISMS OF ANGIOGENESIS

Angiogenesis occurs by the budding of new blood vessels from existing vessels (Fig. 37-1). Inflammation and hypoxia are the two major stimuli for new vessel growth. Hypoxia regulates angiogenesis predominantly by activating a transcription factor, hypoxia-inducible factor-1, which activates the angiogenesis gene expression program. Inflammation stimulates angiogenesis mainly by the secretion of inflammatory cytokines derived primarily from macrophages. In either event, the result is production of vascular endothelial growth factor (VEGF) and other potent angiogenic peptides. VEGF interacts with specific receptors on endothelial cells that, in turn, activate pathways to break down the extracellular matrix, proliferate, migrate toward an angiogenic stimulus, and recruit pericytes and smooth muscle cells to establish the three-dimensional structure of a blood vessel. After making appropriate connections with the vascular system, the newly formed vessel is capable of maintaining blood flow and providing oxygen to the tissue in need.

Angiogenesis occurs in numerous circumstances. During development, the formation of every organ system is dependent on angiogenic events; in fact, the cardiovascular system is the first organ system to function during embryogenesis. In adults, the menstrual cycle is dependent on cyclical angiogenesis that is stimulated in part by reproductive hormones. Beyond this, however, most angiogenesis in adults occurs in pathologic conditions or as a response to injury. Tumor growth and metastasis, diabetic vascular disease (including retinopathy), inflammatory arthritides, and wound healing are some of the processes that depend on angiogenesis. In addition, the invasion of ischemic tissues with new capillaries and the development of a collateral circulation to supply occluded vessels, as may occur in chronic obstructive coronary disease, are angiogenic processes (see angiogram in Fig. 37-2).

ANGIOGENESIS AND ATHEROSCLEROSIS

The response to ischemia in organs such as the heart involves angiogenic events that increase perfusion to the compromised tissue; thus, it is ironic that atherosclerosis (the most common cause of myocardial ischemia) is itself an angiogenesis-dependent process. The media of blood vessels remains avascular until a critical width is achieved, beyond which vascularization is necessary for medial nutrition. Increased medial blood flow in atherosclerotic lesions is due to new growth of medial vessels rather than to dilation of existing vessels. New vessels in atherosclerotic lesions form primarily by branching from the adventitial vasa vasorum. The possibility that neovascularization contributes to the pathophysiology of atherosclerosis surfaced

Figure 37-1

Mechanisms of Angiogenesis

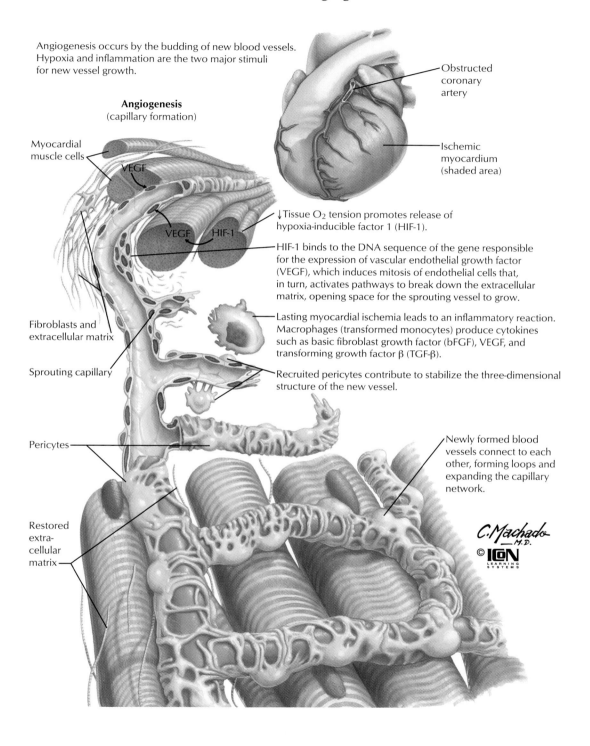

Angiogenesis occurs by the budding of new blood vessels.
Hypoxia and inflammation are the two major stimuli
for new vessel growth.

Angiogenesis
(capillary formation)

Obstructed
coronary
artery

Myocardial
muscle cells

VEGF

Ischemic
myocardium
(shaded area)

VEGF   HIF-1

↓Tissue O_2 tension promotes release of
hypoxia-inducible factor 1 (HIF-1).

HIF-1 binds to the DNA sequence of the gene responsible
for the expression of vascular endothelial growth factor
(VEGF), which induces mitosis of endothelial cells that,
in turn, activates pathways to break down the extracellular
matrix, opening space for the sprouting vessel to grow.

Fibroblasts and
extracellular matrix

Lasting myocardial ischemia leads to an inflammatory reaction.
Macrophages (transformed monocytes) produce cytokines
such as basic fibroblast growth factor (bFGF), VEGF, and
transforming growth factor β (TGF-β).

Sprouting capillary

Recruited pericytes contribute to stabilize the three-dimensional
structure of the new vessel.

Pericytes

Newly formed blood
vessels connect to each
other, forming loops and
expanding the capillary
network.

Restored
extra-
cellular
matrix

C. Machado
M.D.
© ICON
LEARNING
SYSTEMS

Figure 37-2

Mechanisms of Arteriogenesis and Development of Collateral Vessels

Stenotic coronary artery

The presence of a significant stenotic lesion in a coronary artery increases the blood flow in the low-resistance peripheral arteriolar network that connects the pre- and poststenosis segments of the given artery. This leads to elevation of blood shear stress against the wall of the arterioles, triggering the development of collateral vessels.

Myocardium supplied by the branches of the stenotic artery

Stages of the development of collateral vessels

Arteriole

Fluid shear stress

MCP-1

ICAM-1

GM-CSF

EC

1st stage: Endothelial cells (EC) activated by augmented shear stress express on their surface monocyte chemoattractant protein 1 (MCP-1), intercellular adhesion molecule 1 (ICAM-1), and macrophage colony-stimulating factor (GM-CSF).

2nd stage: Monocytes adhere to the endothelial cell surface

3rd stage: Monocytes become macrophages and produce fibronectin, proteoglycans, vascular growth factors, and proteases that digest the extra-cellular matrix. Platelets also adhere to the vascular wall and release interleukin 4 (IL-4), which stimulates adhesion molecules.

IL-4

SMC

Myocardium

5th stage: To open space for the growing collateral vessels, macrophages and lympho-cytes attracted to the site attack and destroy the myocardium and the extracellular matrix

4th stage: Vascular growth factors produced by the macrophages initiate mitosis of smooth muscle cells (SMC) and endothelial cells. At this point, the walls of the vessel during the remodeling process become considerably thinner and leaky.

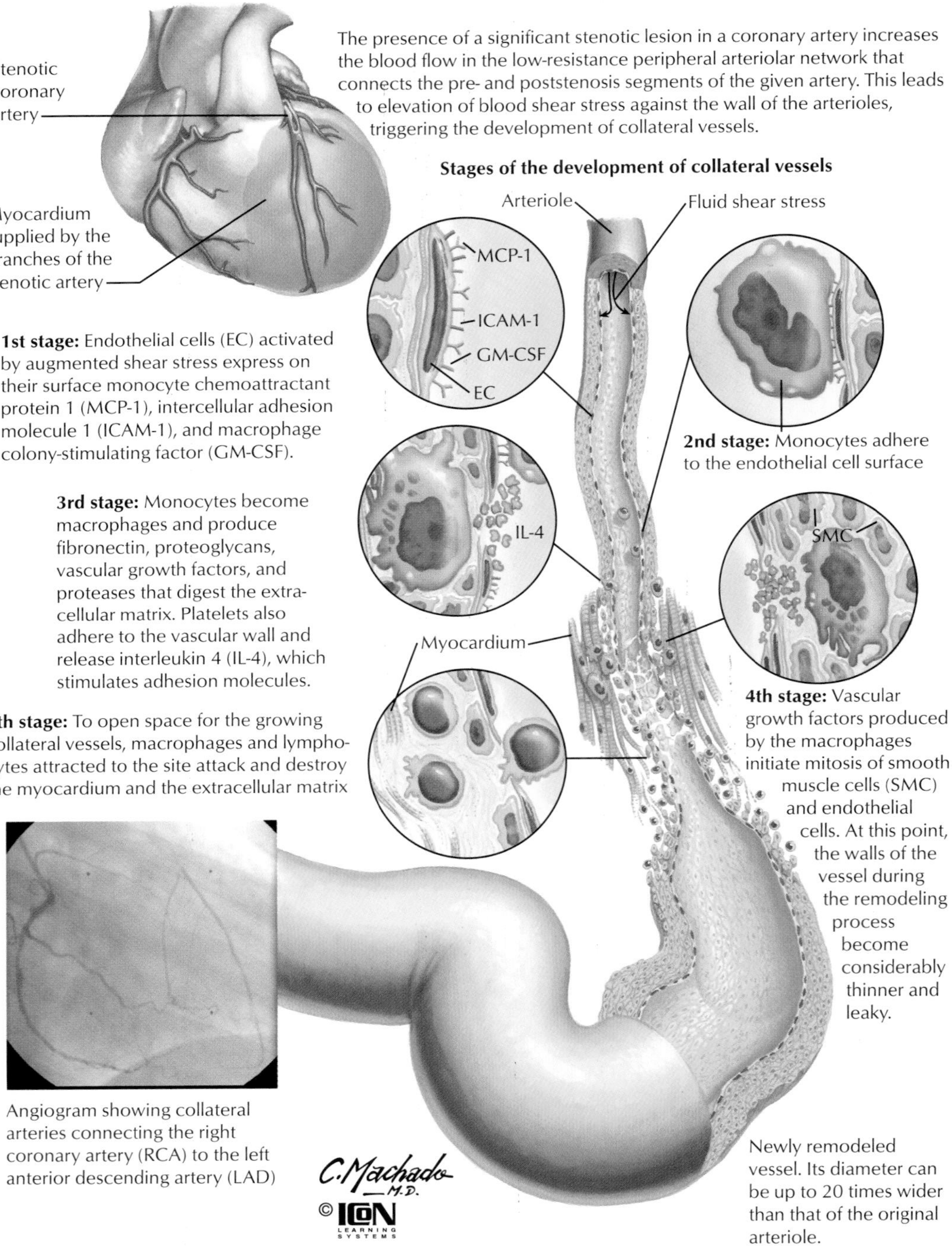

Angiogram showing collateral arteries connecting the right coronary artery (RCA) to the left anterior descending artery (LAD)

C. Machado
M.D.

© ICON
LEARNING
SYSTEMS

Newly remodeled vessel. Its diameter can be up to 20 times wider than that of the original arteriole.

when cinefluorography demonstrated the presence of rich networks of vessels surrounding human atherosclerotic plaques.

Neovascularization may contribute to the clinical consequences of atherosclerosis by several mechanisms. Neovascularization provides a source of nutrients, growth factors, and vasoactive molecules to cells within the media and the neointima, which is evident from the association between neovascularization of atherosclerotic lesions and proliferation of adjacent smooth muscle cells. Intimal hemorrhage, associated with plaque instability, is due to rupture of the rich network of friable new capillaries surrounding lesions. Regulation of blood flow through plaque microvessels may contribute to the pathophysiology of vasospasm in advanced lesions. Vascular wall remodeling also seems to be related to neovascularization. Finally, neovascularization within human atherosclerotic lesions is associated with expression of adhesion molecules, which is strongly related to neointimal inflammatory cell recruitment.

ANGIOGENESIS AND ISCHEMIC HEART DISEASE

Refractory coronary ischemia, particularly in patients with decreased LV function who may not be candidates for revascularization, remains a difficult clinical problem. Recognition of angiogenesis as an endogenous mechanism for perfusion of ischemic tissues raises the possibility that angiogenic factors in general, and VEGF in particular, might be therapeutic tools for patients with refractory ischemia. VEGF gene therapy may induce angiogenesis and improve perfusion in a wide spectrum of ischemia models. Angiogenesis has seemed amenable to gene therapy approaches. New vessel growth is a process that occurs over weeks to months (precluding single-dose therapies), but after new vessels form, they are not likely to regress if they are conduit vessels; therefore, long-term therapy is not necessary. Gene delivery by plasmids and adenoviruses occurs within this "angiogenic window," raising hope for angiogenic gene therapies in chronic ischemic syndromes.

Gene therapy approaches to deliver VEGF in patients with ischemic coronary and peripheral vascular diseases have progressed rapidly. The use of angiogenic gene therapy has tremendous potential for patients with refractory ischemic heart disease who otherwise have no options. Because angiogenesis is a new mechanism for treating this disease, it should be additive to the effects of pharmacologic agents (β blockers, aspirin, and nitrates). The possibility of the creation of new, long-lived conduit vessels raises the possibility of a "cure" because the new vessels should provide relief long after the effects of VEGF or other angiogenic factors have dissipated.

However, it is not yet clear that angiogenesis, which predominantly involves the formation of new capillaries, creates vessels with the capacity to significantly increase blood flow to ischemic tissues. Uncontrolled capillary growth may cause hemangioma formation, which would not be beneficial and might well be deleterious. Few data are available that allow prediction of the appropriate dose, location, and duration of angiogenic gene therapy. In therapy for myocardial ischemia, required invasive approaches are associated with appreciable morbidity. Despite predictions of side effects based on diseases with known angiogenic components, little is known about side effects of angiogenic therapies in humans. Of greatest concern is the possibility that angiogenic therapies will accelerate or unmask occult tumors or metastases, as it is well known that tumor growth is an angiogenesis-dependent process. Worsening diabetic neovascular complications, especially diabetic retinopathy, are also a concern, given the prevalence of diabetes in patients with severe atherosclerotic disease.

Early clinical trials in angiogenesis have produced results that are variably interpreted, depending on the views of those reviewing these studies. Small, but statistically significant, improvements in pain-free exercise duration have been demonstrated in angiogenesis trials involving the coronary vasculature (with chest pain as the limiting symptom) as well as the peripheral vasculature (in patients with limiting claudication). These data support the concept of clinical angiogenesis. An opposing view is that these studies are far from demonstrating an important clinical benefit because the improvements are modest, and to date no studies have shown an effect on mortality or major morbidity.

Still under investigation are whether this is an effective approach, how and when to apply angiogenic agents, and the possible side effects of angiogenic stimulants. Long-term studies are necessary to definitively exclude adverse consequences such as tumor promotion.

VASCULOGENESIS AND ARTERIOGENESIS: ALTERNATIVES TO ANGIOGENESIS

New vessel growth in chronic ischemic syndromes is an attractive idea. Fortunately, more than one mechanism exists to create new blood vessels. Angiogenesis is the creation of blood vessels from sprouts off existing vessels. In contrast, vasculogenesis is the creation of blood vessels de novo by differentiation of new blood cells. Endothelial cell precursors in the bone marrow and circulating in the blood stream can incorporate into developing vessels and contribute to vessel growth in a manner very similar to the vasculogenesis of embryonic development. The therapeutic potential of these cells has not been tested, but they can be recruited from bone marrow and may be a means to accelerate endogenous revascularization in patients with ischemia.

In contrast to angiogenesis, arteriogenesis is the recruitment of existing vessels to increase their capacity and consequent blood flow to ischemic tissue (Fig. 37-2). In a sense, arteriogenesis represents the maturation of vessels that exist but may not contribute significantly to regional blood flow until properly stimulated. Most collateral vessels visualized by arteriography are likely to represent vessels that have undergone arteriogenesis rather than angiogenesis. Because arteriogenesis creates capacitance vessels, this process is more likely to increase blood supply in a way that substantially affects tissue perfusion. Interestingly, the proteins that affect arteriogenesis are distinct from those that regulate angiogenesis—VEGF does not seem to be important for arteriogenesis, whereas macrophage-derived factors are necessary. The therapeutic potential of arteriogenesis has not been tested, but given the role of arteriogenesis in collateral formation in patients with chronic myocardial ischemia, this represents another potential therapeutic tool for the creation of new blood vessels in patients with refractory angina.

FUTURE DIRECTIONS

Despite the range of therapies for patients with coronary atherosclerosis, there is still a large population that is not adequately treated. Many of these patients have severe LV dysfunction from ischemic disease, and, either because of coronary anatomy or because of other comorbidities, are not good candidates for revascularization. The creation of new blood vessels to increase tissue perfusion is one way to alleviate myocardial ischemia. The challenge is to determine the best way to increase tissue perfusion with minimal side effects. Angiogenic agents such as VEGF have the lead in drug development, although their overall benefit remains unproven. It is likely that other therapies designed to stimulate vasculogenesis and arteriogenesis will be evaluated for this patient population. Treatments designed to enhance blood vessel growth are being tested on patients with otherwise refractory disease, but eventually, these approaches could be applied to any patient with ischemic heart disease and could even obviate the need for revascularization procedures in a significant cohort of patients.

REFERENCES

Asahara T, Murohara T, Sullivan A, et al. Isolation of putative progenitor endothelial cells for angiogenesis. *Science* 1997;275:964–967.

Barger AC, Beeuwkes R, Lainey LL, Silverman KJ. Hypothesis: Vasa vasorum and neovascularization of human coronary arteries. *N Engl J Med* 1984;310:175–177.

Folkman J. Angiogenesis in cancer, vascular, rheumatoid and other disease. *Nature Med* 1995;1:27–31.

Freedman SB, Isner J. Therapeutic angiogenesis for coronary artery disease. *Ann Intern Med* 2002;136:54–71.

Koestner W. Endarteritis and arteritis. *Berl Klin Wochenschr* 1876;13:454–455.

O'Brien KD, McDonald TO, Chait A, Allen MD, Alpers CE. Neovascular expression of E-selectin, intercellular adhesion molecule-1, and vascular cell adhesion molecule-1 in human atherosclerosis and their relation to intimal leukocyte content. *Circulation* 1996;93:672–682.

Schaper W. Arteriogenesis, the good and bad of it. *Cardiovasc Res* 1999;43:835–837.

Shweiki D, Itin A, Soffer D, Keshet E. Vascular endothelial growth factor induced by hypoxia may mediate hypoxia-initiated angiogenesis. *Nature* 1992;359:843–845.

Chapter 38

Diagnostic Techniques in Vascular Disease

Alan L. Hinderliter and Walter A. Tan

Peripheral arterial diseases encompass a spectrum of disorders that compromise tissue perfusion and result in ischemia. Two principal morphologic changes can affect blood vessels: stenoses and aneurysms. Although arteriography is the traditional diagnostic gold standard for evaluation and offers superior spatial resolution, particularly for small vessels, angiographic techniques are invasive and offer limited information about the vessel wall and adjacent tissues and organs. Noninvasive methods have assumed an increasingly important role in the assessment of vascular disease. This chapter reviews diagnostic techniques used to evaluate the most commonly encountered occlusive and aneurysmal clinical disorders—stenoses of the carotid, renal, and lower extremity arteries and aneurysms of the abdominal aorta—and investigational imaging techniques used to assess atherosclerotic burden.

ETIOLOGY AND PATHOGENESIS

A wide range of pathologic processes can result in arterial occlusive disease. Most commonly, peripheral vascular disease is a manifestation of systemic atherosclerosis. Clinical manifestations depend on the location and severity of stenoses and the presence of collateral circulation. The pathogenesis of atherosclerosis is described in chapter 37.

LOWER EXTREMITY PERIPHERAL ARTERIAL DISEASE

Clinical Presentation

The prevalence of peripheral arterial disease depends on the age and characteristics of the cohort studied; population studies suggest that about 15% of patients older than 55 years of age have lower extremity arterial disease.

Symptoms of peripheral arterial disease of the lower extremity range from intermittent claudication—discomfort that develops with exercise and is relieved with rest—to pain at rest. Stenoses of the superficial femoral and popliteal arteries result in calf claudication, whereas disease of the distal aorta or iliac arteries may cause pain in the buttocks or thighs, as well as in the legs. Less than 20% of patients with symptomatic lower extremity arterial occlusive disease progress to critical leg ischemia, that is, ischemia that jeopardizes viability of the extremity. More importantly, the presence of peripheral vascular disease is evidence of systemic atherosclerosis and is associated with a threefold increased risk of cardiovascular mortality.

Diagnostic Approach

Evaluation of the lower extremity arterial circulation is designed to establish the presence of peripheral arterial disease, quantify the severity of disease, localize disease, and determine the temporal progression of disease.

Ankle–Brachial Index

With increasingly severe arterial stenoses, there is a progressive decrease in SBP distal to the occlusive lesion. This decrease in BP can be quantified and localized using pneumatic cuffs and either continuous wave Doppler or plethysmographic sensors. The ankle–brachial index (ABI) is determined by measuring SBP in the tibial and brachial arteries. Normally, SBP is amplified in the distal limb by pulse-wave reflection, and the ABI exceeds 1. An ABI of 0.80 to 0.90 is considered to be mildly diminished; 0.50 to 0.80, moderately diminished; and less than 0.50, severely diminished.

The ABI is a valuable office screening tool. A severely decreased ABI identifies an individual at high risk of death or development of critical limb ischemia and at increased risk of cardiovascular morbidity. The value of this index is limited in patients with diabetes mellitus, in whom calcification of the tibial and peroneal arteries develops and may render them noncompressible.

Segmental Pressure Measurements

Measuring pressures at multiple levels along the leg can estimate the location of an arterial occlusion. Cuffs are usually placed on the upper and lower thighs, as well as on the upper and lower calves. A gradient greater than 10 to 15 mm Hg between adjacent sites suggests physiologically significant stenosis. Pressure measurements after treadmill exercise may unmask hemodynamically significant disease that is inapparent on resting studies.

Duplex Ultrasonography

Duplex ultrasonography, using imaging and Doppler waveform analysis, is an accurate method for defining arterial lesion location and severity. Although atherosclerotic plaques can be identified on B-mode images, the resolution is insufficient to quantify the degree of narrowing. Significant arterial stenoses alter the pattern of flow velocity as assessed by continuous wave Doppler, and a change in the flow velocity waveform—an increase in peak systolic velocity at the site of the lesion, turbulence, loss of the reverse flow component, or a decrease in pulse velocity distal to the lesion—is diagnostic of a flow-limiting lesion. Color Doppler imaging identifies the arteries of interest and provides a rough index of disease severity. Critical (>50%) stenoses are characterized by poststenotic turbulence on color imaging (Fig. 38-1) and a doubling of the peak systolic velocity by continuous wave Doppler.

Computed Tomographic or Magnetic Resonance Angiography

Noninvasive contrast-based imaging of arteries has improved, though the diagnostic accuracy still lags behind other methods in most centers, with higher false-positive rates observed. Other disadvantages include availability, cost, and, for computed tomographic angiography (CTA), the necessity for iodinated contrast injection. Visualization of smaller vessels is still inferior to arteriography. Finally, patient factors such as claustrophobia, inability to cooperate (motion during image acquisition), or the presence of incompat-

ible metallic prostheses occasionally limit applicability of these methods (Fig. 38-2).

Lower Extremity Arteriography With Runoff

This invasive test is performed when revascularization is indicated. Detailed anatomic information is needed, including lesion length, presence of total occlusions, collateral flow, and the vessel "outflow" or runoff to the calves and feet. These are critical in determining feasibility or futility of revascularization and for planning the type of procedure (bypass grafting, angioplasty and stenting, or both).

CAROTID ARTERY DISEASE
Clinical Presentation

Close to 700,000 new or recurrent strokes occur each year in the United States, and approximately 4.6 million stroke survivors are alive today. However, stroke is a leading cause of disability, with roughly one of every five victims requiring institutional care. An important cause of preventable stroke is large-vessel or carotid atherosclerosis, which may account for 15 to 20% of ischemic strokes.

Patients with cerebrovascular disease may present with an asymptomatic bruit, a transient ischemic attack, or a stroke. The risk of stroke increases with greater degrees of carotid plaque burden, particularly for those with recent ischemic neurological events. The 5-year stroke risk in these patients can be as high as 35%. However, despite the availability of multiple natural history studies of asymptomatic carotid lesions, it is still difficult to predict which patients will have a neurological event, with or without antiplatelet therapy.

Diagnostic Approach

The goal of evaluation of the carotid arteries is to define the location, laterality, and extent of carotid disease.

Duplex Ultrasonography

The mainstay of noninvasive assessment of carotid disease is duplex ultrasonography. The combination of two-dimensional ultrasound imaging and Doppler interrogation is a safe, convenient, and accurate means of localizing and determining the hemodynamic significance

Figure 38-1

Types of Arterial Noninvasive Tests

Characteristics of normal arterial examination

Pulsatile, laminar flow pattern

Normal waveform analysis

Systolic | Diastolic

Systolic forward flow

Diastolic forward flow

Flow reversal due to high resistance of vascular bed

Pulsatility index

Frequency

Time

A

B

A

0

Normal triphase Doppler velocity waveform. Flow direction varies with cardiac cycle. Pulsatility index derived by dividing the peak-to-peak frequency by mean forward frequency.

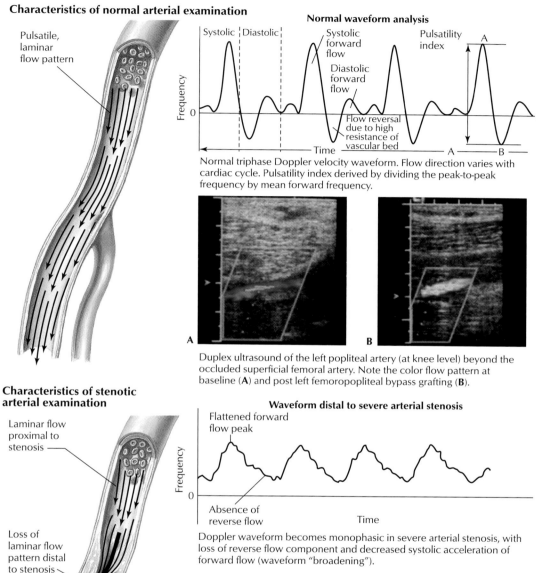

A   B

Duplex ultrasound of the left popliteal artery (at knee level) beyond the occluded superficial femoral artery. Note the color flow pattern at baseline (**A**) and post left femoropopliteal bypass grafting (**B**).

Characteristics of stenotic arterial examination

Laminar flow proximal to stenosis

Loss of laminar flow pattern distal to stenosis with turbulence

High-jet velocity

JOHN A. CRAIG—MD

C. Machado—M.D.

© ICON

Waveform distal to severe arterial stenosis

Flattened forward flow peak

Frequency

Absence of reverse flow

Time

0

Doppler waveform becomes monophasic in severe arterial stenosis, with loss of reverse flow component and decreased systolic acceleration of forward flow (waveform "broadening").

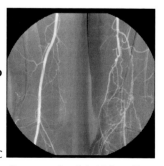
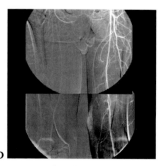

C   D

Corresponding left thigh and knee arteriograms at baseline (**C**) and post left femoropopliteal bypass grafting (**D**).

Figure 38-2   **Diagnostic Techniques in Vascular Disease**

MRA angiography

CT angiography

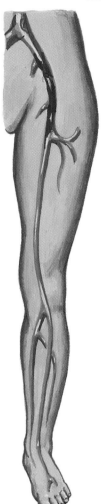

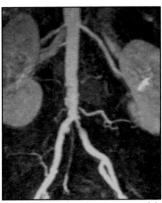

Angiography showing stenosis of the
left proximal iliac artery

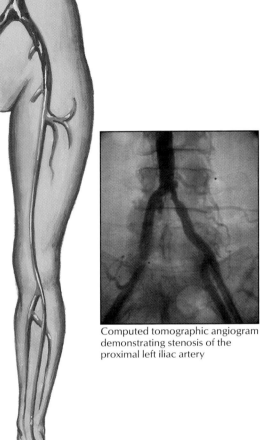

Computed tomographic angiogram
demonstrating stenosis of the
proximal left iliac artery

of carotid lesions. However, the sensitivity and specificity of this approach is lessened in patients with increased carotid wall calcification and/or subocclusive stenoses, and in the hands of less experienced operators (Fig. 38-3).

*Computed Tomographic
or Magnetic Resonance Angiography*

Advantages of these noninvasive imaging techniques include the capacity to visualize the aortic arch, as well as the brachiocephalic trunks

and intracranial arteries (see previous section).

Four-Vessel Cerebral Arteriography

This invasive procedure can provide additional details to influence the decision to proceed with surgery. Two angiographic subsets in a large randomized clinical trial derived significantly greater benefit from endarterectomy instead of drug therapy alone—those with either ulcerative lesions or those with synchronous intracranial artery stenoses. Both occur in 20 to

Figure 38-3

Noninvasive Evaluation of Carotid Arteries
Duplex Ultrasound Evaluation of the
Carotid Arteries in a Patient With Significant
but Asymptomatic Right Carotid Artery Stenosis

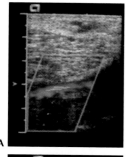

A

B

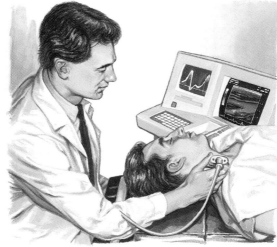

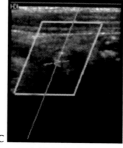

C

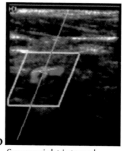

D

Duplex ultrasound of the left carotid artery that did not have significant narrowing: (**A**) proximal common carotid, (**B**) external carotid, (**C**) mid-internal carotid segments

Duplex (B-mode and Doppler) and color Doppler studies are used to evaluate extracranial carotid arterial circulation.

Severe right internal carotid artery stenosis (**D**)

Normal left carotid artery

Doppler flow waveform analysis

Stenotic right carotid artery

External carotid (ECA)

Spike

0

Normal
Pulsatile triphasic high resistance waveform

0

Stenotic
Monophasic, Dopplered waveform

Internal carotid (ICA)

0

Normal
Low-resistance antegrade flow

0

Stenotic
High peak systolic velocity and spectral broading of waveform

Common carotid (CCA)

0

Normal
Common carotid combines flow pattern characteristics of ECA and ICA

Doppler studies detect waveform and velocity abnormalities characteristic of stenosis.

50% of patients with extracranial carotid disease and can be diagnosed best by angiography. Another limitation of other diagnostic methods is distinguishing between subtotal versus total occlusion. Patients who have even a small channel of flow through the internal carotid artery are still candidates for surgical or endovascular therapy, whereas complete occlusions are treated medically (see chapter 41). Finally, angiography provides superb delineation of collateral channels in the setting of occlusive disease.

RENAL ARTERY STENOSIS
Clinical Presentation
See chapter 40 for a discussion of clinical presentation.

Diagnostic Approach
The objectives of noninvasive evaluation of renovascular disease are to determine the location and severity of renal arterial lesions and to assess the functional significance of these stenoses.

Evaluation for renal artery stenosis should be based on the clinical index of suspicion of disease, as outlined in Table 38-1.

Captopril Renal Scan

In patients with functionally significant renal artery stenosis, high levels of angiotensin II maintain glomerular filtration and renal blood flow. Administration of captopril causes an abrupt decrease in filtration pressure in the ischemic kidney, resulting in reduced uptake of ^{99}Tc DTPA or delayed secretion of ^{131}I-hippurate or ^{99}Tc MAG$_3$. Captopril renography is an accurate diagnostic technique in patients with a moderate likelihood of renovascular hypertension and normal renal function, with sensitivities and specificities approaching 90%. It is less reliable, however, in patients with a creatinine concentration greater than 2.0 mg/dL or in patients with bilateral renal artery stenosis (Fig. 38-4).

Doppler Ultrasonography

In selected centers, use of Doppler ultrasonography for detection of changes in renal arterial flow characteristics and detection of significant renal arterial stenoses is a highly sensitive and specific technique. In addition, Doppler

Table 38-1
Testing for Renovascular Hypertension

Low Index of Suspicion (Should Not Be Tested)

· Stage 1 or 2 hypertension, in the absence of clinical clues

*Moderate Index of Suspicion
(Noninvasive Tests Should Be Considered)*

· Severe hypertension (DBP >120 mm Hg)
· Hypertension refractory to standard therapy
· Abrupt onset of sustained stage 2 or 3 hypertension at <20 years of age or >50 years of age
· Stage 2 or 3 hypertension with a suggestive abdominal or flank bruit
· Stage 2 or 3 hypertension in a patient with established vascular disease, unexplained increase in serum creatinine concentration, or history of tobacco use
· Normalization of BP by an ACE-inhibitor or an ARB in a patient with stage 2 or 3 hypertension (particularly a smoker or a patient with recent onset of hypertension)

*High Index of Suspicion
(May Consider Proceeding Directly to Arteriography)*

· Severe hypertension (DBP >120 mm Hg) with either progressive renal insufficiency or refractoriness to aggressive treatment (particularly in a patient with established vascular disease or a history of tobacco use)
· Accelerated or malignant hypertension
· Hypertension with recent increase of serum creatinine concentration, either unexplained or reversibly induced by an ACE-inhibitor or an ARB
· Stage 2 or 3 hypertension with incidentally detected asymmetry of renal size

ACE indicates angiotensin-converting enzyme; ARB, angiotensin II receptor blocker; DBP, diastolic blood pressure.

With permission from Mann SJ, Pickering TG. Detection of renovascular hypertension. State of the art: 1992. *Ann Intern Med* 1992; 117:845–853.

indices of structural alterations of the renal microvasculature (resistive index and pulsatility index) are predictors of the BP response to revascularization. Although technical advances have significantly enhanced the diagnostic accuracy of this technique, it remains operator dependent and is not sensitive in detecting disease in accessory renal arteries.

Figure 38-4

Abnormal Captopril Renal Scan
and Angiogram in a Patient With Renal Artery Stenosis

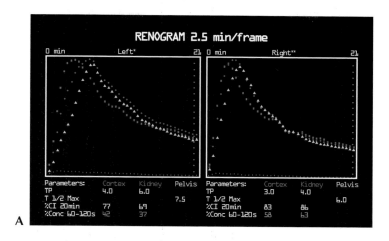

A

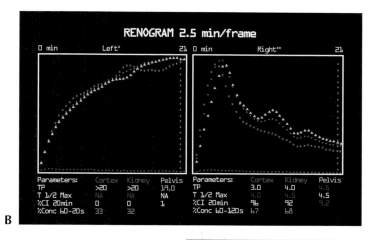

B

Uptake and excretion of ^{99m}Tc MAG$_3$, given IV, by the left and right kidney before (**A**), and after (**B**), oral administration of 50 mg of captopril. (**B**) Shows slow uptake and no excretion of the radiopharmaceutical, suggesting functionally significant stenosis of the left renal artery. (**C**) Shows a high-grade atherosclerotic stenosis of the left renal artery with poststenotic dilation in the same patient. The right renal artery is normal. Note the atherosclerotic changes of the abdominal aorta.

* Left kidney
** Right kidney

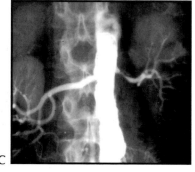

C

Magnetic Resonance Angiography

Gadolinium-enhanced magnetic resonance angiography (MRA) provides excellent images of the main renal arteries and perirenal aorta; however, evaluation of accessory arteries is less accurate. It is a useful technique in patients with mild renal insufficiency. Stents (for prior treatment of renal artery stenosis) result in significant imaging artifacts, essentially precluding the use of this technique.

Spiral Computed Tomographic Angiography

Spiral CTA visualizes the renal arteries and accessory vessels in three dimensions and is highly accurate in detecting anatomic stenoses. The large volume of contrast agent necessary for this technique, however, is potentially nephrotoxic and must be considered in patients with impaired renal function.

ABDOMINAL AORTIC ANEURYSMS

Clinical Presentation

Abdominal aortic aneurysm (AAA) rupture is an important cause of unheralded deaths in people older than 55 years. Although atherosclerotic changes accompany almost all AAAs, classic coronary risk factors seem to be less predictive for this disease, and abnormal collagen, elastin, matrix metalloproteinases, and inflammatory changes causing vessel wall weakness appear to have important contributory roles.

Diagnostic Approach

The best independent predictor of rupture rate is maximal aneurysm diameter. Elective surgical or endovascular treatment is therefore contingent on accurate measurements and is recommended for AAAs 5 cm or greater in diameter, or for aneurysms greater than 4 cm that are enlarging at a rate of 0.5 cm or more per year.

Ultrasonography

Two-dimensional ultrasonography is competitive with CT or MRI for the detection (>95% sensitivity) of an AAA. Ultrasonography availability and reproducibility make it an ideal method for serial follow-up. Obesity, excessive bowel gas, and recent abdominal surgery can limit examinations.

Computed Tomography and Magnetic Resonance Imaging

CT and MRI provide information about the wall of the aorta and delineate the presence of thrombus. They provide detail about surrounding abdominal structures and their relation to the AAA. The occasional finding of perianeurysmal fibrosis, venous anomalies (e.g., retroaortic left renal vein, circumaortic venous collar), or

horseshoe kidney is important for surgical planning. Additional helical or spiral CTA allows reasonable visualization of aortic branches in the context of surrounding structures.

Angiography

Digital subtraction angiography gives a high spatial resolution of the lumen of the vascular tree and defines aberrant vessels. However, it is a poor method for assessing AAA size because laminated or mural thrombus may give the false arteriographic impression of normal luminal diameter. Angiography may be important if mesenteric or renal artery stenosis is suspected.

NONINVASIVE ASSESSMENT OF ENDOTHELIAL DYSFUNCTION AND SUBCLINICAL ATHEROSCLEROTIC DISEASE

The traditional risk factors for atherosclerosis identified by the Framingham Study—age; history of diabetes mellitus, hyperlipidemia, hypertension, and/or tobacco use; and family history of premature coronary disease—can be used to predict an individual's risk of a cardiovascular event. Among those with similar risk profiles, however, there is a broad spectrum of disease. These observations have stimulated interest in the development of noninvasive methods of assessing atherosclerotic burden and detecting preclinical disease. Measurements of carotid intima–media thickness, brachial arterial flow-mediated dilation, and arterial stiffness have been used widely in clinical research.

Intima–Media Thickness

High-frequency B-mode ultrasound can identify the lumen–intima and media–adventitia interfaces of the carotid arteries, permitting quantification of the thickness of the intima and the media, the two layers of the arterial wall involved in atherosclerosis. Cross-sectional studies have demonstrated associations between common carotid intima–media ratio (the relative thickness of the two layers of the arterial wall), various cardiovascular risk factors and the prevalence of cardiovascular disease. The carotid intima–media ratio is an independent predictor of coronary events and stroke. Serial studies may be used to assess the effect of therapeutic interventions. The clinical applicability of this technique is limited, however, by the considerable training needed to acquire and quantify images with a high degree of reproducibility.

Flow-Mediated Dilation of the Brachial Artery

The vascular endothelium plays a critical role in the prevention of atherosclerosis. Elaboration of nitric oxide by endothelial cells inhibits adhesion of leukocytes and platelets to the vessel wall, inhibits proliferation of smooth muscle cells, and causes arterial vasodilation. High-frequency ultrasound imaging can quantify the endothelium-dependent vasodilatory response of medium arteries, such as the brachial artery, to stimuli that enhance nitric oxide production.

Ischemia-induced hyperemia, resulting in increased flow and shear stress in the brachial artery, can be used to stimulate nitric oxide production by the endothelium. The resultant increase in brachial arterial diameter can be quantified by ultrasonography and used as an index of endothelial function. Flow-mediated dilation is impaired in patients with established coronary artery disease or with traditional coronary risk factors and is predictive of future coronary events. Although this method is promising, it is labor intensive and requires a skilled operator for accurate assessments; measurement techniques have not been standardized for its application in clinical laboratories.

Vascular Stiffness

Arterial stiffening is responsible for the increase in SBP associated with aging. It is a key factor in the development of LV hypertrophy and CHF, and contributes to atherosclerosis and coronary heart disease. Noninvasive methods and devices have been developed to evaluate global, regional, or local indices of stiffness. Most use one of three methods: measurement of pulse transit time, analysis of the arterial pulse contour, or direct measurements of vascular diameter change and distending pressure. Additional prospective research is necessary to determine which methods will have a role in the clinical management of patients with cardiovascular disease or risk factors for atherosclerosis.

FUTURE DIRECTIONS

Dramatic developments in noninvasive imaging techniques have revolutionized the evaluation of patients with peripheral vascular disease, and angiography is generally not necessary unless an intervention is anticipated. Technical advances in CT, MRI, and other methods will undoubtedly further improve image quality, and clinical research will better define the roles of these techniques in patient evaluation. Methodologies that provide not only anatomic information, but also assessments of the functional significance of vascular lesions will be valuable in guiding therapy. Finally, techniques to refine the risk stratification provided by evaluation of traditional coronary risk factors may help to identify patients most likely to benefit from aggressive therapies.

REFERENCES

Anonymous. Beneficial effect of carotid endarterectomy in symptomatic patients with high-grade carotid stenosis. North American Symptomatic Carotid Endarterectomy Trial Collaborators [see comments]. *N Engl J Med* 1991;325:445–453.

Hollier LH, Taylor LM, Ochsner J. Recommended indications for operative treatment of abdominal aortic aneurysms. Report of a subcommittee of the Joint Council of the Society for Vascular Surgery and the North American Chapter of the International Society for Cardiovascular Surgery. *J Vasc Surg* 1992;15:1046–1056.

Pannier BM, Avolio AP, Hoeks A, Mancia G, Takazawa K. Methods and devices for measuring arterial compliance in humans. *Am J Hypertens* 2002;15:743–753.

Pearson TA. New tools for coronary risk assessment, what are their advantages and limitations? *Circulation* 2002;105:886–892.

Safian RD, Textor SC. Renal–artery stenosis. *N Engl J Med* 2001;344:431–442.

Tan WA, Yadav JS, Wholey MH. Endovascular options for peripheral arterial occlusive and aneurysmal disease. In: Topol EJ, ed. *Textbook of Interventional Cardiology*. 4th ed. Philadelphia: WB Saunders; 2003.

Young JR, Olin JW, Bartholomew JR, eds. *Peripheral Vascular Diseases*. 2nd ed. St. Louis: Mosby; 1996.

Weitz JI, Byrne J, Clagett GP, et al. Diagnosis and treatment of chronic arterial insufficiency of the lower extremities: A critical review. *Circulation* 1996;94:3026–3049.

Chapter 39
Hypertension

Alan L. Hinderliter and Romulo E. Colindres

Hypertension is a major risk factor for atherosclerotic cardiovascular disease (Table 39-1). Despite advances in the understanding of the pathophysiology, epidemiology, and natural history of hypertension, as well as improvements in therapy, many patients with hypertension are undiagnosed or inadequately treated. High BP remains an important contributor to coronary events, congestive heart failure (CHF), stroke, and end-stage kidney disease.

Blood pressure is a continuous variable, and any BP level chosen to define hypertension is arbitrary. Nevertheless, an operational definition of hypertension has been advocated as a treatment guideline. The Seventh Joint National Committee on the Prevention, Detection, Evaluation, and Treatment of High Blood Pressure (JNC VII) recommended the classification of BP for adults shown in Table 39-2.

Approximately 50 million people in the United States have hypertension, and BP is controlled in only about one third. The percentage of patients with controlled hypertension is even lower in some Western countries (i.e., Canada and England), and is less than 10% in developing countries—a disappointing figure given the available medications and education of the public and physicians about the risks of high BP. Because hypertension is a worldwide problem and a major cardiovascular risk factor, its prevention and treatment should be prioritized.

ETIOLOGY AND PATHOGENESIS

Hypertension is a disorder of BP regulation that results from an increase in cardiac output or, most often, an increase in total peripheral vascular resistance. Cardiac output is usually normal in essential hypertension, although increased cardiac output plays an etiologic role. The phenomenon of autoregulation explains that an increase in cardiac output causes persistently elevated peripheral vascular resistance,

Table 39-1
Hypertension as a Risk Factor for Cardiovascular Disease

· High BP accelerates atherogenesis and increases the risk of cardiovascular events by two- to threefold.

· Levels of SBP and DBP are associated with cardiovascular events in a continuous, graded, and apparently independent fashion. This relation is closer for SBP than for DBP.

· Between a DBP of 110 mm Hg and 70 mm Hg, a persistently lower DBP of 5 mm Hg is associated with at least a 40% decrease in the incidence of stroke and an approximately 20% decrease in the incidence of CHD.

· Hypertension often occurs in association with other atherogenic risk factors, including dyslipidemia, glucose intolerance, hyperinsulinemia, and obesity.

· The association of hypertension with other cardiovascular risk factors increases the risk of cardiovascular events in a multiplicative rather than an additive fashion.

CHD indicates coronary heart disease.

Table 39-2
Classification of BP for Adults Aged 18 Years and Older

Category	Systolic (mm Hg)	Diastolic (mm Hg)
Normal	<120	<80
Prehypertension	120–139	80–90
Hypertension		
Stage 1	140–159	90–99
Stage 2	>160	>100

With permission from Chobanian VA, Bakris GL, Black AR, et al. The seventh report of the Joint National Committee on Prevention, Detection, Evaluation, and Treatment of High Blood Pressure: The JNC 7 report. *JAMA* 2003;289:2560–2572.

with a resulting return of cardiac output to normal. Figure 39-1 shows mechanisms that can cause hypertension. Inappropriate activation of the renin–angiotensin system, decreased renal sodium excretion, or increased sympathetic nervous system activity, individually or in combination, is likely involved in the pathogenesis of all types of hypertension. Hypertension has genetic and environmental causes, including excess sodium intake, obesity, and stress. The inability of the kidney to optimally excrete sodium, and thus regulate plasma volume, leads to a persistent increase in BP regardless of etiology.

Many elderly patients with elevated BP have isolated systolic hypertension—a systolic pressure that exceeds 140 mm Hg with a normal diastolic pressure. Stiffening of large arteries and increased systolic pulse wave velocity elevate systolic BP, increase myocardial work, and decrease coronary perfusion.

CLINICAL PRESENTATION

Most patients with early hypertension have no symptoms attributable to high BP. Long-term BP elevation, however, frequently leads to hypertensive heart disease, atherosclerosis of the aorta and peripheral vessels, cerebrovascular disease, and renal insufficiency.

Left ventricular hypertrophy (LVH) is the principal cardiac manifestation of hypertension. Echocardiography can identify increased left ventricular (LV) mass in nearly 30% of unselected hypertensive adults, and in the majority of patients with longstanding, severe hypertension. LVH is more prevalent in males and more common in black individuals than in white individuals with similar BP values. Increasing age, obesity, high dietary sodium intake, and diabetes are also associated with cardiac hypertrophy.

Mechanical forces—increased ventricular afterload from elevated peripheral vascular resistance and arterial stiffness—are considered the principal determinants of myocardial hypertrophy in patients with hypertension. Hemodynamic overload stimulates increases in myocyte size and the synthesis of contractile elements. Fibroblast proliferation and deposition of extracellular collagen accompany these cellular changes, which contribute to ventricular stiffness and myocardial ischemia. A growing body of evidence suggests that angiotensin II and aldosterone, independent of pressure overload, stimulate this interstitial fibrosis (Fig. 39-2).

Clinical consequences of hypertensive heart disease include CHF and coronary heart disease (CHD). More than 90% of patients with heart failure have hypertension, and data from the Framingham Heart Study suggest that high BP accounts for almost half of the population burden of this disorder. Treating hypertension reduces the risk of heart failure by nearly 50%. Heart failure develops because of the myocyte hypertrophy and ventricular fibrosis that characterize hypertensive LVH. As illustrated in Figure 39-3, the early functional manifestations of LVH include LV impaired relaxation and decreased compliance. Although the ejection fraction (EF) is preserved initially, diastolic dysfunction may increase filling pressures, leading to pulmonary congestion. This mechanism accounts for the symptoms observed in about 40% of hypertensive patients with heart failure. If excessive BP levels persist, myocyte loss and fibrosis contribute to ventricular remodeling and contractile dysfunction. Compensatory mechanisms, including remodeling of the peripheral vasculature and activation of the sympathetic nervous and renin–angiotensin systems, accelerate the deterioration in myocardial contractility. Ultimately, decompensated cardiomyopathy and heart failure from systolic dysfunction develop (Fig. 39-4).

Coronary heart disease is approximately twice as prevalent in hypertensive as in normotensive persons of the same age. CHD risk increases in a continuous and graded fashion, with both SBP and DBP. A 5-mm Hg reduction of diastolic BP with drug therapy decreases the incidence of myocardial infarction (MI) by about 20%. Multiple factors contribute to the enhanced risk of CHD associated with high BP: atherosclerotic narrowing of the epicardial coronary arteries is accelerated; coronary arteriolar hypertrophy, reduced myocardial vascularity (rarefaction), and perivascular fibrosis limit coronary arterial flow reserve and predispose the left ventricle to ischemia; and impaired coronary endothelial function increases coronary tone. MI and chronic ischemia contribute to LV dysfunction, increasing the risk of heart failure and cardiovascular death.

Figure 39-1   Factors Involved in the Control of Blood Pressure

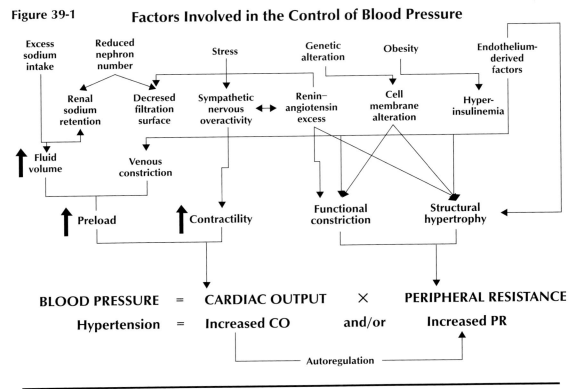

With permission from Kaplan NM. *Kaplan's Clinical Hypertension.* 8th ed. Philadelphia: Lippincott Williams & Wilkins; 2002.

Occasionally, hypertension may enter a phase called malignant or accelerated hypertension, characterized by markedly elevated SBP and DBP and acute target organ damage. Cardiac manifestations can include acute CHF, coronary insufficiency, and aortic dissection.

DIFFERENTIAL DIAGNOSIS

Approximately 95% of patients with elevated arterial pressure have essential hypertension. The remaining 5% have an identifiable cause of secondary hypertension (Table 39-3). Although few patients have secondary hypertension, identification of these patients is important because the hypertension can often be cured or significantly improved by an interventional procedure, a specific drug therapy, or stopping a culprit drug.

Identifiable causes of hypertension should be sought in the initial history, physical examination, and laboratory studies. Further diagnostic evaluation for secondary hypertension causes are pursued when the presentation is atypical for essen-

tial hypertension, or when the initial evaluation suggests an identifiable cause (Table 39-4).

DIAGNOSTIC APPROACH

Objectives of the initial evaluation of a hypertensive patient include confirmation of the presence of hypertension, evaluation of the presence and extent of target organ disease, identification of cardiovascular risk factors and coexisting conditions that influence prognosis and therapy, and exclusion or detection of identifiable causes of elevated BP. These goals can usually be achieved with a comprehensive history, a thorough physical examination, and a few laboratory studies (Table 39-5).

The physical examination focuses on determining the level of BP and evidence of target organ disease or identifiable causes of hypertension. The detection and diagnosis of hypertension begin with the accurate measurement of BP. Measurements should be acquired at each encounter, with follow-up determinations at intervals based on the initial level. Accurate

Figure 39-2

Myocardial Fibrosis

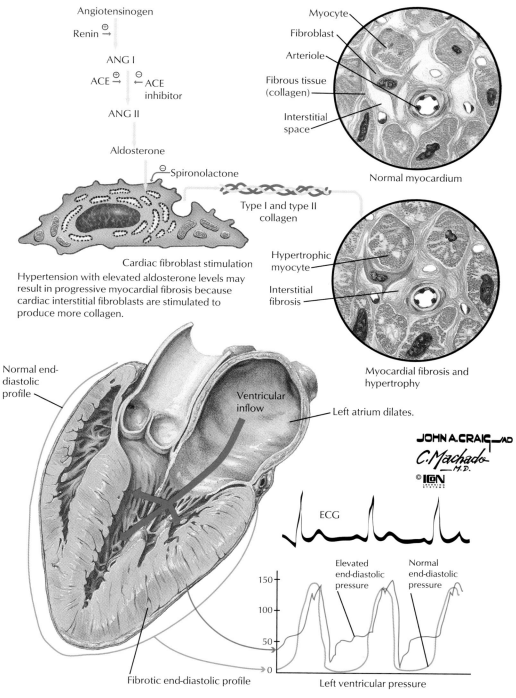

Angiotensinogen

Renin $\xrightarrow{\oplus}$

ANG I

ACE $\xrightarrow{\oplus}$ | $\xleftarrow{\ominus}$ ACE inhibitor

ANG II

Aldosterone

$\xrightarrow{\ominus}$ Spironolactone

Type I and type II collagen

Cardiac fibroblast stimulation

Hypertension with elevated aldosterone levels may result in progressive myocardial fibrosis because cardiac interstitial fibroblasts are stimulated to produce more collagen.

Myocyte

Fibroblast

Arteriole

Fibrous tissue (collagen)

Interstitial space

Normal myocardium

Hypertrophic myocyte

Interstitial fibrosis

Myocardial fibrosis and hypertrophy

Normal end-diastolic profile

Ventricular inflow

Left atrium dilates.

JOHN A. CRAIG —MD

C. Machado —M.D.

© ICON

ECG

Elevated end-diastolic pressure

Normal end-diastolic pressure

150

100

50

0

Fibrotic end-diastolic profile

Left ventricular pressure

Progressive fibrosis stiffens myocardial walls of both ventricles, resulting in decreased compliance (diastolic failure).

Figure 39-3

Hypertension and Congestive Heart Failure

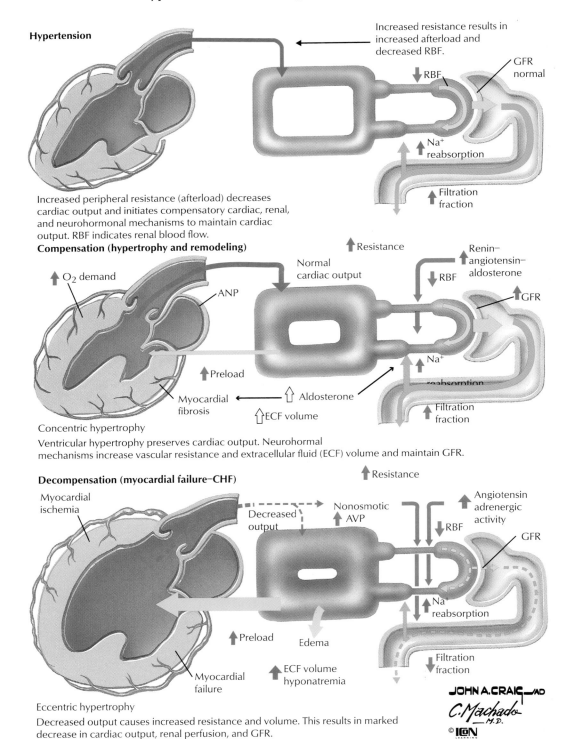

Hypertension

Increased resistance results in increased afterload and decreased RBF.

↓RBF

GFR normal

Na⁺ reabsorption

Filtration fraction

Increased peripheral resistance (afterload) decreases cardiac output and initiates compensatory cardiac, renal, and neurohormonal mechanisms to maintain cardiac output. RBF indicates renal blood flow.

Compensation (hypertrophy and remodeling)

↑Resistance

↑O₂ demand

Normal cardiac output

Renin–angiotensin–aldosterone

↓RBF

ANP

↑GFR

↑Preload

Na⁺ reabsorption

Myocardial fibrosis

⇧Aldosterone

⇧ECF volume

Filtration fraction

Concentric hypertrophy

Ventricular hypertrophy preserves cardiac output. Neurohormal mechanisms increase vascular resistance and extracellular fluid (ECF) volume and maintain GFR.

Decompensation (myocardial failure–CHF)

↑Resistance

Myocardial ischemia

Nonosmotic AVP

Decreased output

Angiotensin adrenergic activity

↓RBF

GFR

↑Preload

Edema

Na⁺ reabsorption

↑ECF volume hyponatremia

Myocardial failure

Filtration fraction

Eccentric hypertrophy

Decreased output causes increased resistance and volume. This results in marked decrease in cardiac output, renal perfusion, and GFR.

JOHN A. CRAIG—MD

C. Machado—M.D.

©ICN

Figure 39-4

The Development of Congestive Heart Failure (CHF) in Patients With Hypertension

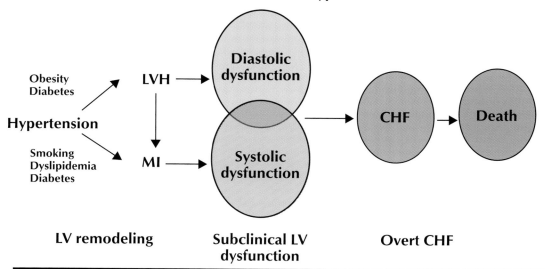

LV indicates left ventricular; LVH, left ventricular hypertrophy; MI, myocardial infarction.

With permission from Vasan RS, Levy D. The role of hypertension in the pathogenesis of heart failure. A clinical mechanistic overview. *Arch Inter* 1996;156:1789–1796.

equipment and a standardized technique are critical. In many patients, home BP monitoring may establish baseline levels or evaluate the response to therapy. In some circumstances, 24-hour ambulatory BP monitoring is useful: when there is unusual variability of BP over the same or different visits, for office hypertension ("white coat" hypertension) in subjects with low cardio-vascular risk, when symptoms suggest hypoten-sive episodes, and when hypertension is resist-ant to drug treatment.

MANAGEMENT AND THERAPY

The principal goal of hypertension treatment is to reduce the risk of cardiovascular morbidity and death. The treatment approach is deter-mined by the absolute risk of a cardiovascular event based on the major cardiovascular risk fac-tors, clinical cardiovascular disease, and target organ damage. In patients at highest risk—espe-cially those with diabetes or renal disease—phar-macologic therapy should be considered when BP is mildly elevated or in the upper prehyper-tension range, with a goal value of less than 130/80 mm Hg. Lower risk patients may benefit from a period of observation and lifestyle modi-fication, using medical therapy if the average

SBP exceeds 140 mm Hg or if the DBP exceeds 90 mm Hg over months of monitoring.

Quantitative assessments of cardiovascular risk may guide treatment decisions in patients with high–normal BP or mild uncomplicated hypertension. Predictive equations use age, sex, systolic BP, total and high-density lipoprotein cholesterol (HDL-C), smoking history, and pres-ence of diabetes or LVH to estimate the chances of a cardiovascular event. Computer programs, Web sites, and risk calculation tables utilizing these predictors enable providers to accurately and efficiently calculate the risk of stroke or MI in an individual patient. Although this approach is attractive, consensus does not exist on the absolute cardiovascular risk that should prompt antihypertensive therapy. The British Hyperten-sion Society advocates treatment for those with a coronary disease risk 15% or more over 10 years. This threshold leaves untreated many patients with stage I hypertension in whom ther-apy is recommended by the JNC VII report.

Lifestyle modifications are an important com-ponent of high-BP therapy. All patients with hypertension, high–normal BP, or a strong family history of hypertension should be encouraged to adopt the measures outlined in Table 39-6. These

Table 39-3
Identifiable Causes of Hypertension

Renal
    Renal parenchymal disease
    Renal vascular disease

Endocrine
    Hypo- or hyperthyroidism
    Adrenal disorders
    Primary hyperaldosteronism
    Cushing's syndrome
    Pheochromocytoma

Exogenous hormones
    Glucocorticoids
    Mineralocorticoids
    Sympathomimetic agents
    Erythropoietin

Coarctation of the aorta

Sleep apnea

Neurological disorders
    Elevated intracranial pressure
    Quadriplegia

Acute stress
    Perioperative
    Hypoglycemia
    Alcohol withdrawal

Drugs and medications
    Alcohol
    Cocaine
    Nicotine

Nonsteroidal anti-inflammatory agents

Immunosuppressive agents (cyclosporine, tacrolimus)

Table 39-4
Indications for Considering Testing for Identifiable Causes of Hypertension

· Onset of hypertension at age <20 years or onset of diastolic hypertension at age >50 years

· Target organ damage at presentation
    Serum creatinine concentration >1.5 mg/dL
    LV hypertrophy determined by electrocardiography

· Presence of features indicative of secondary causes
    Hypokalemia
    Abdominal bruit
    Labile pressures with tachycardia, sweating, and tremor
    Family history of renal disease

· Poor response to generally effective therapy

LV indicates left ventricular.

lifestyle changes are proven to lower BP and may reduce the need for drug therapy, enhance the effectiveness of antihypertensive drugs, and favorably influence other cardiovascular risk factors. Other measures, including smoking cessation and reduced intake of saturated fats, may further reduce cardiovascular risk.

Pharmacologic treatment of hypertension reduces the incidence of stroke and coronary artery disease (CAD), and decreases mortality rate from cardiovascular causes in middle-aged and older adults. Drug therapy is indicated if lifestyle modifications do not bring BP into the desired range. Thiazide diuretics, β-adrenergic receptor blockers, angiotensin-converting enzyme (ACE) inhibitors, angiotensin-receptor blockers (ARBs), and calcium antagonists are appropriate first-line agents. Thiazide diuretics are effective, well tolerated, and inexpensive. They are recommended by expert panels as the drugs of choice in uncomplicated hypertension, and recent data from the Antihypertensive and Lipid-Lowering Treatment to Prevent Heart Attack Trial (ALLHAT) suggest that they are at least as effective as newer agents are in preventing cardiovascular complications of hypertension. In many patients, however, the choice of an agent is influenced by comorbid conditions. Table 39-7 lists agents that are preferred or relatively contraindicated in specific circumstances.

Many patients with hypertension have established cardiovascular disease, and their treatment regimen should include medications that control symptoms, retard disease progression, and prevent cardiovascular events. Treatment strategies for patients with ischemic heart disease or CHF are addressed in chapters 7 and 17. In brief, β-blockers and ACE inhibitors improve symptoms and prolong survival rates in patients with CAD or LV dysfunction. ARBs are an effec-

Table 39-5
Appropriate History, Physical Examination, and Laboratory Tests

Comprehensive History

- Assessment of the duration and severity of elevated BP and the results of prior medication trials
- Evaluation for the presence of diabetes, hypercholesterolemia, tobacco use, and other cardiovascular risk factors
- Identification of a history or symptoms of target organ disease, including CHD and CHF, cerebrovascular disease, peripheral vascular disease, and renal disease
- Assessment of symptoms suggesting identifiable causes of hypertension
- Identification of the use of drugs or substances that may raise BP
- Evaluation of lifestyle factors, such as diet, leisure-time physical activity, and weight gain, that may influence BP control
- Assessment of psychosocial and environmental factors, such as family support, income, and educational level, that influence the efficacy of antihypertensive therapy
- Identification of family history of hypertension or CVD

Physical Examination

- Careful measurement of BP
- Measurement of height and weight
- Fundoscopic examination for hypertensive retinopathy
- Examination of the neck for carotid bruits, elevated jugular venous pressure, and thyromegaly
- Examination of the heart for abnormalities of the apical impulse or the presence of extra heart sounds or murmurs
- Examination of the abdomen for bruits, enlarged kidneys, and other masses
- Examination of the extremities for diminished arterial pulsations or peripheral edema

Laboratory Studies

- Complete blood count
- Serum concentrations of potassium, calcium, creatinine, thyroid-stimulating hormone, fasting glucose, triglycerides, and HDL-C and total LDL-C
- Urinalysis for blood, protein, glucose, and microscopic examination
- Electrocardiography

CHD indicates coronary heart disease; CHF, congestive heart failure; CVD, cardiovascular disease; HDL-C, high-density lipoprotein cholesterol; LDL-C, low-density lipoprotein cholesterol.

tive alternative in patients with heart failure who cannot tolerate ACE inhibitors. Aldosterone antagonists are beneficial in patients with LV systolic dysfunction or a history of MI. Calcium antagonists are useful adjuncts in patients with angina or hypertension that cannot be controlled by β-blockers and ACE inhibitors. The optimal therapy for patients with heart failure but a normal EF is not well established and is under investigation; agents that treat LV systolic dysfunction appear to be useful. Lowering BP

with any of the first-line therapy drugs leads to LVH regression.

The goal of therapy in elderly patients with systolic hypertension and low DBP is not well established. Treatment of isolated systolic hypertension reduces cardiovascular morbidity and mortality rates. In theory, however, antihypertensive drugs that lower systolic BP may compromise coronary perfusion if DBP is lowered excessively. Several studies have suggested a J-shaped relation between DBP and coronary

Table 39-6
Lifestyle Modifications for Prevention and Treatment of Hypertension

· Weight loss if overweight. All overweight hypertensive patients should be enrolled in a monitored weight-reduction program.

· Moderation of alcohol intake. Patients with high BP who drink alcohol should be counseled to limit their intake to 1 oz alcohol for men and 0.5 oz for women.

· Regular aerobic physical activity. Sedentary individuals should be encouraged to engage in regular aerobic exercise.

· Dietary restrictions. Moderate reduction in sodium intake (<100 mmol [2.5 g] and adequate intake of potassium (>90 mmol/d) from food sources such as fruits and vegetables are recommended.*

---

* A diet rich in fruits and vegetables and dairy products, low in saturated fat and total fat results in significant BP reduction, especially when combined with sodium restriction. Sacks FM, Svetkey LP, Vollmer WM, et al. Effects on blood pressure of reduced dietary sodium and the dietary approaches to stop hypertension (DASH) diet. *N Engl J Med* 2001;344:3–10.

---

risk, with an increase in events as DBP is lowered below 80 mm Hg. These observations have led some experts to caution against aggressive BP lowering in elderly patients with isolated systolic hypertension and low DBP.

In general, therapy should be initiated at low doses to minimize side effects. Based on patient response, the dose of the initial agent can be slowly titrated upward, or a small dose of a second agent can be added. Effective drug combinations use medications from different classes and result in additive BP-lowering effects, while minimizing dose-dependent adverse effects. Diuretics potentiate the effect of β-blockers, ACE inhibitors, and ARBs; other useful combinations include dihydropyridine calcium antagonists and β-blockers, or calcium antagonists and ACE inhibitors. Long-acting formulations with 24-hour efficacy are preferred over shorter acting agents because of greater patient adherence to once-daily dosing regimens and more consistent BP control throughout the day.

Prevention of cardiovascular morbidity and death is usually achieved with slow, gradual reduction of BP, maintained over many years.

Table 39-7
Choice of Antihypertensive Agent Based on Coexistent Illnesses

	Specific Drugs
Indications	
Diabetes mellitus	ACE inhibitor or ARB
CHF	ACE inhibitor or ARB, β-blocker, diuretic, aldosterone antagonist
MI	ACE inhibitor, β-blocker, aldosterone antagonist
Chronic CAD	ACE inhibitor, β-blocker
Renal insufficiency	ACE inhibitor or ARB
Contraindications	
Pregnancy	ACE inhibitor, ARB
Renal insufficiency*	Potassium-sparing agent
Peripheral vascular disease	β-Blocker
Gout*	Diuretic
Depression*	β-Blocker, central α agonist
Reactive airway disease	β-Blocker
2nd- or 3rd-degree heart block	β-Blocker, non-dihydropyridine calcium antagonist
Hepatic insufficiency	Labetalol, methyldopa

*Relative contraindications.
ACE indicates angiotensin-converting enzyme; ARB, angiotensin-receptor blockers; CAD, coronary artery disease; CHF, congestive heart failure; MI, myocardial infarction.

Urgent reduction of BP with intravenous medications, however, is necessary in patients with malignant hypertension (Table 39-8).

FUTURE DIRECTIONS

Future research and public health initiatives should more accurately define treatment thresholds and optimal target BP in patients at high risk of cardiovascular events, including elderly individuals and patients with diabetes mellitus or target organ damage; determine the agents most useful in alleviating symptoms and improving longevity in patients with hypertension and heart failure from diastolic dysfunction; and provide better strategies to improve

Table 39-8
Agents Used for Intravenous Drug Therapy of Hypertensive Emergencies

Agent	Use
Nitroprusside	Preferred agent in most instances except acute coronary syndromes or pregnancy. Should be combined with a β-blocker in some instances, such as acute aortic dissection.
Nitroglycerine	Use in combination with a β-blocker for acute coronary syndromes.
Labetalol	Use as adjunctive therapy with nitroprusside or nitroglycerine. Use alone in less intensely monitored situation or treatment of postoperative hypertension.
Enalaprilat	Use for sclerodermal crisis or as adjunctive therapy in some high-renin states.
Hydralazine	May use for treatment of preeclampsia, eclampsia.
Fenoldopam	Same indication as for nitroprusside. Useful in postoperative or postprocedure hypertension in closely monitored situations.
Esmolol	Use in case of need for immediate, very-short-acting β-blocker effect. Use for supraventricular tachycardia.

patient awareness and compliance with lifestyle modifications and medication regimens.

REFERENCES

1999 World Health Organization–International Society of Hypertension Guidelines for the Management of Hypertension. Guidelines Subcommittee. *J Hum Hypertens* 1999;17:151–183.

The ALLHAT Officers and Coordinators for the ALLHAT Collaborative Research Group. Major outcomes in high-risk hypertensive patients randomized to angiotensin-converting enzyme inhibitor or calcium channel blocker vs diuretic: The Antihypertensive and Lipid-Lowering Treatment to Prevent Heart Attack Trial (ALLHAT). *JAMA* 2002;288:2981–2997.

Kannel WB. Blood pressure as a cardiovascular risk factor. *JAMA* 1996; 275:1571–1576.

Kaplan NM. *Clinical Hypertension*. 8th ed. Philadelphia: Lippincott Williams & Wilkins; 2002.

Lorell BH, Carabello BA. Left ventricular hypertrophy: Pathogenesis, detection, and prognosis. *Circulation* 2000;102: 470–479.

Med-Decisions.com. Available at: www.med-decisions.com.

Ramsay LE, Williams B, Johnston GD. Guidelines for management of hypertension: Report of the third working party of the British Hypertension Society. *J Hum Hypertension* 1999;13:569–592.

Seventh Report of the Joint National Committee on Prevention, Detection, Evaluation, and Treatment of High Blood Pressure: The JNC 7 Report. *JAMA* 2003;289:2560–2572.

Chapter 40
Renal Artery Stenosis

George A. Stouffer, Christopher R. Kroll, and Walter A. Tan

Obstructive disease in the renal arteries can decrease blood flow to the kidneys, which can result in activation of the renin–angiotensin system, hypertension, ischemic nephropathy, and other pathologic changes. Technologic advances, including intra-arterial stenting, have generated enthusiasm for revascularization as a treatment for hypertension and progressive renal dysfunction caused by renal artery stenosis (RAS). However, outcomes improve in only approximately 50% of patients who undergo successful revascularization, underlining the limited understanding of this disease and the importance of careful patient selection.

ETIOLOGY AND PATHOGENESIS

The predominant cause of obstructive RAS is atherosclerosis (Fig. 40-1). The atherosclerotic process can involve the renal artery or the aorta, with involvement of the latter leading to disease involving the ostium of the renal artery. Rarely, obstructive RAS is caused by fibromuscular dysplasia (FMD; <10% of cases of RAS).

Fibromuscular disease is a collection of vascular diseases characterized by intimal or medial hyperplasia. It is commonly bilateral and affects women more often than men. The middle and distal portions of the vessel are the most commonly involved sites, with a typical angiographic appearance of "beads on a string." FMD can cause hypertension but rarely leads to major loss of renal function, although progressive renal impairment has been described in smokers.

Regardless of its underlying pathologic cause, decreased renal perfusion results in compensatory activation of the renin–angiotensin system (Fig. 40-2), which can cause systemic hypertension, salt retention, and activation of the neurohormonal system. RAS also causes ischemic changes within the kidney (ischemic nephropathy) and increased systemic markers of oxidative stress. Other pathologic effects have been postulated but not proven to result from RAS.

Natural History

Renal artery stenosis is a rapidly progressive disease. Studies of patients with documented RAS have shown that progression of atherosclerotic disease in renal arteries occurs in approximately 25% of patients at 1 year, in 35% at 3 years, and in 50% at 5 years. The risk of progression increases with diabetes mellitus, SBP greater than 160 mm Hg, and obstructive lesions greater than 60% at the time of enrollment. The rate of progression to total occlusion at 5 years was 10% in arteries with lesions less than 60%. In another study, in which the average stenosis at the time of enrollment was 72%, 16% of the patients randomly assigned to receive medical treatment had total occlusion at 1 year. The 2-year incidence of renal atrophy was 21% for kidneys supplied by an artery with more than 60% stenosis. These studies suggest that patients with significant RAS merit consideration for revascularization at the time of diagnosis.

CLINICAL PRESENTATION

The vast majority of patients with hypertension have essential hypertension. Overall, renovascular disease is the etiology in 0.5 to 2% of patients with hypertension (Fig. 40-3) but is more common in patients who present with new-onset, severe hypertension. RAS is more common in white individuals than in black individuals, and the prevalence increases with age. Clinical factors that increase the likelihood of RAS include age, recent onset or sudden worsening of hypertension, and presence of abdominal bruit. The prevalence of RAS is also higher in patients with atherosclerosis in other vascular beds. Significant RAS is found in 6 to 23% of patients with hypertension who are undergoing cardiac catheterization. Significant RAS has been found in 10.4% of patients at autopsy after a cerebrovascular accident.

Figure 40-1

Renal Artery Disease Causing Hypertension

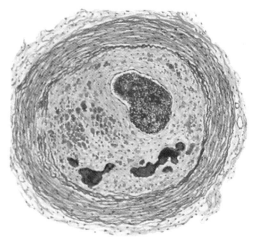

Severe concentric atherosclerosis with lipid deposition and calcification complicated by thrombosis (composite, × 12)

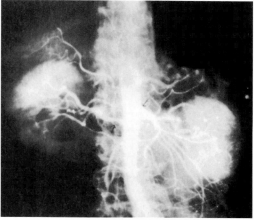

Aortorenogram showing atherosclerotic narrowing and poststenotic dilatation of both renal arteries

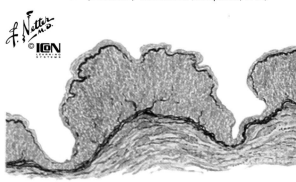

Medial fibroplasia (longitudinal section) with variation in mural thickness, chiefly of media, and aneurysmal evaginations (Verhoeff-Van Gieson stain, × 20)

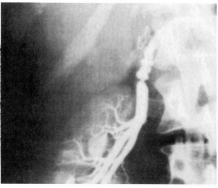

Renal arteriogram showing characteristic beaded appearance caused by alternate stenoses and aneurysmal dilatations

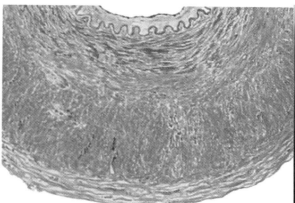

Subadventitial fibroplasia with concentric ring of dense collagen between media and adventitia (Masson's trichrome stain, × 80)

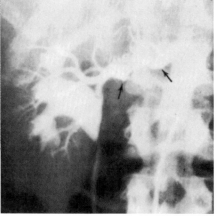

Arteriogram showing extensive, varied stenosis of right renal artery

Figure 40-2

Renin–Angiotensin System

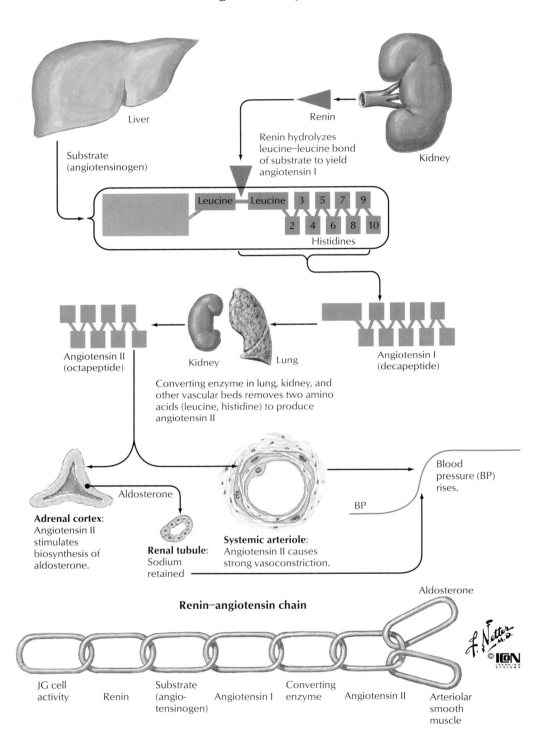

Liver

Renin

Renin hydrolyzes
leucine–leucine bond
of substrate to yield
angiotensin I

Kidney

Substrate
(angiotensinogen)

Leucine — Leucine — 3 5 7 9

2 4 6 8 10

Histidines

Angiotensin II
(octapeptide)

Kidney

Lung

Angiotensin I
(decapeptide)

Converting enzyme in lung, kidney, and
other vascular beds removes two amino
acids (leucine, histidine) to produce
angiotensin II

Blood
pressure (BP)
rises.

Aldosterone

BP

Adrenal cortex:
Angiotensin II
stimulates
biosynthesis of
aldosterone.

Renal tubule:
Sodium
retained

Systemic arteriole:
Angiotensin II causes
strong vasoconstriction.

Aldosterone

Renin–angiotensin chain

JG cell
activity

Renin

Substrate
(angio-
tensinogen)

Angiotensin I

Converting
enzyme

Angiotensin II

Arteriolar
smooth
muscle

Atherosclerotic renovascular disease is estimated to cause renal failure in 5 to 15% of adult patients undergoing dialysis for end-stage renal disease. The mortality associated with this group is staggering; survival rates reported at 2, 5, and 10 years are 56%, 18%, and 5%, respectively.

DIFFERENTIAL DIAGNOSIS

The primary differential diagnosis is essential hypertension (chapter 39), although a number of other less common causes of hypertension must be considered (Fig. 40-3). The point at which renal artery atherosclerosis becomes physiologically significant and leads to increased BP and ischemic nephropathy is incompletely understood. Recognition of lesions that compromise blood flow to the kidney is essential to identify patients whose conditions will improve with renal revascularization. This is especially important given the demographics of patients with RAS because it is common for other etiologies of hypertension (primarily essential hypertension) to coexist in this group.

Several different approaches have attempted to identify physiologically significant lesions. One study found that the only clinical factors that predicted a beneficial BP response to renal artery revascularization were a preprocedure mean arterial pressure greater than 110 mm Hg and bilateral RAS. Measurement of split-vein renin levels may be a means to determine who will benefit from renal artery revascularization (Fig. 40-4). A renal vein renin ratio of 1.5:1 correlates with BP improvement in some studies. Captopril scintigraphy may be of value in identifying patients who will benefit from renal artery revascularization, with a sensitivity of approximately 75% and a specificity of 90%.

Doppler ultrasonography, although technologically demanding, is a promising technique; its measurement of the resistive index can be used as a predictive tool. Patients with resistance index values greater than 80 show much poorer results (no improvement in BP, worsening renal function) after revascularization than do those patients whose values are less than 80.

DIAGNOSTIC APPROACH

The renal arteries can be visualized with arteriography, magnetic resonance angiography (MRA), and spiral CT. Arteriography, the direct injection of contrast dye into the renal artery, remains the gold standard for identifying and quantifying obstructive lesions (Fig. 40-5). MRA and spiral CT are noninvasive methods with excellent sensitivity and good, but not optimal, specificity for identifying RAS.

MANAGEMENT AND THERAPY
Renal Artery Revascularization

Renal artery obstructive disease can be treated by means of surgery or percutaneous approaches. Surgical renal artery revascularization generally involves aortorenal bypass with use of hypogastric artery, saphenous vein, or polytetrafluoroethylene grafts. If severe aortic disease precludes aortorenal bypass, splenorenal (for left RAS) or hepatorenal (for right RAS) approaches are used (Fig. 40-6). Results of surgical renal artery revascularization show operative mortality rates of 2 to 6%, with improvement of hypertension observed in 79 to 95% of patients.

Percutaneous balloon angioplasty for RAS, first reported by Gruntzig et al. in 1978, has resulted in varying rates of improvement in hypertension (36 to 100% of patients in uncontrolled studies) (Fig. 40-7). Success rates with balloon angioplasty are better for nonostial as opposed to ostial stenoses. Restenosis is reported in 10 to 47% of cases. In a randomized trial of 106 patients with hypertension and a renal artery lesion of 50% or greater, there were no significant differences in average BP between patients treated with medical therapy and patients treated with balloon angioplasty at 1 year in an intention-to-treat analysis. Criticism of this study included the lack of physiologic evaluation of the significance of the RAS, the high crossover rate from the medical group to the balloon angioplasty group (>40%), and the conclusion that the treatments had equal efficacy despite the fact that 68% of the angioplasty group had improved BP versus 38% of the medical therapy group.

Percutaneous intervention is generally preferred over medical management in patients with FMD because it improves hypertension in approximately 75% of patients. Balloon angioplasty is successful in 82 to 100% of patients, with restenosis in 10 to 11%.

Figure 40-3

Etiology of Hypertension

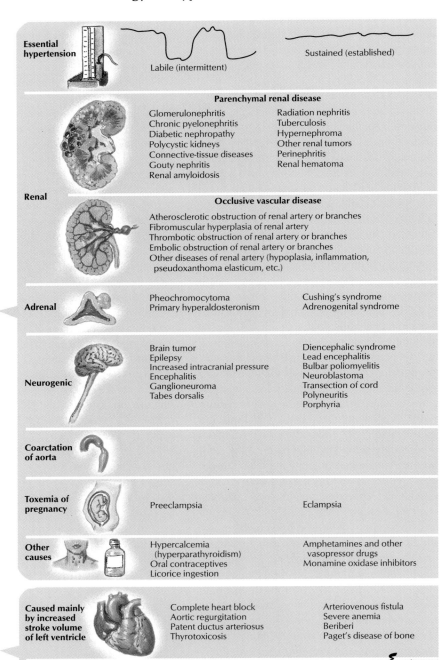

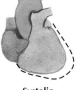

Essential hypertension — Labile (intermittent) — Sustained (established)

Renal

Parenchymal renal disease

Glomerulonephritis
Chronic pyelonephritis
Diabetic nephropathy
Polycystic kidneys
Connective-tissue diseases
Gouty nephritis
Renal amyloidosis

Radiation nephritis
Tuberculosis
Hypernephroma
Other renal tumors
Perinephritis
Renal hematoma

Occlusive vascular disease

Atherosclerotic obstruction of renal artery or branches
Fibromuscular hyperplasia of renal artery
Thrombotic obstruction of renal artery or branches
Embolic obstruction of renal artery or branches
Other diseases of renal artery (hypoplasia, inflammation, pseudoxanthoma elasticum, etc.)

Adrenal

Pheochromocytoma
Primary hyperaldosteronism

Cushing's syndrome
Adrenogenital syndrome

Neurogenic

Brain tumor
Epilepsy
Increased intracranial pressure
Encephalitis
Ganglioneuroma
Tabes dorsalis

Diencephalic syndrome
Lead encephalitis
Bulbar poliomyelitis
Neuroblastoma
Transection of cord
Polyneuritis
Porphyria

Coarctation of aorta

Toxemia of pregnancy

Preeclampsia

Eclampsia

Other causes

Hypercalcemia (hyperparathyroidism)
Oral contraceptives
Licorice ingestion

Amphetamines and other vasopressor drugs
Monamine oxidase inhibitors

Diastolic hypertension

Caused mainly by increased stroke volume of left ventricle

Complete heart block
Aortic regurgitation
Patent ductus arteriosus
Thyrotoxicosis

Arteriovenous fistula
Severe anemia
Beriberi
Paget's disease of bone

Systolic hypertension

Caused mainly by decreased distensibility of aorta

Arteriosclerosis of aorta
Coarctation of aorta (see above)

Figure 40-4

Differential Renin/Aldosterone

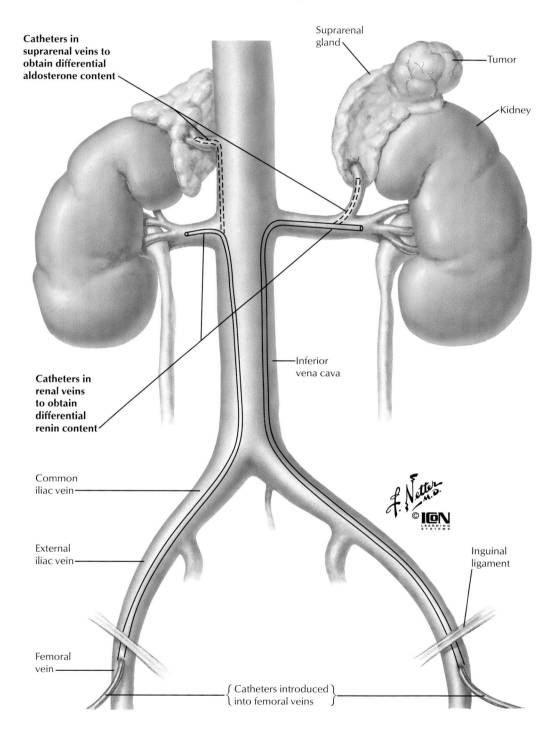

Catheters in suprarenal veins to obtain differential aldosterone content

Suprarenal gland

Tumor

Kidney

Catheters in renal veins to obtain differential renin content

Inferior vena cava

Common iliac vein

External iliac vein

Inguinal ligament

Femoral vein

Catheters introduced into femoral veins

Figure 40-5
Aortorenal and Selective Renal Angiography
(Transfemoral Approach)

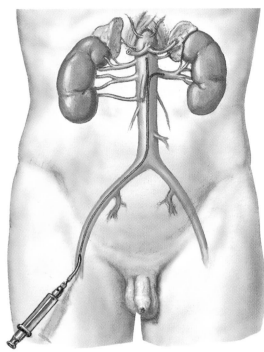

Seldinger technique for catheterization of femoral artery

1: Needle introduced into artery

2: Guide wire passed through needle

3: Needle withdrawn

4: Catheter introduced over wire

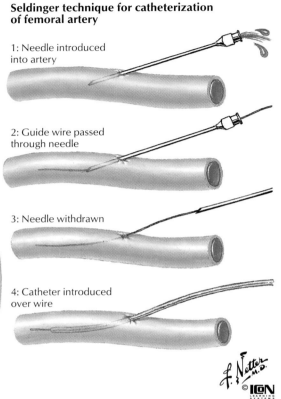

Catheter introduced via femoral artery to desired level of aorta, and contrast medium injected, which then flows into normal and accessory renal arteries and possibly also into other aortic branches (aortorenal angiography, 1); or catheter may be made to enter renal arteries for direct injection (selective renal angiography, 2)

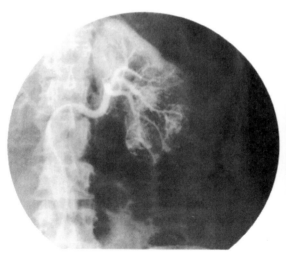

Selective left renal arteriogram. Multiple tumor vessels in lower pole of left kidney suggestive of highly vascular tumor (hypernephroma)

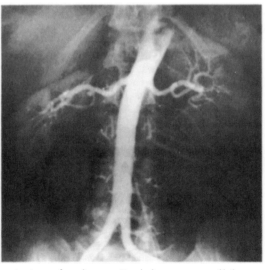

Aortorenal angiogram. Beaded appearance of left renal artery is evidence of fibromuscular hyperplasia; aneurysm at bifurcation of right renal artery

Figure 40-6

Renal Revascularization

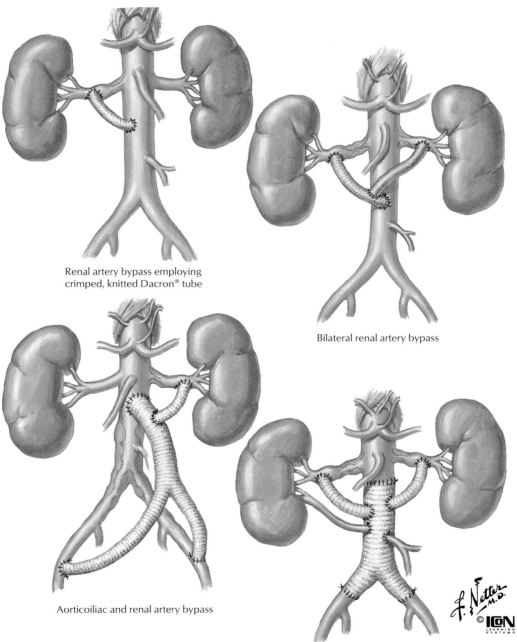

Renal artery bypass employing crimped, knitted Dacron® tube

Bilateral renal artery bypass

Aorticoiliac and renal artery bypass

Aortic graft replacement with bilateral renal artery bypass and preservation of an accessory renal artery

Figure 40-7

Transluminal Renal Angioplasty

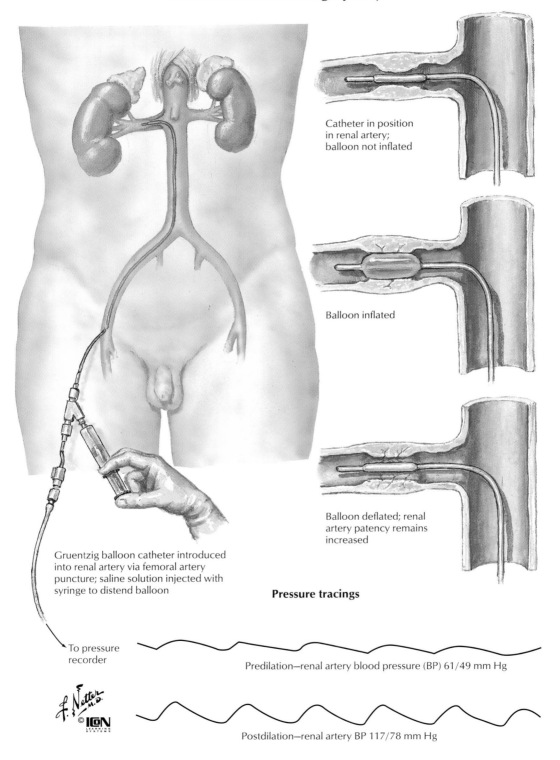

Catheter in position
in renal artery;
balloon not inflated

Balloon inflated

Balloon deflated; renal
artery patency remains
increased

Gruentzig balloon catheter introduced
into renal artery via femoral artery
puncture; saline solution injected with
syringe to distend balloon

Pressure tracings

To pressure
recorder

Predilation—renal artery blood pressure (BP) 61/49 mm Hg

Postdilation—renal artery BP 117/78 mm Hg

Figure 40-8

Percutaneous Revascularization
of Stenotic Renal Arteries

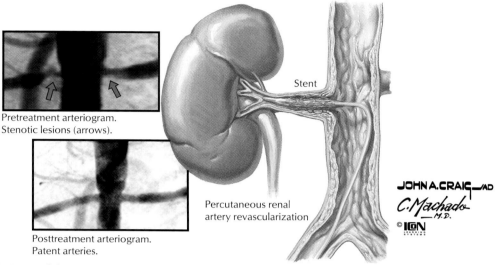

Pretreatment arteriogram.
Stenotic lesions (arrows).

Posttreatment arteriogram.
Patent arteries.

Stent

Percutaneous renal
artery revascularization

JOHN A.CRAIG—MD

C.Machado—M.D.

© ICN

Patients with hypertension and atherosclerotic renal artery stenosis most likely to respond to balloon angioplasty percutaneous renal artery revascularization are those with onset of hypertension within the past 5 years, those without primary renal disease, and middle-aged men with atherosclerotic renal artery stenosis and malignant hypertension not caused by primary renal disease. A positive captopril renogram predicts cure or improvement of hypertension after revascularization.

Stenting has been advocated as the preferred percutaneous treatment for RAS, especially when the lesion is ostial (Fig. 40-8). The use of stenting, as opposed to balloon angioplasty, is associated with higher rates of technical success and lower rates of restenosis. Procedural success rates are generally greater than 95%, with long-term angiographic patency rates of 86 to 92%. Major complications occur in approximately 2% of patients and include parenchymal perforation, cholesterol emboli, embolized stents, and aortic dissection.

Indications for Revascularization in Atherosclerotic RAS

Hypertension

The most common indication for renal artery revascularization is to improve BP control. Improvement occurs in the majority of patients, but complete resolution of hypertension is uncommon. Factors that predict improvement include pretreatment BP (mean level >110 mm Hg) and the presence of bilateral RAS. Because renovascular and nonrenovascular hypertension coexist in an elderly population with atherosclerotic disease, patient selection is critical in deciding whether to undertake renal artery revascularization.

Renal Preservation

Renal artery revascularization can stabilize and even reverse progressive decreases in renal function in selected patients. In a small study of patients with severe hypertension and either bilateral RAS or stenosis in an artery supplying a single functioning kidney, medical therapy resulted in worsening azotemia despite improved BP control, whereas surgical revascularization improved BP control in all patients. Another study showed that renal function improved in 58% and stabilized in 35% of 232 hypertensive patients with elevated creatinine levels who underwent surgical renal revascularization. Results are similar with percutaneous approaches. For example, one study of 25 patients with bilateral RAS and elevated creatinine levels showed that renal artery stenting interrupted progressive renal insufficiency in 18 patients and improved the slope of renal decline in 7.

Pulmonary Edema

Acute pulmonary edema with respiratory failure and death can occur in patients with RAS, especially in patients with bilateral (but usually not unilateral) RAS. Successful revascularization can virtually eliminate recurrent episodes.

FUTURE DIRECTIONS

Important areas of future study include identifying characteristics that predict which patients will benefit from renal artery intervention, determining whether RAS has deleterious effects independent of hypertension and ischemic nephropathy, and optimizing renal artery revascularization.

REFERENCES

Caps MT, Perissinotto C, Zierler RE, et al. Prospective study of atherosclerotic disease progression in the renal artery. *Circulation* 1998;98:2866–2872.

Gruntzig A, Kuhlmann U, Vetter W, et al. Treatment of renovascular hypertension with percutaneous transluminal dilatation of a renal-artery stenosis. *Lancet* 1978;1: 801–802.

Olin JW, Novick AC. Renovascular disease. In: Young JR, Olin JW, Bartholomew JR, eds. *Peripheral Vascular Diseases*. 2nd ed. St. Louis: Mosby; 1996:321–342.

Radermacher J, Chavan A, Bleck J, et al. Use of Doppler ultrasonography to predict the outcome of therapy for renal-artery stenosis. *N Engl J Med* 2001;344:410–417.

Rocha-Singh KJ, Mishkel GJ, Katholi RE, et al. Clinical predictors of improved long-term blood pressure control after successful stenting of hypertensive patients with obstructive renal artery atherosclerosis. *Catheter Cardiovasc Interv* 1999;47:167–172.

Safian RD, Textor SC. Renal-artery stenosis. *N Engl J Med* 2001;344:431–442.

van Jaarsveld BC, Krijnen P, Pieterman H, et al. The effect of balloon angioplasty on hypertension in atherosclerotic renal-artery stenosis. Dutch Renal Artery Stenosis Intervention Cooperative Study Group. *N Engl J Med* 2000;342:1007–1014.

Chapter 41

Interventional Approaches for Peripheral Arterial Disease

Walter A. Tan and Matthew A. Mauro

First introduced in 1964 by Charles Dotter and Melvin Judkins, catheter-based recanalization of arterial atherosclerotic obstruction has expanded in scope and sophistication, benefiting millions of patients with stroke, myocardial infarction (MI), and claudication. Percutaneous interventions have greatly expanded therapeutic options, often complementing and occasionally replacing drugs or surgery. This chapter reviews the indications for endovascular therapy for relatively common extracardiac arterial diseases.

CEREBROVASCULAR AND CARDIOEMBOLIC DISEASE

Carotid Artery Stenosis

More than 600,000 strokes occur annually, and disability as a consequence of stroke is estimated to affect more than 1 million Americans. An important cause of preventable stroke is large-vessel or carotid atherosclerosis. The 2-year risk of stroke ipsilateral to an asymptomatic carotid artery stenosis of 60% or greater is approximately 5% despite drug therapy. This risk increases to 20% in the presence of a previous transient ischemic attack (TIA) or stroke. Carotid endarterectomy (CEA) is highly effective for the primary and secondary prevention of stroke (see chapter 42). The risks of CEA—perioperative death and stroke rates of approximately 3 and 6%, respectively—have led to consideration of percutaneous approaches for the treatment of carotid artery stenosis.

The Carotid and Vertebral Artery Transluminal Angioplasty Study was the first randomized trial to establish the general equivalency of endovascular therapy for carotid stenosis. The 3-year death and stroke rates in the predominantly balloon angioplasty group (only 24% received stents) were similar to those in the CEA group. The trade-off was a higher rate of incidentally detected restenosis: 18% in the balloon angioplasty group compared with 5% for CEA. Carotid stenting was evaluated in a single-center randomized controlled trial of 104 lower-risk patients with a recent TIA or stroke. No statistical difference in death or stroke was found. Of 51

CEA patients, there was 1 death due to postoperative MI and 4 (8%) cranial nerve palsies, compared with 1 intraprocedural TIA and 3 retroperitoneal hemorrhages in the stented group.

Improvements in equipment and operator experience and technique continue to lower the procedural risk. In particular, the development of devices to protect against embolization represents an important step toward improving outcomes in carotid artery stenting. The Stenting and Angioplasty With Protection in Patients at High Risk for Endarterectomy (SAPPHIRE) study, another randomized controlled trial, showed the superiority of carotid stenting in conjunction with cerebral emboli protection in high-risk patients (Fig. 41-1). At 30 days, the primary composite end point of death, stroke, or MI was higher in the CEA group compared with the stented group (12.6% vs. 5.8%, $P < 0.05$).

An important caveat is that procedural experience is a critical determinant of outcome because excessive complication rates occur with operators who have performed fewer than 10 carotid interventions. Although cerebral emboli protection devices generally increase the safety of catheter manipulations within the diseased aortic arch and brachiocephalic arteries, further study will be needed before broad application can be recommended.

Present recommendations are to consider carotid artery stenting for patients who need surgery but are at increased risk because of medical comorbidities or unfavorable anatomic characteristics. These include symptomatic

Figure 41-1

Cerebrovascular Emboli Protection Device

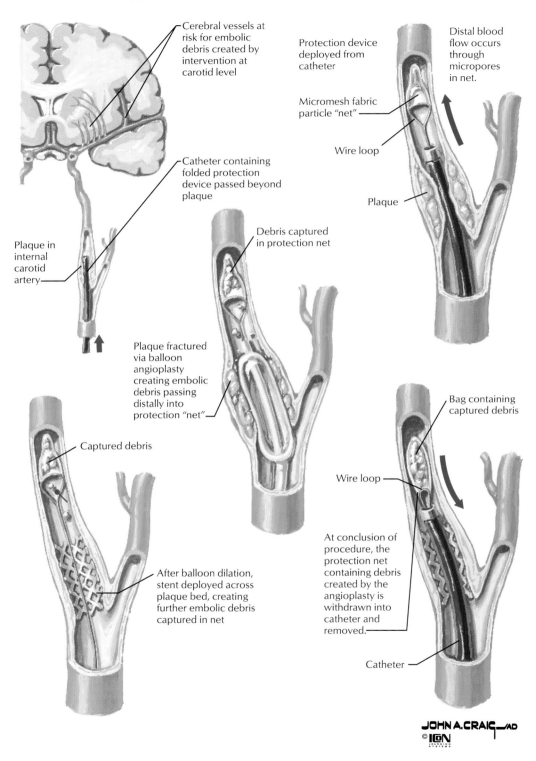

Cerebral vessels at risk for embolic debris created by intervention at carotid level

Protection device deployed from catheter

Distal blood flow occurs through micropores in net.

Micromesh fabric particle "net"

Wire loop

Catheter containing folded protection device passed beyond plaque

Plaque

Debris captured in protection net

Plaque in internal carotid artery

Plaque fractured via balloon angioplasty creating embolic debris passing distally into protection "net"

Captured debris

Bag containing captured debris

Wire loop

After balloon dilation, stent deployed across plaque bed, creating further embolic debris captured in net

At conclusion of procedure, the protection net containing debris created by the angioplasty is withdrawn into catheter and removed.

Catheter

JOHN A. CRAIG—AD
© ICON

patients with more than 50% carotid stenosis and asymptomatic patients with a lesion greater than 80% (SAPPHIRE criteria) who have at least one high-risk feature: age older than 80 years, congestive heart failure, severe coronary artery disease, severe chronic obstructive pulmonary disease (COPD), previous CEA presenting with restenosis, previous radical neck surgery or radiation therapy, or a carotid lesion that is behind the jaw or within the thoracic cavity.

Cerebral Arterial Occlusive Disease

Although angioplasty and stenting of stenoses involving cerebral or vertebral arteries have been performed in patients who do not respond to standard therapy, few randomized data exist to aid in clinical decision making. However, several randomized controlled trials have assessed different fibrinolytics for the treatment of acute stroke. The time window for successful rescue of cerebral tissue is narrow. One trial sponsored by the National Institutes of Health used treatment with IV tissue plasminogen activator within 3 hours after the onset of ischemic stroke and reported improved clinical outcome (death and disability) at 3 months despite an increased incidence of in-hospital intracerebral hemorrhage. Extension of this therapeutic window—to up to 6 hours after stroke onset—is probably feasible with use of catheter-based fibrinolytic therapy which allows local delivery of the fibrinolytic agent. Studies are assessing multiple drug and device strategies to address this problem.

Cardioembolic Stroke

As many as 120,000 strokes per year are attributed to atrial fibrillation. In people 80 years of age and older, atrial fibrillation accounts for nearly 40% of strokes. Although the efficacy of long-term warfarin therapy is established for stroke prevention, a significant number of individuals have contraindications to or complications with anticoagulation or have breakthrough events despite therapeutic concentrations of warfarin. Emerging nonpharmacologic options include percutaneous ablation of arrhythmogenic atrial foci, implantable atrial defibrillators, and percutaneous left atrial appendage transcatheter occlusion (Fig. 41-2, lower).

In young people (<55 years of age), causes of stroke are more variable and approximately 40% of strokes of undetermined origin. It has been proposed that venous-to-systemic (or paradoxical) embolization through a patent foramen ovale (PFO) may account for a significant number of these cryptogenic strokes. Evidence in support of this hypothesis includes the finding that the 4-year risk of recurrent stroke or TIA in patients with no known cause and found to have a PFO estimated to be 2 to 15%, even with anticoagulation therapy. The risk is virtually none after surgical closure of the PFO. Features that predispose patients with PFO to neurologic events are concurrent atrial septal aneurysm, hypercoagulable states, fat or air embolism (e.g., during or following orthopedic surgery or at delivery), and conditions that increase right atrial pressures (e.g., COPD, recurrent pulmonary embolism). Other high-risk markers for subsequent stroke include previous TIA or stroke, large PFO, and higher transatrial bubble counts on echocardiography. Low rates of stroke recurrence have been observed in relatively large case series with transvenous PFO closure devices (Fig. 41-2, upper), and randomized controlled trials comparing this strategy to anticoagulation therapy are currently in progress.

UPPER EXTREMITY DISEASE

The innominate and subclavian arteries supply blood flow to the arms and to the brain via the carotid and vertebral arteries. In patients who have undergone coronary artery bypass grafting using the internal thoracic (mammary) artery, coronary blood flow relies on the innominate and subclavian arteries. Thus, in addition to presenting with arm coolness and claudication, or embolization to the fingers, patients with lesions in the innominate and subclavian arteries can present with angina and symptoms of cerebral hemispheric and vertebrobasilar insufficiency, depending on the specific location of occlusive disease.

Contemporary studies on percutaneous transluminal angioplasty and stenting for brachiocephalic and subclavian stenosis show consistent relief of symptoms and resolution of blood pressure differences between the right and left arms. Complete occlusions are technically more difficult because more manipulations and force

Figure 41-2   ## Interventional Approaches to Peripheral Arterial Disease

Closure of patent foramen ovale (PFO)

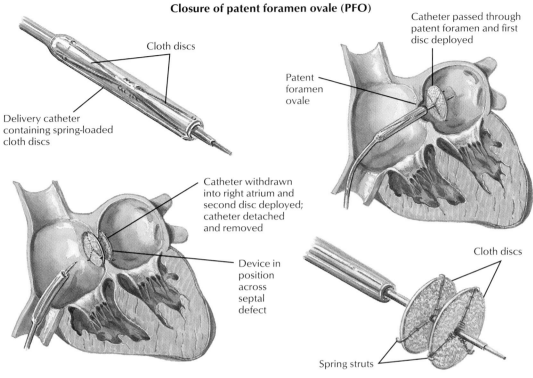

Cloth discs

Delivery catheter containing spring-loaded cloth discs

Catheter passed through patent foramen and first disc deployed

Patent foramen ovale

Catheter withdrawn into right atrium and second disc deployed; catheter detached and removed

Device in position across septal defect

Cloth discs

Spring struts

Percutaneous left atrial appendage transcatheter occlusion (PLAATO)

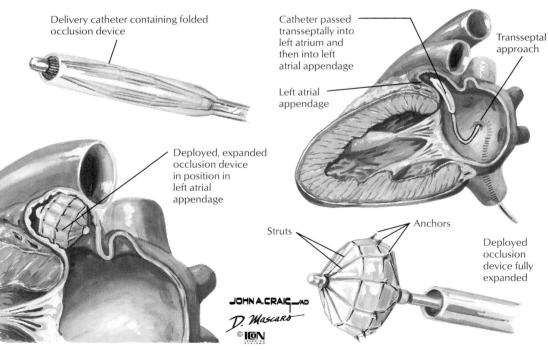

Delivery catheter containing folded occlusion device

Catheter passed transseptally into left atrium and then into left atrial appendage

Transseptal approach

Left atrial appendage

Deployed, expanded occlusion device in position in left atrial appendage

Struts

Anchors

Deployed occlusion device fully expanded

JOHN A. CRAIG_MD
D. Mascaro
© ICN

are needed for recanalization and clinical outcomes are more variable.

There are no available randomized comparisons of surgical and percutaneous revascularization for occlusive diseases involving the aortic arch vessels. Nevertheless, technical success rates for both strategies are close to 97% in the short term, and patency rates are up to 97% at a mean follow-up of 20 months for percutaneous approaches and 84 to 88% at 51 months for surgery. Surgical revascularization seems to be associated with a higher risk of mortality (approximately 2%) and stroke (approximately 3%), events that are rarely seen with percutaneous transluminal angioplasty and stenting. Vascular access bleeding and stent embolization necessitating surgical retrieval have been reported with percutaneous approaches, and dissection, thrombosis, or embolization involving the cerebrovascular arteries, internal thoracic artery, and upper extremity territories are possible, but rare.

Symptomatic extrinsic compression of the subclavian or axillary artery or vein as it crosses the thoracic outlet is a separate clinical entity. Associated anomalies include a cervical rib or fusion of the first and second ribs. Surgical revascularization is the definitive treatment in severe cases of thoracic outlet syndrome or venous (often presenting as superior vena cava) thrombosis. Balloon-expandable stents are relatively contraindicated because of the extrinsic compression risk.

DISEASES OF THE VISCERAL ARTERIES*

The classic presentation of mesenteric ischemia is abdominal pain or bloating 30 to 60 minutes after a meal and weight loss from avoidance of food intake, or "food fear." Symptomatic mesenteric ischemia is rare because multiple collateral pathways connect the three major intestinal branches of the abdominal aorta: the celiac artery and the superior and inferior mesenteric arteries. The differential diagnosis includes atherosclerosis, cardioembolic disease, aortic dissection, celiac artery compression from the median arcuate ligament, and nonocclusive etiologies, such as heart failure with low

---

*See chapter 40 for a discussion of renal artery stenosis.

cardiac output and visceral artery vasospasm from cocaine, ergot, or vasopressors.

Surgery for mesenteric ischemia is highly successful, with nearly a 100% short-term success rate and a primary patency rate of 89% at 6 years. However, the perioperative mortality rate ranges from 4 to 12%. The short-term procedural success rates of visceral artery percutaneous transluminal angioplasty (PTA) are reported to be approximately 79 to 95% and up to 92 to 100% when stents are used. The few procedural failures have been associated with occult malignancy or extrinsic arterial compression by the median arcuate ligament. However, major complications can occur, and restenosis is not rare. A comparison of chronic mesenteric ischemia treated by percutaneous approaches versus historic surgical controls in which the percutaneous group was significantly older (68 vs. 62 years) and had more coronary disease (68% vs. 33%) showed no statistically significant differences in death. Two periprocedural deaths after percutaneous transluminal angioplasty or stenting were related to bowel gangrene and subsequent multisystem organ failure; the third death resulted from MI. There were more than twice as many systemic complications (cardiac, pulmonary, gastrointestinal, or renal) after surgery than after percutaneous revascularization (40% vs. 19%, $P = 0.034$). However, there was almost a threefold difference in cumulative symptom recurrence by 3 years: 34% after percutaneous revascularization and only 13% after surgery.

Poor results are often seen with acute mesenteric ischemia primarily because of associated bowel infarction or necrosis, and exploratory laparotomy should be the main strategy.

LOWER EXTREMITY DISEASE

Clinical results of percutaneous transluminal angioplasty (PTA) are generally comparable to those of surgical bypass for above-knee (iliac or femoropopliteal) arterial disease that does not include multiple serial stenoses or long occlusions. One randomized controlled trial of older patients, 40% of whom had rest pain or gangrene, found no differences between PTA or surgery treatment groups with regard to 1-year primary and secondary patency rates. Complication rates were likewise statistically similar, with a 1-year death rate of 9.8% and a reocclusion rate of 5%. The major amputation rate was 5.7% versus 16% for PTA and surgery, respectively, and the hematoma rates were 7.5% versus 4.1%. In the surgical group, there was an 8% infection rate and an 8% embolization rate, but none of these events were associated with PTA. The Veterans Administration Cooperative controlled trial randomized 255 male patients with claudication or rest pain. There were three study-related deaths, all in the surgery group (n = 126). Of the 129 patients randomized to receive PTA, there were 20 procedural failures (15.4%). Seventeen of these patients who had PTA failure subsequently underwent successful surgical revascularization. A median follow-up of 2 years showed no statistically significant differences between the PTA and surgery groups with regard to death and major amputations. However, the 2-year target limb repeat revascularization was close to 40% after PTA and less than 25% after surgery. It should be noted that no stents were used in this study.

With regard to PTA compared with medical and exercise therapy, the study of Whyman et al. showed a clear advantage exists with PTA up to 6 months' follow-up in terms of improvement in ability to walk up to 1 kilometer and the distance that could be traversed prior to claudication, on a standard treadmill test. Moreover, twice as many patients had lower pain scores on the Nottingham Health profile after undergoing PTA compared with patients who received medical therapy alone. Unfortunately, these benefits were not maintained and there was no statistically significant benefit in the PTA group compared with the control group by 2 years' follow-up. PTA and supervised exercise achieved different but complementary goals in one study. PTA resulted in statistically significant improvement in ankle–brachial pressure index score immediately and up to 15 months after the procedure (mean increase of 0.21), but maximum walking distances improved only modestly. However, the maximum walking distance increased progressively for patients randomized to exercise. In the PTA group, the failure to double the walking distance was due to contralateral (untreated) claudication in five patients and angina or dyspnea in two patients. Although

PTA definitely improves perfusion to the feet, which can confer protection particularly for populations at higher risk for limb loss, such as diabetic patients, supervised exercise improves functional outcome, simultaneously enhances global cardiovascular conditioning, and therefore should be the initial therapeutic approach.

The subset of patients with stenosis confined to the iliac arteries gains the most from PTA or stenting (Fig. 41-3). In one study in which 37% of the randomized patients had iliac artery stenosis, the 1-year patency rate was 90% for the iliac subgroup but diminished to 61% when patients with infrainguinal disease were included. Although surgery seems to confer better long-term patency, complication rates are higher especially in patients with significant comorbidities. In a nonrandomized series of patients who underwent iliac stenting (n = 65) or surgical reconstruction (n = 54), documented surgical complications included death in one patient (due to MI and CHF); pneumonia in three patients; arrhythmias in two patients; and acute renal failure, stroke, ileus, nonspecific colitis, cholecystitis, diverticulitis, and urinary tract infection in one patient each. Vascular complications necessitating treatment in surgical patients included two instances of acute occlusion (one in an aortobifemoral graft and one in an old femoropopliteal graft) and one superficial femoral artery dissection. The corresponding complications for the stent group were acute iliac artery thrombosis in five patients (antiplatelet regimen not specified), retroperitoneal bleeding necessitating transfusion and distal embolization each in two patients, and stent infection in one patient. Based on these findings, it appears that the major advantages of percutaneous therapy are the elimination of the need for general anesthesia, absence of intraperitoneal manipulation, and minimization of postprocedural incisional pain.

FUTURE DIRECTIONS

Atherosclerosis is a systemic disease that involves many arterial territories (Fig. 41-4). Life expectancy estimates for patients with intermittent claudication are decreased by 10 years. Almost one third of these patients die within 5 years after their diagnosis, predominantly as a

Figure 41-3

Interventional Approaches to Peripheral Arterial Disease

Lower extremity arterial disease (PTA or PTAS)

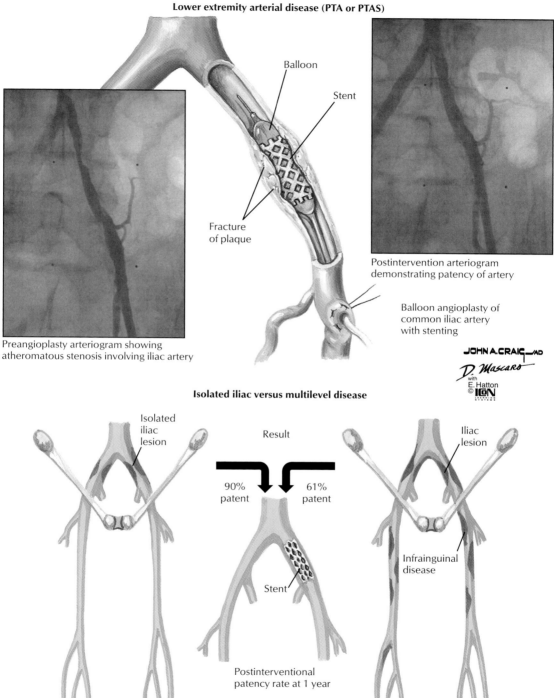

Balloon

Stent

Fracture of plaque

Preangioplasty arteriogram showing atheromatous stenosis involving iliac artery

Postintervention arteriogram demonstrating patency of artery

Balloon angioplasty of common iliac artery with stenting

JOHN A. CRAIG AD
D. Mascaro
with
E. Hatton
© ICN

Isolated iliac versus multilevel disease

Isolated iliac lesion

Result

90% patent

61% patent

Stent

Iliac lesion

Infrainguinal disease

Postinterventional patency rate at 1 year

Clinical results of percutaneous transluminal angioplasty are comparable to those of surgical bypass for above-knee (iliac of femoropopliteal) arterial disease that does not include multiple serial stenoses or long occlusions. The subset of patients with stenosis confined to iliac arteries benefits most from PTA or stenting.

Figure 41-4

Multiterritorial Disease

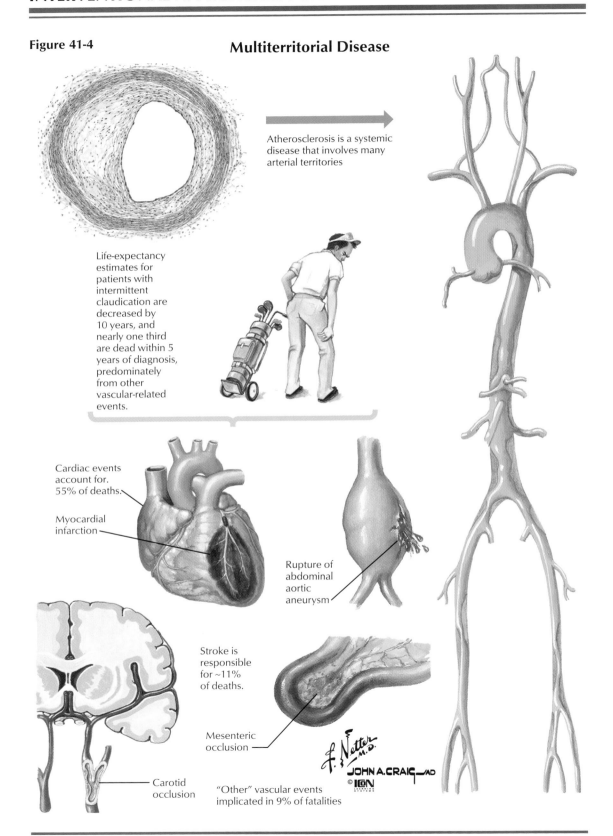

Atherosclerosis is a systemic disease that involves many arterial territories

Life-expectancy estimates for patients with intermittent claudication are decreased by 10 years, and nearly one third are dead within 5 years of diagnosis, predominately from other vascular-related events.

Cardiac events account for. 55% of deaths.

Myocardial infarction

Rupture of abdominal aortic aneurysm

Stroke is responsible for ~11% of deaths.

Mesenteric occlusion

Carotid occlusion

"Other" vascular events implicated in 9% of fatalities

result of cardiac events (approximately 55%), stroke (approximately 11%), and other vascular events (approximately 9%), including ruptured aortic aneurysms. These elderly patients with multiple comorbidities need interspecialty communication and collaboration among primary care providers, geriatricians, cardiologists, interventional radiologists, endocrinologists, neurologists, surgeons, and other healthcare team members. Multidisciplinary care that maximizes prevention, health maintenance, and optimal selection of patients and procedures (diagnostic and therapeutic) with rapid advances in peripheral vascular equipment (coated stents, miniaturized and customized wires and catheters), adjunctive drug therapy (new-generation antiplatelets and anticoagulants), clinical trial methodology and infrastructures, the establishment of training and credentialing standards, and the creation of excellent vascular centers will result in enhanced quantity and quality of life.

REFERENCES

2002 Heart and Stroke Statistical Update. Dallas: American Heart Association; 2001:1–39.

Endovascular versus surgical treatment in patients with carotid stenosis in the Carotid and Vertebral Artery Transluminal Angioplasty Study (CAVATAS): A randomised trial. *Lancet* 2001;357:1729–1737.

Hadjipetrou P, Cox S, Piemonte T, Eisenhauer A. Percutaneous revascularization of atherosclerotic obstruction of aortic arch vessels. *J Am Coll Cardiol* 1999;33: 1238–1245.

Hertzer NR, Beven EG, Young JR, et al. Coronary artery disease in peripheral vascular patients: A classification of 1000 coronary angiograms and results of surgical management. *Ann Surg* 1984;199:223–233.

Mas JL, Arquizan C, Lamy C, et al. Recurrent cerebrovascular events associated with patent foramen ovale, atrial septal aneurysm, or both. *N Engl J Med* 2001;345: 1740–1746.

Wilson SE, Wolf GL, Cross AP. Percutaneous transluminal angioplasty versus operation for peripheral arteriosclerosis: Report of a prospective randomized trial in a selected group of patients. *J Vasc Surg* 1989;9:1–9.

Whyman MR, Fowkes FG, Kerracher EM, et al. Is intermittent claudication improved by percutaneous transluminal angioplasty? A randomized controlled trial. *J Vasc Surg* 1997;26:551–557.

Yadav JS. Late breaking clinical trials: The Stenting and Angioplasty With Protection in Patients at High Risk for Endarterectomy (SAPPHIRE) study. Presented at: American Heart Association Scientific Sessions 2002; November 17–20, 2002; Chicago, Ill.

Chapter 42

Surgery for Peripheral Vascular Diseases

Robert Mendes, Mark A. Farber, and Blair A. Keagy

Peripheral vascular disease (PVD) encompasses pathology of both the arterial and the venous circulations. Advanced disease of either system can be debilitating and disabling. The scope of PVD is extensive. This chapter focuses on the more common problems that require surgical intervention.

Aneurysmal disease usually involves large arteries, most commonly the infrarenal aorta and iliac arteries. Aneurysmal disease less often involves other major arteries, including the thoracic aorta and the femoral and popliteal arteries. Although small aneurysms have been reported to rupture, the risk of rupture is thought to rise exponentially with increasing diameter. Atherosclerosis involving the infrarenal aorta, iliac, and infrainguinal arteries is a common cause of arterial insufficiency of the lower extremities. PVD can be subdivided into categories based on location: inflow (infrarenal aorta, iliac), outflow (femoral, popliteal), and runoff (tibial, peroneal) vessels. These categories help define the risks and the benefits of intervention and treatment options.

A detailed history and physical examination can identify the anatomic distribution of vascular pathology. Invasive and noninvasive imaging augment clinical findings and aid decision making. Several open surgical and endovascular interventions, discussed later herein, provide significant benefits to patients with PVD.

Other vascular system areas affected by occlusive disease include the carotid arteries and the visceral vessels. Surgical options for the treatment of these areas are also discussed. Although PVD includes venous pathologies, because these are less likely to result in serious morbidity and mortality, this chapter focuses on arterial pathologies.

ETIOLOGY AND PATHOGENESIS

For many years, the etiology of aneurysmal disease was felt to be primarily related to atherosclerosis, largely because aneurysmal disease occurs predominantly in elderly hypertensive individuals and is associated with tobacco use.

The etiology is now thought to be multifactorial. Genetic predisposition may be involved in up to one third of patients with aneurysms. Microscopic analysis indicates that deficiencies in elastin, collagen, or both may be crucial factors. Collagen-degrading matrix metalloproteinases are likely culprits in aneurysm formation, and current research focuses on their role in the pathogenesis of aneurysmal disease. Elastin and collagen breakdown, which may be accelerated based on a genetic predisposition to produce matrix metalloproteinases, may precipitate an inflammatory reaction. This inflammatory reaction contributes to weakening of the arterial wall and eventual dilatation. Embolic disease, thrombosis, or trauma may also cause arterial occlusion (Fig. 42-1). However, the most common cause of lower extremity arterial occlusion is atherosclerosis. The etiology and pathogenesis of atherosclerosis are discussed in chapter 37.

ABDOMINAL AORTIC ANEURYSMS
Clinical Presentation

Abdominal pain may indicate rapid enlargement or impending rupture of an abdominal aortic aneurysm (AAA). Ruptured abdominal aortic aneurysms are the 13th leading cause of death in the United States, despite advances in diagnostic imaging, screening programs, and heightened awareness. Other symptoms of AAA include nausea, early satiety, and back pain from compression of adjacent structures; however, approximately 75% of patients are asymptomatic at presentation.

Management and Therapy

Management guidelines center on evaluation of rupture risk. When the risk of rupture exceeds

Figure 42-1

Atherosclerosis, Thrombosis, and Embolism

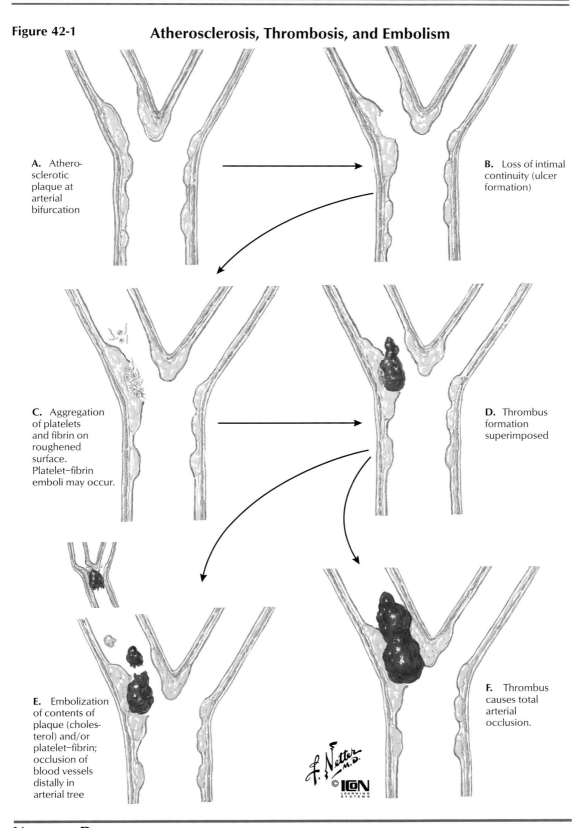

A. Athero-sclerotic plaque at arterial bifurcation

B. Loss of intimal continuity (ulcer formation)

C. Aggregation of platelets and fibrin on roughened surface. Platelet–fibrin emboli may occur.

D. Thrombus formation superimposed

E. Embolization of contents of plaque (choles-terol) and/or platelet–fibrin; occlusion of blood vessels distally in arterial tree

F. Thrombus causes total arterial occlusion.

the risk of surgical repair, replacement of aneurysmal segment of the artery is indicated. For asymptomatic AAA, the risk of rupture varies with the diameter of the aneurysm; an AAA of 5 cm has a 5% rupture risk per year, and an AAA of 6 cm has an estimated 10 to 15% rupture risk per year. Patients with saccular aneurysms, patients with COPD, and patients with hypertension are thought to have a higher than average risk of aneurysm rupture. Treatment is indicated for aneurysms that are greater than twice the normal artery diameter, that are enlarging rapidly (>0.5 cm/6 months), or that are symptomatic—the major symptoms being pain or evidence or distal emboli potentially related to the aneurysm.

During the past 50 years, the technique for AAA repair has remained essentially unchanged, with outcome improvements resulting from advances in preoperative screening and risk stratification, improved anesthetic practice, and intensive care management. In addition, the use of a homograft for AAA repair has been replaced by the use of more durable synthetic grafts (Fig. 42-2, upper). Aneurysmorrhaphy involves mobilization and exposure of the aneurysm and the normal artery above and below the diseased section. Blood flow through the artery is arrested for inline replacement of the diseased artery with an artificial one, resulting in major cardiovascular stress during the procedure and for several days after. The combination of cardiovascular stress and the advanced age and comorbid conditions of the patient increases the procedure-associated morbidity and mortality rates. Patients usually require 7 to 10 days of hospitalization and 6 to 8 weeks to recover. However, once patients fully recover from the procedure, long-term follow-up indicates that few patients need further intervention. When further intervention is needed, generally it is because progression of the disease has occurred in adjacent arteries. Ongoing research focuses on the identification of mechanisms to arrest the disease process to prevent spread and inhibit the inflammatory process.

As general medical care and nutrition have improved, the mean age in the United States and industrialized countries has increased, and with this, there is an increasing number of individuals with AAAs. As the age and medical comorbidities of patients with AAA increased, interest in less invasive procedures for treatment increased, resulting in the development of minimally invasive techniques for the treatment of aneurysmal disease. AAA endovascular repair techniques involve the insertion of a new lining into the diseased artery with the use of hooks or stents to secure the lining to the arterial wall. Four devices are approved by the Food and Drug Administration for the treatment of infrarenal AAA. The indications for treatment with endovascular devices are identical to those for open surgical repair. The procedure can be performed under local, regional, or general anesthesia and typically involves exposure of the common femoral arteries for device insertion. Although insertion has been accomplished with percutaneous techniques, most devices are too large for insertion by routine percutaneous treatment methods. Once the aorta is accessed, imaging methods guide device implantation just below the renal arteries, where the aorta and its endothelium are the healthiest. Most patients are hospitalized for 1 day and are fully recovered from the procedure within 1 week. Successful implantation is accomplished in more than 98% of patients.

Patient selection is crucial to outcomes with endovascular aneurysm repair. Seal failures (endoleak) are more likely to occur in patients with short, angled, or diseased proximal infrarenal arteries. During follow-up, complications associated with endoleaks or migration develop in 6 to 15% of patients. Many of these complications can be treated with secondary endovascular interventions and do not necessitate conversion to open repair and removal of the device. Iliac artery access issues (smaller or diseased artery) may also create complications associated with implantation. Although new design techniques and lower-profile devices have overcome many of these problems, complications occur in 1 to 2% of patients.

Prospective studies have not shown a reduction in the mortality rate associated with endovascular aneurysm repair procedures compared to open surgery; yet most studies show the rate of major morbidity reduced by approximately 50%. Blood loss and time to return to an active lifestyle are also significantly reduced. The

Figure 42-2

Surgical Management of Aortic Aneurysms

Abdominal aortic aneurysm (infrarenal)

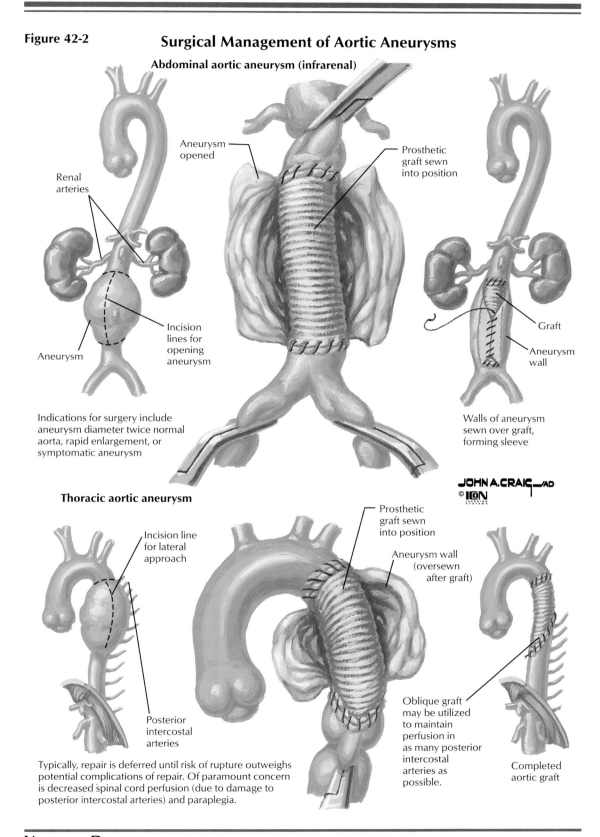

Aneurysm opened

Prosthetic graft sewn into position

Renal arteries

Incision lines for opening aneurysm

Aneurysm

Graft

Aneurysm wall

Indications for surgery include aneurysm diameter twice normal aorta, rapid enlargement, or symptomatic aneurysm

Walls of aneurysm sewn over graft, forming sleeve

JOHN A. CRAIG_AD
©ICON

Thoracic aortic aneurysm

Incision line for lateral approach

Prosthetic graft sewn into position

Aneurysm wall (oversewn after graft)

Posterior intercostal arteries

Oblique graft may be utilized to maintain perfusion in as many posterior intercostal arteries as possible.

Completed aortic graft

Typically, repair is deferred until risk of rupture outweighs potential complications of repair. Of paramount concern is decreased spinal cord perfusion (due to damage to posterior intercostal arteries) and paraplegia.

midterm data suggest that patient survival is greater after endovascular aneurysm repair than after traditional open surgical treatment, and this has resulted in the increased use of this approach. Of all aneurysms treated in 2002, 30% were treated with use of endovascular repair techniques. As branched designs and other innovations are incorporated and durability concerns are addressed, the use of endovascular aneurysm repair technology will increase. It is expected that by 2008, more than 50% of aneurysms will be treated by an endovascular approach.

THORACIC ANEURYSMS
Clinical Presentation

Thoracic aneurysms are less prevalent than AAAs. The clinical presentation of thoracic aneurysms is similar to that of AAAs in that most patients are asymptomatic. Compression of adjacent structures can produce chest pain, hoarseness from recurrent laryngeal nerve injury, back pain, or pulmonary problems from compression of bronchial structures.

Management and Treatment

As is the case for surgical repair of infrarenal disease, surgical repair of thoracic aneurysms usually requires replacement of the diseased artery. However, the risks associated with surgical repair of thoracic and thoracoabdominal aneurysms are significantly higher than those of AAA repair. One major risk associated with thoracoabdominal aneurysm repair is paraplegia, because perfusion to the spinal cord must be interrupted during the repair. Several approaches are used to limit the amount of ischemia, including the use of barbiturates, hypothermia, and spinal cord drainage to increase perfusion pressure via collaterals. Even with these protective approaches, for extensive aneurysms involving the area from the left subclavian artery to the aortic bifurcation, the risk of paraplegia may be as high as 25%. For small aneurysms involving a short section of the aorta, the risk of paraplegia is not negligible (2–8%). Because of the high risk, treatment is delayed until the risk of rupture is greater than the risk of repair, typically when an aneurysm is 6 cm in diameter (Fig. 42-2, lower). Individuals with Marfan's disease or other collagen vascular diseases represent an important

subset, in whom the risk of dissection and/or rupture is increased even at smaller aneurysm diameters, requiring earlier surgical intervention.

The results of endovascular therapy trials being conducted for the treatment of thoracic diseases are promising. Although an association between endovascular therapy and paraplegia exists in patients with a concomitant or previous infrarenal repair, no association is recognized with the length of aorta covered by the endograft. Other thoracic aortic pathologies being treated include aortic dissections, aortic transections, penetrating ulcers, and ruptured plaques, all with promising results. The issues of graft migration and durability are very important in the thoracic aorta and are a major concern for technology development.

FEMORAL AND POPLITEAL ANEURYSMS
Clinical Presentation

Femoral and popliteal artery aneurysms are also associated with AAAs. Most patients present with embolic or thrombotic complications in the form of "blue toes" or lower extremity ischemia, respectively. Popliteal aneurysm thrombosis can result in critical leg ischemia and limb loss. Some patients with popliteal aneurysms may present with posterior knee complaints from compression of adjacent structures. The risk of rupture for either a femoral or a popliteal aneurysm is low; however, there are reports of ruptures related to direct trauma.

Management and Treatment

Because of the superficial location and easy surgical access of femoral artery aneurysms, these aneurysms are treated with aneurysmorrhaphy and, if necessary, reconstruction of the femoral bifurcation. Complication rates are low, usually involving recurrence, intimal hyperplastic issues, or graft infection. Endovascular techniques are not necessary because of the location of the aneurysm and the ease of repair, excellent outcome, and low morbidity with surgical intervention. Surgical bypass is mainly employed for popliteal aneurysms, with aneurysm ligation to prevent further embolization. Reports of successful endovascular therapy for popliteal aneurysms exist but usually involve isolated aneurysms in a proximal or distal arterial section without involvement of the joint space or areas of increased flexibility and mobility. As endovascular device technology improves, it may become an attractive method of treatment, although comparison to the surgical outcome standard will be necessary.

LOWER EXTREMITY ATHEROSCLEROSIS
Clinical Presentation

With the development of collateral circulation, patients are often asymptomatic despite moderate lower extremity atherosclerosis. Comorbid conditions, such as cardiac disease, may restrict patient activity and obviate the need for increased oxygen above baseline levels. For individuals who can ambulate, claudication—muscle "cramping" or discomfort after walking a specific distance, with relief of the pain upon resting—is often the chief complaint. This pain is reproducible and consistent with pathophysiology that limits muscular blood supply during exertion, causing lactic acid accumulation.

Claudication of the proximal muscles of the leg, buttock, or hip usually indicates inflow disease, commonly referred to as *aortoiliac occlusive disease*. In some patients with severe disease, Leriche syndrome may develop; patients with Leriche syndrome exhibit the characteristic triad of sexual dysfunction, buttock claudication, and absent femoral pulses. The association between aortoiliac occlusive disease and proximal muscle complaints is variable, and some patients complain of calf claudication despite the presence of significant occlusion more proximally. Atheromatous embolization from aortoiliac lesions can lodge in the distal vessels, creating localized ischemia of the digits with resulting cyanosis. Because this is an embolic process, patients with the "blue toe syndrome" often have palpable distal pulses and may, depending on the degree of involvement, experience resolution of their clinical symptoms with time or therapy.

Patients with atherosclerosis involving the femoropopliteal (outflow) vessels or with multilevel distribution of the disease can present with complaints ranging from claudication, the mildest presentation, to the most severe symptoms of rest pain and tissue loss. Often, patients with mild complaints never seek medical attention because they attribute symptoms to arthritis or "old age." However, as the disease worsens and rest pain ensues, a persistent "burning" or "aching" sensation over the dorsum of the foot often prompts the individual to seek help. Although usually of little benefit, patients may keep the ischemic limb in a dependent position, in an attempt to allow gravity to aid in blood flow. Other signs characteristic of severe ischemia include dependent rubor, muscle atrophy, skin changes, lower extremity alopecia, ulcerations, and the lack of palpable distal pulses. Although these symptoms and signs of severe ischemia occur in nondiabetic individuals, diabetes is increasingly a contributing comorbidity (Fig. 42-3). Isolated lesions at a single-level rarely result in lower extremity rest pain and nonhealing ulcerations. Patients who present with concomitant lower extremity infections and persistent ulcerations despite medical therapy should be thoroughly evaluated for significant arterial insufficiency. In many instances, these patients require lower extremity revascularization to salvage limbs.

Management and Therapy

All patients should undergo aggressive evaluation and treatment for hyperlipidemia and other genetic disorders associated with progressive atherosclerosis. The alteration of risk factors, most importantly cessation of smoking, may slow disease progression. In addition, patients should integrate diet modification, encouragement of collateral circulation with exercise regimens, and prevention of lower extremity trauma and infection into their lifestyles. Drug therapy with an antiplatelet or hemorheologic agent such as pentoxifylline or cilostazol can provide some benefit.

Ischemic rest pain, ulceration, and gangrene of the digits are indications for arterial reconstruction if anatomically feasible. Decisions about operations for lifestyle-impairing claudication must be based on patient comorbidities and the anatomic distribution of the disease. The decision of which operative approach, if any, is best for an individual is based on the natural history of the disease, the overall condition of the patient, and the risks and benefits of the

Figure 42-3   Complications of Diabetic Vasculopathy and Neuropathy

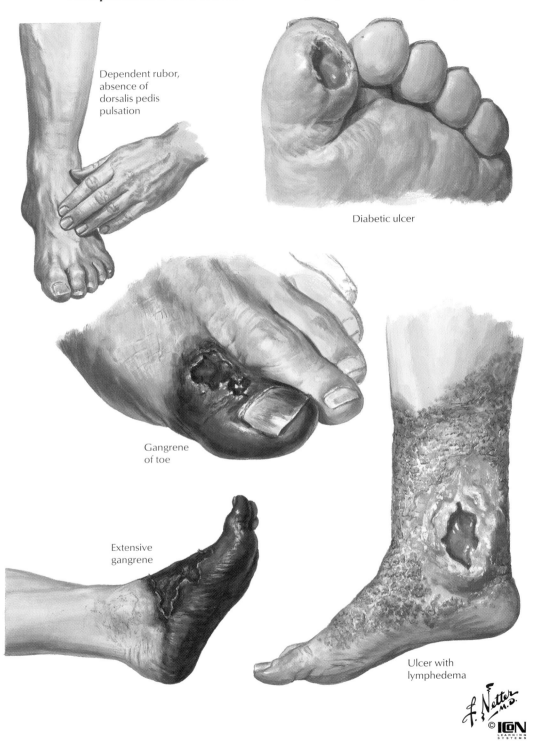

Dependent rubor, absence of dorsalis pedis pulsation

Diabetic ulcer

Gangrene of toe

Extensive gangrene

Ulcer with lymphedema

intervention (Fig. 42-4). Goals for the procedure outcome (limb salvage, wound healing, relief of rest pain, exercise tolerance, etc.) must be determined before surgical intervention. Endovascular procedures increase the options for therapy and are discussed in chapter 41.

Inflow disease should be addressed first; this can often relieve symptoms and obviate the need for the less successful infrainguinal bypasses. Patients with symptomatic inflow disease can be treated with endovascular therapies, inline arterial reconstructions, or extra-anatomic bypass. In making the decision about surgical therapy, consideration of both the patient's perioperative risk and the influence of his/her anatomy and comorbidities on graft survival are important. For instance, comorbidities may exclude one approach or another. Other issues, such as cigarette smoking, may also influence the therapeutic decision. Many vascular surgeons will not perform reconstructive surgery on patients who are still smoking, because smoking lowers bypass patency rates dramatically.

Bilateral aortoiliac disease is best treated with aortobifemoral grafting, using a prosthetic graft. The patency of this graft approximates 80 to 90% at 5 years and about 70% at 10 years. The mortality risks for this procedure are less than 5%. In patients with a history of abdominal infection, prior irradiation, abdominal stomas, or multiple abdominal operations (all of which increase operative morbidity rates), the descending thoracic aorta can be used as an alternative inflow source. The thoracobifemoral bypass achieves patency rates of 75 to 85% at 5 years, with perioperative mortality rates below 5% when the bypasses are performed by experienced vascular surgeons. Extra-anatomic bypasses (grafts that course through a significantly different anatomic pathway from the native arteries) should be performed in patients who would not tolerate major aortic reconstructive surgery because of comorbidities. The most common extra-anatomic procedures are axillobifemoral and femorofemoral bypass grafts. The axillobifemoral reconstruction, used for aortoiliac occlusive disease, has 5-year patency rates of 50 to 60%. For patients with unilateral iliac disease not amenable to angioplasty, femorofemoral bypass has a 5-year patency rate of 50 to 80%.

Critical ischemia or tissue loss from infrainguinal occlusive disease is best treated with arterial reconstruction. With respect to patency and resistance to infections, autologous vein grafts are superior to other conduits, especially when reconstruction below the knee is necessary. Availability, quality, and length requirements may necessitate a search for alternate sites for veins, such as the arms (basilic, cephalic) or the posterior leg (lesser saphenous vein). If possible, an autologous graft rather than synthetic material should be used for infrainguinal bypasses. Prosthetic material in lower extremity bypass procedures is reserved mainly for patients without other conduit options. In some cases, prosthetic material may be used for reconstructions above the knee.

Comparison of autologous saphenous vein with polytetrafluoroethylene grafts in above-the-knee (femoropopliteal) and below-the-knee (distal femoropopliteal and femorodistal) bypass procedures showed equivalent 2-year patency rates in grafts to the same level, but patency diverged to a significant difference at 4 years. The differences at 4 years were significant for infrapopliteal bypasses but not for above-the-knee procedures. Of course, prosthetic graft material for distal bypasses is a better option than primary amputation in patients with suboptimal autologous vein options.

CAROTID DISEASE
Clinical Presentation
Most patients with carotid artery stenosis are asymptomatic (see also chapters 38 and 41). For patients with symptoms, complaints range from contralateral extremity weakness, ipsilateral facial weakness, slurred speech, or temporary monocular blindness (amaurosis fugax) to fully developed stroke deficits.

Management and Treatment
Carotid endarterectomy has been the mainstay of treatment of carotid artery disease for decades. Large multicenter trials (Asymptomatic Carotid Atherosclerosis Study and North American Symptomatic Carotid Endarterectomy Trial) validated the safety and efficacy of carotid endarterectomy in treating and preventing strokes in patients with carotid artery stenosis.

Figure 42-4

Surgical Management of Peripheral Arterial Disease of Lower Extremity

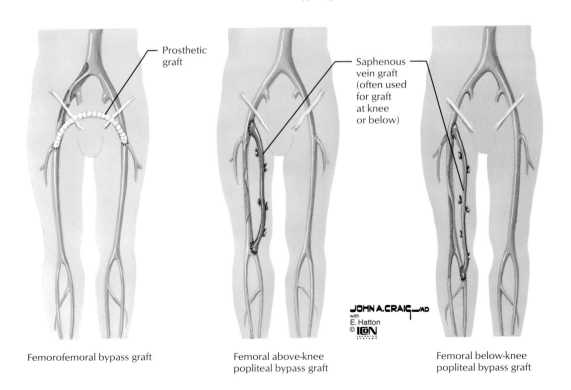

Prosthetic graft
(prosthetic graft material often
used for infrainguinal grafts)

Axillary artery

Inguinal ligament

Aortobifemoral bypass graft

Thoracobifemoral bypass graft

Axillobifemoral bypass graft

Prosthetic graft

Saphenous vein graft
(often used for graft at knee or below)

JOHN A.CRAIG—AD
with
E. Hatton
© ICON

Femorofemoral bypass graft

Femoral above-knee popliteal bypass graft

Femoral below-knee popliteal bypass graft

Surgical therapy involves exposure of the carotid bifurcation under general or regional anesthesia. After arresting flow and removing the intima and the media of the diseased section, the artery is closed. The procedural stroke rate is 1 to 2%. Adjacent nerve injuries and hematomas are the most common complications. With the use of routine carotid patch closure, long-term restenosis rates are significantly reduced. Patients recover quickly from this procedure (1 week) and hospitalizations are routinely less than 24 hours.

VISCERAL DISEASE
Clinical Presentation

Patients with atherosclerotic lesions involving the visceral section typically present with end-organ ischemia. Although abdominal bruits are often detected, the natural history of the disease indicates that patients rarely become symptomatic. With the newer antihypertensive medications, fewer patients present with uncontrollable hypertension. There is considerable debate about whether asymptomatic disease should be treated, with the goal of preserving renal function (see chapter 40).

Management and Treatment

In patients with mesenteric ischemia, collateral flow can come from a number of vascular distributions, including the iliac arteries, the supraceliac aorta, and the thoracic aorta. Because of the low prevalence of the disease, individual series are small and results difficult to compare. After surgical repair, long-term patency is difficult to assess without follow-up angiography. Based on relief of symptoms, surgical approaches are highly successful; symptom-free disease is experienced by 80 to 100% of patients. Because of the limited involvement of the thoracic aorta in atherosclerotic disease, many surgeons prefer the bypass originate from the thoracic aorta. Graft failures are unusual with this approach in patients followed up longitudinally by duplex ultrasonography. Surgical mortality and morbidity rates are low. Bypass techniques for the renal arteries typically utilize a replacement aortic graft or, for inflow, the splenic or hepatic artery. With advances in endovascular therapies, fewer open surgical procedures are being performed on visceral arteries.

AORTIC DISSECTIONS
Clinical Presentation

Aortic dissections typically occur in a younger subset of patients, who present with back pain and uncontrollable hypertension. Management is based largely on the location of disease. The acute and long-term morbidity and mortality rates in patients with ascending aortic arch dissections are very high. Patients presenting with acute aortic regurgitation, cardiac tamponade, and coronary ischemia usually have ascending arch involvement. Fortunately, 80% of aortic dissections involve the descending thoracic aorta.

Management and Treatment

Dissections involving the ascending arch require emergent repair to prevent or correct a rupture into the mediastinum or the pericardium and to prevent or correct coronary artery dissection. In many cases, replacement of the ascending aortic arch and the aortic valve is necessary, with reimplantation of the coronary arteries from their normal ostia into the aortic graft. Management of descending dissections has largely been medical, with blood pressure reduction and expectant management of ischemic complications involving the branch vessels (mesenteric, renal, spinal cord, and lower extremities). When malperfusion exists, reperfusion via bypass or endovascular techniques is necessary to reestablish flow. Improvement in endovascular techniques has decreased the use of open surgical treatment. When surgical intervention is required, it is associated with a greater than 50% mortality rate. In general, surgical correction is most successful for treating patients with descending aortic dissection when the major issue is lower extremity ischemia. In this case, the use of extra-anatomic bypasses, such as axillobifemoral or femorofemoral bypasses, is effective and reasonably safe. When necessary, fenestration with or without aortic stent grafts is used to improve hemodynamics. Stent grafts can exclude acute aortic ruptures resulting from dissections. Multimodality treatment including intravascular ultrasonography is critical for accurate assessment and for identifying the best intervention.

FUTURE DIRECTIONS

As the development of endovascular devices continues, more than 50% of traditional surgical vascular procedures will be replaced with minimally invasive procedures, because of both patient preference and outcomes. The minimally invasive techniques will include branched devices for aneurysmal disease and the use of drug-eluting stents or other devices (analogous to those currently used in coronary artery disease, see chapter 10) to inhibit intimal hyperplasia and arrest the aneurysmal disease process in adjacent arteries. Standard surgical management algorithms will center on endovascular therapies with combined open and endovascular treatments for patients with complex problems not amenable to solely endovascular approaches. Until treatment options involve only endovascular percutaneous therapies—

with proven long-term success rates comparable to the success rates of surgical treatments— physicians trained to perform both endovascular and surgical treatments are best suited to provide care.

REFERENCES

Burnham SJ, Jaques P, Burnham CB. Noninvasive detection of iliac artery stenosis in the presence of superficial femoral artery obstruction. *J Vasc Surg* 1992;16:445–452.

Veith FJ, Gupta SK, Ascer E, et al. Six year prospective multicenter randomized comparison of autologous saphenous vein and expanded polytetrafluoroethylene grafts in infrainguinal arterial reconstructions. *J Vasc Surg* 1986;3:104–114.

Weiss NS. Cigarette smoking and arteriosclerosis obliterans: An epidemiologic approach. *Am J Epidemiol* 1972; 95:17–25.

Section VIII

CONGENITAL HEART DISEASE

Chapter 43

An Approach to Children With Suspected Congenital Heart Disease

G. William Henry

Birth defects occur in approximately 2% of all births. Congenital heart disease comprises almost half of such defects, occurring in approximately 8 in 1000 newborn infants. Many classifications exist for congenital heart disease, and two variations based on a simple physiologic approach follow.

Congenital heart defects can be classified into those that result in cyanosis and those that do not. Acyanotic defects include those with a left-to-right shunt and increased pulmonary blood flow and obstructive defects without associated shunting. Left-to-right shunts occur at various anatomic levels: atrial (e.g., atrial septal defect), ventricular (e.g., ventricular septal defect [part of the complex defect depicted in Fig. 43-1]), or arterial (e.g., patent arterial duct). Obstructive lesions without any associated shunts include pulmonary stenosis, aortic stenosis, and coarctation of the aorta.

Cyanotic defects are generally characterized by a right-to-left shunt and may be classified into two broad categories. In the first group, with intracardiac defects and obstruction to pulmonary flow, cyanosis results from decreased pulmonary blood flow and the intracardiac mixing of oxygenated and desaturated blood. In the second group, cyanosis results from the admixture of pulmonary and systemic venous returns despite normal or increased pulmonary blood flow. In most cardiac malformations classified in this group, a single chamber receives the total systemic and pulmonary venous returns. The admixture lesion can occur at any intracardiac level: venous (e.g., total anomalous pulmonary venous connection), atrial (e.g., single atrium), ventricular (e.g., single ventricle), and great vessel (e.g., persistent truncus arteriosus). Near-uniform mixing of the venous returns usually occurs. Complete transposition of the great arteries (Fig. 43-2) can be included in this group, although only partial admixture of the two venous returns occurs, leading to severe hypoxemia.

CLINICAL INDICATIONS FOR MEDICAL OR SURGICAL INTERVENTION

The interdisciplinary approach that is needed clinically to optimally care for children with congenital heart disease includes accurate assessment of anatomic defects and their physiologic consequences and effective communication of these findings. The consequences of altered blood flow induced by congenital heart disease and the effects of therapeutic interventions invariably influence the pulmonary circulation by increasing pulmonary blood flow (e.g., left-to-right shunting through intracardiac septal defects), decreasing pulmonary blood flow (e.g., right-sided obstructive heart lesions, such as tetralogy of Fallot) (Fig. 43-3), altering the pathway of pulmonary blood flow (e.g., Fontan-Kreutzer repair), or altering the hemodynamics to which pulmonary blood flow (e.g., pulmonary hypertension) is subjected. Successful management can often depend on the ability of the clinician to monitor pulmonary hemodynamics and assess pulmonary vascular impairment.

Critically important to an understanding of the physiologic consequences of these defects are the maturational differences that occur in cardiopulmonary function. For example, cardiac function is subject to maturational changes occurring at the cellular level in a variety of processes, including those in the neurocardiac functional unit: changes in neurotransmitter content, the receptor system, innervation, the effector/transducer systems, and the cellular components affected by autonomic stimulation (Fig. 43-4).

Figure 43-1

Interrupted Aortic Arch Complex

A. Pathophysiology

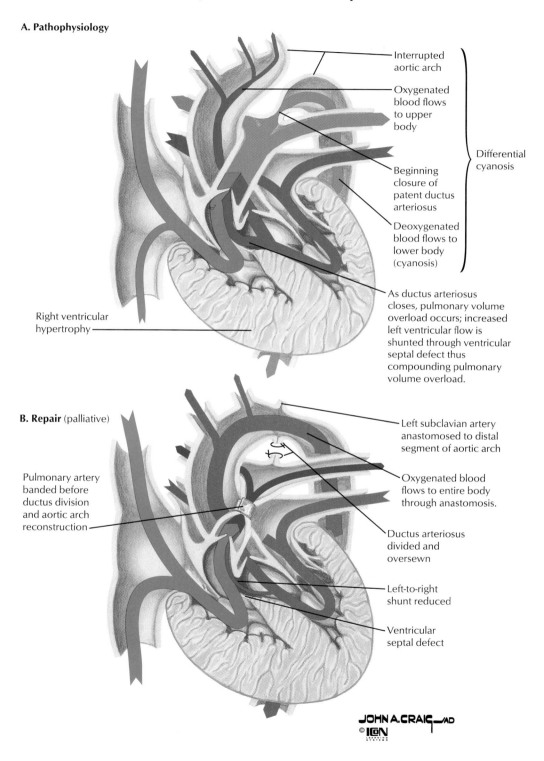

Interrupted aortic arch

Oxygenated blood flows to upper body

Beginning closure of patent ductus arteriosus

Deoxygenated blood flows to lower body (cyanosis)

Differential cyanosis

As ductus arteriosus closes, pulmonary volume overload occurs; increased left ventricular flow is shunted through ventricular septal defect thus compounding pulmonary volume overload.

Right ventricular hypertrophy

B. Repair (palliative)

Pulmonary artery banded before ductus division and aortic arch reconstruction

Left subclavian artery anastomosed to distal segment of aortic arch

Oxygenated blood flows to entire body through anastomosis.

Ductus arteriosus divided and oversewn

Left-to-right shunt reduced

Ventricular septal defect

JOHN A. CRAIG ᴍᴅ
© ICN
LEARNING SYSTEMS

Figure 43-2

Transposition of Great Arteries

Balloon Atrial Septostomy (Technique)

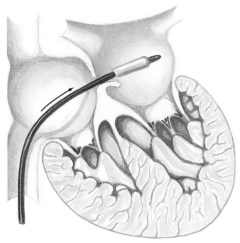

1. Balloon-tipped catheter introduced into left atrium through patent foramen ovale

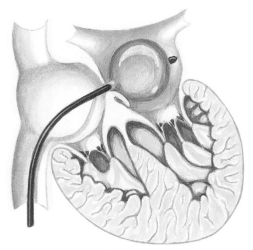

2. Balloon inflated

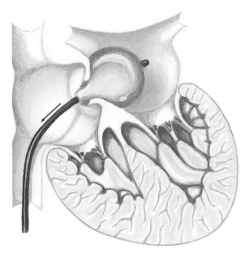

3. Balloon withdrawn producing large septal defect

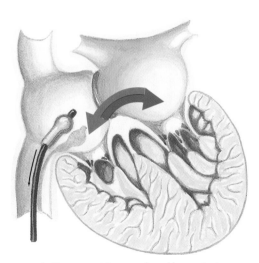

4. Common atrium produced by septostomy allows mixing of oxygenated and deoxygenated blood

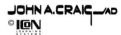

JOHN A. CRAIG—AD
© ICON
LEARNING
SYSTEMS

Regardless of the anatomic defects, the physiologic consequences necessitating medical intervention, surgical intervention, or both fall into three broad categories—heart failure, hypoxemia/hypoxia, and risk of pulmonary vascular disease—and represent a second approach to children with suspected congenital heart disease (by risk stratification).

Heart failure is defined as the inability of the heart to supply an adequate cardiac output

Figure 43-3

Tetralogy of Fallot

Pathophysiology

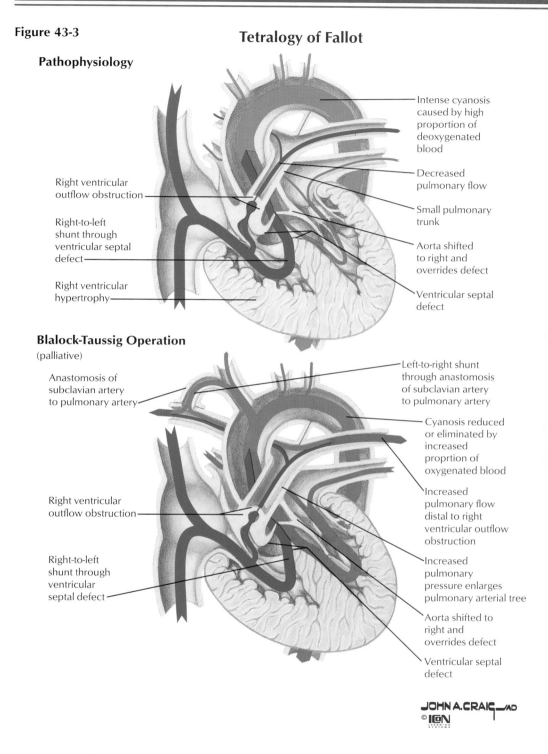

Intense cyanosis caused by high proportion of deoxygenated blood

Decreased pulmonary flow

Small pulmonary trunk

Aorta shifted to right and overrides defect

Ventricular septal defect

Right ventricular outflow obstruction

Right-to-left shunt through ventricular septal defect

Right ventricular hypertrophy

Blalock-Taussig Operation
(palliative)

Anastomosis of subclavian artery to pulmonary artery

Left-to-right shunt through anastomosis of subclavian artery to pulmonary artery

Cyanosis reduced or eliminated by increased proprtion of oxygenated blood

Increased pulmonary flow distal to right ventricular outflow obstruction

Right ventricular outflow obstruction

Right-to-left shunt through ventricular septal defect

Increased pulmonary pressure enlarges pulmonary arterial tree

Aorta shifted to right and overrides defect

Ventricular septal defect

JOHN A. CRAIG__MD
© ICN

(CO) to meet the aerobic metabolic demands of the body, including those incurred by growth; inefficiency of the heart to meet the metabolic demands can also be included in a more liberal definition of heart failure. An alteration in one or more physiologic determinants of ventricular

Figure 43-4

Innervation of Heart: Schema

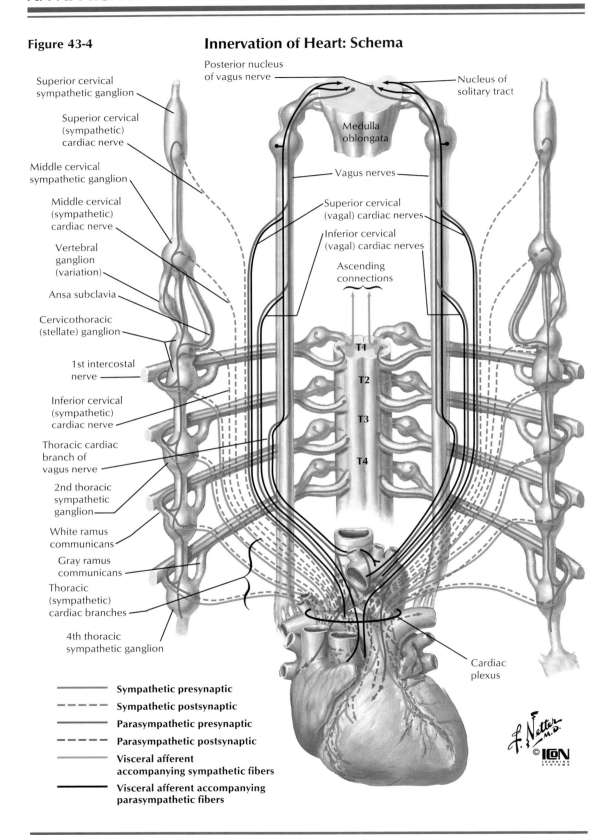

Superior cervical sympathetic ganglion

Superior cervical (sympathetic) cardiac nerve

Middle cervical sympathetic ganglion

Middle cervical (sympathetic) cardiac nerve

Vertebral ganglion (variation)

Ansa subclavia

Cervicothoracic (stellate) ganglion

1st intercostal nerve

Inferior cervical (sympathetic) cardiac nerve

Thoracic cardiac branch of vagus nerve

2nd thoracic sympathetic ganglion

White ramus communicans

Gray ramus communicans

Thoracic (sympathetic) cardiac branches

4th thoracic sympathetic ganglion

Posterior nucleus of vagus nerve

Nucleus of solitary tract

Medulla oblongata

Vagus nerves

Superior cervical (vagal) cardiac nerves

Inferior cervical (vagal) cardiac nerves

Ascending connections

T1
T2
T3
T4

Cardiac plexus

— Sympathetic presynaptic
--- Sympathetic postsynaptic
— Parasympathetic presynaptic
--- Parasympathetic postsynaptic
— Visceral afferent accompanying sympathetic fibers
— Visceral afferent accompanying parasympathetic fibers

function—preload, afterload, contractility, and HR or rhythm—can adversely affect cardiac performance beyond the compensatory mechanisms, particularly in fetuses or newborn infants, where cardiac function occurs much higher (and hence less efficiently) on the Frank-Starling curve because of maturational aspects. As a physiologic consequence, fetuses and infants are more dependent on mechanisms that increase HR rather than those that increase stroke volume to increase CO in response to increased metabolic demands.

The etiology of hypoxemia (abnormal reduction in the arterial oxygen tension) must be established to determine whether therapeutic intervention is necessary immediately. Hypoxia (inadequate tissue perfusion) is always a medical emergency because high morbidity and mortality are associated with uncorrected metabolic acidosis. Hypoxemia is most often associated with defects characterized by right-to-left intracardiac shunting in which effective pulmonary blood flow is reduced. Pulmonary blood flow may be entirely dependent on the patency of the arterial duct. The arterial duct begins to close shortly after birth, at which time the hypoxemic (and hypoxic) consequences of ductal dependency manifest. Since the 1970s, pharmacologic manipulation of the arterial duct to maintain or reestablish patency by constant intravenous infusion of prostaglandin E1 or E2 has dramatically improved the care of affected children by diminishing hypoxia during transport to a center where diagnostic and therapeutic interventions can more safely take place.

Defining the pathophysiology of pulmonary vascular disease remains a fertile area for research. The primary approach is to study therapeutic interventions to eliminate the risk factors for pulmonary vascular disease (Fig. 43-5) in all children identified at high risk because knowledge of the pathogenesis of these arteriolar changes remains incomplete. Three principal risk factors should be characterized by noninvasive and invasive techniques described subsequently: increased pulmonary blood flow from left-to-right, intracardiac or extracardiac shunting or an abnormal cardiac connection (e.g., septal defect, patent arterial duct, arteriovenous fistula, transposition of the great arteries);

increased pulmonary artery pressure from increased pulmonary blood flow or increased pulmonary venous pressure; and hyperviscosity as a consequence of hypoxemia from decreased pulmonary blood flow in right-sided obstructive heart lesions (e.g., tetralogy of Fallot, tricuspid atresia, pulmonary atresia) or hypoxemia from inadequate mixing (e.g., transposition of the great arteries).

Increased pulmonary blood flow can be distinguished physiologically with the concept of independent or obligatory flow, where dependency is defined relative to pulmonary vascular resistance (or impedance). For example, in children with unrestricted ventricular septal defects, the magnitude of the left-to-right shunting, and therefore pulmonary blood flow, depends on the relative difference between pulmonary and systemic vascular resistances (or impedances). As physiologic influences change this relative difference, the ratio of pulmonary to systemic flow changes proportionally. Therefore, this type of shunting depends on the status of the pulmonary vascular bed. In contrast, in children with atrioventricular (AV) septal defects with unrestricted left ventricular (LV)–right atrial (RA) shunting via the abnormal left AV valve, a significant difference in the resistances determining this flow (e.g., LV systolic pressure compared with simultaneous RA pressure) always exists. Therefore, increased flow occurs across the tricuspid and pulmonary valves, independent of the pulmonary vascular resistance. The magnitude of such a shunt is modulated more by ventricular function. Commonly in this clinical setting, pulmonary hemodynamics are further impaired by pulmonary hypertension, increasing the burden on ventricular function and subjecting the child to higher risks of heart failure and accelerated development of pulmonary vascular disease.

Timing for medical or surgical intervention becomes more evident by examining the actuarial consequences of these three risk factors for pulmonary vascular disease: increased pulmonary blood flow, pulmonary hypertension, and hyperviscosity. Increased pulmonary blood flow alone contributes to the risk of development of pulmonary vascular disease, but the time course for irreversible pulmonary vascular

Figure 43-5   Pulmonary Vessel Complications of Left-to-Right Shunts

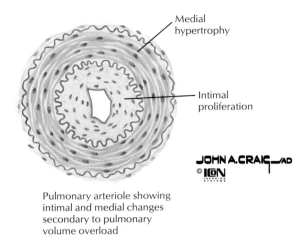

Medial hypertrophy

Intimal proliferation

JOHN A.CRAIG—AD
©ICON

Pulmonary arteriole showing
intimal and medial changes
secondary to pulmonary
volume overload

changes is measured in years. In contrast, pulmonary hypertension is a more significant risk, with irreversible changes observed in months to 1 to 2 years. Severe hyperviscosity states and pulmonary hypertension in children with cyanotic heart disease contribute to an extremely high risk of irreversible changes as early as 3 months of age. An optimal time for intervention to decrease the risk associated with the natural history can be determined by overlaying the actuarial experience for specific medical and surgical interventions.

INITIAL NONINVASIVE ASSESSMENT OF CHILDREN WITH CONGENITAL HEART DISEASE

History

The history is critically important for children with suspected congenital heart disease. Because congenital heart disease is most often diagnosed in early infancy, a chronologic approach is simple but effective. The history of pregnancy, labor, and delivery is often helpful (e.g., perinatal asphyxia) with age and developmentally appropriate attention to expected activity. For example, inquiry into the feeding history may be disproportionately important in infants, whereas inappropriate fatigue or exercise tolerance may be important in older children. One issue that cannot be overemphasized in the pediatric age group is growth. Growth is a

cardiovascular stress, and absence of growth may be the only manifestation of heart failure.

The family history is often benign but may alert the clinician to relevant issues, such as the incidence of and the genetic predisposition to congenital heart disease. Information about gene-specific etiologies of specific defects (or risk of such expression) will increase the importance of family history and inquiry into genetic predisposition in the near future.

Physical Examination

The physiologic features associated with altered pulmonary artery hemodynamics that are discernible by physical examination can be generally ascribed to features associated with pulmonary hypertension and decreased or increased pulmonary blood flow. Cardiac situs must first be established by means of palpation.

Children with decreased pulmonary blood flow secondary to congenital heart disease present clinically with cyanosis. Cyanosis necessitates approximately 5 g of circulating deoxygenated hemoglobin; therefore, in children with relative anemia, cyanosis may not be as obvious as expected, even in cyanotic congenital heart disease. Despite cyanosis, children with congenital heart disease often seem comfortable, without evidence of respiratory distress—an important distinction to differentiate hypoxemia as a consequence of a parenchymal disorder (leading to a ventilation/perfusion defect of perfused but underventilated portions of the lungs). Children with congenital heart disease who are cyanotic because of obstruction to pulmonary blood flow have alterations in the second heart sound with a diminished or absent pulmonary component resulting from diminished or absent flow across the pulmonary valve. Despite the most astute clinical efforts, the diagnosis of specific congenital heart defects by means of physical examination is often disappointing and can only be regarded as an initial screening procedure.

The physical diagnosis of pulmonary hypertension is rarely difficult. The cardiac examination predictably consists of a prominent right ventricular (RV) impulse that is either visible or easily palpable at the lower left sternal border or in the subxiphoid area (when present with normal cardiac situs). On auscultation, a single, loud or narrowly split second heart sound with a loud pulmonary component is present. Pulmonary systolic ejection clicks are also common in severe pulmonary hypertension, arising from a dilated, hypertensive proximal main pulmonary artery. Systolic murmurs at the lower left sternal border consistent with tricuspid insufficiency are sometimes present, although tricuspid insufficiency is common and usually presents without a murmur being noted on auscultation. In severe, long-standing pulmonary hypertension, a decrescendo, high-pitched, early diastolic murmur of pulmonary insufficiency may be present along the mid left sternal border. When pulmonary hypertension is accompanied by RV failure, findings of systemic venous engorgement are present, including hepatosplenomegaly and peripheral edema. Abnormal v and a waves may be found during examination of the neck veins.

Features associated with increased pulmonary artery flow are typically related to auscultatory findings from excessive flow crossing normal heart valves (Fig. 43-6). Because the semilunar valves have approximately one half the cross-sectional area of the AV valves, early diastolic murmurs associated with increased flow across the AV valves require more flow than midsystolic flow murmurs associated with flow across the semilunar valves. This point can be a distinguishing feature in quantifying a left-to-right shunt with

normal ventricular function because flow across the AV valves must be approximately doubled to auscultate such diastolic murmurs.

Chest Radiography

Although more sophisticated imaging modalities exist to provide anatomic and physiologic information regarding the pulmonary circulation, chest radiography is still used routinely as a screening method to determine the status of the pulmonary vasculature, pulmonary parenchyma, and cardiac situs, size, and morphology. Although its role in cardiopulmonary assessment when compared with cross-sectional echocardiographic techniques is challenged, its availability, speed, and usefulness in providing information about pulmonary features suggest that its future as an imaging modality remains secure.

Evaluation of pulmonary hemodynamics by chest radiography includes assessment of pulmonary ventilation and perfusion. Evaluation of perfusion by pulmonary vasculature assessment in chest radiographs is useful to distinguish the pathophysiology of altered pulmonary hemodynamics in children with congenital heart disease. For example, specific diagnostic entities can be considered by evaluating the pulmonary vascularity. Pulmonary vascularity on a posteroanterior chest radiograph can be classified as normal, increased (Fig. 43-7), decreased (Fig. 43-8), or abnormally redistributed and for which each lung field must be compared with the other fields. For pulmonary arterial vasculature to be identified as increased by chest radiography, an increase in pulmonary blood flow of approximately 100% is required. This helps to evaluate children with left-to-right shunting and correlate physical examination findings. An increase in CO of a similar amount (approximately 100%) is necessary to auscultate an early diastolic ventricular filling murmur across either AV valve.

Diminished pulmonary vasculature typically represents obstruction of blood flow to the lungs and is an ominous radiographic finding in newborns. Central dilation and peripheral pruning of pulmonary arterial vessels is noted in more advanced pulmonary vascular disease and is found with evidence for RV hypertrophy as defined by retrosternal filling on the lateral chest radiograph with the cardiac silhouette.

Figure 43-6   **Clinical Characteristics of Too Much Pulmonary Flow
(Pulmonary Volume Overload)**

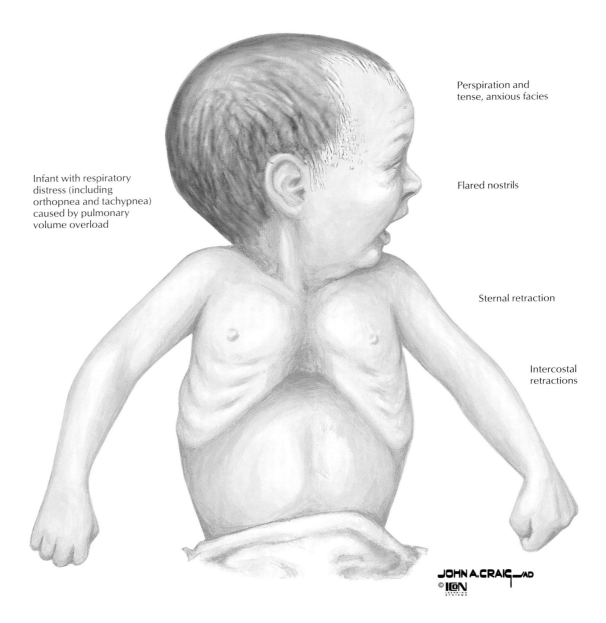

Perspiration and
tense, anxious facies

Flared nostrils

Sternal retraction

Intercostal
retractions

Infant with respiratory
distress (including
orthopnea and tachypnea)
caused by pulmonary
volume overload

JOHN A. CRAIG—AD
©ICN

Pulmonary edema presents a more distinctive pattern of haziness in the lung fields that warrants immediate investigation about etiology because significantly increased morbidity and mortality are associated with this finding. Specific assessment of the size of the main pulmonary artery is possible by means of the chest radi-ograph. Because the pulmonary artery is thin walled, it dilates readily when exposed to increased flow or pressure. Dilation of the main pulmonary artery is readily visible on the chest radiograph, and differentiating radiographic features are then sought to determine the physiologic etiology.

Figure 43-7

Anomalies of the Ventricular Septum

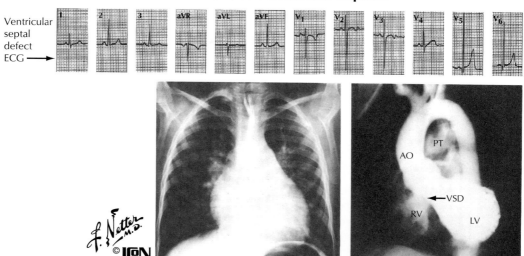

Ventricular septal defect ECG →

X-ray: Ventricular septal defect in a 5-year-old boy

L. ventricular angiocardiogram: AO, aorta; PT, pulmonary trunk; LV, left ventricle; RV, right ventricle; VSD, ventricular septal defect

Figure 43-8

Anomalies of the Right Ventricular Outflow Tract

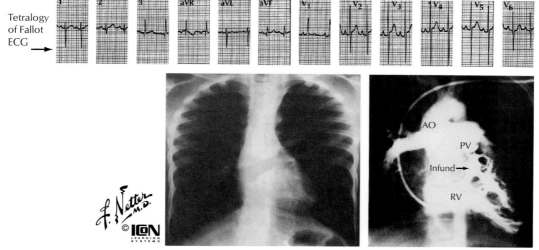

Tetralogy of Fallot ECG →

X-ray: Tetralogy of Fallot in a 6-year-old boy

R. ventricular angiocardiogram: AO, aorta; PV, pulmonary valve; RV, right ventricle; Infund, infundibulum

Evaluation of lung ventilation by assessment of conducting airways and lung parenchyma, including lobar and lung volumes, provides information about pulmonary physiology. Evaluation of the cardiac situs and chamber enlarge-ment by cardiac contour evaluation can greatly aid in the assessment of altered pulmonary hemodynamics. Because the right ventricle is affected by altered pulmonary hemodynamics, attention must be given to changes in shape and size. However, defining changes in RV function by means of chest radiography is less sensitive and specific than by means of evaluation of pulmonary perfusion.

Additional noninvasive assessment of children with congenital heart disease includes application of echocardiographic techniques (chapter 44). Less frequently, an invasive approach, involving cardiac catheterization, is required (chapter 45).

FUTURE DIRECTIONS

Clinical emphasis has focused on optimizing diagnosis and treatment of children with congenital heart disease and including fetuses as patients. In the future, the clinical focus will include the prevention of congenital heart disease through a more complete understanding of the influence of cardiac development. Completion of the initial mapping phase of the Human Genome Project in 2003 will result in accelerated investigations into the control and modulation of gene expression in the development of the human heart. This expanded understanding of cardiac development may allow interventions

to augment specific structural and functional deficiencies and to prevent maldevelopment of the human heart.

REFERENCES

Denfield S, Henry GW. Postoperative cardiac intensive care. In: Long WA, ed. *Neonatal and Fetal Cardiology*. Philadelphia: WB Saunders; 1990:812–829.

Ha B, Henry W, Lucas C, et al. Pulmonary artery blood flow and hemodynamics. In: *Advances in Hemodynamics and Hemorheology*. Vol 1. Greenwich, CT: Jai Press; 1996:230–324.

Henry GW. Perioperative management of the child with pulmonary hypertension and congenital heart disease. In: Harned HS Jr, ed. *Pediatric Pulmonary Heart Disease*. Boston: Little Brown; 1990:355–375.

Hoffman JIE. Incidence, mortality and natural history. In: Anderson RH, Baker EJ, Macartney FJ, et al., eds. *Paediatric Cardiology*. 2nd ed. London: Churchill Livingstone; 2002:111–139.

Keith JD. History and physical examination. In: Keith JD, Rowe RD, Vlad P. *Heart Disease in Infancy and Childhood*. 3rd ed. New York: Macmillan; 1987:14–15.

Long WA, Henry GW. Autonomic and central neuroregulation of fetal cardiovascular function. In: Polin RA, Fox WW, eds. *Fetal and Neonatal Physiology*. 2nd ed. Philadelphia: WB Saunders; 1998:943–961.

Rudolph AM. *Congenital Disease of the Heart*. Chicago: Yearbook Medical Publishers; 1974:29–48.

Chapter 44

Echocardiography in Congenital Heart Disease

John L. Cotton and G. William Henry

Multiple-plane cardiac imaging by echocardiography can noninvasively define the anatomy of the heart and the great vessels by delineating the configuration and the position of the cardiac structures and the spatial interrelations of these structures. The information obtained can be used to accurately diagnosis and for prognosis in complex congenital heart disease. In many pediatric cardiac tertiary care centers, echocardiography is the only diagnostic test performed before neonatal congenital heart surgery. With advances such as pulsed and color Doppler echocardiography and improvements in the size and capabilities of transducers and other imaging equipment, pediatric echocardiography has gained rapid acceptance. The technology allows real-time three-dimensional imaging, assessment of myocardial function, and precise definition of cardiac anatomy from the fetal stage through adulthood. For all of these reasons, echocardiography has become the standard noninvasive diagnostic imaging modality for pediatric cardiology.

Transthoracic multiplane imaging by two-dimensional (2-D) echocardiography defines the anatomy of the heart and the great vessels. Analysis of each cardiac segment allows complete definition of the configuration and the position of the cardiac structures and their spatial interrelations. The cardiac chambers and the intracardiac valves are shown with high resolution. Because tortuous vessels may be difficult to define by a "slice" technology such as echocardiography or magnetic resonance imaging, color Doppler echocardiography is customarily used to provide a map of blood velocity and direction that complements the 2-D image. Small septal defects and fistulous connections may be recognized only by perturbations in blood flow when the anomaly is too small to be visualized clearly. Pulsed and continuous wave Doppler echocardiography provide excellent time resolution that allows precise quantification of blood velocity. Positional and velocity information are combined to assess the presence and the severity of a valvular obstruction or insufficiency, the position and the size of jets associated with septal defects, and abnormal flow in large vessels in congenital lesions such as anomalous systemic and pulmonary venous return, coarctation of the aorta, and patent ductus arteriosus.

Transesophageal echocardiography (TEE) allows imaging planes different from those obtained in a standard transthoracic study. Miniaturization of transducer components now allows TEE to be performed in infants who weigh as little as 2.5 kg. Structures not well visualized by transthoracic echocardiography (TTE), primarily those located posteriorly are well visualized by TEE. In the older child or a child in whom there are poor transthoracic windows, TEE can also be very useful in the evaluation of congenital heart disease. Oftentimes during cardiac surgery it is important to address specific issues. The presence of abnormalities such as anomalous pulmonary venous return, pulmonary vein stenosis, and the presence of atrial baffle flow can be determined with intraoperative TEE. In addition, an immediate intraoperative or postoperative assessment of the adequacy of surgical repair is possible. These perioperative examinations are usually targeted, however, and are not a substitute for a complete preoperative transthoracic evaluation.

Fetal echocardiography is the newest frontier in pediatric echocardiographic imaging. With the use of transvaginal transducers, detailed fetal cardiac anatomy can be seen as early as 12 weeks of gestation. Transabdominal imaging can be performed by 16 weeks, although the optimal time for fetal echocardiography is approximately 18 weeks. Abnormalities detected at 18 weeks by echocardiography may be important in the decision for further imaging, chromosomal testing, or even termination of the pregnancy. As with TTE of infants, fetal echocardiography can identify intracardiac anatomy, blood flow across all the valves in the heart, size and orientation of the great vessels, cardiac function, and cardiac rhythm. The order and the windows used in a fetal echocardiogram depend on the position of the fetus, the amount of fluid in the uterus, and the size and motion of the baby.

TRANSTHORACIC IMAGING IN PEDIATRICS

Each pediatric echocardiography laboratory has a specific protocol for acquiring a complete study of the cardiac anatomy in children. Because patient cooperation is needed, in young children and infants all images may not be obtained using standardized positions. Some centers use conscious sedation for all patients under a certain age to ensure uniformity of studies. Another option is "video sedation": child-friendly videos played during the study to distract the patient and allow time to obtain diagnostic images. As long as clear pictures are obtainable, scanning can be performed with the patient sitting in a parent's lap, feeding, or even in a stroller. This approach substantially decreases the number of patients who must be sedated.

The protocol for a complete study includes views from the four major echocardiographic windows: parasternal, apical, subxiphoid, and suprasternal. Each window provides the image of the heart from a different angle, allowing multiple, corroborating views of the same structures. The image from each window begins from a standard reference view; then a sweep of the heart is made, first with 2-D scanning and then with color Doppler. The color Doppler mapping defines the location for pulsed Doppler scanning in each plane. Once the pertinent information is obtained, the transducer is rotated 90° to perform an orthogonal sweep. The sonographer and the interpreting physician can reconstruct multiple 2-D images into a three-dimensional representation of the cardiac anatomy.

Cardiac function and blood flow are calculated from Doppler mapping and from the 2-D images obtained. For example, pulmonary and aortic flow are calculated from the mean velocity and diameter of the vessel at the area of interest as follows:

Blood flow = (mean flow velocity) × (time) × (cross-sectional area of vessel)

Peak instantaneous gradients are calculated from a simplified Bernoulli equation, using peak flow velocity within the stenotic jet in the following formula, where V is the peak flow velocity measured by spectral Doppler scanning:

Peak pressure gradient = $4V^2$

This gradient is used to estimate pressures in the different cardiac chambers. Several different methods can be used to quantify left ventricular (LV) function. LV fractional shortening (FS) is a measurement of the percentage of change in LV diameter:

FS = (LV end-diastolic dimension − LV end-systolic dimension) / (LV end-diastolic dimension)

Ejection fraction is similarly calculated, using measured LV volumes.

In the discussion that follows, echocardiographic examinations are described for some common congenital heart lesions, with emphasis on the information needed to plan surgical intervention and the best techniques to obtain this information.

ATRIAL SEPTAL DEFECT

Transthoracic echocardiography is often sufficient to define the size and the location of an atrial septal defect (Fig. 44-1). Pulsed and color Doppler echocardiography identify the direction and the amount of shunting at the atrial level. Other findings can confirm the presence of a hemodynamically significant shunt. For instance, RV volume overload can produce diastolic bowing of the ventricular septum to the left during diastole, with the left ventricle assuming an elliptical shape. Partial anomalous pulmonary

Figure 44-1

Atrial Septal Defect

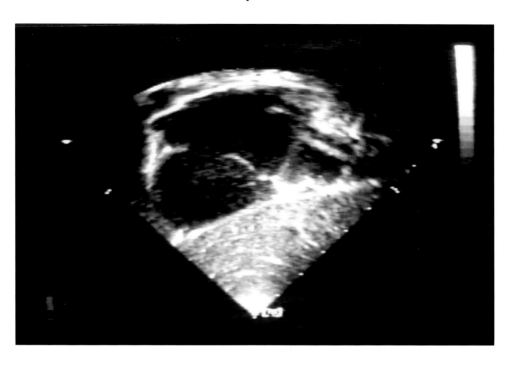

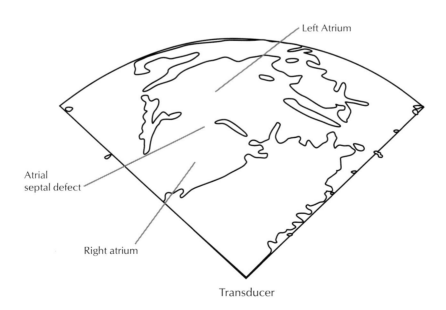

Left Atrium

Atrial
septal defect

Right atrium

Transducer

veins can be identified by 2-D echocardiography and should be sought in patients with an atrial septal defect so that they can be corrected at the time of surgery. The flow of these veins can be traced by color Doppler. TTE and subxiphoid echocardiography are usually sufficient to define the anatomy of the atrial septum and the pulmonary veins in infants and small children. For older children and adults, TTE may be needed for full anatomic definition. Cardiac catheterization is not usually needed in the evaluation of atrial septal defects.

VENTRICULAR SEPTAL DEFECT

Multiple views are needed to visualize the entire interventricular septum. TTE with 2-D imaging will usually demonstrate the size and the location of the interventricular communications. Color Doppler can be used to determine the direction of shunting across the ventricular septal defect (VSD) (Fig. 44-2). By measuring the direction and the velocity of flow across the defect, pulsed and continuous wave Doppler can be used to estimate the pressure gradient across the defect. Cardiac catheterization is not required before surgery unless the physical and noninvasive findings are atypical or contradictory.

ATRIOVENTRICULAR SEPTAL DEFECT

Echocardiography is also an important tool for the preoperative assessment of atrioventricular septal defects (AVSDs) (Fig. 44-3). 2-D imaging defines atrioventricular (AV) valve morphology. If the superior bridging leaflet is divided and has attachments to the crest of the ventricular septum, it is considered a type A valve. Straddling of central superior bridging leaflet attachments to a papillary muscle in the right ventricle defines a type B valve. If the superior bridging leaflet has no attachments to the crest of the interventricular septum and the valve leaflet is free-floating, it is considered a type C valve. Superior bridging leaflet septal attachments can obstruct the ventricular portion of the defect restricting shunting or cross the LV outflow tract—either of which can cause obstruction to aortic blood flow. Anterolateral papillary muscle insertions tend to be rotated counterclockwise in AVSDs and sit much closer to the posteromedial papillary muscle, which may create a "parachute"-like defor-

mity of the left portion of the AV valve. Any significant length of suturing of the superior and inferior leaflets during surgical repair risks creating LV inflow obstruction. In the intermediate form of AVSD, it is not uncommon to find shortened and immobile leaflets with thick, chordal attachments that limit the ability to properly fashion a functioning AV valve. Echocardiographic findings can sometimes anticipate this insufficiency of valvular tissue.

Color, continuous wave, and pulsed Doppler echocardiography assess potential gradients across the outflow tracts and show the direction of shunting across the septal defect. Color Doppler interrogation of the AV valve usually reveals some degree of insufficiency. A double-orifice mitral valve, present in about 5% of AVSDs, can be identified by echocardiography. The usual ostium primum atrial septal defect (with or without a shunt at the ventricular level) is also well visualized with 2-D echocardiography. The VSD component of AVSDs is usually single and in the inlet position; however, multiple defects can be ruled out with close color Doppler interrogation of the septum.

COARCTATION OF THE AORTA

Echocardiography can be valuable in making the diagnosis of coarctation of the aorta (Fig. 44-4). The characteristic narrowing of the aorta with a "posterior ledge" can be identified with 2-D imaging but may be difficult to appreciate if a patent ductus arteriosus is present. When a pressure gradient is present, a high-velocity jet will be present at the coarctation site. At the distal transverse arch, there is diastolic and systolic forward flow. Damped pulsatile flow is seen in the thoracic aorta. Often some degree of hypoplasia of the distal transverse aortic arch exists. 2-D echocardiography can usually distinguish coarctation of the aorta from interrupted aortic arch, but angiography may be necessary if the findings are ambiguous. It is also important to evaluate the patient for other anomalies that commonly present with coarctation of the aorta. As noted previously, VSDs can be well defined with echocardiography. Bicuspid aortic valve and mitral valve abnormalities should be carefully examined by 2-D imaging, color flow, and pulsed Doppler probing. LV outflow tract

Figure 44-2

Ventricular Septal Defect

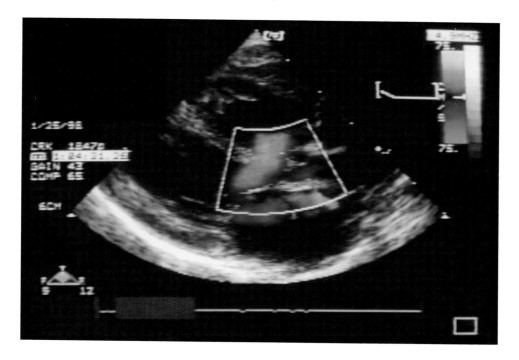

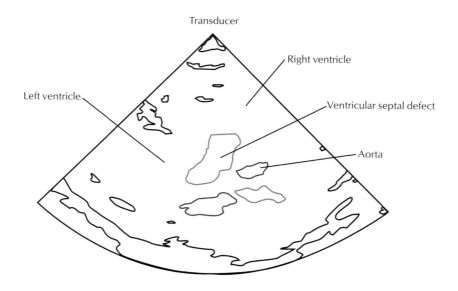

Figure 44-3   ## Atrioventricular Septal Defect

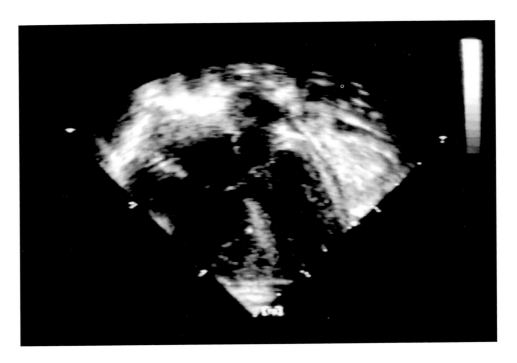

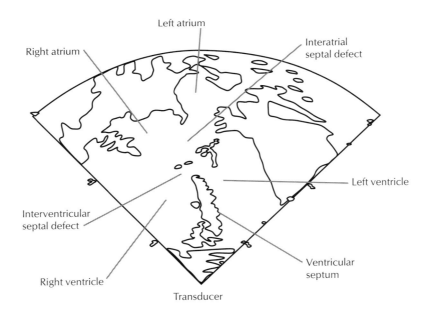

Figure 44-4

Coarctation of the Aorta

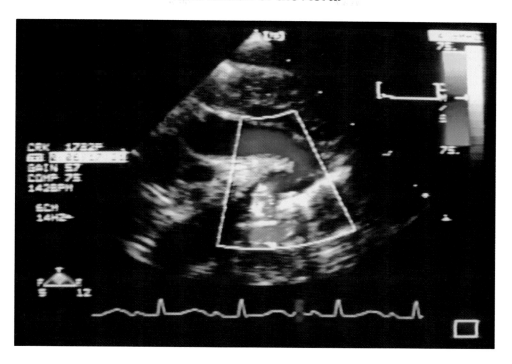

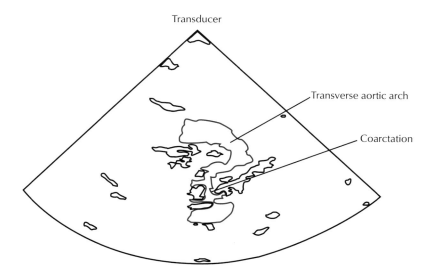

obstruction and other forms of subaortic obstruction can be seen, including posterior infundibular malalignment in the presence of a VSD.

TRANSPOSITION OF THE GREAT ARTERIES

Echocardiography can provide a definitive diagnosis of transposition of the great arteries by demonstrating the origin of the aorta from the right ventricle and the pulmonary artery from the left ventricle. Cross-sectional imaging can determine the presence and size of the interatrial communication. Echocardiography can often define the origins of the coronary arteries, but considerable experience is needed to confidently assess more distal branching patterns. Pulsed and color flow Doppler will identify a patent ductus arteriosus and delineate the magnitude of shunting at the atrial and ventricular levels. Ventricular mass and volumes can be quantified with both 2-D and M-mode echocardiography. The shape of the interventricular septum in systole indicates the differential pressures between the right and the left ventricles because the septum will bow toward the chamber with the least wall stress. In addition, the LV outflow tract can be interrogated with pulsed and color flow Doppler for signs of obstruction.

TETRALOGY OF FALLOT

Diagnosis of tetralogy of Fallot requires delineation of the structures listed in Table 44-1. Since most of these structures are well visualized with echocardiography, many infants do not need catheterization before repair of tetralogy of Fallot with a patent main pulmonary artery and continuity between the branches (Fig. 44-5). The RV outflow tract is usually well visualized by imaging in a combination of different echocardiographic planes. The diameters of the pulmonary valve annulus and the proximal pulmonary arteries are measured from parasternal, subxiphoid, and suprasternal views. Careful interrogation of the ventricular septum using both color flow and pulsed Doppler techniques can reveal any additional septal defects, which are seen with the greatest frequency in patients less than 1 year of age. Both the origins and the proximal branches of the right and left coronary arteries must be visualized because the origin of

Table 44-1
Diagnosis of Tetralogy of Fallot

· Levels and severity of right ventricular outflow tract obstruction
· Pulmonary valve annulus size
· Main and branch pulmonary artery size
· Ventricular septal defect (single vs. multiple)
· Origin of the left anterior descending coronary artery
· Aortopulmonary collaterals
· Aortic arch anatomy

the left anterior descending coronary from the right coronary artery and the presence of a prominent conal branch are infrequent associations that may significantly influence the surgical management of the RV outflow tract in patients who require an outflow patch. There is an increased incidence of right aortic arch in patients with tetralogy of Fallot. The presence of a right aortic arch is usually clearly demonstrated by a combination of plain chest radiography and TTE. Knowledge of this anomaly is critical before a staged shunt operation is considered.

PULMONARY ATRESIA

When an initial echocardiographic examination determines that pulmonary atresia with an intact ventricular septum is present (Fig. 44-6), it is very important to define the level of the RV outflow tract obstruction and the RV morphology, including the inlet, the outlet, and the trabecular components. The nature of the interatrial communication must be known in order to rule out existing or potential restriction to essential right-to-left shunting. Subxiphoid views of the interatrial septum will demonstrate the size and the position of the foramen ovale or of the septal defect. The flap valve of the foramen ovale is usually deviated toward the left atrium, but the flap valve moves back and forth during the cardiac cycle unless there is an obstructive communication. The flow dynamics across the atrial septum can be further defined by color flow and pulsed wave Doppler. Nonpulsatile flow with a velocity in the range of 2 m/sec is strongly suggestive of obstructive atrial communication, especially if the patient has hepatomegaly and evidence of a low-output state.

Figure 44-5

Tetralogy of Fallot

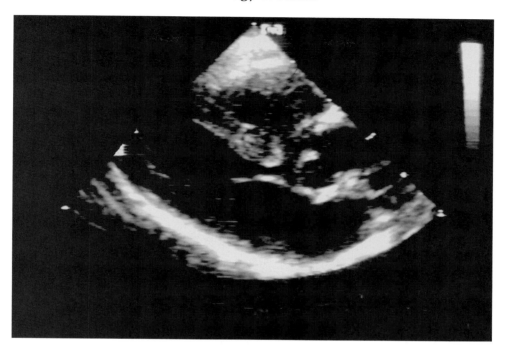

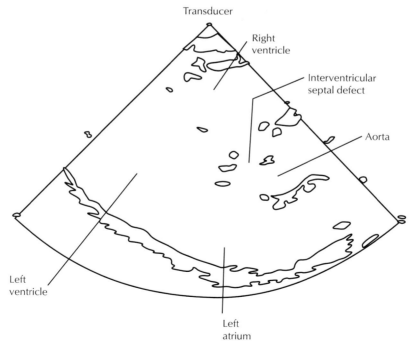

Figure 44-6   **Pulmonary Atresia**

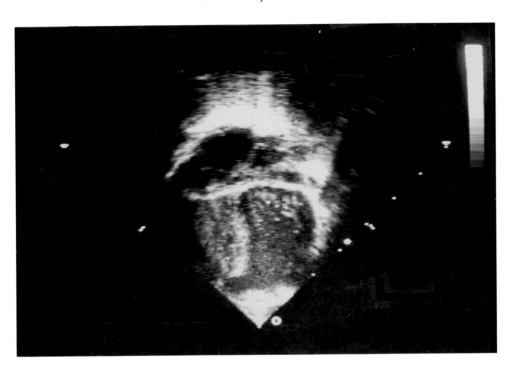

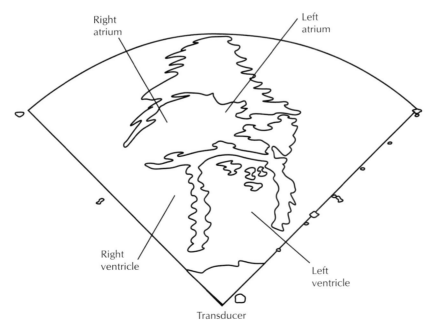

TOTAL ANOMALOUS PULMONARY VENOUS RETURN

Two-dimensional echocardiography will accurately delineate pulmonary venous anatomy in circumstances in which total or partial anomalous pulmonary venous return is present. Color and pulsed Doppler examinations are necessary to confirm the presence of obstruction. Turbulent, nonpulsatile venous flow with a velocity of at least 2 ms signifies hemodynamically significant obstruction. The intracardiac anatomy should also be assessed by echocardiography because other significant congenital lesions occur approximately 30% of the time, including patent ductus arteriosus, atrial isomerism, VSD, single ventricle, transposition of the great arteries, and systemic venous anomalies. Total anomalous pulmonary venous return is strongly associated with complex congenital heart disease and asplenia.

SINGLE VENTRICLE

Echocardiography is a powerful tool in defining the anatomy of the univentricular heart (Fig. 44-7). Both the interatrial and interventricular communications are measured and obstructions noted with color-directed pulsed Doppler. If an outflow chamber (hypoplastic ventricle) is found to communicate with a dominant ventricle via a bulboventricular foramen (VSD), the dimensions of the interventricular communication must be obtained with two orthogonal views. With these dimensions, a prediction can be made about whether the connection may become obstructive in the future. This prediction is made on the basis of the cross-sectional area of the connection, normalized to the body surface area and its boundaries, muscular or membranous. Doppler examination of the subarterial outflow can detect even mild obstruction by an increase in blood flow velocity. When the aorta arises from the hypoplastic chamber, detection of even mild obstruction is particularly important because of the danger that subaortic obstruction will develop. Hence, serial studies are necessary, particularly following interventions that reduce ventricular preload or afterload (including medication use or surgical procedures).

The anatomy of the AV valve is most clearly defined by echocardiographic imaging, and any stenosis or regurgitation should be quantified via color and pulsed Doppler flow imaging. In patients with a pulmonary artery band, echocardiography evaluates the band position, the morphology of the proximal pulmonary artery branches, and gradients at either level.

Ventricular function can be estimated using echocardiography, but the accuracy of echocardiography in this circumstance may be limited by nonuniform ventricular geometry, particularly in patients with a single morphologic right ventricle. Because of large differences in preload and afterload in patients with a single ventricle, measures of contractility that are less load-independent, such as the velocity of circumferential fiber shortening, are of greater value than a simple ejection fraction. However, even these indices are not reliable with subaortic obstruction or when the ventricular geometry does not conform to a prolate ellipsoid, and alternate means for assessment of ventricular function (MRI or radionuclide ventriculography) are sometimes needed. A reliable means for assessing ventricular function serially is needed in order to optimally time the stages of surgical correction and/or palliation (see chapter 50).

TRUNCUS ARTERIOSUS

Echocardiography can visualize the large truncal root overlying a subarterial VSD (Fig. 44-8). The origin of the pulmonary arteries may be seen as a single trunk, or the arteries may be seen arising separately from the proximal truncal root. The number of truncal valve leaflets can be determined by a combination of 2-D imaging and Doppler echocardiography. The presence of valvular regurgitation or stenosis, or stenosis at the origin of the pulmonary artery or branches, can, and should, be evaluated by TTE. The appearance of a small ascending aortic portion and a larger pulmonary portion of the common truncus should prompt a careful examination of the aortic arch from the suprasternal, high parasternal, and subxiphoid transducer positions to determine whether an associated coarctation of the aorta or an interrupted aortic arch is present.

FUTURE DIRECTIONS

Refinements in pediatric echocardiographic techniques produce a highly accurate picture of

Figure 44-7   **Hypoplastic Left Heart**

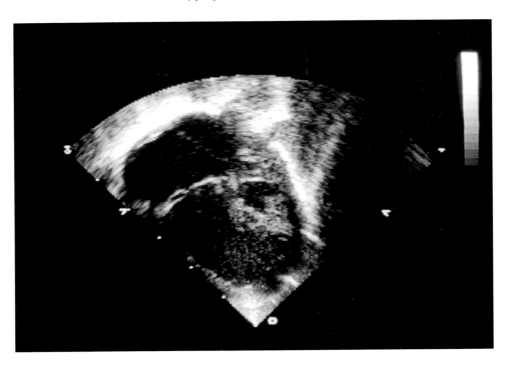

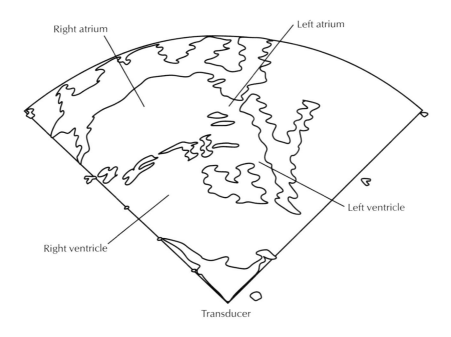

Figure 44-8

Truncus Arteriosus

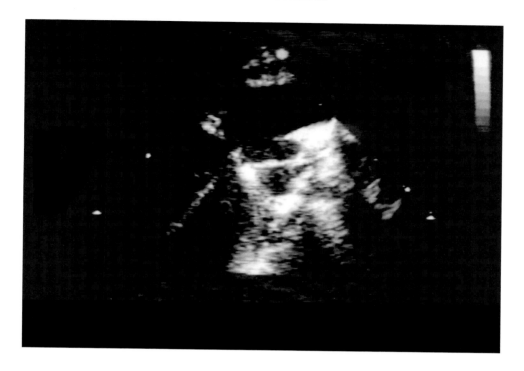

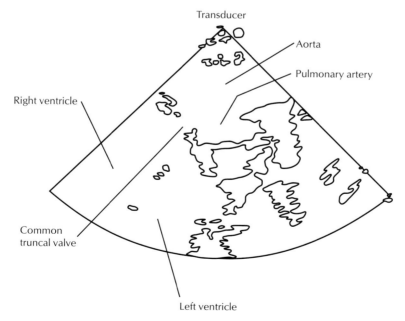

the anatomy and the evolving physiology of congenital cardiac lesions. For many straightforward lesions, invasive studies may be eliminated entirely. In some lesions, such as atrial septal defect, coarctation of the aorta, and patent ductus arteriosus, more often than not surgery is performed on the basis of a noninvasive perioperative evaluation. A variety of complex lesions, such as AVSDs, single ventricle, and complex conotruncal anomalies, have also been surgically palliated or repaired without cardiac catheterization, although the approaches used vary locally by the experience of the diagnostic and surgical team with each abnormality. Even for complex lesions requiring cardiac catheterization, advances in echocardiography have reduced the number of cardiac catheterizations needed in the lifetime of a single patient. As the use of echocardiography has become dominant in the preoperative evaluation of cardiac lesions, cardiac catheterization has taken on a more therapeutic role, being used in the closure of patent ductus arteriosus and septal defects, the occlusion of vascular structures, and the relief of outflow obstructions (see chapter 45). These advances are closely interrelated with the evolution of cardiac surgery toward the repair of increasingly complex lesions at increasingly earlier ages (chapter 46).

REFERENCES

George B, Disessa TG, Williams RG, Friedman WF, Laks H. Coarctation repair without catheterization in infants. *Am Heart J* 1987;114:1421–1425.

Leung MP, Mok CK, Hui PW. Echocardiographic assessment of neonates with pulmonary atresia and intact ventricular septum. *J Am Coll Cardiol* 1988;12:719–725.

Murphy DJ, Ludomirsky A, Huhta JC. Continuous wave Doppler in children with ventricular septal defect: Noninvasive estimation of intraventricular pressure gradient. *Am J Cardiol* 1986;57:428–432.

Pasquini L, Sanders SP, Parness IA, Colan SD. Diagnosis of coronary artery anatomy by two-dimensional echocardiography in patients with transposition of the great arteries. *Circulation* 1987;75:557–564.

Sanders SP, Bierman FZ, Williams RG. Conotruncal malformation: Diagnosis in infancy using subxiphoid two dimensional echocardiography. *Am J Cardiol* 1982;50:1361–1367.

Shimazaki Y, Maehara T, Blackstone EH, Kirklin JW, Bargeron LM. The structure of the pulmonary circulation in tetralogy of Fallot with pulmonary atresia. *J Thorac Cardiovasc Surg* 1988;95:1048–1058.

Smallhorn JF, Freedom RM. Pulsed Doppler echocardiography in the pre-operative evaluation of total anomalous pulmonary venous connection. *J Am Coll Cardiol* 1986;8:1413–1420.

Snider AR, Serwer GA, Ritter SB. *Echocardiography in Pediatric Heart Disease.* St. Louis: Mosby; 1997:23–75.

Chapter 45

Cardiac Catheter Interventions for Congenital Heart Disease

Gregory H. Tatum and Elman G. Frantz

The goals and techniques of cardiac catheterization for patients with congenital heart disease have evolved rapidly. For diagnostic purposes, cardiac catheterization has often been replaced by echocardiography. In contrast, the value of cardiac catheter interventional procedures continues to increase. In some cases, these procedures are important adjuncts to surgery, eliminating the need for early operation in a growing child or the need for reoperation after primary surgical correction. In many cases, these cardiac catheter interventions substitute for open-chest surgical procedures, resulting in reductions in length of hospitalization, cost, and patient discomfort.

BALLOON ATRIAL SEPTOSTOMY

Interventional pediatric cardiology can trace its roots to the 1966 introduction by Rashkind of balloon atrial septostomy as a palliative procedure for patients with transposition of the great arteries (Fig. 45-1). A large balloon is passed transvenously across the foramen ovale and pulled forcefully across the atrial septum, tearing the thin tissue in the floor of the oval fossa, creating a larger atrial septal defect and thus improving intracardiac mixing and systemic oxygen delivery. Although prostaglandin and improved surgical techniques have eliminated the need for this procedure in many infants, balloon atrial septostomy remains a lifesaving palliative procedure for some. Initially, balloon atrial septostomy was performed in the cardiac catheterization laboratory, but it is now safely and effectively performed at the bedside under echocardiographic guidance.

BALLOON VALVULOPLASTY
Pulmonary Stenosis

Balloon pulmonary valvuloplasty has become the standard of care for pulmonary stenosis (Fig. 45-2). The procedure is indicated for symptomatic infants and for older children in whom the systolic pressure gradient exceeds 30 to 35 mm Hg. After performing preliminary hemodynamic measurements and angiography, an end-hole catheter and wire are placed transvenously across the stenotic valve. The catheter is then replaced with a dilating balloon catheter

with a diameter 20 to 40% greater than the diameter of the valve annulus and the balloon is inflated until a "waist" is seen to disappear. Balloon valvuloplasty of the pulmonary valve compares well with surgery. Balloon valvuloplasty of the pulmonary valve provides equal relief of right ventricular outflow tract obstruction with less pulmonary valve insufficiency, has a lower rate of complications, does not require extended hospitalization, and is a more comfortable procedure for the patient. In the neonate with critical pulmonary stenosis, balloon valvuloplasty is more technically challenging and the complication rate is higher. However, it remains the procedure of choice, with definitive results in most patients. The long-term outcome of this procedure is excellent, except occasionally in patients with dysplastic pulmonary valves or in neonates with a hypoplastic valve annulus. The procedure can also be applied to infants with pulmonary atresia and an intact ventricular septum after initial perforation of the atretic valve.

Aortic Stenosis

Two distinct groups of patients with congenital valvular aortic stenosis are candidates for balloon dilation of the aortic valve via catheter intervention: infants with critical aortic stenosis who are symptomatic shortly after birth and older children with moderately severe aortic stenosis who are usually asymptomatic (Fig. 45-3). Children with congenital valvular aortic stenosis generally undergo intervention when they are symptomatic

Figure 45-1

Transposition of Great Arteries
Balloon Atrial Septostomy (Technique)

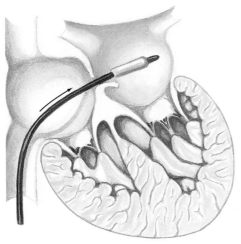

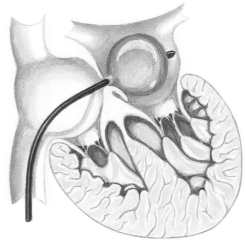

1. Balloon-tipped catheter introduced into left atrium through patent foramen ovale

2. Balloon inflated

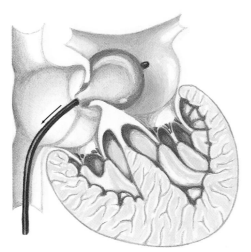

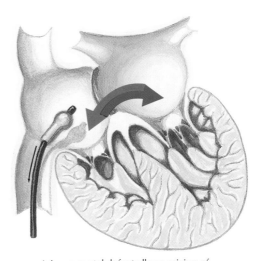

3. Balloon withdrawn producing large septal defect

4. Large septal defect allows mixing of oxygenated and deoxygenated blood

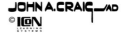

JOHN A. CRAIG—AD
© ICN
LEARNING SYSTEMS

or when the peak systolic pressure gradient exceeds 60 mm Hg. The peak pressure gradient is most commonly estimated by Doppler echocardiography. The valve is usually crossed retrograde, and an exchange wire is looped in the left ventricular apex. A balloon dilation catheter with a diameter 90 to 100% of the diameter of the valve annulus is passed over the wire and inflated several times to abolish the waist formed by the valve on the balloon.

Balloon aortic valvuloplasty is considered the initial treatment of choice for congenital aortic stenosis, albeit a palliative procedure with future interventions anticipated. Many patients require

Figure 45-2

Pulmonary Valvular Stenosis and Atresia

Pulmonary valvular
stenosis with intact
septum; hypertrophy
of right ventricle

Stenotic pulmonary valve viewed
from above: Poststenotic dilatation
of pulmonary trunk

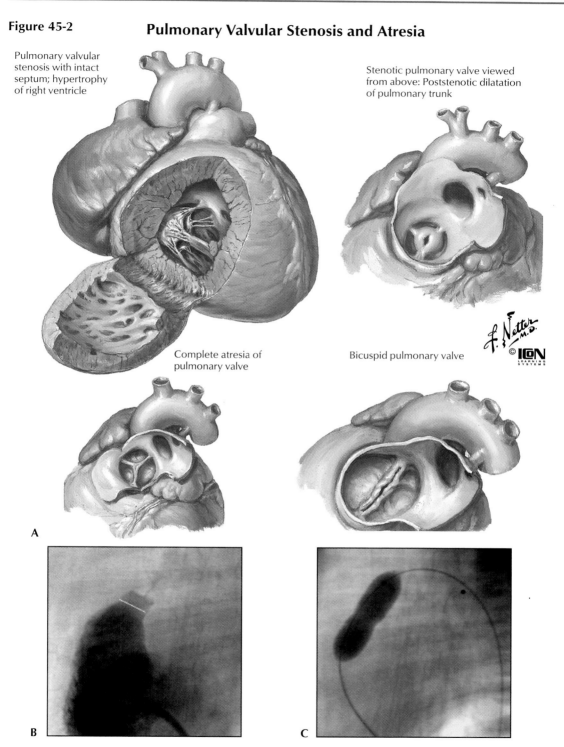

Complete atresia of
pulmonary valve

Bicuspid pulmonary valve

A

B

C

(A) The anatomic features of congenital pulmonary stenosis and atresia are illustrated. (B) A lateral-view right ventricular angiogram in a neonate with critical pulmonary valve stenosis shows the doming valve with an annulus diameter of 5.9 mm and a tiny poststenotic jet. (C) A lateral view of an 8-mm-diameter balloon dilation catheter fully inflated across the annulus. The balloon has been passed over a guide wire that had been placed across the ductus to the descending aorta.

Figure 45-3

Congenital Aortic Stenosis

Congenital bicuspid aortic valve

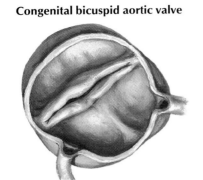

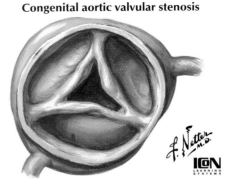

Congenital aortic valvular stenosis

A

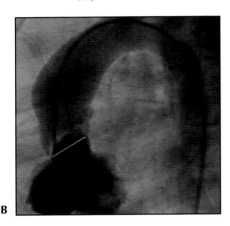

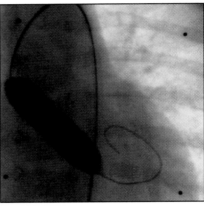

B

C

(A) The anatomic features of congenital aortic stenosis are illustrated. **(B)** A lateral-view left ventricular angiogram shows the doming aortic valve with a valve annulus diameter of 9.6 mm and poststenotic dilation of the ascending aorta. **(C)** Anteroposterior view of a 9-mm-diameter balloon dilation catheter fully inflated across the annulus. The balloon has been passed over a guide wire that had been placed retrograde across the valve and looped in the left ventricular apex.

repeat intervention within 5 to 10 years of undergoing the procedure, but less than half require surgical aortic valve replacement after 10 years of follow-up. Catheter and surgical intervention have been found to be equally effective in relieving left ventricular outflow obstruction and have a similar incidence of subsequent aortic insufficiency, repeat intervention, valve replacement, mortality, and preserved functional status.

BALLOON ANGIOPLASTY AND ENDOVASCULAR STENT PLACEMENT

Pulmonary Artery Stenosis

Peripheral pulmonary artery stenosis is common, occurring as a native lesion and as a complication of previous surgeries. Unfortunately, this

stenosis is difficult to treat. Surgery achieves limited success, and restenosis is common. Despite the less than ideal results, angioplasty has become the initial procedure of choice, particularly in smaller, growing patients. A catheter and wire are positioned across the stenotic vessel, and a balloon dilation catheter is advanced to the site and inflated until a waist disappears. Low-pressure balloons were used initially but were modestly successful in only about half of the patients. The introduction of high-pressure balloons has improved the success rate, although restenosis remains a problem. Cutting balloons have produced encouraging early success, but larger and long-term follow-up studies are still needed.

Balloon expandable stents represent a major advance over angioplasty in the treatment of

Figure 45-4

Pulmonary Artery Stenosis

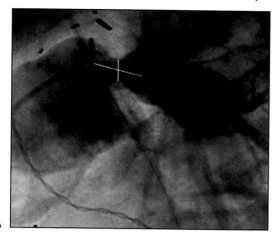 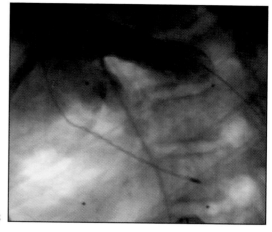

A   B

(A) A lateral-view pulmonary arteriogram in a patient with late postoperative tetralogy of Fallot, showing discrete proximal left pulmonary artery stenosis with a minimum diameter of 6 mm over a length of 13.4 mm. **(B)** A lateral-view pulmonary arteriogram showing no residual stenosis after expansion of a commercial stent using a 12-mm-diameter balloon.

pulmonary artery stenosis (Fig. 45-4). The use of stents has increased the acute success rate and results in a greater increase in arterial size than does balloon dilation. The stent is mounted and hand-crimped onto a high-pressure balloon dilation catheter. The stent-balloon complex is then advanced over a wire through a long, large-caliber sheath, previously positioned across the stenosis. After careful positioning of the stent and test angiograms, the stent is expanded by inflating the balloon. The main limitation to the use of stents is patient size. Although modest late further expansion of stents has been reported, placing a stent in a small child is technically challenging and often commits that child to surgery in the future. Improvements in stent design have facilitated the delivery of stents to remote sites, but sites with stents less than 6 to 8 mm in final diameter frequently become stenotic again or develop local thromboses. Complications unique to stent placement include obstruction of side branches or nonlinear balloon rupture or misplacement of the stent, necessitating surgical removal.

Coarctation of the Aorta

Native *coarctation of the aorta* is a congenital discrete narrowing of the juxtaductal aorta and, in the critical neonatal form, is often associated with proximal aortic hypoplasia (Fig. 45-5).

Recurrent coarctation of the aorta occurs after primary surgical repair and is particularly common after neonatal repair. Intervention is undertaken urgently in symptomatic infants and electively for upper extremity hypertension or an estimated systolic pressure gradient across the coarctation of greater than 20 mm Hg.

Balloon coarctation angioplasty was initially applied to children with recurrent coarctation because repeat surgery was technically difficult, carried an increased complication rate, and had a mortality rate in some series as high as 10 to 20%. The procedure involves passing a catheter and wire retrograde across the coarctation site to the ascending aorta, where the wire is looped. A balloon dilation catheter with a diameter 2 to 4 times the coarctation diameter but not more than 2 mm greater than the diameter of the proximal aorta is passed over the wire and inflated several times until the waist is abolished. Follow-up pressures are obtained, and angiography is performed to ensure that an adequate result was obtained and that no dissection is present (Fig. 45-6). Balloon dilation has been widely accepted for recurrent coarctation; the procedure has a success rate of 80 to 90% in achieving a residual coarctation gradient of less than 20 mm Hg and carries a low risk of complications.

Angioplasty for native coarctation is less wide-

Figure 45-5

Anatomic Features of Aortic Coarctation in Older Children and Neonates

Coarctation of the Aorta

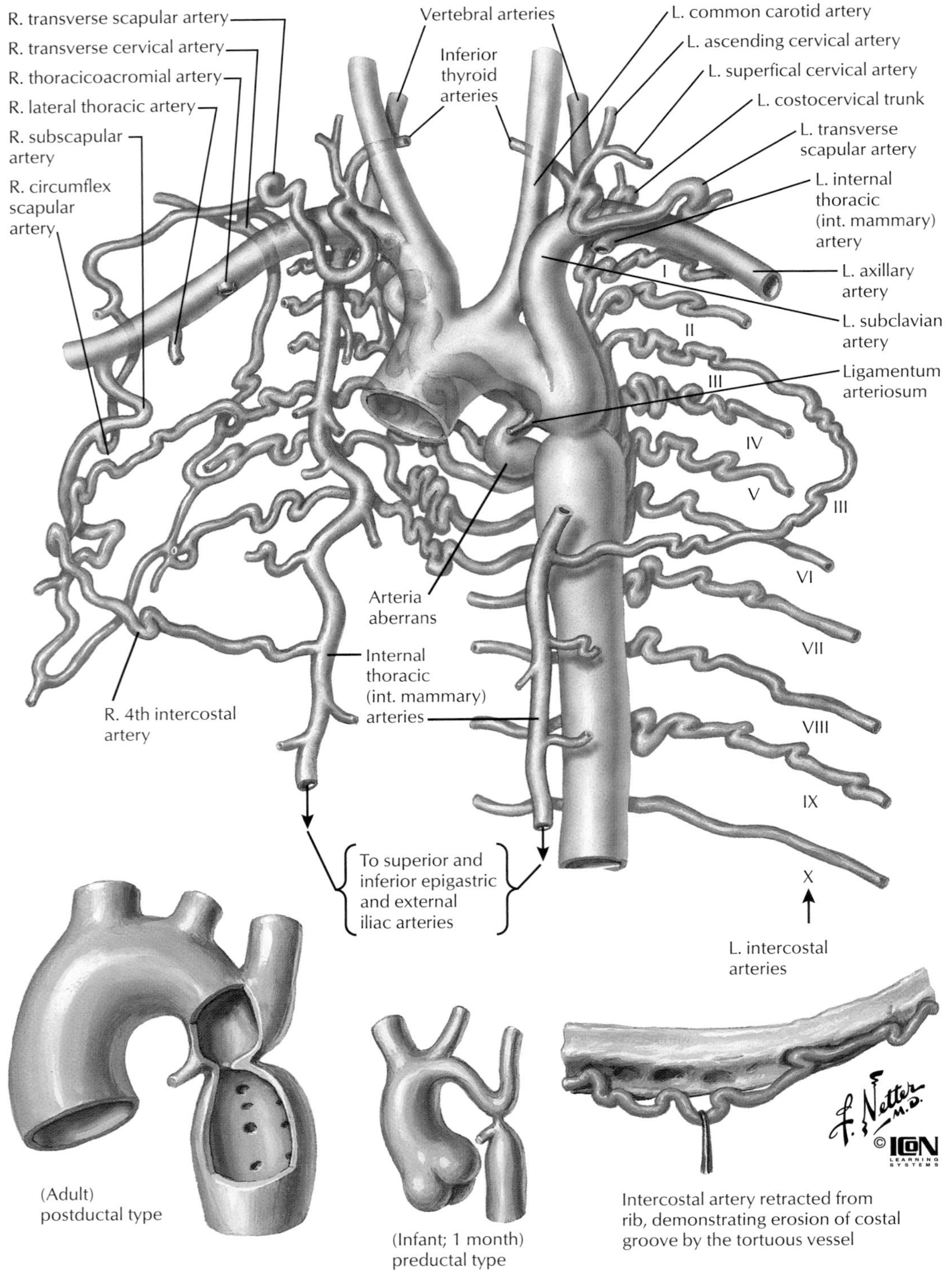
R. transverse scapular artery
R. transverse cervical artery
R. thoracicoacromial artery
R. lateral thoracic artery
R. subscapular artery
R. circumflex scapular artery
Vertebral arteries
Inferior thyroid arteries
L. common carotid artery
L. ascending cervical artery
L. superfical cervical artery
L. costocervical trunk
L. transverse scapular artery
L. internal thoracic (int. mammary) artery
L. axillary artery
L. subclavian artery
Ligamentum arteriosum
I
II
III
IV
V
III
VI
VII
VIII
IX
X
Arteria aberrans
Internal thoracic (int. mammary) arteries
R. 4th intercostal artery
To superior and inferior epigastric and external iliac arteries
L. intercostal arteries
(Adult) postductal type
(Infant; 1 month) preductal type
Intercostal artery retracted from rib, demonstrating erosion of costal groove by the tortuous vessel
F. Netter M.D.
© ICON LEARNING SYSTEMS

Figure 45-6

Coarctation of the Aorta

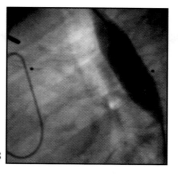
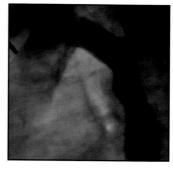

(A) A lateral-view angiogram showing a recurrent aortic coarctation distal to the left subclavian artery. **(B)** A balloon dilation catheter fully inflated in the site of narrowing, guided by a wire looped in the ascending aorta. **(C)** Follow-up angiogram showing marked improvement in the caliber of the aorta in the site of coarctation, without aneurysm formation or residual stenosis.

ly accepted, primarily because of concerns about restenosis and aneurysm formation at the site of dilation. Predictors of restenosis are young age, a hypoplastic arch, a coarctation diameter of less than 3.5 mm, and a postdilation gradient greater than 20 mm Hg. Because of the high rate of restenosis in neonates, the procedure is palliative rather than curative in this age group. In contrast to early reports, recent studies report a low incidence of aneurysm development, similar to the rate of aneurysm development observed in surgical patients. In an increasing number of centers, balloon angioplasty for native coarctation is favored in patients who are more than 6 months of age or who weigh more than 8 kg.

Stents have also been used in the treatment of recurrent and native coarctation. In patients with coarctation of a long segment without a focal stenosis, stenting may have a more favorable outcome than angioplasty. Although stents can be reexpanded later, there is a significant risk of acquired stenosis in the growing child. For this reason, the use of stents has been limited primarily to fully grown patients, but the results are encouraging in this group of patients, many of whom have undergone several surgical procedures.

TRANSCATHETER CLOSURE OF CONGENITAL SHUNT LESIONS
Persistent Ductus Arteriosus

Although the ductus arteriosus is a necessary vascular channel in fetal life, in postnatal life the persistently patent arterial duct can cause congestive heart failure or pulmonary hypertension, and is a lifelong risk of endarteritis. When the ductus arteriosus persists beyond infancy and is of clinical significance based on physical examination and echocardiography, it should be closed to prevent such morbidity. Surgical ligation and division through a thoracotomy has been extremely successful and mostly free of complications but requires hospitalization, is painful, leaves a scar, and may occasionally lead to scoliosis. The standard method of percutaneous transcatheter closure using Gianturco spring coils was introduced in the 1990s. These preformed stainless steel coils of varying caliber, diameter, and length have strands of Dacron attached to increase their thrombogenicity. The ductus arteriosus is usually conical or tubular in intraluminal shape, with a larger aortic ampulla and a smaller diameter near the pulmonary end (Fig. 45-7). This ductal morphology allows selection of a Gianturco coil with a loop diameter at least twice the minimum internal diameter of the ductus and placement of this coil such that most of the loops and coil mass fit into the aortic ampulla. Numerous modifications of the technique allow delivery of coils antegrade, retrograde, "freehand," or assisted by a snare or a bioptome through 4 French delivery catheters. If necessary, multiple coils can be delivered to achieve complete closure. In most patients (with a minimum ductus diameter <4 mm), this coil closure method is successful in achieving com-

Figure 45-7

Patent Ductus Arteriosus

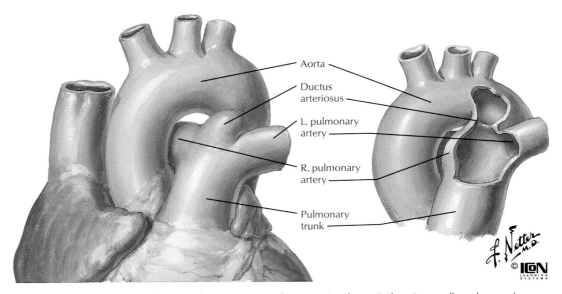

Aorta

Ductus arteriosus

L. pulmonary artery

R. pulmonary artery

Pulmonary trunk

The internal anatomy of a typical "type A" ductus arteriosus, demonstrating the conical aortic ampulla and narrowing near the pulmonary end, making coil placement feasible

plete closure, has a minimal rate of complications, and can be performed as an outpatient procedure without general anesthesia. This technique can also be applied to other abnormal vascular channels, such as aortopulmonary collateral arteries. Figure 45-8 shows a residual ductal leak years after placement of a Rashkind occluder and closure of this leak with Gianturco coils.

Another occlusion device, the Amplatzer® Duct Occluder, (AGA Medical Corp., Golden Valley, MN) is useful for transcatheter closure of the larger ductus and other vascular channels. The Amplatzer® Duct Occluder is a mushroom-shaped plug of nitinol wire mesh with polyester patches sewn into the framework. The device, which is screwed onto a delivery cable, can be delivered through 5–7 French delivery systems in a controlled fashion. When the device is deployed, the outer walls of the expanded plug "stent" the lumen of the vessel, securing the device in position and achieving complete closure.

Atrial Septal Defect

Deficiencies of the interatrial septum can involve all regions of the septum, and all but the secundum, or oval fossa, defect require surgical correction (Fig. 45-9). Unrepaired atrial septal defects can lead to pulmonary hypertension, atrial arrhythmias, or right-sided heart failure. Defects large enough to produce right-sided heart volume overload should be closed early in life to prevent these associated morbidities.

Attempts to develop a highly successful and low-risk transcatheter method for closure of secundum atrial septal defects have led to the invention of the Amplatzer® Septal Occluder, approved by the Food and Drug Administration in 2001. This device consists of a self-expanding double-disk nitinol frame with a central waist sized to "stent" the rims of the atrial septal defect. Three polyester patches are sewn to the framework to aid closure and endothelialization (Fig. 45-10). After performing routine hemodynamic measurements and with transesophageal echocardiographic monitoring, a balloon sizing catheter is passed across the defect over a wire in a left pulmonary vein. The stretched diameter of the defect is measured echocardiographically and fluoroscopically by the waist of the rims of the defect on the balloon. The stretched diameter is often twice the unstretched diameter, as measured by transthoracic echocardiography, and 50% larger than that measured by trans-

Figure 45-8

Patent Ductus Arteriosus

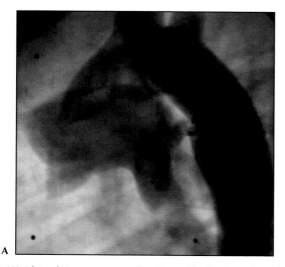 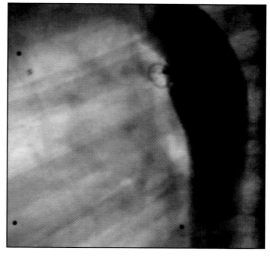

A   B

(A) A lateral-view aortogram showing residual leakage through a patent ductus arteriosus that had been partially closed with a Rashkind umbrella occluder years previously. Three platinum markers can be seen on the aortic umbrella of the Rashkind device. (B) Follow-up lateral-view aortogram after snare-assisted coil delivery showing complete closure.

esophageal echocardiography. A device with a central waist equal to or slightly larger than the stretched diameter is selected and is attached to a delivery cable by a screw-eye mechanism. The device is then delivered through a 7–12 French delivery sheath in the left atrium. After deployment of the device, the device position is carefully evaluated by transesophageal echocardiographic monitoring; the device can be recaptured and repositioned or completely retrieved and removed if necessary. Once proper positioning and function are confirmed, the device is then released by unscrewing the delivery cable.

In properly selected patients, the Amplatzer® Septal Occluder achieves complete closure in 99% of cases, with a very low rate of complications (about 1% embolization and 1% transient neurologic symptoms). Although surgical results are excellent, the transcatheter technique avoids cardiopulmonary bypass, longer hospitalization and recovery time, cosmetic concerns, and patient discomfort.

Ventricular Septal Defect

The precise anatomy of ventricular septal defects determines whether transcatheter clo-

sure is feasible (Fig. 45-11). The proximity of perimembranous defects to the aortic valve makes device closure impossible or at least challenging. The CardioSeal® double-umbrella occluder has been approved by the Food and Drug Administration for closure of muscular ventricular septal defects. These defects are often difficult to treat surgically because of their remote location; therefore, a transcatheter method is appealing. However, the technique is challenging to perform, operator experience is crucial, and the patient population is small. Despite the anatomic limitations, a uniquely designed perimembranous ventricular septal defect occluder has been developed and initial results in small numbers of patients are encouraging.

FUTURE DIRECTIONS

Continued refinements and advances in catheter-based therapy for congenital heart disease are likely. Fetal interventions for critical right- and left-sided heart obstructive disease are in their early stages but may become standard. Preliminary efforts to use catheter-delivered covered stents to "complete" the Fontan operation nonsurgically have been initiated. Miniaturization and improvements in stent design will

Figure 45-9

Atrial Septal Defects

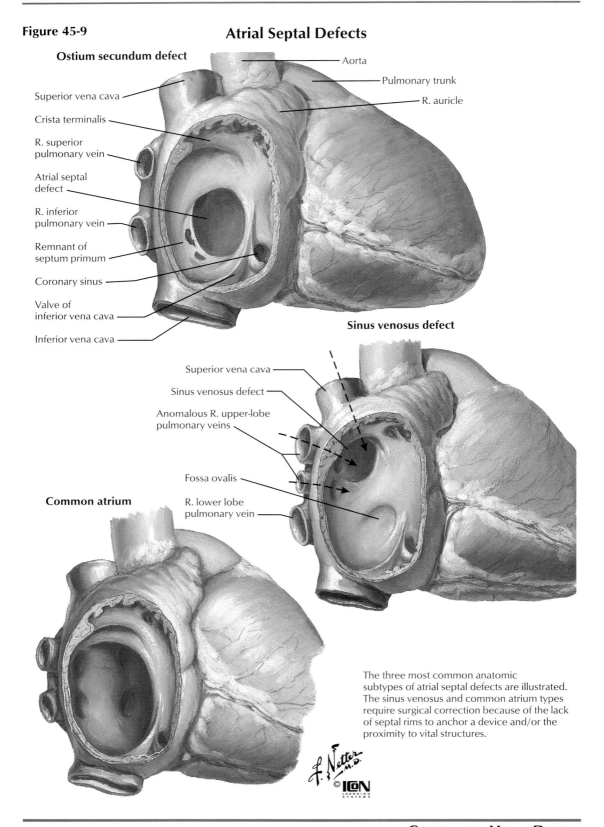

Ostium secundum defect

Aorta

Pulmonary trunk

Superior vena cava

R. auricle

Crista terminalis

R. superior
pulmonary vein

Atrial septal
defect

R. inferior
pulmonary vein

Remnant of
septum primum

Coronary sinus

Valve of
inferior vena cava

Inferior vena cava

Sinus venosus defect

Superior vena cava

Sinus venosus defect

Anomalous R. upper-lobe
pulmonary veins

Fossa ovalis

Common atrium

R. lower lobe
pulmonary vein

The three most common anatomic
subtypes of atrial septal defects are illustrated.
The sinus venosus and common atrium types
require surgical correction because of the lack
of septal rims to anchor a device and/or the
proximity to vital structures.

Figure 45-10

Amplatzer® Septal Occluder

The Amplatzer® Septal Occluder is deployed from its delivery sheath forming two disks, one for either side of the septum, and a central waist available in varying diameters to seat on the rims of the atrial septal defect.

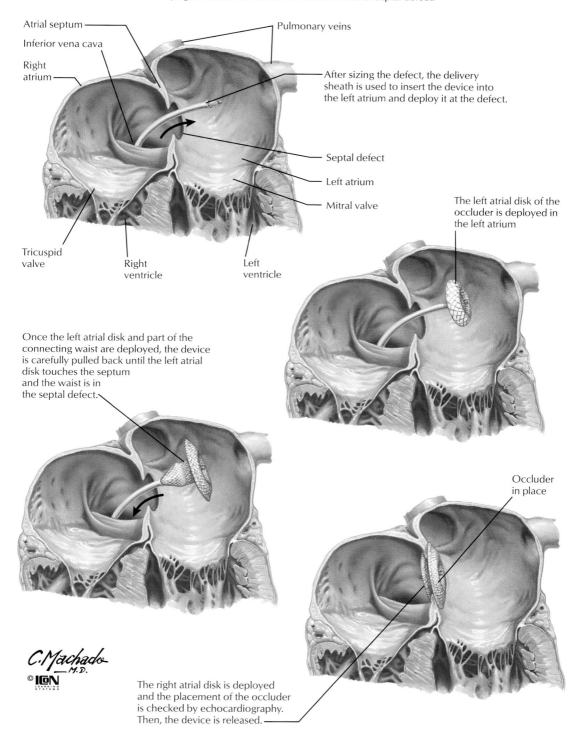

Atrial septum

Inferior vena cava

Right atrium

Pulmonary veins

After sizing the defect, the delivery sheath is used to insert the device into the left atrium and deploy it at the defect.

Septal defect

Left atrium

Mitral valve

Tricuspid valve

Right ventricle

Left ventricle

The left atrial disk of the occluder is deployed in the left atrium

Once the left atrial disk and part of the connecting waist are deployed, the device is carefully pulled back until the left atrial disk touches the septum and the waist is in the septal defect.

Occluder in place

The right atrial disk is deployed and the placement of the occluder is checked by echocardiography. Then, the device is released.

C.Machado
M.D.
© ICON
LEARNING
SYSTEMS

Figure 45-11

Anatomic Features of Perimembranous and Muscular Ventricular Septal Defects

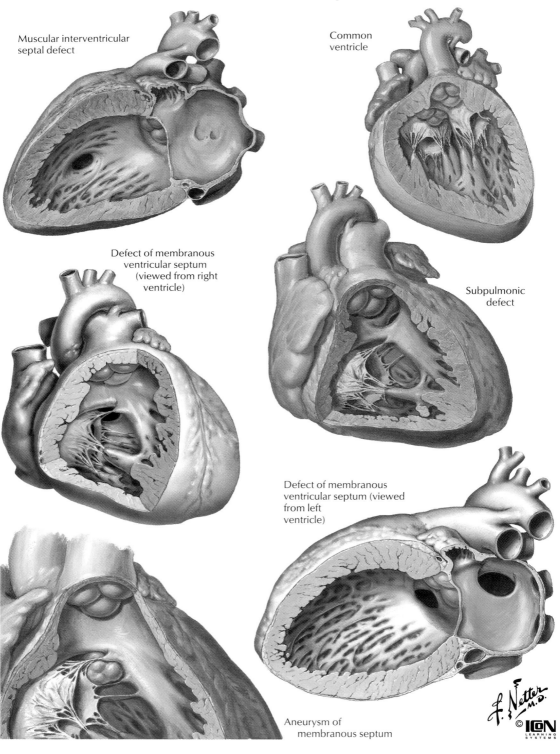

Muscular interventricular septal defect

Common ventricle

Defect of membranous ventricular septum (viewed from right ventricle)

Subpulmonic defect

Defect of membranous ventricular septum (viewed from left ventricle)

Aneurysm of membranous septum

expand the indications to smaller patients. Despite advances in catheter-based therapy, surgical intervention will remain the primary treatment method for many complex forms of congenital heart disease.

REFERENCES

Cambier PA, Kirby WC, Wortham DC, Moore JW. Percutaneous closure of the small (less than 2.5 mm) patent ductus arteriosus using coil embolization. *Am J Cardiol* 1992;69:815–816.

Du ZD, Hijazi ZM, Kleinman CS, Silverman NH. Comparison between transcatheter and surgical closure of secundum atrial septal defect in children and adults: Results of a multicenter nonrandomized trial. *J Am Coll Cardiol* 2002;39:1836–1844.

Kan JS, White RIJ, Mitchell SE, Gardner TJ. Percutaneous balloon valvuloplasty: A new method for treating congenital pulmonary valve stenosis. *N Engl J Med* 1982;307:540–542.

Lababidi Z, Wu JR, Walls TJ. Percutaneous balloon aortic valvuloplasty results in 23 patients. *Am J Cardiol* 1984;53:194–197.

Lock JE, Bass JL, Amplatz K, Fuhrman BP, Castaneda-Zuniga WR. Balloon dilatation angioplasty of aortic coarctation in infants and children. *Circulation* 1983;68:109–116.

O'Laughlin MP, Perry SB, Lock JE, Mullin CE. Use of endovascular stents in congenital heart disease. *Circulation* 1991;83:1923–1939.

Ovaert C, McCrindle BW, Nykanen D, et al. Balloon angioplasty of native coarctation: Clinical outcomes and predictors of success. *J Am Coll Cardiol* 2000;35:988–996.

Rashkind WJ, Miller WW. Creation of an atrial septal defect without thoracotomy: A palliative approach to complete transposition of the great arteries. *JAMA* 1966;196: 991–992.

Chapter 46

Surgical Interventions for Congenital Heart Disease

Alden M. Parsons, G. William Henry, and Michael R. Mill

Our understanding of the complexities of congenital heart disease, a deviation from normal cardiac anatomic development that affects 8 in 1000 births, has progressed immensely since the establishment of the Board of Pediatric Cardiology (and hence the subspecialty) in 1961. Advances have paralleled improvements in diagnostic imaging, such as echocardiography and cardiac angiography, and innovations in surgical repair techniques. Basic scientific investigation has led to greater comprehension of the patterns of embryologic development and of the aberrancies that cause the common congenital anomalies. This chapter gives a broad overview of the genesis of congenital heart disease with a focus on the role of corrective surgical interventions.

Embryologic development of the heart begins with the fusion of angiogenetic cell clusters within the splanchnic mesoderm layer of the primitive embryo to form the heart tube at 18 to 21 days of gestation. The cardiac tube surrounds a core of cardiac jelly, which serves as an extracellular matrix, and plays a key role in the complex intracellular signaling and feedback mechanisms that regulate cardiac morphogenesis. The cardiac tube consists of a myocardial mantle three to five layers thick and an inner single layer of endocardial cells. The endocardial cells play a role in the formation of endocardial cushions, as well as in cellular signaling. The heart begins to rhythmically contract as early as day 17, once the functional units of the myocytes begin to form. Myocardial growth proceeds with segmentation and looping of the heart tube and cellular differentiation and migration along the embryologic axes, with the establishment of laterality and the organization of the primitive cells into a sophisticated organ.

The fetal circulation adapts to placental gas exchange and nutritional support. The right side of the heart is responsible for about two thirds of the fetal cardiac output, which is shunted through the ductus arteriosus into the descending aorta. During development, pulmonary vascular resistance is high and pulmonary blood flow is low. Closer to term, pulmonary blood flow slowly increases and, as new arterioles develop and increased pulmonary arterial cross-

sectional area increases, pulmonary vascular resistance decreases. At birth, with the entrance of air into the lungs and alveolar expansion, pulmonary vascular resistance falls and pulmonary blood flow rapidly increases 8- to 10-fold. The ductus arteriosus changes from a right-to-left conduit to a left-to-right shunt after birth, until it closes within the first hours to days of life. Pulmonary arterial blood pressure is thought to reach adult levels by 2 to 6 weeks after birth. Increased pulmonary venous return to the left atrium elevates left-sided intracardiac pressures relative to the right-sided pressures, and the valve of the foramen ovale closes.

Deviations from this complex process of cardiac development lead to congenital cardiac anomalies, with presentations that vary from the immediate postnatal period to adulthood. Congenital cardiac lesions can be broadly divided into cyanotic and acyanotic lesions. The clinical manifestations of congenital heart disease in the neonatal period usually result in cyanosis, respiratory distress, and/or hypoperfusion with evidence of cardiogenic shock. Congenital heart disease is suspected when a history and physical examination, a chest radiograph, and an ECG show one or more of these clinical findings. Further evaluation by Doppler echocardiography is routine and an integral part of the noninvasive evaluation of congenital heart disease (see also chapter 44). Echocardiography can determine the basic anatomic configuration of the heart, and Doppler studies provide information about patterns and disturbances in blood flow. Angiography can further elucidate the cardiopulmonary defects. Indications for angiography may include inconsistencies in the noninvasive findings, the need for images of the branch pulmonary arteries, or suspected complex ventricular septal defects (VSDs). Abnormalities of the aortic arch, such as coarctation or vascular rings, are best evaluated by magnetic resonance imaging.

Therapy for congenital heart disease has evolved with surgical and nonsurgical innovations. The development of transcatheter procedures has made therapeutic cardiac catheterization a viable alternative to surgery for specific congenital cardiac lesions (see chapter 45). In addition, advances in imaging and prenatal diagnosis have spurred the development of antenatal surgical intervention for congenital heart disease.

INTERVENTIONAL CARDIOLOGY

Early management of congenital heart lesions was largely surgical. With the development of angiography, initially a diagnostic modality, interventional catheter-based techniques for management of congenital heart disease became possible. Definitive treatment with device closure now exists for amenable lesions such as fossa ovalis (secundum type) atrial septal defect (ASD), muscular VSD, and patent ductus arteriosus. Balloon valvuloplasty for pulmonic or aortic stenosis and balloon angioplasty with stenting for branch pulmonary artery stenosis and coarctation of the aorta are other common catheter-based interventions that have been used with some success. Studies on transcatheter perforation and pulmonic valvuloplasty in pulmonary atresia with intact ventricular septum have reported an 81% initial success rate; however, more than 50% of patients may need a systemic-to-pulmonary shunt to augment pulmonary blood flow or are better suited for definitive surgical repair.

SURGICAL TREATMENT

The development of pediatric cardiac surgery has led to the survival of many children with complex congenital heart disease. These successes have depended on improved diagnoses, advances in surgical technique, and the development of a means for extracorporeal circulation—cardiopulmonary bypass (CPB). Complex repairs for previously fatal lesions such as transposition of the great arteries and hypoplastic left-sided heart syndrome (HLHS) have become routine, with declining mortality rates and improved long-term outcomes.

Surgically Correctable Lesions: Common Congenital Anomalies

Ventricular Septal Defects

Ventricular septal defect is the most common congenital cardiac anomaly, occurring in 20% of patients with congenital heart disease (Fig. 46-1). Interventricular communication occurs with the failure of the ridges of tissue to fuse to form the septum. VSDs are traditionally classified as perimembranous, muscular, and doubly committed subarterial, with the perimembranous and muscular types further classified on the basis of anatomic location as inlet, outlet, or trabecular. Of surgically repaired defects, 80% are perimembranous. Of patients with VSDs, 50% have other associated cardiac anomalies. The flow across a VSD is related to the size of the VSD. "Restrictive" VSDs are small to medium-sized, with a pressure gradient across the defect. "Nonrestrictive" VSDs are large, with equal left ventricular and right ventricular (RV) pressures. Congestive heart failure can develop with significant left-to-right shunting and increased volume load to the pulmonary vasculature, the left atrium, and the left ventricle. Persistent elevation in pulmonary vascular resistance (PVR) can lead to equalization of PVR and systemic vascular resistance (SVR) and irreversible changes to the pulmonary vasculature. *Eisenmenger's complex* (reversal of the shunt to right to left and subsequent cyanosis) can result if the VSD is left untreated. Surgical repair is performed by means of a median sternotomy and exposure via the right atrium, right ventricle, or pulmonary artery, depending on the location of the lesion.

Atrial Septal Defect

An interatrial communication accounts for 10 to 15% of congenital cardiac anomalies. The term ASD refers to a spectrum of anomalies that are broadly classified into four categories: oval fossa or "secundum" defect, ASD of the atrioventricular

Figure 46-1   ## Transatrial Repair of Ventricular Septal Defect (VSD)

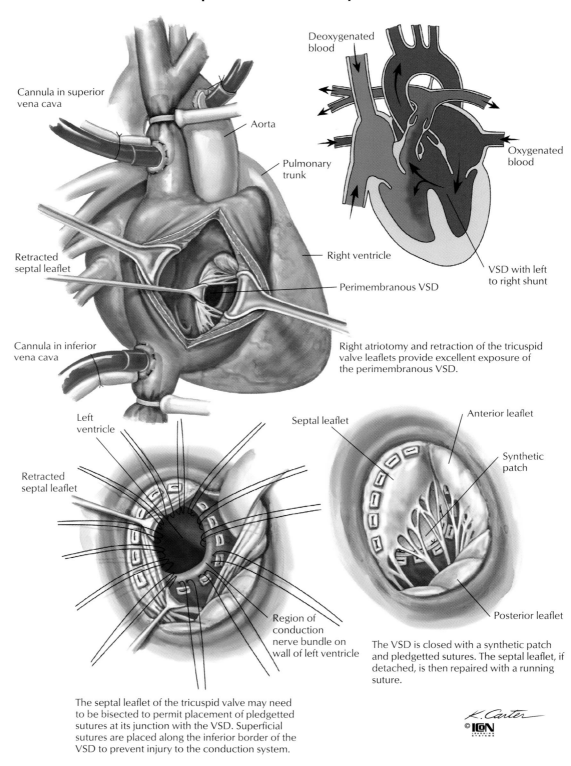

Cannula in superior vena cava

Deoxygenated blood

Aorta

Pulmonary trunk

Retracted septal leaflet

Right ventricle

Perimembranous VSD

Oxygenated blood

VSD with left to right shunt

Cannula in inferior vena cava

Right atriotomy and retraction of the tricuspid valve leaflets provide excellent exposure of the perimembranous VSD.

Left ventricle

Retracted septal leaflet

Septal leaflet

Anterior leaflet

Synthetic patch

Posterior leaflet

Region of conduction nerve bundle on wall of left ventricle

The VSD is closed with a synthetic patch and pledgetted sutures. The septal leaflet, if detached, is then repaired with a running suture.

The septal leaflet of the tricuspid valve may need to be bisected to permit placement of pledgetted sutures at its junction with the VSD. Superficial sutures are placed along the inferior border of the VSD to prevent injury to the conduction system.

K. Carter

©ICON

septal defect (AVSD) type or partial AVSD or "ostium primum" defect, superior or inferior sinus venosus defects, and coronary sinus defects. ASDs often coexist with other anomalies, such as partial anomalous venous drainage. The degree of hemodynamic disturbance is related to the size of the defect and the amount of blood flow shunting. Indications for closure are a significant left-to-right shunt, leading to a ratio of pulmonary blood flow to systemic blood flow (also known as shunt fraction, Qp:Qs) of greater than 1.5:1, or known venous thrombosis (because of the risk of paradoxical embolization and cerebrovascular accident). Device closure can be performed for simple oval fossa ASDs. Surgical repair is most often performed via a median sternotomy with CPB and bicaval cannulation via a right atriotomy.

Patent Ductus Arteriosus

Patent ductus arteriosus is a vascular connection postnatally between the main pulmonary trunk or proximal left pulmonary artery and the descending thoracic aorta. This anomaly occurs in about 1 in 2000 to 2500 births and accounts for 10% of congenital heart lesions. In full-term infants, the ductus arteriosus is usually functionally closed by 10 to 15 hours after birth. Persistent blood flow through this vessel is often associated with other congenital anomalies, and depending on the vascular connections, pulmonary blood flow may be dependent on patency of the ductus, as in lesions of RV outflow obstruction. In this case, the vessel may be kept open with prostaglandin E_1 therapy until an aortopulmonary connection is surgically created. When no other associated anomalies exist, and ductus closure has not occurred after medical therapy with indomethacin for 48 to 72 hours, direct surgical ligation or division via a left posterolateral thoracotomy or, alternatively, catheter-based device closure is indicated. Surgical closure before 10 days of age reduces the duration of ventilatory support, the length of hospital stay, and the overall morbidity rate.

Atrioventricular Septal Defects

Atrioventricular septal defects are defects involving deficiencies in the AV septum and abnormalities of the AV valves (mitral and tricuspid), commonly referred to as "endocardial cushion defects." AVSDs account for 4 to 5% of congenital heart disease, and 7 to 25% of AV septal defects are associated with other cardiac defects. There is a wide spectrum of lesions, with a partial AVSD being limited to a deficiency in the atrial portion of the atrioventricular septum and a common atrioventricular valve (ostium primum ASD) and a complete AVSD referring to a deficiency of the entire atrioventricular septum with a common atrioventricular valve. Complete AVSDs are commonly seen in patients with Down's syndrome and can occur in combination with tetralogy of Fallot (TOF) in this patient population. The mortality rate for unrepaired complete AVSDs at 2 years of age is as high as 80% because of progressive congestive heart failure and pulmonary vascular disease. Surgical repair is performed via a median sternotomy with CPB and with the use of a right atriotomy. The interatrial and/or interventricular communication is closed, and valvular competency is restored.

Tricuspid Atresia

Tricuspid atresia, a congenital lesion with an absent right-sided AV connection, occurs in up to 3.7% of patients with congenital heart disease. Left ventricular preload is dependent on interatrial blood flow via an ASD. Often, there is an associated VSD with left-to-right shunting, the degree of which depends on the size of the VSD and the right ventricle or infundibular chamber, and the right- and left-sided pressures. The physiology of the lesion varies by the amount of pulmonary blood flow. The original surgical repair, the classic Fontan procedure, involved a direct connection between the right atrium and the main pulmonary artery. Present-day conversion to the Fontan circulation usually requires a two-stage surgical approach after early palliation. A cavopulmonary anastomosis can be performed as early as 3 months of age but is usually created between 4 and 9 months, followed by the Fontan procedure, which is performed between 18 months and 3 years. The modern Fontan procedure includes a total cavopulmonary connection using a bidirectional Glenn shunt and an extracardiac conduit connection between the inferior vena cava and the pulmonary artery. The bidirectional Glenn shunt is a connection between the divided end of the superior vena cava and the right pulmonary artery that shunts venous return from the superior vena cava directly to both lungs. This modification reduces associated morbidity and mortality rates, including a lowered incidence of early failure and a reduction in early and late arrhythmias.

Surgically Correctable Lesions: Complex Congenital Anomalies

Double-Outlet Right Ventricle

Double-outlet right ventricle is a conotruncal malformation with both great arteries arising from the right ventricle and an associated VSD. This anomaly has a wide spectrum of presentations depending on the location of the VSD, its relation to the great vessels, and the degree of arterial overriding of the interventricular septum. Classifications are based on the relationship of the VSD to the great vessels: subaortic VSD with or without pulmonary stenosis, subpulmonary VSD with or without subaortic stenosis, doubly committed VSD, and noncommitted or remote VSD. The degree of hemodynamic compromise of this lesion depends on the variable degree of subvalvar stenosis and the size and precise position of the VSD. The surgical approach also depends on the nature of the lesion.

Hypoplastic Left Heart Syndrome

Hypoplastic left heart syndrome (HLHS), a congenital lesion with univentricular physiology, involves an atretic left ventricle, an underdeveloped mitral or aortic valvular apparatus, or both, and hypoplasia of the ascending aorta. Systemic blood flow is usually ductal-dependent, and the appearance of symptoms in the neonatal period usually correlates with spontaneous ductal closure. Thus, early management with prostaglandin E_1 to maintain ductal patency is life-sustaining. The appropriate balance between pulmonary and systemic blood flow (Qp:Qs) is critical. HLHS accounts for 25% of cardiac mortality during the first week of life. The major neonatal palliative approach is the Norwood procedure, in which an aortopulmonary connection is created (Figs. 46-2 and 46-3). This procedure involves the enlargement of the aortic arch with a homograft patch, and a shunt to provide pulmonary blood flow. The surgery is usually performed during the neonatal period and carries a

20 to 40% risk of mortality. The Norwood procedure is followed by a bidirectional Glenn shunt at 3 to 6 months of age and a Fontan procedure at 2 to 3 years of age. Alternatively, cardiac transplantation is favored for HLHS at some centers. The operative risk of cardiac transplantation in the neonatal period is 10%, but there is a high mortality rate (25%) for patients on the waiting list.

Tetralogy of Fallot

Classically, TOF refers to four major congenital defects: VSD, infundibular pulmonary stenosis, dextroposition of the aorta, and RV hypertrophy (Fig. 46-4). The common anatomic abnormality responsible for all features is posterior malalignment of the outlet septum. TOF can present with a range of clinical findings: from cyanosis at birth to oxygen desaturation without cyanosis ("the pink tetralogy"). The degree of compromise is determined by the severity of the RV outflow obstruction and the size and location of the VSD. The reported mortality rate for unrepaired TOF is 30% by 6 months of age, 50% by 2 years, and up to 84% by 5 years. Infants with severe forms of TOF are often maintained on prostaglandin E_1 to support pulmonary blood flow until repair. Studies reviewing early palliative procedures versus complete repair show lower overall mortality rates for early complete repair of uncomplicated TOF relative to a two-stage approach to TOF repair. Total correction is accomplished on CPB. Closure of the VSD and provision of unobstructed flow from the right ventricle are the main goals of surgery.

Total Anomalous Pulmonary Venous Return

There are three types of total anomalous pulmonary venous return: supracardiac (most common, 50%), with pulmonary venous drainage into the innominate vein through a vertical vein; intracardiac, with drainage into the coronary sinus or the right atrium (least common); and infracardiac, with drainage into the inferior vena cava. Total anomalous pulmonary venous return may present with total pulmonary venous obstruction and pulmonary edema, requiring urgent surgical intervention. Without surgery, the mortality rate is 100% in the first year of life. Surgical repair with direct anastomosis of the

Figure 46-2   ## Norwood Correction of HLHS

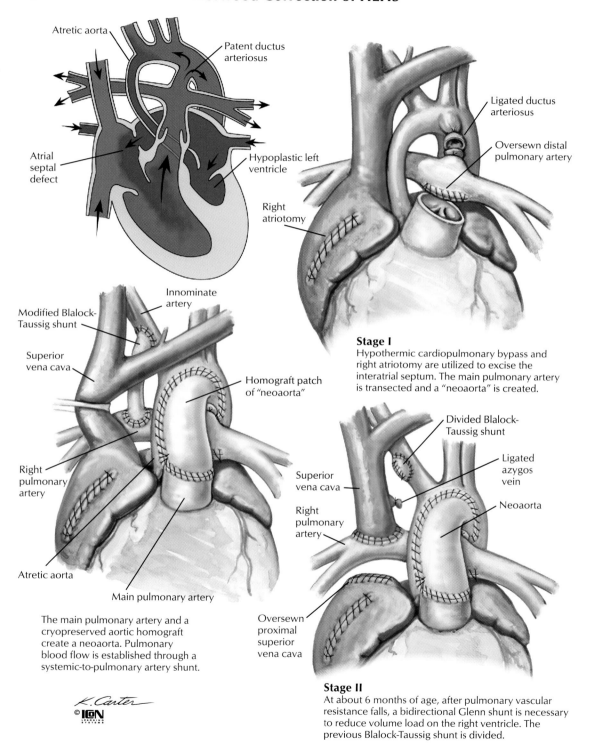

Atretic aorta

Patent ductus arteriosus

Atrial septal defect

Hypoplastic left ventricle

Right atriotomy

Ligated ductus arteriosus

Oversewn distal pulmonary artery

Stage I
Hypothermic cardiopulmonary bypass and right atriotomy are utilized to excise the interatrial septum. The main pulmonary artery is transected and a "neoaorta" is created.

Modified Blalock-Taussig shunt

Innominate artery

Superior vena cava

Homograft patch of "neoaorta"

Right pulmonary artery

Atretic aorta

Main pulmonary artery

The main pulmonary artery and a cryopreserved aortic homograft create a neoaorta. Pulmonary blood flow is established through a systemic-to-pulmonary artery shunt.

Divided Blalock-Taussig shunt

Ligated azygos vein

Superior vena cava

Neoaorta

Right pulmonary artery

Oversewn proximal superior vena cava

Stage II
At about 6 months of age, after pulmonary vascular resistance falls, a bidirectional Glenn shunt is necessary to reduce volume load on the right ventricle. The previous Blalock-Taussig shunt is divided.

K. Carter

© ICON
LEARNING
SYSTEMS

Figure 46-3

Norwood Correction of HLHS: Fontan Circulation

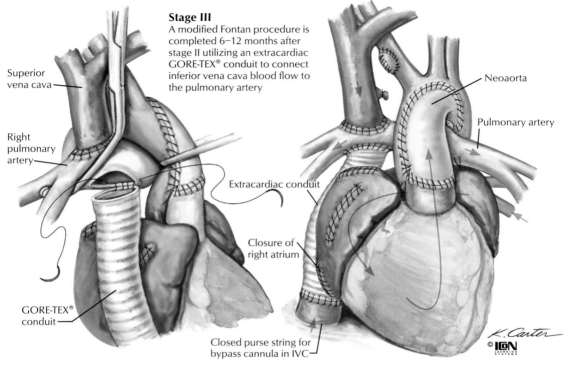

Stage III
A modified Fontan procedure is completed 6–12 months after stage II utilizing an extracardiac GORE-TEX® conduit to connect inferior vena cava blood flow to the pulmonary artery

Superior vena cava

Right pulmonary artery

Neoaorta

Pulmonary artery

Extracardiac conduit

Closure of right atrium

GORE-TEX® conduit

Closed purse string for bypass cannula in IVC

Systemic venous blood bypasses the right heart directly to the pulmonary arteries and lungs. Oxygenated blood is pumped from the left to right atrium through a septotomy. The "neoaorta" directs oxygenated systemic blood flow from the right ventricle.

common pulmonary venous channel to the right atrium is accomplished under circulatory arrest or low-flow continuous CPB and carries a mortality rate of approximately 16%.

Transposition of the Great Arteries

The neonate with discordant ventriculoarterial connections is dependent on intracardiac mixing for survival and typically presents with cyanosis at birth. Initial management of transposition of the great arteries with prostaglandin E_1 and balloon septostomy to increase atrial mixing is life-sustaining, but the mortality rate without surgical repair is very high. Initial complete repair is optimal if it can be done within the first 30 days of life. Correction involves the redirection of systemic venous blood to the pulmonary circulation and pulmonary venous blood to the systemic arterial circulation. Over the years, numerous

surgical approaches have been proposed for correction of transposition of the great arteries. Based on the outcomes obtained at numerous centers, the surgical approach of choice today is the arterial switch procedure (Fig. 46-5). Mortality rates have steadily declined since the arterial switch procedure has become widely accepted.

Truncus Arteriosus

Truncus arteriosus, a relatively uncommon defect (0.21–0.34% of those with congenital heart disease), consists of a single semilunar valve (the truncal valve) that regulates outflow from the single arterial trunk (rather than normally separate LV and RV outflow tracts) to the aorta, pulmonary arteries, and coronary circulation. The single arterial trunk overrides the interventricular septum. Left-to-right shunting occurs via a VSD and the aortopulmonary connection.

Figure 46-4

Tetralogy of Fallot

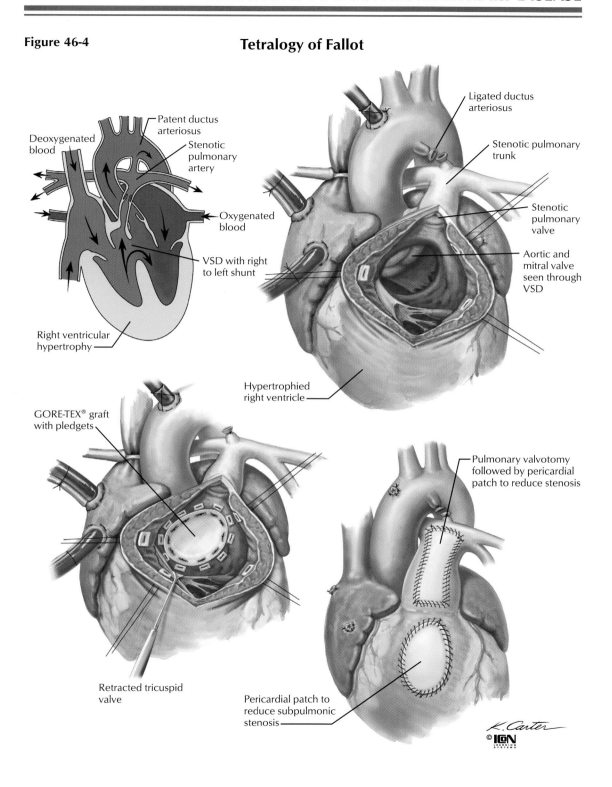

Patent ductus arteriosus

Deoxygenated blood

Stenotic pulmonary artery

Oxygenated blood

VSD with right to left shunt

Right ventricular hypertrophy

Ligated ductus arteriosus

Stenotic pulmonary trunk

Stenotic pulmonary valve

Aortic and mitral valve seen through VSD

Hypertrophied right ventricle

GORE-TEX® graft with pledgets

Retracted tricuspid valve

Pulmonary valvotomy followed by pericardial patch to reduce stenosis

Pericardial patch to reduce subpulmonic stenosis

K. Carter

© ICON
LEARNING
SYSTEMS

Figure 46-5   Arterial Repair of Transposition of the Great Arteries

Initial steps

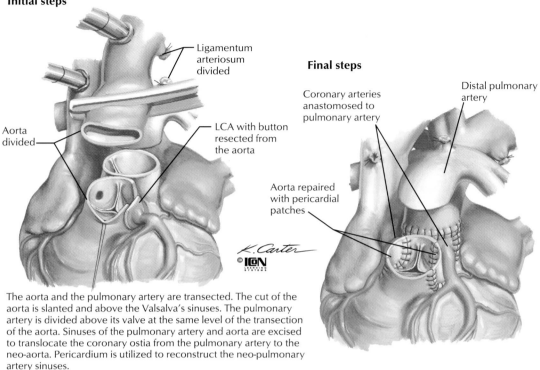

Ligamentum
arteriosum
divided

Aorta
divided

LCA with button
resected from
the aorta

Final steps

Coronary arteries
anastomosed to
pulmonary artery

Distal pulmonary
artery

Aorta repaired
with pericardial
patches

K. Carter
© ICON

The aorta and the pulmonary artery are transected. The cut of the
aorta is slanted and above the Valsalva's sinuses. The pulmonary
artery is divided above its valve at the same level of the transection
of the aorta. Sinuses of the pulmonary artery and aorta are excised
to translocate the coronary ostia from the pulmonary artery to the
neo-aorta. Pericardium is utilized to reconstruct the neo-pulmonary
artery sinuses.

Patients are occasionally cyanotic at birth but most often develop symptoms of CHF within the first weeks of life. Surgical repair can be accomplished safely in the neonatal period (Fig. 46-6). The mortality rate for untreated truncus arteriosus is as high as 65% at 6 months of age and 75% at 1 year.

Pediatric Heart Transplantation

The success of pediatric cardiac transplantation is highest in the neonatal period. For HLHS or primary cardiomyopathies, the 5-year survival rate after transplantation is greater than 80%. Pediatric heart transplantation has been performed in more than 3500 children since the late 1960s. Congenital heart disease indications for transplantation are HLHS, severe Ebstein's anomaly, pulmonary atresia with intact ventricular septum, unbalanced AV canal, single ventricle with subaortic stenosis, complex truncus arteriosus, and double-inlet left ventricle. Of the transplantation rates for the two broad categories of indications for heart transplantation in children,

the rates of transplantation for congenital heart disease have recently reached and surpassed the rates for cardiomyopathy, the previously more common indication for transplantation.

The major drawback to cardiac transplantation as an answer to end-stage disease is the availability of donors, with a potential recipient to donor ratio of approximately 15:1. Two risk factors have been identified for death while waiting on the cardiac transplantation list: status 1 at listing (ICU patients on inotropic agents) and ventilator dependence. An obstacle to long-term survival after cardiac transplantation, besides rejection, is the development of graft coronary disease, which occurs in 2 to 30% of patients at 1 year after transplantation and in up to 50% of patients at 5 years. Rejection accounts for approximately 30% of deaths in children who have undergone heart transplantation. Developments in the field of immunosuppression and improvements in graft preservation and operative techniques have resulted in much improved outcomes, and further advances in these areas are on the horizon.

Figure 46-6

Truncus Arteriosus

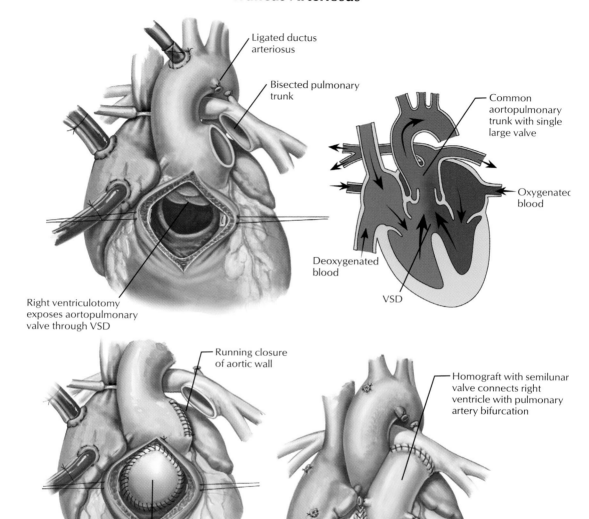

Ligated ductus arteriosus

Bisected pulmonary trunk

Common aortopulmonary trunk with single large valve

Oxygenated blood

Deoxygenated blood

VSD

Right ventriculotomy exposes aortopulmonary valve through VSD

Running closure of aortic wall

Homograft with semilunar valve connects right ventricle with pulmonary artery bifurcation

Care is taken not to damage the cardiac conduction system when sewing GORE-TEX® graft over the inferior rim of the VSD

Pericardial patch over closure of right ventriculotomy

K. Carter
© ICON

FUTURE DIRECTIONS

Research in the field of perinatology and the development of prenatal diagnostic modalities have led to advances in fetal heart surgery. Improvements in fetal Doppler ultrasound now permit diagnosis of fetal heart disease as early as 10 to 14 weeks of life. Antenatal intervention in fetal heart disease is an emerging, but yet unproven field. To date, published information about antenatal interventions has been limited to isolated case reports of balloon valvuloplasty for severe semilunar valvular obstruction, performed with minimal success. There are reports of attempted pulmonic valvular dilatation antenatally in pulmonary atresia with intact ventricular septum and of attempted transuterine percutaneous pacemaker lead placement for congenital complete heart block. Future directions involve further development of transuterine as well as transumbilical approaches to fetal heart disease.

REFERENCES

Allen HD, Gutgesell HP, Clark EB, Driscoll DJ, eds. *Moss and Adams' Heart Disease in Infants, Children, and Adolescents*. Vol 1. 5th ed. Baltimore: Williams & Wilkins; 1995.

Ebert PA, Turley K, Stanger P, Hoffman JI, Heymann MA, Rudolph AM. Surgical treatment of truncus arteriosus in the first 6 months of life. *Ann Surg* 1984;200:451–456.

Kohl T, Sharland G, Allan LD, et al. World experience of percutaneous ultrasound-guided balloon valvuloplasty in human fetuses with severe aortic valve obstruction. *Am J Cardiol* 2000;85:1230-1233.

LeBlanc JG, Russell JL. Pediatric cardiac surgery in the 1990s. *Surg Clin North Am* 1998;78:729–747.

Nichols DG, Cameron DE, Greeley WJ, Lappe DG, Ungerleider RM, Wetzel RC, eds. *Critical Heart Disease in Infants and Children*. St. Louis, MO: Mosby; 1995.

Saiki Y, Rebeyka IM. Fetal cardiac intervention and surgery. *Semin Thorac Cardiovasc Surg Pediatr Card Surg Annu* 2001;4:256–270.

Soto B, Becker AE, Moulaert AJ, Lie JT, Anderson RH. Classification of ventricular septal defects. *Br Heart J* 1980;43:332–343.

Townsend CM, Beauchamp DR, Evers MB, et al, eds. *Sabiston Textbook of Surgery: The Biological Basis of Modern Surgical Practice*. 16th ed. Philadelphia: WB Saunders; 2001.

Wilcox BR, Anderson RH. *Surgical Anatomy of the Heart*. 2nd ed. New York: Gower Medical Publishing; 1992.

Chapter 47

Arrhythmias in Congenital Heart Disease

Scott H. Buck

Advances in medical and surgical care of children with congenital heart disease have dramatically reduced mortality and, consequently, increased the population of children, adolescents, and adults with congenital heart disease. Arrhythmias are an important source of morbidity and mortality among these patients. Arrhythmias can result from congenital anomalies of the conducting system; from effects of chronic cyanosis, chamber distension, hypertrophy, and fibrosis; and from surgical intervention. Although the overall incidence of sudden death related to arrhythmias in congenital heart disease is low, subsets of patients are at considerable risk. Risk stratification continues to evolve, as do strategies for pharmacologic and nonpharmacologic arrhythmia management.

CYANOTIC CONGENITAL HEART DISEASE

Tetralogy of Fallot

Electrocardiographic features of tetralogy typically are RV hypertrophy and right axis deviation. Among patients who have not undergone surgical repair, supraventricular and ventricular arrhythmias are rare in childhood but can increase by adolescence (Fig. 47-1). After repair, right bundle branch block is present in most patients and left axis deviation and PR prolongation are also occasionally seen. Although the long-term survival rate is excellent, nearly 90% at 30 years of age, ventricular arrhythmias are common. Significant ventricular arrhythmias are present in 5 to 10% of patients' ECGs, in 20 to 40% of treadmill exercise recordings, and in 40 to 60% of ambulatory recordings (Fig. 47-2). The severity of ventricular arrhythmias increases with age at repair, RV pressure, and duration of follow-up. Electrophysiologic testing usually demonstrates a monomorphic macroreentry circuit involving the scarred RV outflow tract or the conal septum. The incidence of sudden cardiac death among long-term tetralogy survivors is 1.5 to 5%; however, the ability to identify those patients at highest risk is limited. Although some studies suggest that ambulatory recordings and/or invasive electrophysiology testing is useful, other reports are less compelling. One finding that is almost always useful is marked QRS prolongation. QRS duration of greater than 180 ms indicates a risk of sustained ventricular arrhythmias and sudden cardiac death. In addition to ventricular arrhythmias, supraventricular arrhythmias are common in long-term follow-up, with atrial flutter or fibrillation being present in as many as 25% of patients.

D-Transposition of the Great Arteries

Electrocardiographic findings of unoperated D-transposition of the great arteries (D-TGV) primarily reflect the ventriculoarterial discordance of D-TGV (i.e., the right ventricle serving as the systemic ventricle, resulting in RV hypertrophy). Children with D-TGV require surgical repair. Atrial baffle (Mustard and Senning) procedures to direct pulmonary venous blood to the systemic (morphologic right) ventricle and systemic venous blood to the pulmonary (morphologic left) ventricle were for several decades the "repair of choice" for D-TGV (Fig. 47-3). Atrial baffle repair of D-TGV frequently produces direct trauma to the sinus node or its blood supply and creates conduction barriers by suture lines and scars—essentially substrates for atrial reentry rhythms. There is progressive loss of sinus rhythm; 5 to 10 years after atrial baffle surgery, only 20 to 40% of patients remain in sinus rhythm, 7 to 35% are in junctional rhythm, up to 40% are in slow ectopic atrial rhythm, and 10% have intra-atrial reentry. At longer follow-up, nearly half of these patients have supraventricular tachycardia, predominantly intra-atrial reen-

Figure 47-1

Tetralogy of Fallot

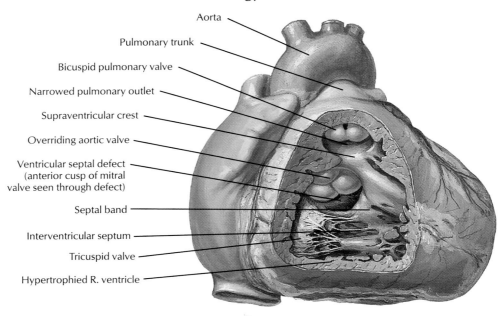

Aorta

Pulmonary trunk

Bicuspid pulmonary valve

Narrowed pulmonary outlet

Supraventricular crest

Overriding aortic valve

Ventricular septal defect
(anterior cusp of mitral
valve seen through defect)

Septal band

Interventricular septum

Tricuspid valve

Hypertrophied R. ventricle

**Corrective operation
for tetralogy of Fallot**

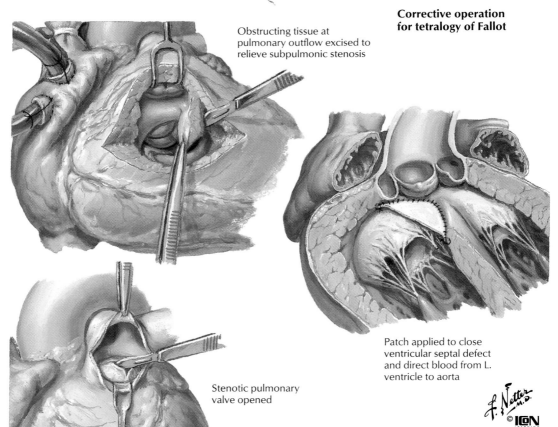

Obstructing tissue at
pulmonary outflow excised to
relieve subpulmonic stenosis

Stenotic pulmonary
valve opened

Patch applied to close
ventricular septal defect
and direct blood from L.
ventricle to aorta

Figure 47-2

Tetralogy of Fallot

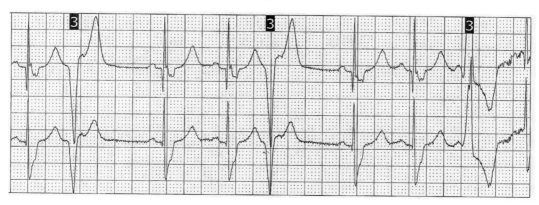

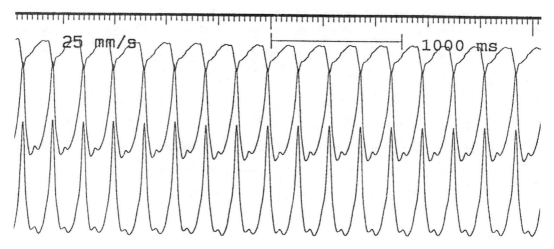

Sample ambulatory recording of adolescent patient s/p repair of tetralogy of Fallot in childhood (**upper**) and lead I, II, and III recordings from another patient s/p tetralogy repair with inducible ventricular tachycardia at electrophysiologic study (**lower**).

try. Loss of sinus rhythm and development of junctional rhythm is associated with an increased risk of development of symptomatic bradycardia. Ten years after atrial baffle surgery, approximately 8% of patients need cardiac pacing, which increases to approximately 20% of patients at 20 years' follow-up. Sudden cardiac death occurs in 3 to 15% of patients after atrial baffle repair, with the risk seeming to be greater among patients with decreased right (systemic) ventricular function and among patients with uncontrolled intra-atrial reentry. Since the 1980s, most infants born with D-TGV have undergone the arterial switch procedure, resulting in a significant reduction of complex atrial

arrhythmias. However, simple atrial ectopy is frequently seen, speculated to be related to balloon atrial septostomy, venous cannulation, or atrial defect repair.

Tricuspid Atresia

Electrocardiographic findings of tricuspid atresia (TA) include RA enlargement, left axis deviation, and increased LV forces. A short PR interval is seen occasionally and is usually attributed to enhanced atrioventricular (AV) node conduction rather than to an accessory connection. Initially applied to TA and now increasingly applied to diverse single-ventricle variants, including hypoplastic left-sided heart syndrome, Fontan

Figure 47-3   **Transposition of the Great Vessels**

Mustard operation

The interatrial septum has been widely excised, opening into transverse sinus at upper end. This opening is being sutured and coronary sinus opened into L. atrium.

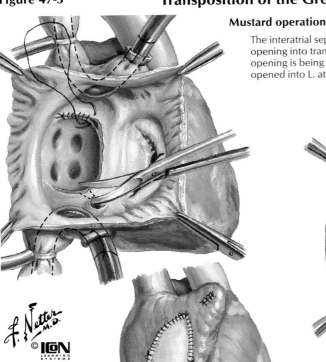

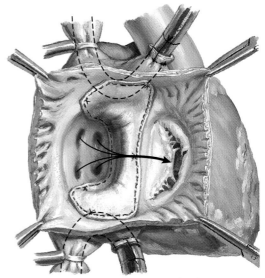

A patch of pericardium has been applied to close incision and enlarge newly formed R. atrium

A patch of pericardium has been applied so as to channel blood from pulmonary veins through tricuspid valve to R. ventricle, then out the aorta. Blood from venae cavae will now pass to L. ventricle and then to pulmonary artery.

palliation (nearly always preceded by superior vena cava-to-pulmonary artery anastomosis or Hemi-Fontan staging) directs systemic venous blood to the pulmonary arteries (Fig. 47-4). In classic or old-style Fontan atriopulmonary connections, the sinus node or its blood supply is often interrupted, and the atria are subjected to increased pressure, resulting in atrial distension, hypertrophy, and fibrosis. Surgical scars and patches produce conduction barriers that support intra-atrial reentry circuits, frequently involving the lateral atrial wall, the perimeter of the ASD patch, and the inferomedial RA isthmus, the latter also being a component of typical atrial flutter in structurally normal hearts. The incidence of late atrial tachycardia after Fontan palliation is 30 to 50% at 5 years, and 5 to 15% of these patients need a pacemaker. Advanced

patient age at follow-up, increased RA size, and increased pulmonary artery pressure are risk factors for atrial arrhythmia development (Fig. 47-5). Late sudden cardiac death occurs in 2 to 3% of patients. Modification of surgical techniques to reduce atrial distension and atrial suture lines (e.g., lateral tunnel and extracardiac conduit modifications) has apparently reduced the incidence of atrial arrhythmias, although long-term follow-up is limited.

Ebstein's Malformation

Electrocardiographic findings of Ebstein's malformation typically include RA enlargement and RV conduction delay. Accessory connection–mediated supraventricular tachycardia is reported in 23% of patients; most prominent are manifest accessory pathways (i.e., Wolff-Parkinson-

Figure 47-4

Tricuspid Atresia

Features of tricuspid atresia

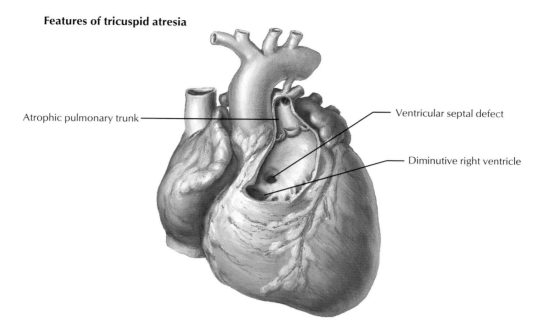

Atrophic pulmonary trunk

Ventricular septal defect

Diminutive right ventricle

Final anatomic aspect of the classic two-stage procedure created by Francis Fontan for ventricularization of the right atrium

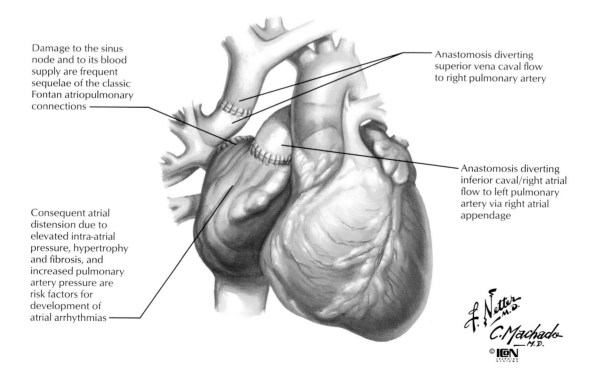

Damage to the sinus node and to its blood supply are frequent sequelae of the classic Fontan atriopulmonary connections

Anastomosis diverting superior vena caval flow to right pulmonary artery

Anastomosis diverting inferior caval/right atrial flow to left pulmonary artery via right atrial appendage

Consequent atrial distension due to elevated intra-atrial pressure, hypertrophy and fibrosis, and increased pulmonary artery pressure are risk factors for development of atrial arrhythmias

Figure 47-5

Tricuspid Atresia

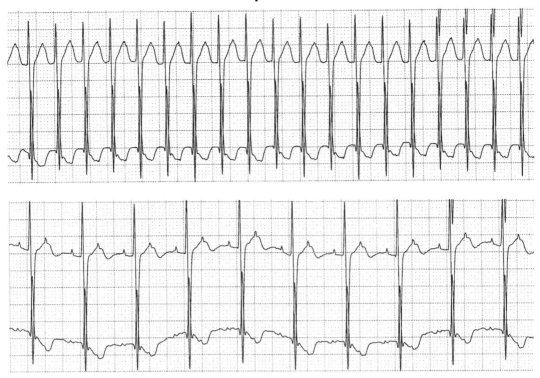

Lead V$_1$ and II recordings of adolescent patient s/p Fontan repair of tricuspid atresia demonstrating intra-atrial reentry tachycardia with 1:1 AV conduction **(upper)** and 2:1 AV conduction **(lower)**.

White [WPW] syndrome) (Fig. 47-6). Concealed accessory connection–mediated tachycardia and AV node reentry tachycardia are less common. Catheter ablation techniques can be very useful in patients with Ebstein's anomaly and WPW syndromes. However, multiple accessory connections can occur, and the altered tricuspid valve architecture results in higher procedural failure and recurrence rates compared with catheter ablation of accessory connections in structurally normal hearts. Surgical advances for improving tricuspid valve and right-sided heart function have dramatically reduced the development of late atrial reentrant tachycardia (Fig. 47-7).

ACYANOTIC CONGENITAL HEART DISEASE

Ventricular Septal Defect

Electrocardiographic findings of VSD generally reflect the hemodynamic impact of the left-to-right shunt, with the smallest defects causing no electrocardiographic changes. Moderate defects are associated with left atrial (LA) enlargement and left ventricular (LV) hypertrophy, and larger defects are associated with biventricular hypertrophy. Compared with the general population, adult patients who have not undergone surgery for their VSD have more frequent premature supraventricular beats, premature ventricular beats, ventricular couplets, and multiform premature ventricular beats by ambulatory monitoring; arrhythmia incidence is related to age and pulmonary artery pressure. In long-term postsurgical follow-up, the prevalence of serious arrhythmias (ventricular couplets, ventricular tachycardia, and multiform premature ventricular contractions) in adults correlates with cardiac functional status. The risk of arrhythmia is eightfold greater among patients with congestive heart failure (New York Heart Association class II–IV) and nearly threefold greater in patients with cardiomegaly compared with patients with

Figure 47-6

Ebstein's Malformation

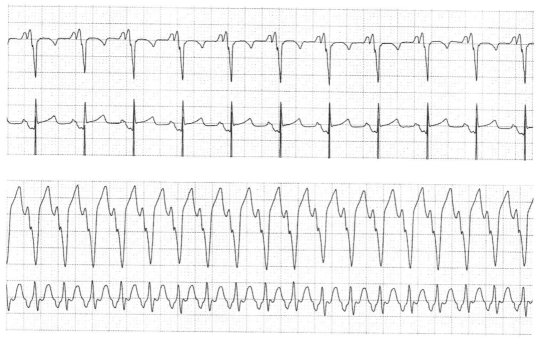

Lead V$_1$ and II recordings of infant with Ebstein's malformation demonstrating sinus rhythm with Wolff-Parkinson-White pattern **(upper)** and supraventricula tachycardia **(lower)**.

normal heart size. Current surgical practices, including earlier age at surgery and minimizing ventriculotomy, are anticipated to reduce the incidence of arrhythmia.

Atrial Septal Defect

ECG findings of secundum ASD typically include a normal P wave, a rightward QRS axis, and a mildly prolonged QRS complex with an rSr' or an rsR' pattern, the latter being attributed to disproportional thickening of the right ventricular (RV) outflow tract. Dilation of the right atrium due to left-to-right shunting is thought to be responsible for mild intraatrial conduction delay, which is manifested as PR prolongation. Sinus node dysfunction based on electrophysiologic testing is an age-related finding in many children with ASD. However, symptomatic sinus node dysfunction requiring therapy is rare. Among adults who have not undergone surgery for their ASD, the incidence of atrial flutter or fibrillation increases with advancing age, and the risk increases with the magnitude of left-to-right shunting, pulmonary artery pressure, and pul-

monary resistance. Sinus node dysfunction complicating ASD repair can result from cannulation for cardiopulmonary bypass (CPB) but is more likely the result of direct trauma to the sinoatrial node or its blood supply and is more common among patients with sinus venosus than secundum ASD. Long-term follow-up of patients undergoing ASD repair reveals development of atrial flutter and fibrillation proportional to the patient's age at repair: from less than 5% of patients undergoing repair at the age of 11 years or younger to 60% of patients undergoing repair at the age of 40 years or older.

Patent Ductus Arteriosus

ECG findings of patent ductus arteriosus (PDA) are typically normal with small left-to-right shunts; with larger shunts, LV hypertrophy and LA enlargement can be present. Arrhythmias are exceedingly rare in young patients with PDA. However, atrial fibrillation is common among patients of advanced age who have not had repair and have long-standing volume loading and congestive heart failure.

Figure 47-7

Ebstein's Malformation

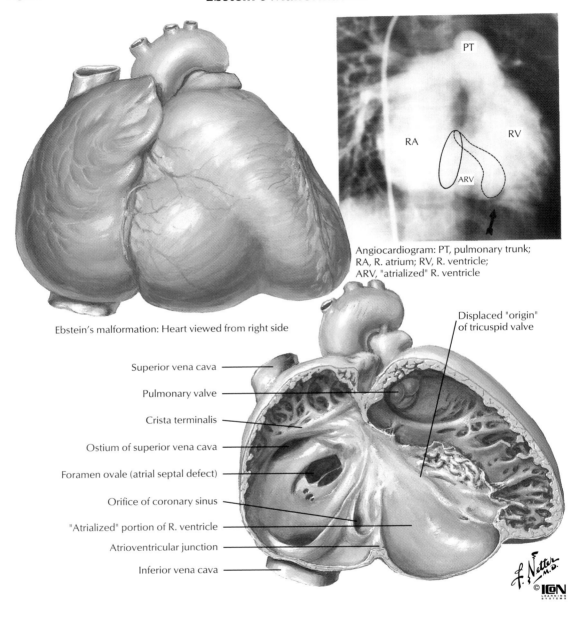

Angiocardiogram: PT, pulmonary trunk; RA, R. atrium; RV, R. ventricle; ARV, "atrialized" R. ventricle

Ebstein's malformation: Heart viewed from right side

Displaced "origin" of tricuspid valve

Superior vena cava

Pulmonary valve

Crista terminalis

Ostium of superior vena cava

Foramen ovale (atrial septal defect)

Orifice of coronary sinus

"Atrialized" portion of R. ventricle

Atrioventricular junction

Inferior vena cava

Atrioventricular Septal Defect

ECG findings of atrioventricular septal defect (AVSD) include left axis deviation and a counterclockwise depolarization pattern. In the presence of a primum ASD or AVSD with a small ventricular component, right atrial (RA) and RV enlargement from left-to-right atrial shunt are present. Among patients with large atrial and ventricular components, biventricular hypertrophy and biatrial enlargement are common, especially with significant atrioventricular (AV) valve insufficiency. Arrhythmias are rare among children with AVSD who have not had surgical repair; however, a mild intra-atrial conduction delay (PR prolongation) is often seen, attributable to atrial dilatation.

After repair of AVSD, atrial arrhythmias are reported in 10% of patients, and ventricular premature beats are observed in 33% by ambulatory monitoring. Arrhythmia incidence is associated with larger patient size, greater RV end-diastolic dimension, larger VSD, and the presence of postoperative right bundle branch block.

Pulmonary Stenosis

ECG features of PS, right axis deviation and RV hypertrophy correlate well with obstruction severity. As observed by ambulatory monitoring, the incidences of premature supraventricular beats, premature ventricular beats, ventricular couplets, and multiform premature ventricular beats are more frequent among adult PS patients without surgical repair compared with the general population. In long-term follow-up of adults after pulmonary valvotomy, the incidence of serious arrhythmias is approximately 25%.

Despite the relative frequency of arrhythmias and regardless of whether patients have undergone surgical repair, sudden death is exceedingly rare, approximately one tenth the rate among patients with aortic stenosis (AS).

Aortic Stenosis

ECG findings do not correlate well with the severity of AS obstruction, particularly in patients aged older than 10 years. The most reliable findings of severe obstruction are ST depression and T-wave inversion in lateral precordial leads. In childhood, AS is rarely associated with arrhythmias except in critical stenosis. However, as observed by ambulatory monitoring, premature supraventricular beats, premature ventricular beats, ventricular couplets, and multiform premature ventricular beats are more frequent among adult AS patients without surgical repair compared with the general population. The incidence of serious arrhythmias (ventricular couplets, ventricular tachycardia, and multiform premature ventricular contractions) approaches 25% of patients with AS. In long-term follow-up of adults after AS repair, the incidence of serious arrhythmias exceeds 40% of valvotomy patients and 60% of patients after aortic valve replacement. Serious arrhythmia risk doubles for every 5-mm Hg increase in LV end-diastolic pressure and increases more than 10-fold in the presence of moderate or severe aortic insufficiency. Sudden death is a well-recognized complication of AS, with incidence as high as 20% at 30 years. Current surgical practices are anticipated to reduce the incidence of arrhythmia and the risk of sudden cardiac death.

L-Transposition of the Great Arteries

Electrocardiographic findings of L-transposition of the great arteries (L-TGV) typically include a normal P wave followed by QRS with reversal of the Q-wave pattern in precordial leads (i.e., presence of the Q wave in right precordial leads and absence in the left). Among patients with L-TGV, 4% have congenital complete AV block. Acquired AV block occurs in approximately 2% of these patients per year; eventually, up to 75% of patients with L-TGV have complete heart block. Associated with Ebstein-like malformation of the tricuspid valve are accessory connection–mediated AV reciprocating tachycardias, seen in 2 to 5% of patients. Additionally, primary atrial arrhythmias increase with increasing patient age, particularly with atrial distension attributed to tricuspid valve regurgitation.

POSTOPERATIVE COMPLETE HEART BLOCK

The most common cause of acquired complete heart block in children is damage of the conduction system during cardiac surgery. It is the most common indication for pacemaker implantation in children. Complete heart block occurs in approximately 3% of operations involving CPB, most frequently among patients undergoing surgery for LV outflow tract obstruction, L-TGV, VSD, and tetralogy of Fallot. Recovery of AV conduction is reported in more than half of children, and nearly all of whom regain AV conduction do so within 10 days. If intact AV conduction is not present within 10 days after surgery, permanent pacemaker implantation is indicated because of the risk of sudden death among patients with junctional rhythm and AV dissociation after congenital heart surgery (Fig. 47-8).

Table 47-1
Congenital Heart Disease and Associated Arrythmias

Condition	Arrythmia Risk	Comment
Atrial septal defect	Atrial flutter, atrial fibrillation, sinus node dysfunction	Arrhythmias rare in children. Arrhythmias increase with age at repair and with age among unoperated patients.
Ventricular septal defect	Ventricular premature beats, ventricular couplets, ventricular tachycardia, premature supra-ventricular beats	Arrhythmias rare among unoperated. Arrhythmias greater among postoperative patients with higher NYHA functional class and with cardiomegaly.
Patent ductus arteriosus	Atrial fibrillation	Arrhythmias very rare in children. Arrhythmias may be seen among unoperated adult patients of advanced age.
Atrioventricular septal defect	Postoperative premature supraventricular beats, ventricular premature beats	Arrhythmias rare among unoperated. Arrhythmias increase with age at repair and with greater VSD, RV size.
Aortic stenosis	Ventricular couplets, ventricular tachycardia, multiform premature ventricular contractions	Arrhythmias increase with elevated LVEDP and with moderate or severe aortic insufficiency. Sudden death as high as 20% at 30 year follow-up.
Pulmonary stenosis	Ventricular couplets, ventricular tachycardia, multiform premature ventricular contractions	Sudden death exceedingly rare.
D-Transposition of the great arteries	Atrial baffle repair: atrial fibrillation/ flutter, sinus node dysfunction, AV block, ventricular tachycardia, pacemaker. Arterial switch repair: premature supraventricular beats	Sudden death 3–15% after atrial repair; increased among patients with depressed RV function and uncontrolled intraatrial reentry. Atrial arrhythmias significantly reduced with arterial switch.
L-Transposition of the great arteries	Acquired AV block in ~2%/year. Atrioventricular reciprocating tachycardia in 2–5% due to accessory pathway.	AV block eventually in up to 75%. AP-mediated tachycardia associated with Ebsteinlike tricuspid valve.
Tricuspid atresia	Atrial fibrillation/flutter, sinus node dysfunction, AV block, pacemaker common among atriopulmonary Fontan single-ventricle repair patients	Arrhythmias increase with follow-up duration, RA size, PA pressure. 30–50% atrial arrhythmias at 5 years. Pacemaker required in 5–15%. Late sudden death in 2–3%.
Ebstein's malformation	Atrioventricular reciprocating tachycardia due to accessory pathway	AP-mediated tachycardia in 23%.
Tetralogy of Fallot	Ventricular premature beats, ventricular couplets, ventricular tachycardia, atrial tachycardia, atrial flutter	90% long-term survival. Severe ventricular arrhythmia and sudden death risk increase with QRS duration >180 ms.
Postoperative complete heart block	Occurs in ~3% of congenital heart repairs involving cardiopulmonary bypass	Permanent pacemaker indicated when AV conduction is absent 10 days following surgery.

Figure 47-8

Postoperative Complete Heart Block

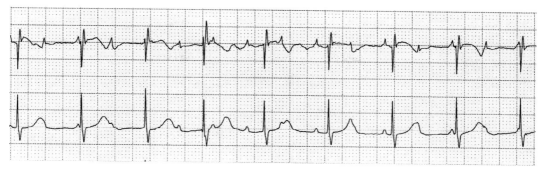

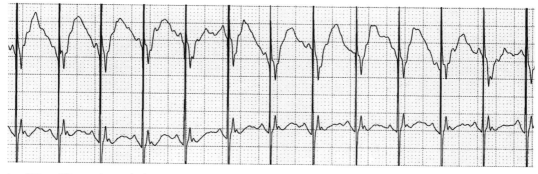

Lead V_1 and II recordings of infant demonstrating postoperative complete heart block **(upper)** and ventricular pacing tracking atrial rhythm **(lower)**.

FUTURE DIRECTIONS

Although most children with congenital heart disease survive into adulthood, the prevalence of arrhythmias poses significant challenges (Table 47-1). Surgical advances are anticipated to decrease the development of arrhythmia. Earlier definitive surgical intervention is being performed to minimize the deleterious effects of chronic hypertrophy, volume loading, fibrosis, and cyanosis in the development of a substrate for arrhythmia. Surgical techniques to minimize ventriculotomy and extensive atrial incisions that result in damage to specialized conduction tissues and to formation of conduction barriers, favoring development of reentrant rhythms, will likely decrease the development of arrhythmias. However, arrhythmias will continue to be a significant source of risk of morbidity and mortality, necessitating pharmacologic and nonpharmacologic therapy.

The goal of drug therapy is to reduce the occurrence of significant atrial and ventricular arrhythmia while minimizing the risks of drug-induced proarrhythmia and adverse effects. Drug treatment is further complicated by negative inotropy and chronotropy of the majority of available antiarrhythmic agents and could be improved by new antiarrhythmic agents. Invasive electrophysiologic studies and radiofrequency ablation or cryoablation are increasingly important in the management of congenital heart disease and arrhythmia. Although the locations of the specialized conducting tissues and the anatomic cardiac connections are complex, short-term procedural success and freedom from arrhythmia after ablation procedures are favorable. New intracardiac geometric mapping techniques have proven to be particularly useful in characterizing arrhythmia circuits in patients with congenital heart disease. Refinements of ablation energy–delivery systems are improving long-term results, including specialized catheters capable of greater ablation lesion depth. Lastly, surgical therapy, such as modifications of the Maze procedure for recurrent atrial reentrant rhythms, will continue to be an important component of arrhythmia management. These therapeutic advances, along with contemporary primary surgical management, will continue to improve the long-term outcome of patients with congenital heart disease.

REFERENCES

Gatzoulis MA, Freeman M, Siu S, et al. Atrial arrhythmias after surgical closure of atrial septal defects in adults. *N Engl J Med* 1999;340:839–846.

Gatzoulis MA, Till JA, Somerville J, et al. Mechanoelectrical interaction in tetralogy of Fallot: QRS prolongation relates to right ventricular size and predicts malignant arrhythmias and sudden death. *Circulation* 1995;92:231–237.

Kanter RJ, Garson A. Arrhythmias in congenital heart disease. In: Topol EJ, ed. *Textbook of Cardiovascular Medicine*. Philadelphia: Lippincott Williams & Wilkins; 2002: Chapter 70.

Silka MJ, Hardy BG, Menashe VD. A population-based prospective evaluation of risk of sudden death after operation for common congenital heart defects. *J Am Coll Cardiol* 1998;32:245–251.

Silka MJ, McAulty JH. Arrhythmias in patients with congenital heart disease. *Cardiac Electrophysiol Rev* 1997; 1/2:237–240.

Triedman JK. Arrhythmias in adults with congenital heart disease. *Heart* 2002;7:383–389.

Walsh EP. Arrhythmias in patients with congenital heart disease. *Card Electrophysiol Rev* 2002;6:422–430.

Weindling SN, Saul JP, Gamble WJ, et al. Duration of complete atrioventricular block after congenital heart surgery. *Am J Cardiol* 1998;82:525–527.

Wolfe RR, Driscoll DJ, Gersony WM, et al. Arrhythmias in patients with valvar aortic stenosis, valvar pulmonary stenosis, and ventricular septal defect. *Circulation* 1993;87:I89–I101.

Chapter 48

Cardiopulmonary Exercise Testing in Children With Congenital Heart Disease

James P. Loehr

Exercise is a common physiologic stress that places demands on multiple organ systems, including skeletal muscle, cardiac muscle, and the pulmonary and systemic circulations. The physiologic responses of the heart and the lungs to this stress are tightly coupled with the metabolic demands of exercising muscle.

The increased skeletal muscle contraction that occurs with exercise increases the demand for oxygen delivery and for the clearance of important by-products of metabolic work, including CO_2, lactate, and heat (Fig. 48-1). Several processes, including increased oxygen extraction from blood perfusing the active muscles, vasodilation of selected peripheral vascular beds, increased cardiac output, and increased pulmonary blood flow and ventilation, mediate this increased demand. The capacity of the body to deliver and utilize oxygen is determined empirically as *maximum oxygen consumption* (Vo_2max). As defined by the Fick principle, the relationship between oxygen consumption (Vo_2), cardiac output (CO), and the arteriovenous oxygen difference (AVo_2 difference) is

$$Vo_2 = CO \times (AVo_2 \text{ difference}).$$

By further describing cardiac output as the product of stroke volume (SV) and heart rate (HR), the relationship becomes

$$Vo_2 = HR \times SV \times (AVo_2 \text{ difference}).$$

Early in exercise, cardiac output is significantly augmented by an increase in stroke volume. Increased venous return and ventricular filling pressure may in part cause increased stroke volume as predicted by the Frank-Starling relationship. Later in exercise, increases in cardiac output are more closely related to increases in heart rate. The heart rate response to exercise is mediated by increased sympathetic tone and decreased parasympathetic (vagal) influence on the heart. Increased heart rate generally parallels increased oxygen uptake and workload and occurs primarily at the expense of diastolic time, which, in some disease states, can result in inadequate ventricular filling time at elevated heart rates. The AVo_2 difference, which normally results in about 23% extraction of oxygen at rest, may increase more than threefold at Vo_2max. Arterial oxygen levels remain essentially normal throughout exercise in individuals with normal cardiopulmonary function.

Mean arterial blood pressure is essentially the product of cardiac output and peripheral resistance. The increased cardiac output that occurs with exercise is associated with a marked decrease in peripheral vascular resistance, resulting in a progressive increase in systolic blood pressure and unchanged or mildly decreased diastolic blood pressure. The expected increase in systolic pressure is positively related to body size and age. Attenuated systolic blood pressure responses to exercise may reflect a limitation of cardiac output or an alteration of vascular resistance control.

The ventilatory response to exercise is tightly coupled with production of CO_2. Both tidal volume and respiratory rate increase during progressive exercise to keep pH and Pco_2 (partial pressure of CO_2) constant over a wide range of metabolic work rates. Acidosis occurs only during heavy exercise because of increased blood lactate concentrations. Dyspnea occurs during moderate exercise from the increased need for CO_2 release and the tight coupling of minute ventilation to CO_2 production. Further increases in CO_2 production with intense exercise result in

Figure 48-1

Exercise Tests

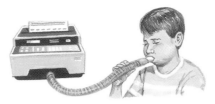

Heart rate
Blood pressure
ECG

A complete exercise evaluation includes, at a minimum, the measurement of heart rate, blood pressure, and evaluation of exercise ECG for pathologic changes or exercise-induced arrhythmias.

Spirometry pre- and postexercise, as well as respiratory gas exchange during exercise, is routinely measured in some laboratories.

Normal and abnormal responses to exercise

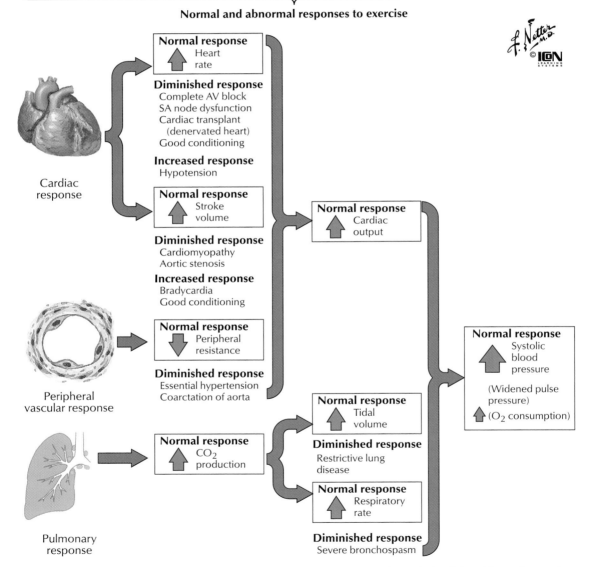

Cardiac response

Normal response
⬆ Heart rate

Diminished response
Complete AV block
SA node dysfunction
Cardiac transplant
(denervated heart)
Good conditioning

Increased response
Hypotension

Normal response
⬆ Stroke volume

Diminished response
Cardiomyopathy
Aortic stenosis

Increased response
Bradycardia
Good conditioning

Normal response
⬆ Cardiac output

Peripheral vascular response

Normal response
⬇ Peripheral resistance

Diminished response
Essential hypertension
Coarctation of aorta

Pulmonary response

Normal response
⬆ CO_2 production

Normal response
⬆ Tidal volume

Diminished response
Restrictive lung disease

Normal response
⬆ Respiratory rate

Diminished response
Severe bronchospasm

Normal response
⬆ Systolic blood pressure

(Widened pulse pressure)

⬆ (O_2 consumption)

The physiologic response to the increased metabolic demands of exercise is multifactorial. The ability of the cardiovascular system to respond to such demands may be diminished by congenital structural or electrical abnormalities, which diminish or restrict stress response.

a decline in serum sodium bicarbonate, a disproportionate increase in hydrogen ion levels, and consequent acidosis, resulting in a hyperventilatory response.

NORMAL RESPONSES OF CHILDREN TO EXERCISE

A complete exercise evaluation includes, at a minimum, the measurement of heart rate and blood pressure and the evaluation of the exercising ECG for pathologic changes and the presence or absence of exercise-induced arrhythmias. In children, the normal response to exercise is for the heart rate to increase to a maximum of 190 to 200 beats/min. Electrocardiographically, one should observe sinus tachycardia, with no evidence of atrioventricular block during exercise. The presence of atrial and/or ventricular ectopy, either of which can to be stimulated by exercise, is considered an abnormal response. ECG intervals follow characteristic changes; the PR interval generally shortens with exercise and the resultant tachycardia, and the QRS duration remains unchanged or shortens slightly. The normal response of the QT interval is to be unchanged or to shorten, but this shortening is often difficult to document because of the merging of the end of the T wave with the following P wave. The interpretation of the ST segment is sometimes difficult because of physiologic J point depression, but the normal slope of the ST segment at peak exercise is upward rather than flat or down.

The normal blood pressure response is dictated by the complex interaction of increased cardiac output, caused by increased heart rate and stroke volume, and vasodilation in the peripheral vascular bed. In normal exercise, systolic blood pressure increases progressively, to levels as high as 230 mm Hg, whereas diastolic pressure changes less dramatically. The anticipated increase in blood pressure is related to the body size and age of the individual. Pathologically high blood pressure responses can occur in individuals with resting hypertension and in individuals with either occult or poorly repaired aortic arch obstruction such as coarctation of the aorta. A diminished blood pressure response is generally attributed to an inadequate exercising cardiac output response, which may be secondary to a variety of factors, including an inadequate heart rate response or a limitation of stroke volume caused by obstructive lesions (such as valvular aortic stenosis) or by diminished contractility (in cardiomyopathic states). Individuals with decreased peripheral vascular resistance may also have a diminished blood pressure response to exercise in spite of adequate cardiac output.

Some pediatric exercise laboratories routinely measure respiratory gas exchange during exercise. The most useful measurement is that of Vo_2max, which is influenced by cardiac output, ventilatory capacity, and the degree of extraction of oxygen by exercising tissue. During incremental exercise, oxygen consumption and CO_2 production increase in parallel to workload; at higher rates of oxygen consumption, there is a disproportionate increase in CO_2 production, resulting in further stress on the respiratory system to compensate for this increase in CO_2. The point at which this phenomenon (disproportionately increased CO_2 production)occurs is called the ventilatory anaerobic threshold. In children in whom the ventilatory anaerobic threshold is reached earlier than anticipated, one should consider both congenital (or acquired) cardiac and pulmonary anomalies, as well as severe deconditioning. Individuals who are especially fit (well conditioned) typically reach their ventilatory threshold later than would be anticipated. An estimate of stroke volume may be derived by dividing oxygen consumption by the heart rate, referred to as the oxygen pulse (oxygen pulse = Vo_2/HR).

The oxygen pulse measurement is probably proportional to changes in stroke volume at low levels of exercise, but this measurement loses that proportionality at more rapid heart rates because of the contribution of increased oxygen extraction from the tissues to oxygen consumption. Nevertheless, lesions associated with poor ventricular function are associated with low maximum oxygen pulse.

Finally, the measurement of ventilation is of some use. Although the rate of change in ventilation is proportional to the change in CO_2 production, the slope of that increase is higher in patients with congestive heart failure. Spirometry performed pre- and postexercise can demonstrate the presence of exercise-induced bronchospasm, which can be relieved by use of an inhaled bronchodilator.

CHARACTERISTIC PATHOLOGIC EXERCISE RESPONSES IN PATIENTS WITH CONGENITAL STRUCTURAL HEART DISEASE

Coarctation of the Aorta

Characteristically, patients with poorly repaired coarctation of the aorta who are essentially asymptomatic have normal exercise capacity but their systolic blood pressure increases excessively with exercise. The increased blood pressure tends to occur at both submaximum and maximum effort. Even after successful repair, exertional hypertension may occur, especially in those who underwent surgery later in life. The potential etiologies of late hypertension include increased aortic stiffness, unusual arch gradients from differential growth of segments of the aortic arch, and, possibly, increased flow acceleration across the aortic valve from increased left ventricular mass.

Left Ventricular Outflow Tract Obstruction

In contrast to coarctation of the aorta, severe obstruction of left ventricular outflow (from either valvular aortic stenosis or subvalvular or supravalvular obstruction) is associated with an attenuated increase, or even a decrease, in blood pressure during exercise. Presyncope or syncope can occur when exertional cardiac output is unable to compensate for the normal peripheral vasodilatory response to activity. Pathologic ST-segment depression can occur during exertion from subendocardial ischemia related to the presence of ventricular hypertrophy, high diastolic ventricular pressures, and low cardiac output. Interestingly, in contrast to adults, ST-segment depression in children is frequently not associated with chest discomfort.

Pulmonary Stenosis

Pulmonary stenosis with an intact ventricular septum is a common anomaly that results in fixed right ventricular outflow tract obstruction, which may limit cardiac output. Exercise tolerance is essentially normal in individuals with mild pulmonary stenosis but may be impaired in those with more severe disease. The impairment resolves with relief of the obstruction in childhood.

Atrial Septal Defect

Individuals with an atrial septal defect who have undergone repair in childhood have normal or near-normal exercise tolerance. A decreased maximum heart rate has been reported, however. Exercise intolerance may be related to poor diastolic compliance of either ventricle. If there is both an unrepaired atrial defect and a significant degree of right ventricular dysfunction, oxygen saturation will occasionally fall during exercise.

Tetralogy of Fallot

A principal concern in the adolescent or the adult who has survived tetralogy of Fallot repair is the association of sudden cardiac death with a poor hemodynamic result and the presence of ventricular arrhythmias. Patients with surgically repaired tetralogy of Fallot routinely undergo exercise testing primarily to examine their cardiac rhythm during maximum activity. The finding of exertional ventricular arrhythmias frequently leads to further evaluation and surgical or medical intervention.

Individuals who have undergone only palliation of tetralogy of Fallot with a systemic-to-pulmonary artery shunt have markedly reduced Vo_2max and an increased ventilatory response to exercise. If complete surgical repair is performed in childhood, however, and the patient has regular physical activity, the resulting exercise capacity is frequently in the normal range. The mean heart rate and oxygen consumption in this group of patients, however, is mildly decreased compared with normal controls.

Transposition of the Great Arteries

In individuals who have undergone the atrial repair of transposition of the great arteries (the Mustard or Senning procedure), the right ventricle functions as the systemic ventricular chamber. Because of this, these individuals are subject to frequent atrial arrhythmias and sinus node dysfunction. Although early in life most report that they are asymptomatic, decreased work performance and Vo_2max are found on formal testing. This finding is generally associated with a decreased maximum heart rate but is likely also due to poor right ventricular stroke volume augmentation with activity.

Physiology of Single-Ventricle Malformation

The heterogeneous group of individuals with single-ventricle malformation usually undergoes the Fontan procedure as palliation. Before the Fontan procedure is performed in this heterogeneous group of patients, exercise capacity is markedly reduced, associated with an increased ventilatory response to exercise and decreased systemic oxygen levels that are presumably the result of decreased pulmonary blood flow and increased intracardiac right-to-left shunting. Performance of the Fontan procedure results in improvement in these parameters, but the exercise capacity of the patient after the Fontan procedure remains decreased. Formal measurements of cardiac output support the inference that the decreased capacity results from a diminished heart rate response and a decreased stroke volume response to exercise.

Cardiac Rhythm Disturbances

Premature ventricular contractions are a frequent finding in normal children. The normal response is for exercise to suppress this arrhythmia, although it may only be suppressed at very elevated heart rates. Conversely, the induction of couplets or ventricular tachycardia with exercise is abnormal and warrants further investigation. Premature atrial contractions are common and usually benign in childhood. Unlike ventricular ectopy, the persistence of premature atrial beats with exercise is not considered to be ominous. Patients with congenital complete atrioventricular block have diminished resting and exertional heart rates and may demonstrate ventricular arrhythmias with exercise.

Patients with Wolff-Parkinson-White syndrome may demonstrate supraventricular tachycardia with exercise. Disappearance of the delta wave may result from exertional sinus tachycardia, suggesting a long refractory period for the accessory connection. Disappearance of the delta wave may be a helpful finding, but it cannot be used as the sole criterion for determining management.

FUTURE DIRECTIONS

Exercise testing provides a unique estimate of the functional capacity of the heart and the response of the heart to important physiologic stress. Although the most common use of exercise testing is in the evaluation of patients for possible coronary artery disease, exercise testing is being used increasingly in the assessment of overall cardiopulmonary function in a variety of disease states. Increasingly, patients facing heart or lung transplantation, patients facing partial lung resection, and patients with a limitation of maximum cardiac output from congenital heart disease are being subjected to exercise testing as part of the overall evaluation. Future investigations of the exercise responses of individuals with inborn errors of metabolism will likely add insight into the physiology of human exercise.

REFERENCES

Braden DS, Carroll JF. Normative cardiovascular responses to exercise in children. *Pediatr Cardiol* 1999;20:4–10.

Driscoll DH, Durongpisitkul K. Exercise testing after the Fontan operation. *Pediatr Cardiol* 1999;20:57–59.

Paul MH, Wessel HU. Exercise studies in patients with transposition of the great arteries after atrial repair operations (mustard/Senning): A review. *Pediatr Cardiol* 1999;20:49–55.

Rowland TW, ed. *Pediatric Cardiology Exercise Testing.* Champaign, IL: Human Kinetics; 1993.

Ruttenberg HD. Pre- and postoperative exercise testing of the child with coarctation of the aorta. *Pediatr Cardiol* 1999;20:33–37.

Steinberger J, Moller JH. Exercise testing in children with pulmonary valvar stenosis. *Pediatr Cardiol* 1999;20:27–31.

Wasserman K, Hansen JE, Sue DY, Whipp BJ, Casaburi R. *Principles of Exercise Testing and Interpretation.* 2nd ed. Philadelphia: Lea and Febiger; 1994.

Wessel HU, Paul MH. Exercise studies in tetralogy of Fallot: A review. *Pediatr Cardiol* 1999;20:39–47.

Chapter 49

Kawasaki Disease

Blair V. Robinson

Kawasaki disease is a multisystem vasculitis, first recognized in 1961 and subsequently described in 1967 by Dr. Tomisaku Kawasaki. Kawasaki disease was initially thought to be a benign, self-limited febrile illness; the association of disease with the development of coronary aneurysms and subsequent mortality did not become evident until the 1970s. Since then, Kawasaki disease has been recognized in all populations and is now reported to be the most common acquired heart disease in U.S. children, replacing rheumatic heart disease.

The incidence of Kawasaki disease varies among ethnic groups. It is highest in children of Asian ancestry (90 per 100,000 in Japan) and lower in Europeans (3 per 100,000 in Britain). The U.S. incidence is 9 to 20 per 100,000. Kawasaki disease usually occurs in children 1 to 2 years of age, with 80% of cases diagnosed in children younger than 4 years of age. However, the diagnosis has been made in children of all ages. Males are more commonly affected than females (ratio 1.5:1).

ETIOLOGY AND PATHOGENESIS

The etiology of Kawasaki disease is unknown. A genetic predisposition to the disease is suggested by the higher incidence in children of Asian ancestry and in siblings. The occurrence of the disease in siblings also suggests exposure to a common causative agent. Various bacteria, viruses, heavy metals, and detergents have come under suspicion as etiologic agents. Recently, a superantigen (toxin)-mediated hypothesis has been proposed. However, large multicenter studies have failed to conclusively identify any single etiologic agent or group.

Kawasaki disease is a nonspecific vasculitis that affects small and medium-sized arteries throughout the body. Its most serious consequences evolve in phases within the coronary arteries (Fig. 49-1).

The **acute febrile phase** of Kawasaki disease lasts 0 to 10 days. Inflammation in the coronary artery walls consisting mostly of polymorphonuclear cells may occur. An increased ratio of T4 (helper) to T8 (suppressor) cells has been found in vessel walls during the acute phase. Pancardi-

tis may also develop during the acute phase. However, the mortality rate during this phase is low, and death is usually the result of myocardial dysfunction or arrhythmias.

The **subacute phase** lasts 10 to 40 days. An accumulation of cytokines, B cells, and T cells in the vessel walls may cause fragmentation of the internal elastic lamina of the coronary arteries and, subsequently, the formation of an aneurysm. Thrombocytosis occurs simultaneously and predisposes patients to acute coronary thrombosis, the leading cause of mortality during this phase of the illness.

The **convalescent phase** (beyond 40 days) consists of healing and fibrosis of the coronary aneurysms formed during the subacute phase. A stenosis may occur at such sites, with resulting ischemia, infarction, and death. Of all deaths, 70% occur in infants younger than 1 year of age, and almost all deaths occur during the convalescent stage of the illness.

The risk factors for the development of coronary artery disease include fever lasting more than 14 days, recurrence of fever or rash, treatment with intravenous immunoglobulin (IVIG) less than 10 days into the acute illness, male gender, and age younger than 1 year.

CLINICAL PRESENTATION

Fever is the cardinal presenting sign and persists for more than 7 days in more than 95% of patients. It responds only temporarily to antipyretic therapy and may last up to 2 weeks in patients who are not treated with IVIG. In 90% of patients, a polymorphous rash develops, predominantly over the trunk (Fig. 49-2). This

Figure 49-1   **Pathogenesis and Clinical Course of Kawasaki Disease**

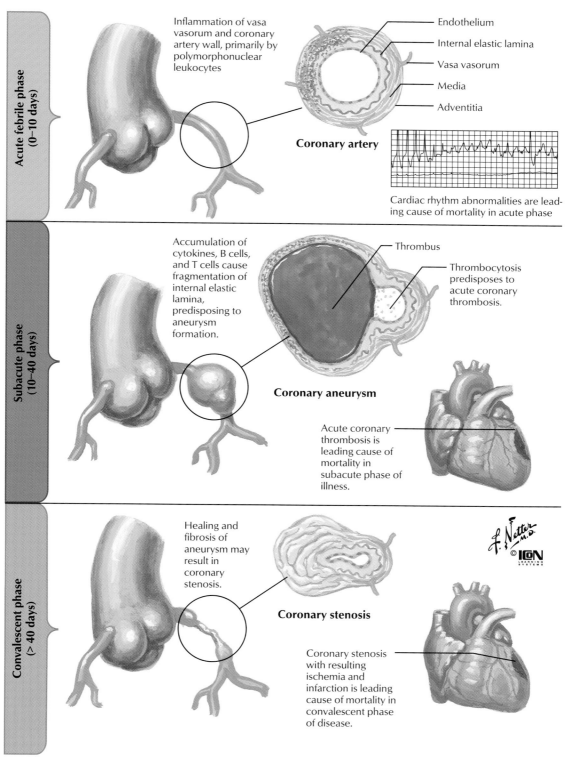

Acute febrile phase (0–10 days)

Inflammation of vasa vasorum and coronary artery wall, primarily by polymorphonuclear leukocytes

Endothelium

Internal elastic lamina

Vasa vasorum

Media

Adventitia

Coronary artery

Cardiac rhythm abnormalities are leading cause of mortality in acute phase

Subacute phase (10–40 days)

Accumulation of cytokines, B cells, and T cells cause fragmentation of internal elastic lamina, predisposing to aneurysm formation.

Thrombus

Thrombocytosis predisposes to acute coronary thrombosis.

Coronary aneurysm

Acute coronary thrombosis is leading cause of mortality in subacute phase of illness.

Convalescent phase (> 40 days)

Healing and fibrosis of aneurysm may result in coronary stenosis.

Coronary stenosis

Coronary stenosis with resulting ischemia and infarction is leading cause of mortality in convalescent phase of disease.

Figure 49-2

Clinical Features of Kawasaki Disease

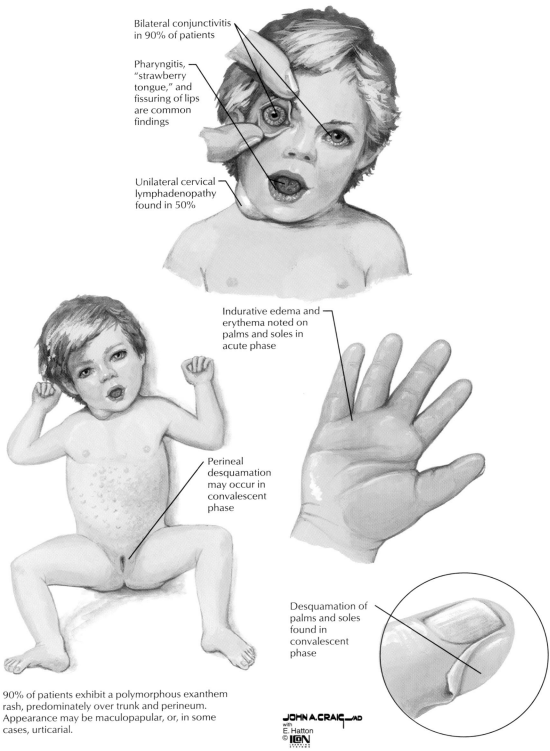

Bilateral conjunctivitis in 90% of patients

Pharyngitis, "strawberry tongue," and fissuring of lips are common findings

Unilateral cervical lymphadenopathy found in 50%

Indurative edema and erythema noted on palms and soles in acute phase

Perineal desquamation may occur in convalescent phase

Desquamation of palms and soles found in convalescent phase

90% of patients exhibit a polymorphous exanthem rash, predominately over trunk and perineum. Appearance may be maculopapular, or, in some cases, urticarial.

JOHN A.CRAIG—MD
with
E. Hatton
© ICON

rash may be a diffuse maculopapular rash, or it may be a more urticarial rash. Rarely, perineal desquamation is seen in the subacute phase. Mucosal changes, erythema, and fissuring of the lips occur in 90% of patients. Pharyngitis and prominent papillae ("strawberry tongue") are also typical signs. Within the first week of the illness, bilateral conjunctivitis, consisting of a discrete vascular injection with absence of corneal clouding or purulent exudates, develops in 90% of patients. The bilateral conjunctivitis persists for 1 to 2 weeks. Anterior uveitis is a common finding on slit-lamp examination. Indurative edema and erythema of the hands and feet occur in 75 to 90% of patients. Desquamation of the fingertips and/or the palms and the soles may occur 2 to 3 weeks after the acute illness. Cervical lymphadenopathy, the least consistent finding, occurs in approximately 50% of patients. It is usually unilateral, and the diameter of the nodes may exceed 15 mm.

Although the diagnosis of Kawasaki disease generally requires fever plus four of the multiple findings described under Differential Diagnosis, some patients with Kawasaki disease may have an atypical presentation that does not fulfill the diagnostic criteria. These patients are usually younger than 1 year or older than 8 years, and their condition is commonly misdiagnosed.

Additional clinical findings include gastrointestinal signs, such as emesis, diarrhea, and jaundice (40%); arthralgias (30%); aseptic meningitis (25%); and pancarditis with myocardial dysfunction, pericardial effusion, and valvar insufficiency (50%). Common laboratory findings include leukocytosis; thrombocytosis (platelet count >450,000 in 50% of patients); elevated acute-phase reactants (ESR, C-reactive protein, immunoglobulin E, α-2-globulin); elevated transaminases; sterile pyuria; and proteinuria.

DIFFERENTIAL DIAGNOSIS AND DIAGNOSTIC APPROACH

Because the etiology of the disease is unknown, "Kawasaki disease" remains a clinical diagnosis. Classically, the diagnosis of Kawasaki disease requires 5 days of fever and four of the following: rash, oral mucosal changes, conjunctivitis, extremity changes, and cervical lymphadenopathy (Table 49-1). Laboratory findings

Table 49-1
Diagnostic Findings of Kawasaki Disease

Fever persisting for more than 5 days *plus four of the following*:
- Bilateral, nonexudative conjunctivitis
- Polymorphous exanthem
- Peripheral extremity changes: indurative edema, erythema of palms and soles
- Oropharyngeal changes: erythema or fissuring of lips, strawberry tongue
- Nonpurulent cervical lymphadenopathy

such as elevated white blood cell counts, ESR, and platelet counts are supportive of the diagnosis of Kawasaki disease but are not pathognomonic. The characteristic pathologic findings in the coronary arteries are not visible during the acute febrile illness and therefore are not useful in differentiating Kawasaki disease from other illnesses with similar clinical presentations.

Because ongoing inflammation is a significant risk factor for the development of coronary artery aneurysms, early diagnosis and treatment are imperative. However, differentiating Kawasaki disease from other illnesses with similar clinical features can be difficult.

The differential diagnosis includes measles, scarlet fever, toxic shock syndrome, staphylococcal scalded skin syndrome, drug hypersensitivity reactions, Rocky Mountain spotted fever, and juvenile rheumatoid arthritis. Distinguishing measles from Kawasaki disease may be difficult, but important differences are typically found. Both illnesses may present with a polymorphous rash and swelling of the hands and feet. However, in measles, conjunctivitis is exudative and oral lesions (Koplik's spots) are diagnostic. In Kawasaki disease, the conjunctivitis is nonexudative and there are no discrete oral lesions. The exanthem of measles typically begins on the face, whereas the rash of Kawasaki disease is found predominantly on the trunk and the extremities. Unlike in Kawasaki disease, the ESR and the white blood cell count are typically low in measles. Furthermore, the immunoglobulin M antimeasles titer can be used to differentiate these clinically similar entities.

Because of the presentation of fever, strawberry tongue, cervical lymphadenopathy, and rash, Kawasaki disease has commonly been misdiagnosed as scarlet fever. However, in scarlet fever, conjunctivitis is absent, desquamation is not limited to the extremities, and these findings all typically resolve with antibiotic therapy. Patients with scarlet fever are typically older than 3 years at presentation.

Young patients (<1 year) with Kawasaki disease may have an atypical presentation that does not fulfill the diagnostic criteria, and therefore the diagnosis of Kawasaki may not be considered. Fever may be the only initial presenting sign, and other clinical signs may be delayed or may not appear at all. After initial treatment with antibiotics, the rash and the conjunctivitis may appear, leading to the incorrect conclusion of a drug hypersensitivity reaction. In the patient with fever of unknown origin who develops desquamation of the fingers and toes 2 to 3 weeks into the illness, it is important to consider the possibility of Kawasaki disease and to evaluate the coronary arteries accordingly.

MANAGEMENT AND THERAPY

Before the use of IVIG, there was a 25% incidence of coronary aneurysm development in patients with Kawasaki disease. Early diagnosis and treatment with IVIG has reduced the incidence of aneurysm formation to less than 2% in those treated.

When the patient initially presents with symptoms, echocardiography is performed to evaluate myocardial function and provide a baseline study of the coronary arteries. ECG is performed in the acute phase to detect conduction abnormalities. Patients are treated with anti-inflammatory doses of aspirin (80–100 mg/kg/day) and given a single dose of IVIG (2 g/kg). If a patient is afebrile 48 to 72 hours after IVIG treatment, the aspirin dose is decreased to antithrombotic levels of 3 to 5 mg/kg/day and this dose is continued throughout the convalescent phase or until the platelet count returns to normal. After the single dose of IVIG, approximately 10% of patients remain febrile beyond 48 hours and repeat dosing of IVIG may be necessary. The use of steroids in "IVIG-resistant" patients is under investigation. Although there does not appear to be an

increase in coronary aneurysms, the efficacy of this approach remains to be proven.

Echocardiography is usually performed again 2 weeks and 6 to 8 weeks after the initial presentation. There is increasing evidence that if coronary aneurysms have not developed within the first 8 weeks of the illness, subsequent aneurysm formation is unlikely. The current American Heart Association guidelines recommend that patients undergo echocardiographic follow-up 6 to 12 months after initial presentation. Patients without aneurysms at this time require no further follow-up.

The development of coronary aneurysms requires close follow-up and long-term anticoagulation therapy. Risk stratification may be based on the size of the aneurysms. Small solitary aneurysms resolve without intervention in more than 50% of patients, and aspirin therapy is generally all that is warranted. However, giant aneurysms (>8 mm in diameter) are associated with a much greater risk of thrombosis. Japanese data show that approximately 50% of deaths occur in patients with giant coronary aneurysms. Therefore, these patients are usually maintained on aspirin and coumadin.

Echocardiography is an excellent screening tool for detecting proximal aneurysms, but distal aneurysms are more difficult to visualize. Coronary angiography (Fig. 49-3) helps delineate more distal aneurysms and the presence of coronary stenoses and should be performed in patients with evidence of ischemia or extensive coronary involvement on echocardiography. Patients developing a coronary stenosis and ischemia may require surgical revascularization or, rarely, heart transplantation. Exercise restrictions are placed on individuals with significant coronary disease.

FUTURE DIRECTIONS

The incidence of Kawasaki disease appears to be increasing; however, the etiology of the disease remains unknown. Despite the unclear mechanism of action of IVIG, the introduction of IVIG therapy has dramatically altered natural history of the disease. Kawasaki disease is self-limited in most cases, and many coronary aneurysms resolve without intervention. However, there may be significant endothelial dysfunction in vessels with previous aneurysms, which raises

Figure 49-3

Cardiac Evaluation in Kawasaki Disease

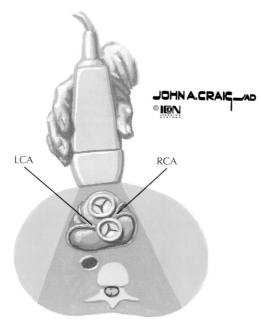

LCA

RCA

JOHN A. CRAIG—AD
©ICN

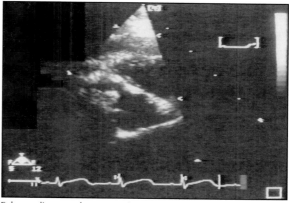

Echocardiogram demonstrating coronary artery aneurysm

Echocardiography is performed at initial presentation to evaluate myocardial function and to provide baseline study of coronary arteries. Repeat studies performed at 2 weeks, 6–8 weeks, and 6–12 months after initial presentation.

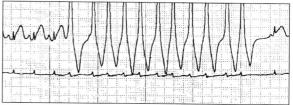

Electrocardiogram performed in acute phase to detect cardiac rhythm disturbances

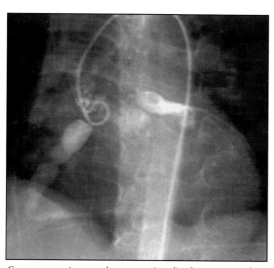

Coronary angiogram demonstrating distal aneurysm of coronary artery

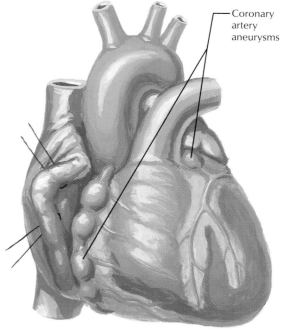

Coronary artery aneurysms

Coronary angiography is useful in detecting distal aneurysms of coronary arteries not easily detected by echocardiography.

the question of whether the children who have had aneurysms may be at increased risk for coronary disease as adults. Future research will be directed at determining etiology, the mechanism of the therapeutic effect of IVIG, other therapies, and long-term patient outcomes.

REFERENCES

Dajani AS, Taubert KA, Takahashi M, et al. Guidelines for long-term management of patients with Kawasaki disease. Report from the Committee on Rheumatic Fever, Endocarditis, and Kawasaki Disease, Council on Cardiovascular Disease in the Young, American Heart Association. *Circulation* 1994;89:916–922.

Kato H, Sugimura T, Akagi T, et al. Heart and vascular disease in the young: Long-term consequences of Kawasaki disease; a 10 to 21 year follow-up study of 594 patients. *Circulation* 1996;94:1379–1385.

Kawasaki T, Kosaki F, Okawa S, Shigematsu I, Yanagawa HJ. A new infantile acute febrile mucocutaneous lymph node syndrome (MLNS) prevailing in Japan. *Pediatrics* 1974;54:271–276.

Leung D, Meissner C, Shulman S, et al. Prevalence of superantigen-secreting bacteria in patients with Kawasaki disease. *J Pediatr* 2002;140:742–746.

Newburger JW, Takahashi M, Burns JC, et al. The treatment of Kawasaki syndrome with intravenous gammaglobulin. *N Engl J Med* 1986;315:341–347.

Chapter 50

Congenital Coronary Anomalies

S. Adil Husain, Brett C. Sheridan, and Michael R. Mill

Congenital coronary anomalies may have a significant impact on myocardial perfusion and secondary ischemia, inducing left ventricular (LV) dysfunction and sudden cardiac death. This clinical relevance underlies the necessity of an understanding of the anatomy and presentation of congenital coronary anomalies and the treatment options for these anomalies. The two primary congenital coronary anomalies, anomalous origin of the left coronary artery from the pulmonary artery (ALCAPA) and anomalous course of a coronary artery between the pulmonary artery and the aorta (ACCBPAA), are reviewed here. Two other entities associated with coronary artery anomalies—coronary artery fistulas and anomalous coronary circulation—are also reviewed in this chapter.

Normally, the two main coronary arteries arise from separate ostia within the sinuses of Valsalva. The left coronary artery (LCA) then divides into the left anterior descending artery, which traverses the anterior interventricular groove, and the left circumflex coronary artery, which courses in the left atrioventricular groove. The right coronary artery (RCA) originates anteriorly from the right aortic sinus and courses along the right atrioventricular groove, commonly giving rise to the posterior descending artery.

ANOMALOUS ORIGIN OF THE LEFT CORONARY ARTERY FROM THE PULMONARY ARTERY

Anomalous origin of the LCA from the pulmonary artery is a rare congenital anomaly, usually an isolated lesion, occurring in 1 in 300,000 live births (Fig. 50-1). The clinical spectrum of ALCAPA is also known as the Bland-White-Garland syndrome. Infants with myocardial ischemia typically present with failure to thrive, profuse sweating, dyspnea, pallor, and atypical chest pain upon eating or crying. Malignant arrhythmias leading to sudden cardiac death are the most extreme presentation of myocardial ischemia in ALCAPA. During the neonatal period, high pulmonary vascular resistance ensures antegrade flow from the pulmonary artery through the LCA. However, as this resistance diminishes, there is eventual reversal of flow, with left-to-right shunting through the pulmonary artery. The result is the phenomenon of "coronary steal," with LV perfu-sion becoming dependent on collateral circulation from the RCA.

Because infantile circulation has little or no coronary collateral development, ALCAPA leads to severe myocardial ischemia, with resultant LV dysfunction and dilation. Because of papillary muscle ischemia, and as the left ventricle dilates, mitral valve regurgitation occurs. Without surgical intervention and correction of the anomaly, patients die within weeks to months after birth. Patients who survive to adulthood, secondary to the presence and formation of collateral circulation, may remain asymptomatic despite subclinical ongoing ischemia. Arrhythmic sudden death purportedly occurs in 80 to 90% of patients by 35 years of age.

Although ALCAPA is rare, a high index of suspicion should be present for infants presenting with signs of myocardial ischemia or dysfunction. The most frequent confounding diagnosis is dilated cardiomyopathy. Both conditions may present with cardiomegaly, a murmur of mitral insufficiency, and ischemic signs on ECG. Two-dimensional echocardiography and coronary angiography typically clarify the diagnosis. Echocardiographic examination alone may be sufficient to achieve diagnosis, if this examination reveals an enlarged RCA with global hypokinesis and dilation of the left ventricle. Pulsed and color flow Doppler examination may delineate a left-to-right shunt. Two-dimensional echocardiographic evaluation may permit the visualization of the anatomic origin of the ALCAPA and the assessment of the degree of mitral insufficiency. Although not

Figure 50-1 ## Congenital Coronary Artery Anomalies

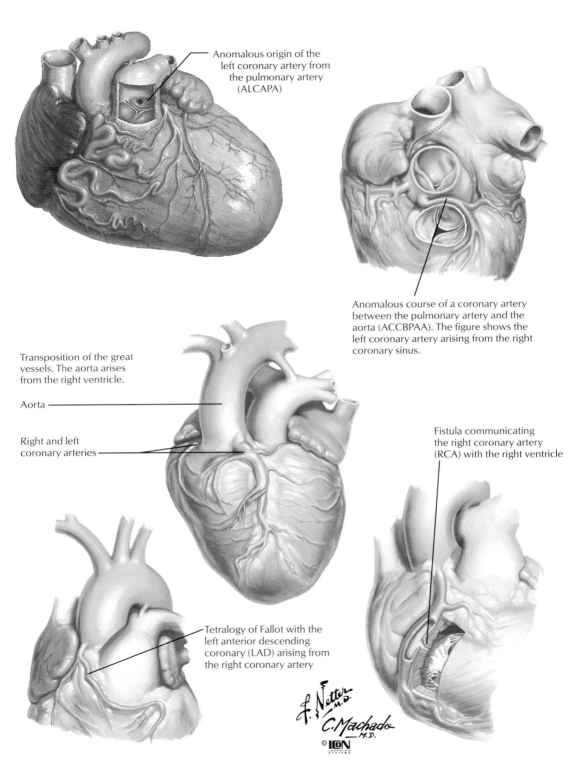

Anomalous origin of the left coronary artery from the pulmonary artery (ALCAPA)

Anomalous course of a coronary artery between the pulmonary artery and the aorta (ACCBPAA). The figure shows the left coronary artery arising from the right coronary sinus.

Transposition of the great vessels. The aorta arises from the right ventricle.

Aorta

Right and left coronary arteries

Fistula communicating the right coronary artery (RCA) with the right ventricle

Tetralogy of Fallot with the left anterior descending coronary (LAD) arising from the right coronary artery

essential, coronary angiography or ventriculography, may be performed if ALCAPA is suspected but not visualized on echocardiography. Coronary angiography also assists in excluding other anatomic etiologies for ischemia and ventricular dysfunction.

Surgical correction remains the gold standard of therapy, but important changes in surgical technique have resulted in improved outcomes. Surgical repair involves direct reimplantation of the anomalous LCA into the aorta by transferring it with a button of pulmonary artery (Fig. 50-2). Variations of this technique are used when it is necessary to overcome anatomic challenges of the length and the course of the LCA for reimplantation. In adults, in whom reimplantation is more technically challenging, bypass grafting with the left internal thoracic artery is an equally effective approach.

After reestablishment of a two-coronary system, the previously dilated RCA returns to normal size, with regression of the intercoronary collateral network. Operative mortality for all surgical techniques has improved dramatically; mortality rates ranging from 75 to 80% in the early 1980s have decreased to 5 to 25%. No differences in LV function or in the late mortality rate have been demonstrated with various reimplantation or revascularization techniques, with one exception: direct ligation of the anomalous coronary was abandoned because of poor outcomes.

ANOMALOUS COURSE OF A CORONARY ARTERY BETWEEN THE PULMONARY ARTERY AND THE AORTA

Anomalous course of a coronary artery between the pulmonary artery and the aorta may result in myocardial ischemia and sudden death (Fig. 50-1). This anomaly presents with two anatomically and therapeutically distinct variations. If the RCA arises from the left aortic sinus and is nondominant, such an entity may be benign. Surgical intervention is undertaken in patients with this form of the anomaly if they have demonstrable ischemia. If the LCA arises from the right coronary sinus and courses between the aorta and the pulmonary artery, however, surgical intervention is indicated because the risk of sudden cardiac death is high in this group.

The incidence and natural history of ACCBPAA are unknown. The most significant review of this abnormality, with 242 patients, described sudden death in 59% of patients. There are no pathognomonic clinical features consistent with ACCBPAA. The diagnosis should be considered in patients with exercise-induced myocardial ischemia or sudden death. Although echocardiographic evaluation may provide valuable information, coronary angiography is essential to accurately delineate the anatomy and exclude other associated coronary disease.

Surgical options to manage this anatomic abnormality include revascularization with an internal mammary artery or a saphenous vein bypass graft or reimplantation alone. With reimplantation, a transverse aortotomy may become essential to assess the coronary ostia. When the anomalous coronary artery arises from the opposite sinus, it is necessary to detach the aortic valve commissure. The slit-like ostium, which is characteristic of ACCBPAA and partially responsible for ischemic symptoms, is opened along its longitudinal axis, and a portion of the common wall between the aorta and the coronary artery is excised, with reapproximation of the intimal surfaces. The valve commissure is subsequently resuspended with a pledgeted suture.

CORONARY ARTERY FISTULAS

Coronary artery fistulas are defined as communications with right-sided (arteriovenous fistula) or left-sided (arterio-arterial fistula) cardiac structures. The most common fistula is the RCA communicating with the right ventricle. Patients rarely present with symptoms during infancy and are frequently diagnosed in early adulthood. Often asymptomatic, a fistula is most commonly discovered during evaluation for a murmur. Echocardiographic examination may reveal evidence of a dilated or enlarged coronary artery, with color flow Doppler demonstrating the fistula. Preoperative coronary angiography ensures accurate anatomic definition for surgical planning.

Intervention prevents ventricular volume overload and resulting congestive heart failure. Although observation and transcatheter coil embolization have been described, these management options are limited to highly selected patients, because surgical treatment of coronary artery fistulas is efficacious, reliable, and durable. If the fistula arises from the distal end of the coronary artery, ligation may be employed without cardiopulmonary bypass. Before permanent ligation, a trial occlusion of the affected coronary artery at the distal site should be performed to observe for signs of ischemia. If signs of myocardial ischemia are absent, ligation may then be performed. If the fistula arises from the midportion of a coronary artery, cardiopulmonary bypass with cardioplegic arrest allows opening of the abnormal coronary artery, where the fistula is oversewn. If coronary artery luminal compromise occurs, bypass grafting may be warranted. In other instances, the fistulous tract may be closed internally via access through the involved cardiac chamber (Fig. 50-2).

CORONARY ARTERY ANOMALIES ASSOCIATED WITH CONGENITAL HEART DISEASE

Several important forms of congenital heart disease are associated with coronary artery anomalies, which can have major implications for surgical repair. Coronary artery anomalies are particularly important in patients with tetralogy of Fallot, transposition of the great arteries, and pulmonary atresia with an intact ventricular septum (Fig. 50-1).

Coronary artery anomalies are reported in 18 to 31% of patients with tetralogy of Fallot and involve the presence of a large coronary artery crossing the right ventricular (RV) outflow tract just below the pulmonary valve. These anomalies include the origin of the left anterior descending artery from the RCA, a large conus branch across the RV outflow tract, a paired anterior descending coronary artery off the RCA, and an origin of both coronary arteries from a single left ostium. In each situation, the potential exists for damage to or severing of the coronary artery during a right ventriculotomy to correct RV outflow tract obstruction.

In pulmonary artery atresia with an intact ventricular septum, embryonic sinusoids within the right ventricle may persist and communicate with the epicardial coronary arteries in several ways. Usually this occurs in patients with diminutive RV chambers and severe RV hypertrophy. The communications may feed one or both coronary arteries and may be associated with proximal or distal coronary stenosis, or both, at the insertion site of the fistulous communications. In some patients with coronary stenosis, the coronary fistulous connections are sufficiently developed to produce an RV-dependent coronary circulation. Angiography of the RV cavity is required to demonstrate retrograde filling of one or more coronary arteries via the fistulous connection. Coronary angiography can determine whether the LV myocardium is normally perfused or whether significant segments are perfused from the right ventricle through myocardial sinusoids. In this circumstance, perfusion of parts of the left ventricle from the right ventricle must be identified before surgical repair. Decompression of the right ventricle to relieve RV outflow tract obstruction reduces RV pressure and therefore coronary artery perfusion, which can result in coronary artery ischemia and infarction during surgery.

Patients who have pulmonary artery atresia with an intact ventricular septum usually require an early systemic-to-pulmonary shunt and, if the tricuspid valve and the RV chamber have growth potential, surgical relief of the pulmonary atresia. If the right ventricle is miniscule, a Fontan procedure is the definitive treatment. However, if the myocardium is perfused via the right ventricle through sinusoids because of stenotic coronary arteries, then a systemic right ventricle must be preserved as part of the Fontan operation. Cardiac transplantation may be the only option for those patients with pulmonary artery atresia with an intact ventricular septum.

The treatment for patients with a simple dextraposed-transposition (D-transposition) of the great arteries or a D-transposition of the great arteries with a ventricular septal defect is an arterial switch operation during the neonatal period (Fig. 50-2). In D-transposition of the great arteries, both in its simple form and with a ventricular septal defect, the aorta arises from the right ventricle and the pulmonary artery rises from the left ventricle. During the arterial switch procedure, the coronary arteries are transferred from the anterior semilunar valve to the posterior valve along with reversing the location of the great vessels to the appropriate ventricles. The success of the operation depends on the transfer of the coronary arteries without compromising

Figure 50-2

Surgical Procedures for Correction of Congenital Coronary Artery Anomalies

Surgical correction of ALCAPA

LCA with button from the pulmonary artery anastomosed to the aorta

Sectioned pulmonary artery showing the site from where the button of the pulmonary artery and the coronary artery were taken

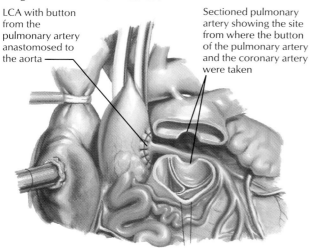

The technique involves direct reimplantation of the anomalous LCA into the aorta by transferring it with a button of pulmonary artery. Seen here: Variation with transection of the pulmonary artery.

Arterial repair of transposition of great the arteries—First steps

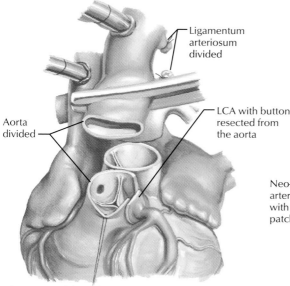

Ligamentum arteriosum divided

Aorta divided

LCA with button resected from the aorta

The aorta and the pulmonary artery are transected. The cut of the aorta is slanted and above the Valsalva's sinuses. The pulmonary artery is divided above its valve at the same level of the transection of the aorta. Sinuses of the aorta and pulmonary artery are excised to translocate the coronary ostia from the pulmonary artery to the neo-aorta. Pericardium is utilized to reconstruct the neo-pulmonary artery sinuses.

Technique to close fistula from RCA to RV and plication of coronary aneurysm

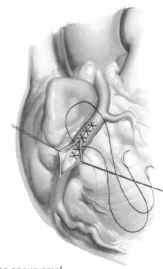

The aneurysmal coronary artery is opened and the fistula is sutured. The coronary artery is closed and the aneurysm is repaired by plication.

Arterial repair of transposition of great the arteries—Last steps

Coronary arteries anastomosed to neo-aorta

Distal pulmonary artery

Neo-pulmonary artery repaired with pericardial patches

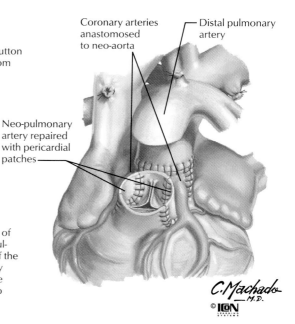

C. Machado
—M.D.
©ICON

the blood supply of the coronary circulation. Seven different coronary artery patterns are recognized in patients with a D-transposition of the great arteries, but normal anatomy is usually present. Although certain unusual coronary artery patterns were previously associated with an increased mortality rate, the specific coronary artery anatomy has become less important as surgical experience with this operation has improved technical approaches and overall outcomes. The presence of an intramural coronary artery, a segment of coronary artery that courses within the wall of the aorta without a separate layer of adventitial tissue between the coronary artery and the aorta, remains a difficult challenge. Although follow-up angiography after the arterial switch operation shows varying coronary artery abnormalities in approximately 10% of patients, most patients are asymptomatic.

FUTURE DIRECTIONS

Several issues of anomalous coronary arteries remain to be explored, including but not limited to the choice of the best noninvasive diagnostic imaging technique, the further pathophysiologic characterization of myocardial perfusion in patients with anomalous coronary arteries, and the definition of the indications for percutaneous intervention in adults who have symptomatic coronary disease in anomalous coronary vessels.

The tools for noninvasive imaging of anomalous coronary arteries include 16-slice multidetector spiral CT and free-breathing, three-dimensional coronary magnetic resonance angiography. Spiral CT, a noninvasive imaging modality, has comparable resolution to magnetic resonance angiography and is faster and less costly. Free-breathing, three-dimensional coronary magnetic resonance angiography is limited by availability, time, cost, and patient comfort. Magnetic resonance angiography studies are challenging to perform because of the enclosed space in which patients must be placed and the length of time to complete an evaluation. Ultimately, the method best suited for defining anomalous coronary vessels will depend on the degree of resolution offered by the technique and other considerations including cost and availability. As imaging techniques improve, noninvasive imaging for anomalous coronary arteries will likely become the standard of care. Rapid advances in imaging technologies have occurred in the last decade and promise to further improve imaging of anomalous coronary circulation in the future.

Further investigation is warranted into regional myocardial flow reserve in survivors of ALCAPA and its underlying pathology (i.e., endocardial and subendocardial fibrosis, damage to the papillary muscles, patchy myocardial necrosis, dilation of the ventricle, mitral incompetence, LCA hypoplasia of the media, distal stenosis and hypoplasia of the RCA). The physiologic issues need further definition in relation to myocardial perfusion after treatment in long-term survivors of this often lethal condition.

Anomalous coronary arteries have a reported frequency of approximately 0.64% in nonselected patients undergoing coronary angiography; it can therefore be predicted that adults who have anomalous coronary arteries will present with symptomatic coronary artery disease in these vessels later in life. Because this anatomy may offer unique challenges for interventional cardiologists, specific indications for percutaneous intervention remain to be defined in this area of improving interventional technology.

REFERENCES

Arciniegas E, Farooki ZQ, Hakimi M, Green EW. Management of anomalous left coronary artery from the pulmonary artery. *Circulation* 1980;62:180–189.

Dodge-Khamati A, Mavroudis C, Backer C. Anomalous origin of the left coronary artery from the pulmonary artery: Collective review of surgical therapy. *Ann Thorac Surg* 2002;74:946–955.

Gaynor JW. Coronary anomalies in children. In: Kaiser LR, Kron IL, Spray TL, eds. *Mastery of Cardiothoracic Surgery*. Philadelphia: Lippincott-Raven; 1998.

Gersony WM and Rosenbaum MS. Congenital anomalies of the coronary circulation. In: Gersony WM, Rosenbaum MS, eds. *Congenital Heart Disease in the Adult*. New York: McGraw-Hill; 2002.

Huddleston CB, Balzer DT, Mendeloff EN. Repair of anomalous left main coronary artery arising from the pulmonary artery in infants: Long-term impact on the mitral valve. *Ann Thorac Surg* 2001;71:1985–1989.

Keith JD. The anomalous origin of the left coronary artery from the pulmonary artery. *Br Heart J* 1959;21:149–161.

Neches WH, Mathews RA, Park SC, et al. Anomalous origin of the left coronary artery from the pulmonary artery: A new method of surgical repair. *Circulation* 1974;50:582–587.

Takeuchi S, Imamura H, Katsumoto K, et al. New surgical method for repair of anomalous left coronary artery from pulmonary artery. *J Thorac Cardiovasc Surg* 1979;78:7–11.

Section IX

SYSTEMIC DISEASES AND THE HEART

Chapter 51

Cardiovascular Disease in Pregnancy

Eileen A. Kelly

As more women delay childbearing into their thirties and forties, the interaction between coronary disease, its risk factors, and pregnancy becomes increasingly important in prenatal care. In addition to traditional cardiovascular risk, more women with congenital heart disease are reaching childbearing age. If disease is identified during pregnancy, a multidisciplinary approach is needed to achieve optimal maternal and fetal outcomes. Normal physiologic adaptations to pregnancy and their potential effect on cardiovascular hemodynamics are central to the management of women with heart disease during pregnancy. Thus, a thorough understanding of the cardiovascular physiologic adaptations to pregnancy is increasingly required for practitioners who care for pregnant women.

PHYSIOLOGIC ADAPTATIONS TO PREGNANCY

Changes During Pregnancy

Two important hematologic parameters that affect the hemodynamic changes during pregnancy are increases in red blood cell mass and plasma volume. Plasma blood volume generally increases by about 50% during pregnancy, and red blood cell mass concomitantly increases by about 20 to 30%. Thus, the rise in total blood volume creates a relative anemia, referred to as the **physiologic anemia** of pregnancy. The etiology of this increase in blood volume is multifactorial and due mainly to activation of the renin-angiotensin-aldosterone system by estrogen. In addition, other pathways responsible for water retention are stimulated by other pregnancy-related hormones (Fig. 51-1).

Cardiac output increases by about 50% during a normal pregnancy, predominantly from an increase in stroke volume (during the first and second trimesters) and an increase in heart rate (during the third trimester). Most of the increase in cardiac output occurs by gestational week 16. This increase is followed by a further, slower increase in cardiac output until week 32. Subsequently, there is a slight decrease in cardiac output owing primarily to decreased stroke volume and increased systemic vascular resistance in the final weeks of pregnancy (Fig. 51-1, middle).

Positional changes have hemodynamically significant effects on the pregnant woman. Of particular importance is the **supine hypotension syndrome** characterized by symptoms of near-syncope/syncope caused by compression or occlusion of the inferior vena cava by the gravid uterus when the patient lies supine. The symptoms can be relieved by assuming another position, particularly lying in the left lateral decubitus position (Fig. 51-1, lower). The **supine hypotension syndrome** is one of the primary reasons to advise pregnant women against exercising in the supine position after the first trimester. This positional effect is especially important if the pregnant woman, particularly in the second or third trimester, needs cardiopulmonary resuscitation. If this unfortunate situation arises, the woman should be placed in the left lateral decubitus position.

Changes During Labor and Delivery

Marked increases in stroke volume, heart rate, and, subsequently, cardiac output occur during labor and delivery. Blood pressure (both systolic and diastolic) and oxygen consumption also increase significantly. The degree of pain and anxiety during labor has a dramatic effect on these parameters, and modulation via analgesia, sedation, or both may help limit the hemodynamic changes.

Significant hemodynamic changes occur with both vaginal delivery and cesarean section (C-section). The decision to pursue cesarean delivery should be individualized and based on the status of the fetus and the hemodynamic state of the mother. Although counterintuitive, vaginal delivery has been demonstrated to cause fewer hemodynamic alterations than C-section and is generally better tolerated even in

Figure 51-1

Cardiovascular Adaptations to Pregnancy

Hematologic changes in pregnancy

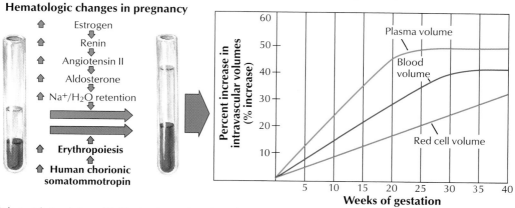

⬆ Estrogen
⬇
⬆ Renin
⬇
⬆ Angiotensin II
⬇
⬆ Aldosterone
⬇
⬆ Na^+/H_2O retention

⬆ **Erythropoiesis**

⬆ **Human chorionic somatommotropin**

Multifactorial stimulation of fluid retention and erythropoiesis in pregnancy results in a 50% increase in plasma volume and a 30% increase in red cell mass, creating a relative "physiologic" anemia and an increased blood volume

Changes in cardiac output

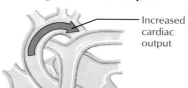

Increased cardiac output

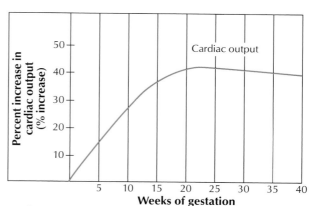

Cardiac output increases 50% in normal pregnancy, predominately from increased stroke volume in first and second trimesters and increased pulse rate in third trimester

Postural changes

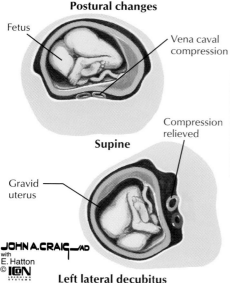

Fetus

Vena caval compression

Supine

Compression relieved

Gravid uterus

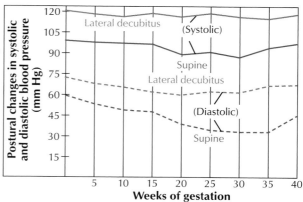

Left lateral decubitus

Positional changes have hemodynamically significant effects on pregnant women. Compression of the inferior vena cava by the gravid uterus in the supine position may cause hypotension and syncope. Condition is relieved by altering position from supine to lateral decubitus to relieve compression and restore venous return and cardiac output.

JOHN A. CRAIG—AD
with
E. Hatton
© ICN

women with heart disease. Therefore, vaginal delivery is the recommended mode of delivery unless there is an obstetric indication for C-section. Exceptions in pregnant women with heart disease include those individuals with a markedly dilated aortic root (>5.5 cm) as seen in Marfan's syndrome (in whom a hypertensive episode might cause aortic dissection), women with severe aortic coarctation with poorly controlled hypertension, and in the setting of acute severe cardiovascular decompensation.

Changes in the Postpartum Period

After delivery, the cardiac output again increases because of increased venous return from relief of vena caval compression, autotransfusion of uterine blood, and fluid mobilization. Most reports show cardiac output returning to prelabor values within 1 hour of delivery and continuing to return toward baseline values within 2 to 6 weeks after vaginal delivery.

Cardiac Examination During Normal Pregnancy

The symptoms of normal pregnancy, often including fatigue, dyspnea, palpitations and even near-syncope, in association with the normal signs of pregnancy, including augmentation of the jugular venous pulsations, normal heart sounds or murmurs, and a modest amount of lower extremity edema, may be misinterpreted as those of cardiac disease. Conversely, pathologic signs and symptoms at times may be attributed to **normal pregnancy**. Thus, knowledge of the normal cardiac examination of pregnancy is crucial (Table 51-1).

Although the presence of an S_3 had been previously thought to be a normal finding in pregnancy, it is rare in the healthy pregnant state. An S_4 is also unusual. Although diastolic murmurs have been reported in normal pregnancy, if a diastolic murmur is identified, further workup via echocardiography should be performed to evaluate for valvular pathology.

PHARMACOLOGIC THERAPY DURING PREGNANCY

Drugs are rarely tested in pregnant women. Consequently, safety information on the vast majority of pharmaceuticals in this population is

Table 51-1
Normal Physical Findings for the Cardiac Examination During Pregnancy

Examination	Findings
Precordial palpation	Laterally displaced left ventricular impulse
	Palpable right ventricular impulse
Heart sounds	Increased intensity of S_1 and S_2
	Splitting of S_1
	Increased physiologic splitting of S_2
Heart murmurs	Midsystolic murmurs (common; usually grade I–II/VI)—heard best at left lower sternal border
	Diastolic murmurs (rare; soft, medium- to high-pitched)—heard best over the pulmonic area and over the left sternal border
	Continuous murmurs Cervical venous hum—heard best over the right supraclavicular fossa Mammary souffle (may also be heard as only a systolic murmur)—heard best in the left 2nd–4th intercostal space; decreased by pressing stethoscope firmly against the chest wall and the upright position

lacking. Most cardiovascular drugs cross the placenta and are also secreted in breast milk. Therefore, when possible, it is advisable to avoid the use of all prescription and over-the-counter drug during pregnancy and during the postpartum period if the mother is breast-feeding.

When this is not possible, every effort should be made to use a medication that has been shown to be safe during pregnancy. The Food and Drug Administration categorizes drugs according to their potential to cause birth defects, based on data from human and animal studies. The categories range from class A drugs (no documented fetal risks) to class X drugs (contraindicated in part or all of pregnancy due to proven teratogenicity). Very few cardiovascular drugs are class B (animal studies suggest risk, but results are unconfirmed in controlled human studies). Examples of class B drugs include methyldopa, lidocaine, and sotalol. The majority of cardiovascular drugs currently in use are actually class C (animal studies have demonstrated adverse fetal effects, but no controlled human studies are available). Examples include labetalol, hydralazine, calcium channel blockers, and most β-blockers.

Concern about the accuracy and ambiguity of the Food and Drug Administration's classification system has prompted the proposal that the Food and Drug Administration abandon the current system and replace it with more evidence-based, narrative statements. Nonetheless, it is important to weigh the risk/benefit ratio of each case individually. If pharmacologic therapy is needed, drugs that have been in use for longer periods prescribed at the lowest possible dosages are recommended.

PREEXISTING DISEASE STATES AND PREGNANCY

Maternal and fetal risks of cardiac disease generally depend on the underlying cardiovascular lesion and the functional class of the mother. Overall, women with functional New York Heart Association class I–II have a low mortality rate, less than 1% during pregnancy, whereas those with New York Heart Association class III and IV carry a much higher associated mortality rate—greater than 7%. An updated **risk index** has been proposed to better risk-stratify pregnant women with heart disease. It includes four predictors of primary events: prior cardiac events or arrhythmia, baseline New York Heart Association class greater than II or cyanosis, significant left heart obstruction (mitral valve area of <2 cm^2, aortic valve area of <1.5 cm^2, or a peak left ventricular outflow tract gradient >30 mm Hg by echocardiography), and reduced systemic ventricular systolic function (ejection fraction <40%).

Congenital heart disease is thought to be multifactorial in origin, arising from a genetic predisposition to the disease combined with environmental factors. In general, the risk to offspring is about 3 to 5%. However, reported rates vary between 1 and 18%, depending on the specific type of maternal lesion and the number of affected siblings.

Ideally, pre-pregnancy counseling provides the patient with information about case-specific maternal and fetal risks to prepare for the safest pregnancy possible. This also allows the physician and the patient to discuss risk factor modification and potential prenatal surgical correction of the underlying defect if pregnancy is desired.

Congenital Heart Disease

Uncomplicated acyanotic lesions, including atrial and ventricular septal defects, patent ductus arteriosus (with left to right shunting), and aortic coarctation, are usually well tolerated during pregnancy. Patients with coarctation who develop severe hypertension are at risk for heart failure, cerebral aneurysm rupture, and aortic dissection. Therefore, modest, but not aggressive, blood pressure control is warranted for this population.

The maternal and fetal outcomes of pregnancy in acyanotic and cyanotic women with congenital heart disease are favorable provided that their New York Heart Association functional class is I–II and the ejection fraction measured at the beginning of pregnancy is normal. However, the outcome of pregnant women with cyanotic or complex lesions depends significantly on the type of lesion, the state of surgical repair (if any), the degree of pulmonary hypertension, the magnitude of hypoxemia, and the functional status of the mother. Hence, it is important to address each case individually.

Valvular Heart Disease

Regurgitant valvular lesions, unless severe, are usually well tolerated in pregnancy. In addition, mild congenital aortic stenosis, mild mitral stenosis, and mild to moderate pulmonic stenosis are also fairly well tolerated. However, pregnant women with stenotic valvular lesions require close monitoring throughout pregnancy, labor, and delivery and prompt intervention on rare occasion. Ideally, women with more significant stenotic valvular lesions should either have their valves replaced before pregnancy or be counseled against becoming pregnant.

Mitral stenosis often becomes symptomatic and is first diagnosed during pregnancy. Symptoms usually develop in the later part of pregnancy from the increase in stroke volume and heart rate. In this instance, institution of modest diuretic therapy and β-blockade are effective. Digoxin may also be of benefit if valvular atrial fibrillation develops. If the stenosis is moderate to severe and medical therapy is unsuccessful, mitral commissurotomy or balloon valvuloplasty should be considered. Valvuloplasty of severe aortic and pulmonic stenosis has also been successfully performed during pregnancy. Infrequently, aortic and mitral valves have been replaced during pregnancy for refractory symptoms or deterioration of functional class. Because of the significant risk this confers to the mother and the fetus, surgical valve replacement should be considered only a last resort.

Pulmonary Vascular Disease and Eisenmenger's Syndrome

The spectrum of pulmonary vascular disease includes primary pulmonary hypertension, secondary vascular pulmonary hypertension, and Eisenmenger's syndrome. Although the morbidity and mortality of these disease states is high in the general population, the coexistence with pregnancy poses an exceptionally high risk of poor maternal and fetal outcomes. Maternal mortality rate varies, based on the etiology of pulmonary vascular disease, but is reported to be in the range of 30–50%; 36% for Eisenmenger's syndrome, 30% for primary pulmonary hypertension, and 56% for secondary vascular pulmonary hypertension. Typically, women with pulmonary vascular disease and Eisenmenger's syndrome die shortly after delivery from sudden or progressive heart failure, arrhythmia, or thromboembolic events. It also appears that late hospitalization, operative delivery, pulmonary vasculitis of a systemic disease, and illicit drug use are risk factors associated with maternal death in the secondary vascular, but not primary, pulmonary hypertension group.

Because of the significant mortality rate, women with pulmonary vascular disease and Eisenmenger's syndrome should be advised against becoming pregnant. If these states are diagnosed in gestation, early termination of the

pregnancy is recommended. If the patient refuses termination or if the pulmonary vascular disease is diagnosed late in pregnancy, physical activity should be limited and the patient must be closely monitored. Early hospitalization has decreased mortality in pregnant women with secondary vascular pulmonary hypertension and Eisenmenger's syndrome.

Standard drug therapies include calcium channel blockers, inhaled nitric oxide, and inhaled or intravenous prostaglandins. Anticoagulation therapy is controversial but usually recommended during the third trimester, to be continued for 4 to 6 weeks postpartum. Spontaneous vaginal delivery is preferred, with attempts to shorten the second stage of labor using forceps or vacuum extraction. The use of pulmonary artery catheters during labor, although advocated by some, remains controversial.

Marfan's Syndrome

Marfan's syndrome is a connective tissue disorder with an autosomal dominant pattern of inheritance. It can have significant cardiovascular involvement, most commonly involving mitral valve prolapse and dilation of the aortic root at the level of the sinuses of Valsalva. Mitral regurgitation, aortic regurgitation, and aortic dissection can develop before or during pregnancy in women with Marfan's syndrome. Otherwise healthy pregnant women are at increased risk for aortic dissection; thus, pregnant women with Marfan's syndrome potentially possess an even greater risk for this devastating event. Pregnant women with Marfan's syndrome and only minor cardiovascular involvement and an aortic root diameter of less than 40 mm usually tolerate pregnancy without difficulty and have little change in aortic root diameter. However, pregnant women with Marfan's syndrome and an aortic root measuring greater than 40 mm, aortic regurgitation, or a history of aortic dissection are at higher risk.

Because of the risks, women with Marfan's syndrome are often advised against becoming pregnant. When pregnant, women with Marfan's syndrome should be advised to avoid vigorous activity. Because β-blockers decrease the rate of aortic root dilation and aortic complications in the general population with Marfan's syndrome, they are routinely administered to all pregnant women with Marfan's syndrome. Serial echocardiograms are usually performed.

CARDIOVASCULAR DISEASE UNIQUE TO PREGNANCY

Hypertension in Pregnancy

In 2000, the National Heart, Lung and Blood Institute issued an update to its Working Group Report on High Blood Pressure in Pregnancy. This NHLBI working group classified high blood pressure during pregnancy into five categories based on the Sixth Report of the Joint National Committee on Detection, Evaluation and Treatment of High Blood Pressure guidelines: chronic hypertension, gestational hypertension, transient hypertension, preeclampsia superimposed on chronic hypertension, and preeclampsia-eclampsia. These categories can help in predicting the course of hypertension and the necessity for treatment. If pharmacologic treatment is required in addition to lifestyle modifications during pregnancy, methyldopa is the preferred first-line therapy. If methyldopa is not tolerated, labetalol is used; other alternatives may be used on the basis of risk/benefit data. Angiotensin-converting enzyme inhibitors and angiotensin receptor blockers are contraindicated in pregnancy.

Chronic hypertension is defined as hypertension diagnosed before pregnancy, before the 20th week of gestation, or during pregnancy that does not resolve postpartum. Most of the increased risk in this population occurs with superimposed preeclampsia.

Gestational hypertension is high blood pressure diagnosed for the first time after midpregnancy with no accompanying proteinuria. If preeclampsia does not develop and blood pressure returns to normal by 12 weeks postpartum, the final diagnosis is **transient hypertension**. However, if postpartum blood pressure remains high, the final diagnosis is chronic hypertension.

Preeclampsia superimposed on chronic hypertension is diagnosed when a patient with hypertension, but without proteinuria before the 20th week of gestation, develops proteinuria. This diagnosis is also made when a patient with hypertension and proteinuria before the 20th week has a sudden increase in proteinuria,

a sudden increase in blood pressure, a platelet count drop to less than 100,000, or an acute elevation in serum transaminases (AST or ALT).

Finally, the classification of **preeclampsia-eclampsia** applies to women who develop increased blood pressure associated with proteinuria, a condition that may occur after the 20th week of gestation (Fig. 51-2). Particularly dangerous signs that help confirm the diagnosis of preeclampsia–eclampsia include systolic blood pressure of 160 mm Hg or higher and/or diastolic blood pressure of 110 mm Hg or higher, proteinuria greater than 2.0 g per 24 hours, increased serum creatinine concentration, platelet count below 100,000, and/or evidence of microangiopathic hemolytic anemia and elevated AST or ALT concentrations. Additional symptoms that should raise concern include persistent epigastric discomfort, persistent headaches, visual disturbances, and other central nervous system complaints.

The etiology of preeclampsia-eclampsia is unknown. This systemic disease is associated with significant increased morbidity and mortality for the mother and fetus. Preeclampsia can progress to eclampsia, a convulsive phase that may be fatal. Cerebral infarction and hemorrhage account for most deaths in preeclampsia-eclampsia. The severity of preeclampsia varies from mild to severe, and it may progress rapidly, a course that can be difficult to predict. In general, patients with mild preeclampsia may be closely supervised. Those with severe preeclampsia should be admitted to a tertiary care center and monitored closely for signs of maternal and/or fetal distress. Intravenous hydralazine, labetalol, and nitroglycerin are commonly used to treat hypertension in patients with eclampsia. Magnesium sulfate is recommended for prevention of seizures in women with severe preeclampsia and should also be given to women with eclampsia for the treatment and prevention of recurrent seizures. Delivery timing should be based on maternal and fetal conditions, including gestational age. Delivery is the cure for preeclampsia, with signs and symptoms usually regressing within 24 to 48 hours postpartum. However, it has been reported to last longer; therefore, it is important to monitor postpartum women with prepartum

Figure 51-2

Preeclampsia–Eclampsia

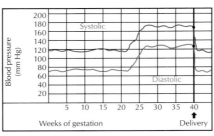

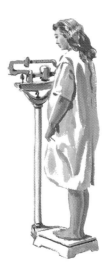

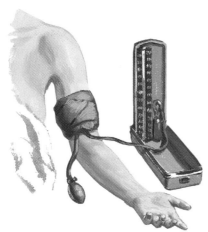

Preeclampsia–eclampsia is characterized by increase in blood pressure above 160 mm Hg systolic and/or 110 mm Hg diastolic after 20th week of gestation, accompanied by proteinuria, elevation of serum transaminases, and additional clinical findings, which usually resolve within 24–48 hours postpartum.

Elevated blood pressure

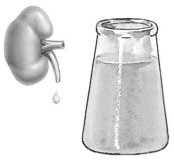

Proteinuria seen in preeclampsia and eclampsia

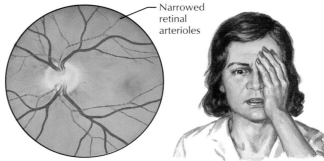

Visual changes and persistent headaches are common complaints.

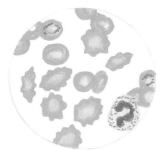

Microangiopathic hemolytic anemia and thrombocytopenia often noted

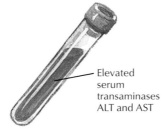

Elevated serum transaminases common in preeclampsia–eclampsia

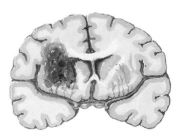

Cerebral infarction or hemorrhage most common cause of death

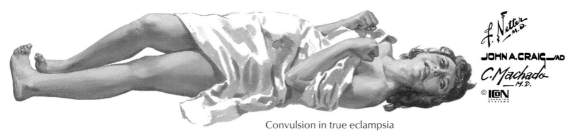

Convulsion in true eclampsia

Table 51-2
Risk Factors for Peripartum Cardiomyopathy

· Advanced maternal age (>30 years of age)
· Multiparity
· Multiple gestation
· Black race
· Preeclampsia

preeclampsia–eclampsia until hypertension has resolved and other abnormal parameters have returned to normal.

Peripartum Cardiomyopathy

Peripartum cardiomyopathy is a rare form of congestive heart failure affecting otherwise healthy young women. Risk factors for its development are shown in Table 51-2. *Peripartum cardiomyopathy* is defined as the onset of cardiac failure without identifiable cause within the last month of pregnancy or within 5 months after delivery in the absence of preexisting heart disease. Recent modifications to the definition of peripartum cardiomyopathy include strict echocardiographic criteria for left ventricular dysfunction (left ventricular ejection fraction <45% or M-mode fractional shortening <30%, or both, and end-diastolic dimension >2.7 cm/m^2).

The etiology of this disorder is unknown. Suggested hypotheses include myocarditis, an autoimmune process, and genetic predisposition. An association with tocolytic therapy (see below) has also been reported. The outcome of patients with peripartum cardiomyopathy is highly variable. Most mortality reports range between 25 and 50%, with the majority of deaths occurring in the first 3 months after diagnosis. In approximately 50%, systolic function returns to normal or near normal within 6 months postpartum. The remaining patients demonstrate persistent cardiac dysfunction or deteriorating function and experience the symptoms and complications associated with chronic heart failure.

Patients who develop peripartum cardiomyopathy should be treated using standard approaches for the treatment of acute and/or chronic systolic dysfunction, including basic sup-

portive care, medical therapy, and even an intra-aortic balloon pump or left ventricular assist device to improve hemodynamic performance (see chapters 12 and 17). The risks and benefits of medications should be reviewed before administration especially if the patient is still pregnant. If the cardiomyopathy is diagnosed before delivery, hydralazine is the afterload-reducing agent of choice (because angiotensin-converting enzyme inhibitors are teratogenic). In addition, because of the increased risk of thromboembolic events in patients with severe left ventricular dysfunction combined with the hypercoagulability of the pregnant state, anticoagulation is often recommended.

There is controversy about the outcome of subsequent pregnancies in women with a history of peripartum cardiomyopathy. In patients with persistent left ventricular dysfunction, future pregnancies should be avoided. However, in patients whose systolic function returned to normal after the initial incident, the recommendations are not as steadfast. Relapse of left ventricular dysfunction does occur in this group, albeit less frequently and perhaps less severely, than in those with persistent systolic dysfunction. Women in this population, however, experience a significant decrease in left ventricular function and clinical deterioration. Mechanistically, impaired contractile reserve, which can be demonstrated by dobutamine echocardiography, may be important. Based on these observations, even for women with peripartum cardiomyopathy in whom systolic function returned to normal, subsequent pregnancy should be considered with caution and consideration of the known risks.

Pulmonary Edema Induced by Tocolytic Therapy

Tocolytic agents are sometimes used to prevent preterm labor. They are commonly β_2 receptor agonists. Although these agents are often successful at preventing labor, they have significant side effects: tachycardia (ventricular tachycardia has been reported), chest pain without ECG changes, electrolyte abnormalities, and noncardiogenic pulmonary edema. The rate of pulmonary edema induced by these agents is low. However, it is important because patients are often misdiagnosed with decompensated heart failure and the question of peripartum cardiomyopathy may also arise. The increased incidence of pulmonary edema seen in women treated with tocolytic therapy is most often associated with short-term (<48 hours) IV infusions. There has been at least one report associating long-term (>4 weeks) oral tocolytic therapy with development of peripartum cardiomyopathy.

FUTURE DIRECTIONS

The increased survival rate of women with coronary heart disease combined with the trend toward delaying childbearing until later years will continue to increase the likelihood that the providers of health care to pregnant women will manage complex cardiovascular disease. Ideally, a multidisciplinary approach to these patients at a tertiary care center is recommended to optimize outcomes for mother and child and to provide data for treatment of other like individuals.

Knowledge of pregnancy-related disease states is rapidly expanding because of the increased awareness of these states, more stringent diagnostic criteria, and data from centers with specific interests. Diagnosis and treatment of peripartum cardiomyopathy and pulmonary hypertension and the optimal treatment of prosthetic valvular disease in pregnancy have benefited from this knowledge. It is hoped that this benefit will translate into therapeutic opportunities and improved outcomes.

REFERENCES

Elkayam U, Tummala PP, Rao K, et al. Maternal and fetal outcomes of subsequent pregnancies in women with peripartum cardiomyopathy. *N Engl J Med* 2001;344: 1567–1571.

Gei AF, Hankins GD. Cardiac disease and pregnancy. *Obstet Gynecol Clin North Am* 2001;28:465–512.

Hibbard JU, Lindheimer M, Lang RM. A modified definition for peripartum cardiomyopathy and prognosis based on echocardiography. *Obstet Gynecol* 1999;94:311–316.

Lampert MB, Lang RM. Peripartum cardiomyopathy. *Am Heart J* 1995;130:860–870.

Lupton M, Oteng-Ntim E, Ayida G, Steer PJ. Cardiac disease in pregnancy. *Curr Opin Obstet Gynecol* 2002;14: 137–143.

Ramsey PS, Ramin KD, Ramin SM. Cardiac disease in pregnancy. *Am J Perinatol* 2001;18:245–265.

Siu SC, Sermer M, Colman JM, et al. Prospective multicenter study of pregnancy outcomes in women with heart disease. *Circulation* 2001;104:515–521.

Weiss BM, Hess OM. Pulmonary vascular disease and pregnancy: Current controversies, management strategies, and perspectives. *Eur Heart J* 2000;21:104–115.

Chapter 52

Aging and the Cardiovascular System

Walter A. Tan

Senescence is a fundamental life process that manifests as a complex combination of physiologic changes resulting from the following: aerobic respiration, with the costs of oxidative metabolism and stress; genetic and cellular damage due to the accumulation of mutations; and lifelong exposure to various environmental stresses. Together, these events outpace endogenous surveillance and repair mechanisms and/or provoke compensatory responses that become maladaptive and cause cellular and organ dysfunction. Although disease should not be misconstrued as an inevitable consequence of aging, distinctions are often arbitrarily defined, and the difference between diminished biologic reserve and overt dysfunction can be simply quantitative rather than qualitative. In addition, the interplay between genetics and environmental effects (see also chapter 62) is important in aging. Although the role of genetics in aging in the broadest spectrum remains poorly understood, examples of hereditary syndromes of premature aging, such as Hutchinson-Gilford syndrome (progeria) and Werner's syndrome (where affected individuals typically die between the second and fourth decades of life), support the notion that aging is, at least in part, genetically programmed.

Although its histologic features vary little across the age spectrum, the presence and severity of atherosclerosis dramatically increases with aging. This atherosclerotic burden, along with maladaptive changes associated with aging, including myocardial changes, account for the high mortality and morbidity rates of myocardial infarction (MI) and heart failure in elderly cohorts. Chronic deconditioning and other confounding comorbidities in elderly persons add yet another layer of complexity in discerning which changes are attributable to age and which to environment (see Table 52-1). This chapter focuses on age-related changes in the cardiovascular system and considers strategies that may decrease the risk of death and disability from cardiovascular diseases in elderly individuals.

CARDIOVASCULAR CHANGES WITH AGE

Myocardial Chambers and Valves

The effects of aging on the myocardium and cardiac valves are dramatic. Deposition of lipids and their peroxidation products occurs throughout the myocardium and the vasculature at the cellular level and in subcellular components such as the mitochondria. DNA denaturization and decreased RNA and protein synthesis result. These changes diminish regenerative and reparative capacity with age.

Cardiac mass increases for several reasons, including the increased size of individual myocytes and an increased abundance of amyloid, collagen, fat, fibrotic foci, and advanced glycation products, even in the absence of myocardial damage from ischemia or infarction. It is thought that myocyte hypertrophy is a compensatory mechanism in response to the myocyte loss (due to apoptosis, necrosis, or both). Myocyte hypertrophy may also be a physiologic response to the increased hemodynamic stress on the myocardium that results from the chronic increase in peripheral vascular resistance that also occurs with aging. The left atrium tends to enlarge with advancing age, increasing the likelihood that atrial fibrillation will develop. Fibrosis and calcification of the aortic valve and the mitral annulus may lead to valvular dysfunction.

Recent investigations have demonstrated that intrinsic myocardial contractility is diminished with age, in large part due to higher vascular afterload and insensitivity to compensatory sympathetic overactivity. Although the normal sitting and submaximal end-systolic volume index

Table 52-1
Cardiovascular Changes in Elderly Individuals Without Overt Disease

Measured Change	Functional Consequence
· Myocardium	
Increased interventricular septal thickness; increased cardiac mass per body mass index in women	Increased propensity for diastolic dysfunction
Prolonged action potential, Ca_i transient, and contraction velocity (in animal models); desensitization of myocardial β-adrenergic receptors	Decreased intrinsic contractile reserve and function
Reduced early and peak left ventricular filling rate and increased pulmonary capillary wedge pressure	Greater dependence on atrial kick, and physiologic S_4 heart sound
· Cardiac Valves	
Fibrosis and calcification of the aortic valve and the mitral annulus	Valvular stiffening
· Vasculature	
Thickening of the media and subendothelial layers; increased vessel tortuosity	Decreased vessel compliance; increased hemodynamic shear stress and lipid deposition in the arterial walls
Large elastic arteries (e.g., aorta, carotid artery) become thicker and more dilated	Increased peripheral vascular resistance and earlier reflected pulse waves, and consequent late augmentation of systolic pressure
· Impulse Formation and Propagation	
Substantial decrease in sinoatrial pacemaker cell population, with separation from atrial musculature due to surrounding fatty tissue accumulation	Diminished intrinsic sinus and resting heart rates
Increase in collagenous and elastic tissue in all parts of the conduction system	Slight PR interval prolongation; increased incidence of ventricular ectopy
Decreased density of bundle fascicles and distal conduction fibers	Propensity toward bundle branch blocks and abnormal conduction
Reduced threshold for calcium overload and for diastolic afterdepolarizations and ventricular fibrillation	Lower threshold for atrial and ventricular arrhythmias; increased fibrosis and myocyte death
· Autonomic System	
Diminished autonomic tone, especially parasympathetic; increased sympathetic nerve activity and circulating catecholamine levels	Decreased spontaneous and respiratory-related heart rate variability

is similar in adults 20 to 85 years old, the response to maximal exercise (seated cycle exercise to ≥100 watt workload) is significantly attenuated in elderly individuals. A young person can increase left ventricular (LV) ejection fraction by almost 50% to accommodate the demands of intense exercise, from a baseline LV ejection fraction of about 62% to 87%, whereas the very old can recruit only about a fifth of this contractile reserve (increasing LV ejection fraction from ~63% to only ~70%) in spite of the compensatory effect of increased preload via the Frank-Starling mechanism. Often, the isovolumic relaxation time is prolonged (the interval increases between the closure of the aortic valve and the opening of the mitral valve) in elderly individuals. Moreover, the peak rate of LV diastolic filling is reduced by about 50%. These changes appear even in those who do not exhibit LV hypertrophy, and may be related to asynchronous relengthening of myocardial segments causing inefficient ventricular relaxation. These changes may help explain the proclivity for diastolic dysfunction in elderly individuals and the increased dependence on atrial contraction ("kick") for augmentation and completion of diastolic LV filling. Elderly individuals with impaired diastolic filling are consequently more vulnerable to the hemodynamic and symptomatic consequences of atrial fibrillation (AF). Reduced LV cavity size in association with hypertension has been observed in some otherwise healthy adults.

Impulse Formation and Conduction

As with cardiac contractility, multiple factors contribute to the progressive dysfunction of the cardiac conduction system in aging. Minor quantities of amyloid deposits exist in nearly half of otherwise healthy individuals over 70 years of age. The sinoatrial node may also separate physically from the atrial tissue as fat accumulates around it. Further, the population of pacemaker cells in the sinus node declines substantially after 60 years of age, with only 10% remaining by 75 years of age. Together, these changes likely account for the increased prevalence of sick sinus syndrome with aging. Other age-related findings include an increase in fibrous tissue in the internodal tracts and a diminished density of left bundle fascicles and distal conducting fibers. Thus, the high prevalence of arrhythmias in elderly individuals relates to increased polyunsaturated fatty acids in cardiac cellular membranes and to changes in ion thresholds and exchange, as well as to myocardial changes that are proarrhythmic.

Large studies support this increase in arrhythmias in elderly individuals. In adults older than 60 years of age the presence of atrial ectopic beats was demonstrated in 6% by resting electrocardiography, in 39% with maximal treadmill exercise, and in 88% of those who underwent 24-hour ambulatory monitoring. Although not known to be associated with any adverse outcome, short runs of paroxysmal supraventricular tachycardia are nearly twice as prevalent in octogenarians as in septuagenarians and are ob-

served in about half of those 65 years of age or older. The prevalence of ventricular ectopic beats rises from 0.5% in those under 40 years of age to 11.5% in those 80 years of age and older, and increases further in those with associated cardiac disease. For instance, one study demonstrated that in individuals older than 85 years of age with normal cardiac function the prevalence of ventricular ectopic beats was 5%, compared to 13 and 28% in those with coronary artery disease and heart failure, respectively. The prognostic significance of isolated ventricular ectopic beats in elderly individuals has not been studied, whether experienced at rest, during continuous 24-hour monitoring, or after treadmill exercise. However, in a recent study of younger subjects with ventricular ectopic beats on a 2-minute rhythm strip they were found to have a 14-fold increase in relative risk of sudden cardiac death in a recent study. Although sinoatrial function slows with age, healthy octogenarians and nonagenarians do not typically have resting heart rates lower than 43 beats/min or sinus pauses longer than 2 seconds. The PR interval is slightly prolonged with age, primarily from delayed conduction proximal to the His bundle, and the prevalence of first-degree atrioventricular block is 6 to 8% in octogenarians.

Vasculature

Vessel wall stiffness increases with age (Fig. 52-1). There is progressive thickening of medial and subendothelial layers and increased calcium deposition, often initially affecting proximal coronary segments. Moreover, blood flow becomes less laminar as vessels become more tortuous and endothelial cells exhibit greater heterogeneity in size, shape, and axial orientation. In response to chronic injurious stimuli, vascular smooth muscle cells phenotypically revert to a proliferative, migratory and secretory mode and produce more collagen and matrix. Arterial conduit vessels have increased elastase activity and degradation of elastin, with resulting increased stiffness. There may also be diminished reparative capacity, as indicated in vitro observations of proliferative senescence in endothelial cells and fibroblasts. These factors, plus the increased presence of inflammatory cytokines and metalloproteinases in the vessel

Figure 52-1 ## Wave Reflection and Isolated Systolic Hypertension

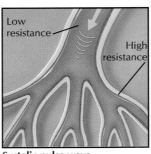

Pulse wave generation

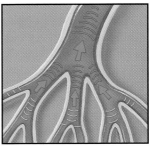

Systolic
pulse
wave

Systole

Systolic pulse wave   **Reflected pulse wave**

Systolic pulse wave reflected at transition from low- and
high-resistance vessels and returned centrally as secondary
pulse wave

Normal diastolic return

Abnormal systolic return

Reflected
(secondary)
pulse
wave

Summation of
systolic and
reflected
pulse waves

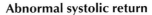

JOHN A. CRAIG—MD

C. Machado
—M.D.

© ICON
LEARNING
SYSTEMS

Pulse wave
velocity

Pulse wave
velocity

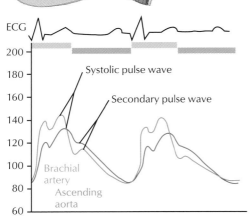

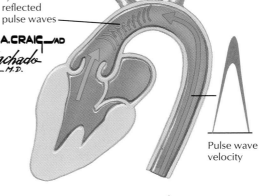

ECG

200
180
160 — Systolic pulse wave
140 — Secondary pulse wave
120
100 — Brachial
80 — artery
      Ascending
60 — aorta

ECG

Arterial pressure (mm Hg)

200 — Systolic
180   hypertension
160
140
120
100 — Brachial
80 — artery
      Ascending
60 — aorta

Amplitude of reflected wave greatest in
periphery, accounting for higher systolic
pressures in extremities than in aorta;
Diastolic return of reflected wave to heart
increases coronary perfusion and decreases
afterload

Stiffening of arterial wall increases pulse wave
velocity and results in systolic return of reflected
wave with increase in systolic pressure (isolated
systolic hypertension), decreased diastolic
pressure, increased afterload, and left ventricular
hypertrophy.

wall, predispose one to vascular occlusive and aneurysmal changes.

The peripheral arterial tree also exhibits morphologic and physiologic decline. The average aortic root size is about 14 mm/m^2 for both sexes in the early twenties, increasing to 17 mm/m^2 in healthy octogenarians. Large-caliber vessels thicken progressively; the intimal–medial wall thickness of carotid arteries is 0.03 mm in the young and doubles by age 80. After the fourth decade of life, renal blood flow per gram of kidney weight decreases progressively, likely because of increased renal arterial resistance.

Peak oxygen utilization (Vo$_2$max), a measure of work capacity and physical conditioning, declines about 50% by 80 years of age compared to the Vo$_2$max of a 20-year-old individual (~10% loss per decade of life). Aside from age-associated decline in cardiac function, up to half of the Vo$_2$max impairment is attributable to poor peripheral oxygen extraction and utilization, largely from inefficient redistribution of blood flow to skeletal muscles.

Neurohormones and Growth Factors

Age-related postsynaptic signaling deficits attenuate β-adrenergic modulation of heart rate variability and vascular tone, decreasing heart rates slightly at rest and substantially during exertion. A lower heart rate ceiling with age substantially affects exercise reserve capacity. The maximum heart rate achieved in 20-year-old persons is about 180 beats/min, but only about 120 beats/min in octogenarians. The maximal cardiac index therefore decreases about 30% over 6 decades (11 and 8 L · min^{-1} · m^{-2}, respectively) due to this phenomenon alone.

Elderly myocytes secrete more stress-related products such as atrial natriuretic factor and opioid peptides. Moreover, ambient plasma catecholamine levels are elevated, whereas the production of nitric oxide is notably lower, all contributing to increased afterload and lowered cardiac output.

CARDIOVASCULAR PATHOLOGY AND AGE

Estimates predict that roughly one in four individuals will be aged 65 years or older by 2025, with 80% of all cardiovascular deaths occurring in this cohort.

Heart Failure

Although congestive heart failure (CHF) is relatively uncommon before 45 years of age, its incidence grows linearly thereafter and geometrically at 85 years of age and older. More than 500,000 hospital admissions per year are for CHF in patients older than 65 years of age. The diagnosis of CHF in elderly individuals can be difficult, the condition sometimes presenting only as altered mental status, anxiety, dyspnea, sleep disturbance, or abdominal discomfort. Even severe LV dysfunction can be occult in sedentary individuals. Conversely, normal or near normal LV systolic function does not exclude heart failure from diastolic dysfunction, which is the underlying cause in almost half of patients older than 65 years of age with CHF symptoms. Further, many comorbidities mimic heart failure symptoms; peripheral edema may result from benign causes such as venous stasis, or it may result from liver or renal failure. Opportunities to treat potentially reversible etiologies such as anemia, aortic stenosis, thyroid dysfunction, bilateral renal artery stenosis, or tachycardia-induced cardiomyopathy should not be missed.

One special therapeutic issue in elderly individuals is polypharmacy. The clinician must be vigilant against agents considered benign by the patient that may actually exacerbate CHF, such as nonsteroidal anti-inflammatory drugs. The potential for drug interactions (e.g., with warfarin or digitalis) or intolerance from altered renal or hepatic metabolism is magnified, particularly with the standard multidrug therapy for CHF.

Finally, because the prognosis of CHF in the very old is worse than the prognosis of most cancers (<20% 5-year survival rate), it may be appropriate for the primary physician to help patients prepare for "end-of-life" issues for their own and their families' benefit.

Coronary Artery Disease

Recognition of angina or acute coronary syndromes can be difficult in elderly individuals, because up to 90% present with symptoms other than classic chest pain. Between the ages of 65 and 85 years, the prevalence of silent or misclassified ischemia increases by 50% in males and by nearly 300% in females. Underdiagnosis is not trivial, because the 30-day mortality for acute MI in elderly persons can exceed 20%. Even non–Q-wave MI has a significant age gradient of 1-year cardiac mortality rate: 29% in those 70 years of age or older, compared to 14% in younger patients. Corresponding all-cause 1-year mortality rates were recently reported to be 36% and 16%, highlighting the hazard from competing comorbidities in geriatric patients.

The absolute risk reduction in mortality for acute MI patients older than 65 years of age who received thrombolytic therapy was 3.5% compared to 2.5% for younger patients. However, this came at the cost of nearly 1% excess bleeding complications, including hemorrhagic stroke. For this reason, in many centers, emergent percutaneous coronary revascularization is preferred over thrombolytic therapy in elderly patients with ST-elevation MI. One study of elective angioplasty showed similar rates of cardiac death or recurrent angina in patients 75 years of age or older to those in their younger counterparts (mean age, 55 years) when complete revascularization was achieved. Randomized clinical trials of angioplasty versus coronary artery bypass grafting showed these results 3 years after angioplasty and coronary artery bypass grafting groups, respectively: 78% versus 100% survival, 15% versus 25% Q-wave MI, 11% versus 0% late coronary artery bypass grafting, and persistent angina in 29% versus 12%. These data should be interpreted with caution because there was unequal randomization in this small elderly cohort, because the PTCA group had a higher prevalence of diabetes and hypertension.

One special consideration for elderly patients undergoing invasive procedures or open heart surgery is the risk of stroke or multiorgan atheroemboli commonly attributed to severe atherosclerosis and calcification of the aortic arch and peripheral vessels. Foreknowledge of the concomitant vascular disease distribution and consequent adaptation of technique may minimize these perioperative complications.

Valvular Heart Disease

The most common valvular diseases requiring treatment in elderly individuals are calcific aortic stenosis and mitral regurgitation from myxomatous degeneration or annular dilatation. Aortic stenosis prevalence in adults older than 62 years of age is reported to be approximately 10% mild, 6% moderate, and 2% severe.

Unfortunately, physical examination and screening for significant valvular disease in elderly individuals are unreliable (see also chapter 1). First, many elderly individuals may be asymptomatic because they are sedentary by nature or as an adaptation to severe valvular and myocardial disease. Second, up to half of geriatric patients have systolic murmurs that are of little clinical consequence. Third, many comorbidities in elderly individuals, including kyphosis, chronic obstructive pulmonary disease, or decreased blood flow velocity across the valves (secondary to decreased cardiac output), may obscure the classic signs of aortic stenosis or mitral regurgitation. Fourth, peripheral pulsus parvus et tardus can be confounded by aortic and carotid arterial stiffening or by heart failure and β-blocker use. Therefore, especially for patients who are in declining health, clinicians should have a lower threshold for suspecting reparable aortic valve disease. Many studies have demonstrated the efficacy of aortic valve replacement even in octogenarians. The clinician should also actively search for significant mitral regurgitation before the onset of irreversible cardiomyopathy.

The relief of aortic stenosis is associated with substantial improvements in quality of life even in very old individuals, with long-term survival rates similar to age-matched individuals who do not require open heart surgery. Of the septuagenarians and older patients who had operations for aortic stenosis in three studies, more than two thirds were in New York Heart Association functional class III–IV at baseline. However, 80 to 90% improved to functional class I status and independent living after surgery. Although the risk-to-benefit ratio is acceptable for individuals who are otherwise healthy, the decision to operate is not trivial. The surgical mortality rate doubles with age older than 75 years (12.4% for patients older than 75 years of age, compared to 6.6% for younger patients). Interestingly, this risk did not continue to increase for those older than 90 years of age, perhaps because of a "survivor effect"; that is, those who survive to old age tend to be healthier. The mortality risk increases substantially when concomitant coronary artery bypass grafting or other procedures are required. Other predictors of increased risk are impaired LV function, diabetes mellitus, non-sinus rhythm, urgency of surgery, or severe renal or lung disease. Determining what is best for an individual includes considering whether surgery should be done, the feasibility of valve repair, the type of valve to be used for replacement, and the risks associated with anticoagulation. Operative mortality with mitral valve surgery is even higher, mostly because of complex underlying etiologies and the likelihood that LV dysfunction resulting from mitral regurgitation will not improve after surgery.

Percutaneous valvuloplasty is a proven therapeutic method for mitral stenosis but offers only short-term relief for aortic stenosis and, generally, is contraindicated. Moreover, for mitral stenosis, the favorable long-term outcomes reported are based predominantly on young cohorts who had rheumatic mitral stenosis. The procedural complication-free success rate is lower for older cohorts with degenerative and calcific valve disease.

Arrhythmias

Atrial fibrillation is the most important supraventricular arrhythmia in elderly individuals because of its high prevalence and associated morbidity. The prevalence is about 3 per 1000 subjects in the general population, but it increases to 3 to 4 per 100 between 60 and 65 years and to 14% in those older than 85 years. Of patients with AF, about 70% are 65 to 85 years of age. Other cardiac comorbidities significantly increase the prevalence of AF; coronary artery disease doubles the risk of AF for men, whereas heart failure increases the risk by 8-fold in men and by 14-fold in women. Although the incidence of stroke is only about 6 to 7% in patients with AF in their sixties, stroke afflicts 26% of nonagenarians with AF, often presenting a therapeutic clinical dilemma because the risk of hemorrhage with anticoagulant therapy increases with age.

Cerebrovascular Disease

Stroke produces 20% of all cardiovascular deaths in elderly individuals and is the leading cause of neurologic disability resulting in institutionalization. Unlike MIs, for which the initial male predominance in rates (up to 4:1 ratio in those younger than 55 years) narrows with age, there is only a 30% higher incidence of atherothrombotic brain infarction in males overall. This mildly increased risk in men is maintained into older age. In brain magnetic resonance imaging studies, almost one in three subjects between the ages of 65 and 84 years has evidence of silent strokes.

With the exception of subarachnoid hemorrhage and embolic stroke, the etiology of stroke is similar across age categories. Comparing those aged 65 and older to those aged 35 to 64 years, the proportion of strokes caused by subarachnoid hemorrhage was about half in elderly individuals, but there were more strokes caused by embolic mechanisms. CHF and heart failure gain increasing importance as risk factors for stroke with age. The attributable risk of stroke from AF is 1.5% in the fifth decade of life, rising exponentially to 23.5% by the eighth decade of life. For CHF, the corresponding attributable risks are 2.3 and 6%.

Unfortunately, the consequences of stroke are more severe in very old individuals. For those aged 85 years or older, in-hospital mortality rate is more than 25% compared to 13.5% for those younger than 85 years of age. Among those who survive to be discharged, only a fifth have minimal or no neurologic deficit compared to a third of a younger cohort. In another study, one third of stroke survivors had dementia (based on Mini-Mental Status Exam score <24), a threefold higher prevalence than stroke-free subjects. Because dementia with or without stroke is the largest contributor to disability in basic activities of daily living (e.g., dressing, bathing, and transfers), the estimated 18.4% population-attributable risk of dementia from stroke is of great importance.

As with other therapies, the risk of treatment is higher in elderly individuals but, oftentimes, interventions reduce risk compared with conservative therapy. For instance, elderly individuals with severe carotid stenosis are at high risk if treated with medications only; but, when carefully selected, carotid endarterectomy reduces the risk of stroke and stroke-related death (Fig. 52-2). Related to stroke risk, isolated systolic hyperten-

Figure 52-2

Endarterectomy for Extracranial of Carotid Artery Atherosclerosis

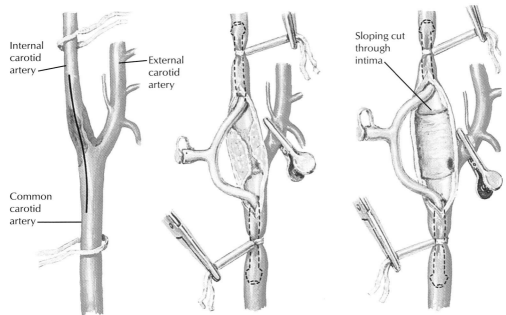

Internal carotid artery

External carotid artery

Sloping cut through intima

Common carotid artery

Longitudinal incision to remove atherosclerotic obstruction at carotid bifurcation

Silastic tube inserted to shunt blood flow during endarterectomy.

Endarterectomy performed

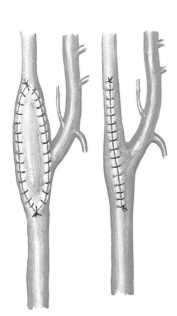

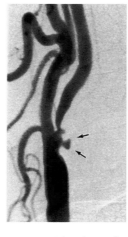

Angiogram (lateral view) showing moderately severe stenosis at origin of left internal carotid artery, with ulceration indicated by protrusion of contrast medium (arrows). Such a case is suitable for endarterectomy.

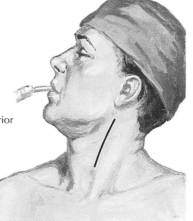

Patient's head turned to side; incision along anterior margin of sternocleido-mastoid muscle

Vein graft or Dacron® velour patch used to widen vessel if necessary. Arteriotomy closed by direct suture.

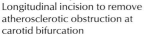

Figure 52-3

Age and PAD Distribution

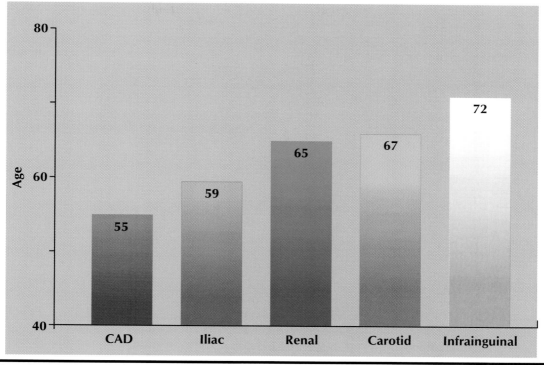

With permission from Tan WA, Yadav JS, Wholey MH. Endovascular options for peripheral arterial occlusive and aneurysmal disease. In: Topol EJ, ed. *Textbook of Interventional Cardiology*. 4th ed. Philadelphia: WB Saunders; 2002.

sion increases with age, most likely because of increased vascular impedance with a recalibration in baroreceptor reflex thresholds (Fig. 52-1). Fortunately, the absolute and relative risk reductions from antihypertensive therapy increase also, with a 50% relative risk reduction in the 5-year stroke rate in those older than 80 years of age, compared to a 30% relative risk reduction with treatment in sexagenarians.

Peripheral Arterial Occlusive and Aneurysmal Disease

Peripheral vascular wall integrity degenerates with age. For example, the incidence of abdominal aortic aneurysms increases fourfold in subjects older than 65 years of age compared to those 55 years of age or younger. Peripheral arterial occlusive disease can be considered a late-stage manifestation of atherosclerosis. Although the mean age in clinical trials of European patients requiring coronary interventions is 55 years of age, the average ages for those with extracoronary occlusive disease are 59, 65, 67, and 72 years, respectively, for those with iliac, renal, carotid, and infrainguinal artery stenoses (Fig. 52-3; see also chapters 41 and 42).

THE THERAPEUTIC WINDOW

Up to 50% of elderly patients do not receive appropriate thrombolytic therapy on the basis of age alone, in spite of data showing large absolute and relative mortality risk reductions for this group. The increasing use of percutaneous coronary interventions in elderly patients with acute MI is beginning to partially offset concerns about stroke risk with thrombolytic therapy. However, the problem of undertreatment extends far beyond the initial therapy. Of Medicare patients with acute MI who had no contraindication to aspirin therapy, only 61% received this proven therapy during hospitalization, and less than 50% were instructed to take aspirin at discharge.

There has also been debate over lipid-lowering therapy in elderly individuals, even though this population is at highest risk for severe cardiovascular catastrophes. Treatment with simple drugs such as chlorthalidone and atenolol where necessary to control isolated systolic hypertension decreases the relative risk of stroke by 29% in sexagenarians, 30% in septuagenarians, and 49% in octogenarians or nonagenarians. Nonetheless, 55% of eligible octogenarians are not on any antihypertensive medications.

FUTURE DIRECTIONS

The narrower physiologic reserve with advancing age elevates risk and narrows the therapeutic window. However, outcomes improve dramatically with advances in medical and interventional therapies, particularly in more vulnerable populations such as elderly patients. A progressive decrease in 30-day acute MI mortality rate has been documented in octogenarians from 55% in the 1970s to 31% in the1980s to 22% by 1991. This represents a 72% decrease after statistical adjustment for comorbidities and MI severity. Better and safer monitoring and anesthetic techniques permit necessary surgery even for high-risk patients. Endovascular therapies are less invasive, offering the very old short- and medium-term outcomes that previously could be obtained only with major surgery (e.g., stent grafting for abdominal aortic aneurysms).

The benefits of prevention and therapy should be extended more aggressively to all age groups, with careful consideration of individual risk profiles and preferences. More important, simply extending life span no longer suffices. The key challenge for health care in the 21st century is extension of the "health span" or quality of later life of the older patient.

REFERENCES

de Boer J, Andressoo JO, de Wit J, et al. Premature aging in mice deficient in DNA repair and transcription. *Science* 2002;296:1276–1279.

Lakatta EG. The cardiovascular system: Circulatory function in younger and older humans in health. In: Hazzard WR, ed. *Principles of Gerontology and Geriatric Medicine.* New York: McGraw-Hill; 1999:645–660.

Mackey RH, Sutton-Tyrrell K, Vaitkevicius PV, et al. Correlates of aortic stiffness in elderly individuals: A subgroup of the Cardiovascular Health Study. *Am J Hypertens* 2002;15:16–23.

National Institute on Aging, NIH. The Baltimore Longitudinal Study of Aging (BLAS). Available at: http:// www.grc. nia.nih.gov/ branches/blsa/blsa.htm. Last updated March 14, 2002.

Tan WA, Yadav JS, Wholey MH. Endovascular options for peripheral arterial occlusive and aneurysmal disease. In: Topol EJ, ed. *Textbook of Interventional Cardiology.* 4th ed. Philadelphia: WB Saunders; 2003:481–522.

Tresch DD, Aronow WS, eds. *Cardiovascular Disease in the Elderly Patient.* New York: Marcel Dekker; 1993:1–662.

Wei JY. Age and the cardiovascular system. *N Engl J Med* 1992;327:1735–1739.

Wenger NK, ed. *Cardiovascular Disease in the Octogenarian and Beyond.* London: Martin Dunitz; 1999:1–439.

Chapter 53

Neuromuscular Diseases and the Heart

Ajmal Masood Gilani and Colin D. Hall

Diseases affecting skeletal muscle may also involve cardiac muscle, and those involving the peripheral nervous system may affect neurologic control of the heart. Cardiovascular manifestations vary in nature and severity in different patients, even those with the same disease. Cardiovascular sequelae can result in greater morbidity and mortality than the neuromuscular manifestations. A comprehensive review of neuromuscular diseases with some degree of cardiac manifestation is beyond the scope of this text; the common disorders likely to have cardiac effects have been included.

Elevation of creatine kinase (CK) in the bloodstream is a hallmark of active muscle disease. CK from postnatal skeletal muscle is composed of MM subunits, but CK from fetal and regenerating skeletal muscle is composed of MB subunits. Therefore, in diseases with attempted muscle regeneration, including inflammatory myopathies and some dystrophies, an elevated MB fraction is not specific for myocardial injury and may, rather reflect skeletal muscle regeneration.

DISEASES OF MUSCLE
Muscular Dystrophies

Traditionally categorized by mode of inheritance, age of onset, severity, and pattern of clinical presentation, these inherited disorders generally present with progressive muscle weakness. However, advances in molecular biology have identified many dystrophies by specific gene or protein abnormalities.

Dystrophinopathies

Duchenne's and Becker's muscular dystrophies (MDs) are X-linked recessive disorders resulting from abnormalities in **dystrophin**, an essential component of the cytoskeleton of skeletal and cardiac muscle. Progressive weakness and pseudohypertrophy of muscles, particularly the calves, is characteristic of both.

Clinical manifestations of Duchenne's MD become obvious at 3 to 5 years of age, with contractures and proximal muscle weakness greater than distal weakness. Gower's maneuver is char-

acteristic (Fig. 53-1). Nonprogressive mental retardation occurs in approximately 70% of patients. Severe scoliosis occurs in 90% by early in the second decade of life. There is steady progression to wheelchair use within 10 years, and death usually occurs in the second or early third decade of life from respiratory or cardiac failure. Cardiovascular manifestations include dilated cardiomyopathy, usually of the posterobasal and posterolateral left ventricle; mitral regurgitation; frequently incomplete right bundle branch block; atrial and ventricular arrhythmias; QT dispersion; and autonomic dysfunction manifested by abnormal heart rate variability.

Becker's MD is less severe, with the age of onset in the second decade of life or later. Progression is slower, with death occurring usually in middle adulthood. Cardiac involvement is independent of the severity of the skeletal muscle disease.

Both conditions result in marked, persistent CK elevation, generally 10 times the upper limit of normal or higher. The diagnosis can be made in more than 90% of patients by confirmation of a deletion or point mutation of the Xp21 gene locus. Analysis of dystrophin content by muscle biopsy is also a reliable diagnostic tool.

Treatment of the muscle weakness is supportive. Selected patients may benefit from surgery to retard scoliosis, respiratory support, and treatment of cardiac complications. Standard therapies are generally used for cardiac failure and dysrhythmias. For drug-refractory ventricular arrhythmias, use of an implantable cardiac

Figure 53-1

Duchenne's Muscular Dystrophy
Gower's Maneuver

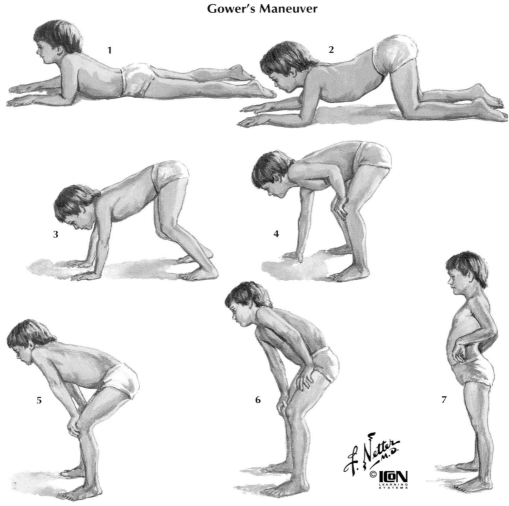

Characteristically, the child arises from prone position by pushing himself up with hands successively on floor, knees, and thighs, because of weakness in gluteal and spine muscles. He stands in lordic posture.

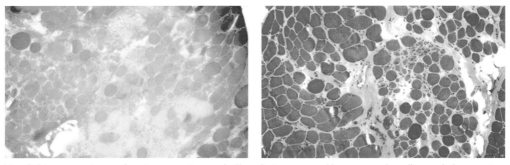

Muscle biopsy specimens showing necrotic muscle fibers being removed by groups of small, round phagocytic cells (**left**, trichrome stain) and replaced by fibrous and fatty tissue (**right**, H and E stain)

defibrillator (ICD) has been reported to be beneficial. In Becker's MD, a number of patients with disproportionate cardiac involvement have successfully undergone cardiac transplantation.

Emery-Dreifuss Muscular Dystrophy

This rare X-linked disorder is characterized by a clinical triad of early contractures of the elbows, ankles, and posterior cervical muscles; slowly progressive muscle weakness in a scapulohumeroperoneal distribution; and dilated or restrictive cardiomyopathy with atrial conduction defects. The genetic defect is at the Xq28 gene locus, with resulting deficiency of the protein emerin—a protein found in the inner nuclear membrane in skeletal and cardiac muscle. Findings include an elevated CK, but generally less than 10 times the normal level, a myopathic EMG, and a dystrophic muscle biopsy result with prominent fibrosis. The diagnosis is confirmed by an absence of emerin in skin or muscle tissue.

Cardiac involvement is invariable, with onset generally between the second and fourth decades of life, and usually including sinus bradycardia, atrial fibrillation and/or flutter and junctional arrhythmias. Syncopal episodes and sudden death are common. Affected males should be monitored carefully for development of abnormalities on ECG. Early pacing can reduce the incidence of sudden death.

Myotonic Dystrophy

Myotonic dystrophy, an autosomal dominant MD, is a multiple-system disease. Its expression is variable within and between affected families. Patients may have facial muscle weakness, especially temporalis, levator palpebrae superioris, and masseters, resulting in a typical "cadaveric" facies. Weakness of the distal muscles of the upper extremity is prominent. Lower limb muscles are less involved. Myotonia results in delayed muscle relaxation after contraction or muscle percussion (Fig. 53-2). Systemic features may include frontal balding, cataracts, hypogonadism, insulin resistance, dysphagia, hypersomnia, Pickwickian syndrome, and mental retardation. Children of affected mothers are more likely to be severely weak and hypotonic and to have mental retardation in infancy. The progression of myotonic dystrophy is variable, with death usually resulting from aspiration pneumonia, respiratory failure, or cardiac involvement.

Cardiac manifestations include conduction defects, atrial and ventricular tachyarrhythmias (occasionally causing sudden death), mitral valve prolapse, and dilated cardiomyopathy. Anesthesia may increase the risk of atrioventricular (AV) conduction block. A yearly ECG is recommended, and in high-risk families or individuals deemed to be at risk, His bundle studies and prophylactic cardiac pacemaker placement is often recommended. β-Adrenergic blockers and angiotensin-converting enzyme (ACE) inhibitors improve cardiomyopathic symptoms. Quinidine, phenytoin, or other antiepileptic agents can sometimes ameliorate the myotonia. Modafinil or methylphenidate may alleviate hypersomnia.

The diagnosis of myotonic dystrophy is confirmed by identification of trinucleotide (CTG) repeats found on the long arm of chromosome 19. The greater the number of repeats, the more severe the clinical manifestations are. Myotonic discharges have a characteristic "dive bomber" sound on EMG, although this feature is not generally present in infants.

Facioscapulohumeral Muscular Dystrophy

Many families affected by this usually autosomal dominant condition show a deletion at the 4q35 gene locus. The prevalence is 1 to 2 in 100,000, and onset varies from the first through fifth decades of life. Facial, scapular, and humeral muscles are involved earliest and most prominently, but there is often progression to extraocular, peroneal, pectoral, and respiratory muscles. The involvement of various muscle groups is often asymmetric. Patients commonly have a transverse smile with poor emotional expression; failure of complete eye closure, particularly in sleep; and dysarthria. Other systemic manifestations may include sensorineural deafness, retinal telangiectasia, epilepsy, and mental retardation. Cardiac manifestations are less common; however, labile hypertension, conduction block, and arrhythmias may occur. The diagnosis is based mainly on clinical appearance but may be supported by elevated CK, EMG, and muscle biopsy. Treatment is primarily

Figure 53-2

Myotonic Dystrophy

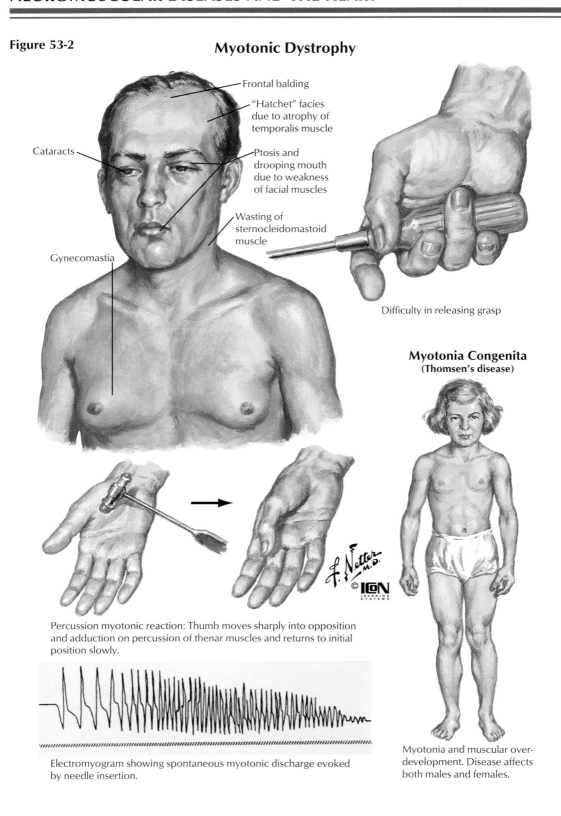

Frontal balding

"Hatchet" facies due to atrophy of temporalis muscle

Cataracts

Ptosis and drooping mouth due to weakness of facial muscles

Wasting of sternocleidomastoid muscle

Gynecomastia

Difficulty in releasing grasp

Myotonia Congenita
(Thomsen's disease)

Percussion myotonic reaction: Thumb moves sharply into opposition and adduction on percussion of thenar muscles and returns to initial position slowly.

Electromyogram showing spontaneous myotonic discharge evoked by needle insertion.

Myotonia and muscular over-development. Disease affects both males and females.

supportive. Approximately 20% of these patients advance to wheelchair use, and some die of respiratory failure, but life expectancy is near normal in most.

Limb Girdle Muscular Dystrophy

Characterized by limb weakness and wasting, limb girdle MD is poorly classified and represents a number of different conditions. Gene mutation identification and resulting protein defects have categorized more than 10 subtypes, and the list continues to grow. Many result from abnormalities in the dystrophin-associated protein complex. The most common forms are autosomal recessive, but dominant and sporadic inheritance patterns occur. Proximal arms or legs may be first affected, with progression to all limbs, sparing the facial muscles. Associated cardiac abnormalities include AV conduction block, atrial and ventricular arrhythmias, and dilated cardiomyopathy. The diagnosis is supported by elevated CK, myopathy seen on EMG, muscle biopsy results, and, in some, molecular genetic analysis. No specific treatment is available. Serial ECG and echocardiographic evaluations are recommended.

Distal Myopathies

This heterogeneous group of muscular dystrophies starts in the distal limbs and usually has a benign course. They include Miyoshi's myopathy, which starts in the feet and the calves, and Welander's myopathy, which starts in the hands. Cardiac conduction abnormalities are common, and periodic ECG is recommended.

Other Hereditary Conditions
Affecting Muscle and the Heart

These conditions include McLeod's syndrome (myopathy with elevated CK, polyneuropathy, movement disorders, psychiatric syndromes, seizures, and dilated or restrictive cardiomyopathy), X-linked dilated cardiomyopathy associated with abnormal taffazin, X-linked vacuolar cardiomyopathy and myopathy (Danon's disease), scapuloperoneal muscular dystrophy with mental retardation and lethal cardiomyopathy, and neuromuscular junction disorders, including familial limb girdle myasthenia and slow-channel syndrome.

Metabolic Disorders Causing Myopathy and Cardiac Disease
Electrolyte Disorders

Hypokalemic periodic paralysis (PP), a calcium channel defect, hyperkalemic PP, a sodium channel defect, and potassium-sensitive PP are autosomal dominant disorders characterized by attacks of weakness of variable severity and duration, generally lasting for hours to days (Fig. 53-3). Precipitants may include exposure to cold and rest after activity. Fasting and supplementation of potassium can trigger attacks of hyperkalemic and ameliorate hypokalemic PP. Ingestion of carbohydrates can precipitate hypokalemic PP and ameliorate hyperkalemic PP. Cardiovascular manifestations, including ventricular bigeminy, bidirectional tachycardias, and increased QT interval, are more common in hyperkalemic PP and potassium-sensitive PP. Although ventricular arrhythmias rarely result in sudden death in these patients, therapeutic decisions should be made, as would be the case in those without PP with ventricular arrhythmias (see chapter 23). The diagnosis is suspected based on familial occurrence of transient attacks of weakness. Abnormalities in potassium and sodium levels during the attacks can often be ascertained, and are diagnostic. Genetic testing is available for some of these conditions.

Mexiletine, calcium gluconate, glucose, and insulin are effective in the treatment of hyperkalemic PP. Administration of oral potassium is effective in hypokalemic PP. Acetazolamide and dichlorphenamide may be helpful in both conditions. Management of the electrolyte imbalance usually improves muscle weakness but not cardiac arrhythmias.

Glycogen Storage Diseases

The autosomal recessive glycogen storage diseases result from deficiency or absence of specific enzymes in the glycogen degradation pathway. At least nine different enzyme abnormalities can result in glycogen-containing vacuoles in muscle. Generally, cardiac involvement is not significant, but acid maltase deficiency (Pompe's disease) is an exception. Infantile, childhood, and adult forms variably feature muscle weakness and hypotonia.

The infantile form of Pompe's disease is most severe, with liver, spleen, and often tongue

Figure 53-3

Myopathies Related to Disorders of Potassium Metabolism

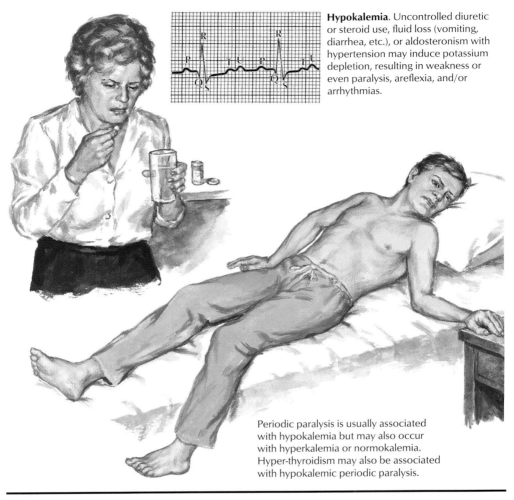

Hypokalemia. Uncontrolled diuretic or steroid use, fluid loss (vomiting, diarrhea, etc.), or aldosteronism with hypertension may induce potassium depletion, resulting in weakness or even paralysis, areflexia, and/or arrhythmias.

Periodic paralysis is usually associated with hypokalemia but may also occur with hyperkalemia or normokalemia. Hyper-thyroidism may also be associated with hypokalemic periodic paralysis.

Hyperkalemia. Addison's disease (primary adrenocortical insufficiency), characterized by bronzing of skin, weakness, weight loss, and hypotension, is associated with elevated serum potassium. Manifestations may be mild in early stages, with weakness predominating.

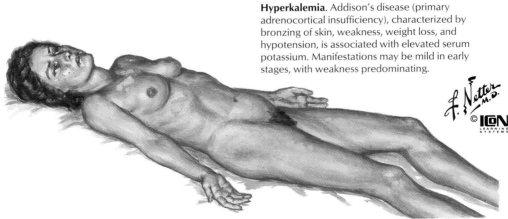

enlargement from abnormal glycogen storage. The ECG typically shows cardiomegaly with high-amplitude QRS complexes. Measurement of acid maltase concentration in leukocytes, muscle, or cultured fibroblasts confirms the diagnosis. Death is generally a result of cardiac or respiratory failure. There is no effective treatment.

Carnitine Deficiency

The lipid storage myopathies are characterized by abnormal fat accumulation in muscle, resulting from many different metabolic defects. Carnitine deficiency is the only one of these resulting in significant cardiac involvement. Most patients who experience this condition have a systemic deficiency associated with enzymatic defects or a secondary deficiency from renal disease or use of drugs such as sodium valproate. Whether an isolated muscle carnitine deficiency is a discrete entity is uncertain. Clinical features may include recurring acute encephalopathy, developmental delay, myopathy, and recurring hypoketotic hypoglycemia. One form manifests as progressive and potentially fatal cardiomyopathy with recurring hypoglycemia, rarely with involvement of other organs. The diagnosis is established by measurement of carnitine levels in plasma, urine, and muscle tissue. Treatment consists of dietary carnitine supplementation and glucose infusion during acute episodes.

Mitochondrial Disorders

Mutations in mitochondrial DNA result in defective energy-generating pathways and oxidative phosphorylation with eventual cellular apoptosis. A variety of different syndromes have been recognized: the Kearns-Sayre syndrome results in progressive external ophthalmoplegia, cardiac conduction defects, and dilated cardiomyopathy; Leber's hereditary optic neuropathy manifests clinically as progressive blindness and may be associated with a shortened PR interval and supraventricular tachycardias; mitochondrial encephalomyopathy with lactic acidosis and stroke and myoclonic epilepsy with ragged red fibers may each be accompanied by hypertrophic cardiomyopathy. Genetic defects are identified for some of these diseases. Skeletal muscle biopsy shows ragged red fibers on Gomori trichrome staining and abnormalities of numbers or structure of mitochondria or both on electron microscopy. Biochemical analysis of mitochondrial activity from muscle tissue is useful.

No accepted treatment regimen exists, but administration of l-carnitine may improve cardiomyopathy, and prophylactic pacing may improve survival rate.

Inflammatory Myopathies

These immune-mediated acquired muscular disorders have a controversial classification because features of inflammatory myopathy accompany all collagen–vascular diseases. Conditions isolated to the muscle are generally categorized as *polymyositis* or *dermatomyositis*. Although they probably have different immune etiologies, the major clinical difference is the presence of a heliotrope rash in dermatomyositis, most frequently found in the periorbital region and over the knuckles, knees, and elbows. Either may be a manifestation of occult neoplasm.

There is progressive symmetric weakness of proximal limb muscles, often with myalgias, but without wasting until late in the course when there may also be distal involvement. Neck flexor weakness is common. Dysphagia may occur secondary to esophageal dysmotility. Respiratory muscle involvement and pulmonary fibrosis may lead to respiratory failure; this may be more common in patients with a positive anti-Jo antibody. Raynaud's phenomenon and joint involvement may be systemic features. Cardiac manifestations include myocarditis, diffuse hypokinesia, and ventricular enlargement with or without heart block. CK is elevated in the active stage of the disease. With effective treatment, the total CK may return toward normal, but the percentage MB fraction may rise.

EMG may show nonspecific but characteristic changes. Muscle biopsy is generally definitive, with perivascular and endomysial inflammatory responses. However, the disease is patchy and can be missed on biopsy. In adults, the diagnostic approach should include evaluation for occult malignancy.

The standard therapy is prednisone administration. High-dose intravenous immunoglobulin infusion may be effective but necessitates periodic administration for months to years. Antimetabolites, including methotrexate azathioprine and cyclosporine, may have a role in steroid-resistant disease. Cardiac and respiratory involvement may prove resistant to these therapies.

Alcoholic Myopathy

Long-term alcohol abuse may be associated with acute necrotizing myopathy, myopathy with hypokalemia, or progressive proximal myopathy. Alcoholic cardiomyopathy may be associated with any of these conditions. Cardiac involvement has been described in three stages: (1) palpitations and vague chest wall pain often accompanied by atrial dysrhythmia, (2) LV hypertrophy, and (3) cardiac dilatation and congestive heart failure (CHF). Advanced alcoholic myopathy has a high mortality rate, even if the patient becomes abstinent.

DISEASES OF NERVE

Many peripheral neuropathies are associated with cardiac disease, although the degree varies among patients with the same disease. Neuropathies with prominent autonomic involvement, such as alcoholic and diabetic neuropathy, are likely to show abnormalities of heart period variability. They may also have clinically obvious cardiac disease, but whether this results from neuropathy, cardiovascular disease, or both is difficult to determine.

Hereditary Diseases

The hereditary motor and sensory neuropathies are the most common inherited neurologic diseases. They rarely involve the heart, but arrhythmias frequently accompany the less common hereditary sensory and autonomic neuropathies.

Friedreich's Ataxia

Friedreich's ataxia is a progressive autosomal recessive degenerative disease. The genetic deficit is a trinucleotide repeat (GAA) linked to chromosome 9, with resulting abnormality of *frataxin*, a mitochondrial protein important in iron homeostasis and intracellular respiratory function. Neurologic features include cerebellar ataxia, dysarthria, a combination of spasticity and lower limb neuropathy, weakness and sensory deficit (particularly vibration and position),

and absence of deep tendon reflexes with extensor plantar responses (Fig. 53-4). Twelve to 15 years after the onset of symptoms, most patients are no longer able to walk. Heart disease, scoliosis, and an increased incidence of diabetes are characteristic. Cardiac manifestations include atrial and ventricular tachyarrhythmias, hypertrophic cardiomyopathy, hypokinetic and dilated left ventricle, and muscular subaortic stenosis.

Diagnosis is confirmed by an expanded repetition of trinucleotide GAA, which encodes for *frataxin*. There is no specific treatment.

Acute Intermittent Porphyria

Generally an autosomal dominant condition, acute intermittent porphyria manifests as acute abdominal pain and a variety of psychiatric and neurologic symptoms. These include axonal neuropathy with a major autonomic component, including marked changes in BP and tachycardia. Treatment consists of respiratory support, use of β-blocking agents if tachycardia and hypertension are severe, and pyridoxine. Use of intravenous glucose and hematin is recommended as the most direct and effective therapy.

Storage Diseases

Amyloidosis

Clinical manifestations of hereditary and acquired amyloidosis depend on the organs involved. Neuropathy is the most common presentation of familial disease but also occurs in acquired systemic amyloidosis. Autonomically mediated orthostatic hypotension is common. The heart is generally infiltrated, with resulting cardiomegaly, CHF, dysrhythmia, and, at times, pericarditis. Treatment is symptomatic.

Abetalipoproteinemia

Symptoms of hereditary storage disease may include acanthocytosis, retinitis pigmentosa, malabsorption, and devastating neurologic features, including mental retardation, spinocerebellar degeneration, and occasionally peripheral neuropathy. Cardiac involvement includes ventricular enlargement, repolarization (T wave) changes, and arrhythmias. Many of the complications may be prevented by use of DL-α-tocopherol.

Figure 53-4

Friedreich's Ataxia

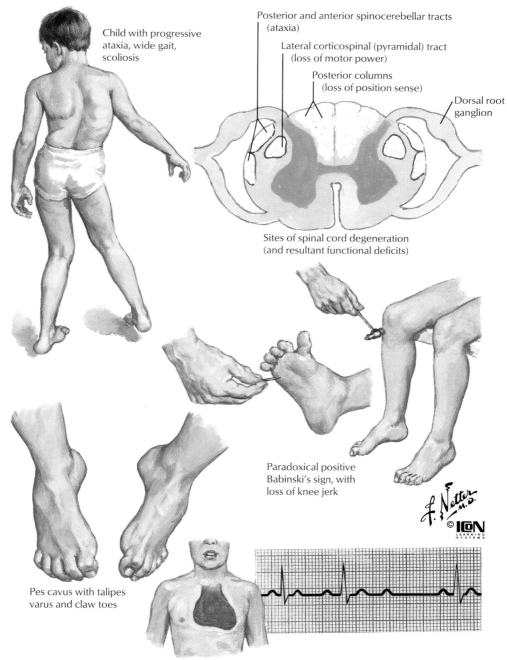

Child with progressive ataxia, wide gait, scoliosis

Posterior and anterior spinocerebellar tracts (ataxia)

Lateral corticospinal (pyramidal) tract (loss of motor power)

Posterior columns (loss of position sense)

Dorsal root ganglion

Sites of spinal cord degeneration (and resultant functional deficits)

Paradoxical positive Babinski's sign, with loss of knee jerk

Pes cavus with talipes varus and claw toes

Death often caused by cardiac abnormalities (interstitial myocarditis, fibrosis, enlargement, arrhythmias, murmurs, heart block)

Refsum's Disease

The result of inadequate oxidation of phytanic acid, *Refsum's disease* manifests with retinitis pigmentosa, cerebellar degeneration, peripheral neuropathy, and, sometimes, ichthyotic skin changes, skeletal changes, and hearing loss. Cardiomegaly, dysrhythmias, and conduction defects may result in sudden death. Phytanic acid levels in serum and alpha oxidation capacity in cultured skin fibroblasts establish the diagnosis. Efforts to reduce dietary phytanic acid are effective in arresting disease progression and improvement of the complications.

Guillain-Barré Syndrome

The Guillain-Barré syndrome, an acute inflammatory neuropathy, is characterized by peripheral, autonomic, and cranial nerve dysfunction. Generally, a history of infection, immunization, or surgical procedure precedes clinical onset by days to weeks.

The first symptoms are usually symmetric lower limb sensory changes, followed by ascending distal weakness. Onset may be in the proximal limb or cranial nerve distribution. Weakness progresses rapidly, with loss of tendon reflexes. Facial diplegia and oropharyngeal and respiratory weakness occur in 30 to 40% of patients. Clinical progression may continue for up to 3 weeks, followed by gradual improvement to normal or near normal over weeks or months in more than 70% of patients. Death is generally a result of respiratory or cardiac disease. Autonomic dysfunction produces cardiac involvement, including orthostatic hypotension, hypertension, ST-segment abnormalities, tachyarrhythmias or bradyarrhythmias, and loss of heart rate variability from reduction of sympathetically mediated peripheral vascular tone, vagal dysfunction, or both. As a rule, severe cardiac involvement only occurs with severe motor weakness.

The laboratory hallmark of the syndrome is elevated protein levels without an increase in cells in the cerebrospinal fluid. This occurs in more than 80% of patients by the second week. EMG and nerve conduction study results may be normal in the first week.

Treatment with plasmapheresis or intravenous immunoglobulin within the first 2 weeks improves outcome. Careful observation of respiratory func-

tion is essential until progression stabilizes; ventilatory support may be necessary. Volume replacement or treatment with pressor agents may be necessary to counter hypotension.

Diphtheric Polyneuropathy

Diphtheria is rare in the United States but does occur in unvaccinated patients. It is estimated that neuropathy develops in 20% of patients. Bulbar paralysis occurs in week 3 or 4. Intact pupillary light response with failure of accommodation is a classic feature of this disease. Generalized peripheral neuropathy may occur from weeks 3 to 15 or later. An initial throat infection may be mild enough to be missed clinically. Cardiac arrhythmias and CHF are the most common causes of death and may occur from the second week to the late convalescent period. In the early period, this may be because of myocardial involvement; later, it may be because of involvement of the vagus nerve. Strict bed rest is recommended in the acute stages, and in later stages if there is cardiac involvement.

Toxin-Induced Neuropathies

Acute muscarinic effects of organophosphate exposure may result in hypotension and bradycardia, and nicotinic effects may result in hypertension and tachycardia. Peripheral neuropathy may occur as a delayed effect. The neuropathy of thallium exposure may be accompanied by subacute hypotension and tachycardia.

FUTURE DIRECTIONS

Linking clinical syndromes with specific genetic and proteomic defects is the subject of intense research activity. Specific genetically oriented treatments may emerge to revolutionize the approach to these degenerative diseases.

REFERENCES

Anders HJ, Wanders A, Kruger K. Myocardial fibrosis in polymyositis. *J Rheumatol* 1999;26:1840–1842.

Dyck PJ, Thomas PK, Lambert EH, eds. *Peripheral Neuropathy.* 2nd ed. Philadelphia: WB Saunders; 1984.

Engel AG, Franzini-Armstrong C, eds. *Myology.* 2nd ed. New York: McGraw-Hill; 1994.

Finsterer J, Stollberger C, Blazek G, Spahits E. Cardiac involvement in myotonic dystrophy, Becker muscular dystrophy and mitochondrial myopathy: A five-year follow-up. *Can J Cardiol* 2001;17:1061–1069.

Flachenecker P, Wermuth P, Hartung HP, Reiners K. Quantitative assessment of cardiovascular autonomic function in Guillain-Barre syndrome. *Ann Neurol* 1997;42:171–179.

Hayashi Y, Shimada K. Secondary cardiomyopathy accompanied by neuromuscular disorders. *Nippon Rinsho Japan J Clin Med* 2000;58:191–195.

Santorelli FM, Tessa A, D'Amati G, Casali C. The emerging concept of mitochondrial cardiomyopathies. *Am Heart J* 2001;141:E1.

Yotsukara M, Yamamoto A, Kajiwara T, et al. QT dispersions in patients with Duchenne-type progressive muscular dystrophy. *Am Heart J* 1999;137(pt 1):672–677.

Chapter 54

Cardiovascular Manifestations of Endocrine Diseases

David R. Clemmons

Endocrine system diseases generally affect multiple organ systems because hormones secreted into the general circulation act on multiple tissues that are distant from their sources of synthesis and secretion. Nearly all hormones and accompanying hormonal disorders are, at times, associated with a pathophysiologic disarrangement of some component of the cardiovascular system. This chapter focuses on the most common disorders and those with the most significant deleterious consequences for cardiovascular function.

PITUITARY GLAND DISORDERS

The seven peptide hormones secreted by the anterior pituitary gland and two secreted by the posterior pituitary gland all affect the cardiovascular system. Most indirectly cause changes in salt or water metabolism or affect vascular tone. A summary of the anterior pituitary hormones and their direct and indirect effects on cardiovascular function are listed in Table 54-1. Three disorders can result in major changes in cardiovascular function: hypopituitarism, acromegaly, and disorders of antidiuretic hormone (ADH) secretion.

Hypopituitarism

Hypopituitarism in adults often results from mass lesions arising in the hypothalamus or the pituitary fossa. Growth hormone (GH) deficiency and gonadotropin deficiencies are often present. If the lesion causing the deficit is extensive, thyrotropin-stimulating hormone (TSH) and adrenocorticotrophic hormone (ACTH) secretion may also be impaired. GH deficiency per se does not lead to cardiomyopathy or loss of vascular tone; however, patients with GH deficiency most commonly present with a lack of energy and stamina. Therefore, cardiac output (CO) may not be adequate to sustain peak exercise activity, and endurance may be moderately impaired. Treatment with GH replacement therapy for periods as long as 3 years improves treadmill performance, suggesting that GH deficiency leads to a decrease in exercise tolerance. However, whether this improvement is due solely to GH stimulation of myocardial function

is not clear because GH also increases red cell mass, which could alter exercise tolerance. TSH and ACTH deficiencies lead to changes in cardiovascular function, as discussed herein the sections on hypothyroidism and hypoadrenalism. Loss of gonadotropin secretion, particularly in men, can lead to extremely low testosterone concentrations. This can lead to impaired exercise performance, loss of skeletal muscle mass, and decreased stamina. Replacement with testosterone improves muscle function and exercise performance.

Acromegaly

The sustained hypersecretion of GH by a pituitary tumor can lead to overgrowth of several tissues, and significant cardiovascular changes (Fig. 54-1). Cardiovascular function is an important determinant of morbidity and mortality in untreated acromegaly. The most common deleterious effect is hypertension, present in 50% of inadequately treated patients. Cardiomegaly can be disproportionate to the changes in size that occurs in other organs in severe acromegaly. The severity of the cardiomyopathy correlates with the duration of exposure to high levels of GH. Mean left ventricular (LV) mass can be significantly increased compared with that of normotensive patients. A concentric ventricular hypertrophic cardiomyopathy unassociated with hypertension but associated with long-standing acromegaly commonly results in both diastolic and systolic dysfunction. Histologic evaluation of the myocardium in patients with

Figure 54-1

Acromegaly

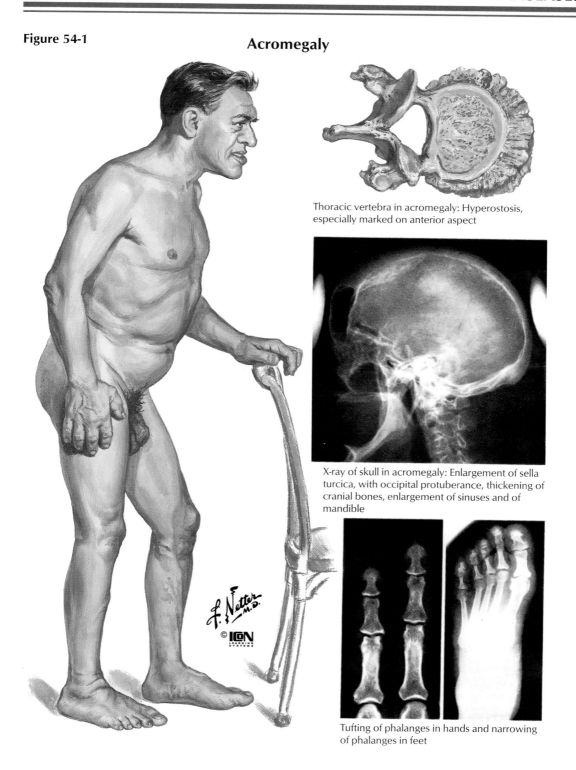

Thoracic vertebra in acromegaly: Hyperostosis, especially marked on anterior aspect

X-ray of skull in acromegaly: Enlargement of sella turcica, with occipital protuberance, thickening of cranial bones, enlargement of sinuses and of mandible

Tufting of phalanges in hands and narrowing of phalanges in feet

Table 54-1
Pituitary Hormones and Their Actions on the Cardiovascular System

Hormone	Direct	Indirect
ACTH	Stimulates cortisol secretion Stimulates aldosterone	Cortisol increases arteriolar tone Aldosterone stimulates Na$^+$ retention and K$^+$ excretion
TSH	Stimulates thyroxine and triiodothyronine synthesis	Thyroxine stimulates HR, pulse pressure, and LV contractility
LH	Stimulates estrogen and testosterone synthesis	Estrogen acts as a vasodilator
ADH	Stimulates water retention, increases plasma volume; acts through a central mechanism to increase vasoconstriction	
GH	Stimulates vasomotor force and LV function	Through IGF-I, it stimulates HR

ACTH indicates adrenocorticotrophic hormone; ADH, antidiuretic hormone; GH, growth hormone; IGF-I, insulin-like growth factor I; LH, lutenizing hormone; LV, left ventricular; TSH, thyrotropin-stimulating hormone.

acromegaly shows interstitial fibrosis, lymphocytic infiltration, and, at times, necrosis. Hypertension in acromegaly is usually mild but can be difficult to manage conventionally. Curing the acromegalic condition is the most effective way to lower BP. Other changes in acromegaly can lead to secondary effects on the cardiovascular system; some patients have sleep apnea that causes chronic recurrent hypoxemia, approximately 25% of patients have diabetes mellitus, and up to 40% of patients have hypertriglyceridemia. Premature mortality is increased in acromegaly, and cardiovascular diseases are the cause of death in 38 to 62% of patients. Normalizing GH and insulin-like growth factor I (IGF-I) levels with conventional treatment restores normal life expectancy, including premature death resulting from cardiovascular disease. Every effort should be made using surgical and medical management to normalize hormone levels in acromegaly.

Disorders of ADH Secretion

Unlike diseases of the anterior pituitary gland, the etiology of ADH deficiency is often hypothalamic lesions (in approximately 60% of patients). Most cases of ADH deficiency are acquired, and many result from attempts to remove the pituitary tumor surgically, damaging the pituitary stalk or the posterior pituitary. Severe ADH deficiency leads to polyuria, polydipsia, and, if untreated, vascular collapse. Hypothalamic causes are usually mass lesions, principally tumors of the hypothalamus, such as craniopharyngioma and dysgerminoma.

Antidiuretic hormone is a potent pressor agent and stimulates direct vasoconstriction of blood vessels. This action is conferred at the level of the regional arterioles, and physiologic concentrations can induce this effect. Loss of ADH leads to a significant increase in serum osmolarity of greater than 295 mOsm/L, with inappropriately dilute urine of less than 300 mOsm/L. The diagnosis is established by detecting abnormally high serum osmolarity with low plasma vasopressin and low urinary osmolarity.

Administering vasopressin quickly reverses the changes in these parameters. Vasopressin acts on the kidney to increase free water clearance. It also affects the brain to maintain central BP control; these brain actions are probably necessary for the maintenance of normal upright BP. The use of ADH antagonists illustrates the importance of endogenous arginine vasopressin for maintaining normal BP.

Syndrome of Inappropriate ADH Secretion

Several central nervous system and primary pulmonary diseases, as well as medications, can cause inappropriately high concentrations of ADH, leading to decreases in plasma osmolarity. In these syndromes, high levels of ADH secretion continue, despite the low osmolarity. Arginine vasopressin concentrations can be increased up to 10 to 20 times greater than normal in this disorder. This does not lead to hypertension per se but rather to water intoxication. Serum sodium continues to decrease because free water clearance is consistently impaired, thus leading to severe hyponatremia, sometimes manifested as seizures. Identification of the source of inappropriate ADH secretion or correction of the underlying lesion is needed for successful treatment. Empiric treatment is undertaken by severely restricting free water intake.

THYROID DISORDERS
Hyperthyroidism

Hyperthyroidism causes some of the most impressive and sustained disarrangements of cardiovascular function. Graves' disease, usually the etiology of hyperthyroidism, is triggered by an autoimmune process whereby thyroid antigens that are recognized as foreign stimulate the production of an autoantibody that stimulates the TSH receptor. The autoantibody directly binds to the TSH receptor on thyroid tissue and stimulates thyroid function. The effect of this stimulating antibody is unremitting and necessitates specific therapy to block thyroid hormone biosynthesis for patients to obtain symptomatic relief.

The symptoms of cardiac dysfunction that occur most commonly in thyrotoxicosis include fatigue, palpitations, dyspnea, heat intolerance, increased sweating, and weight loss. Tachycardia and palpitations occur in 80 to 90% of untreated patients (Fig. 54-2). Elderly patients in whom Graves' disease develops may also experience heart failure. In this circumstance, the failing heart cannot meet metabolic requirements that are raised by increased thyroid hormone, resulting in overt congestive heart failure (CHF). Similarly, angina pectoris may be an important symptom in elderly patients with hyperthyroidism. Myocardial oxygen consumption can increase by as much as 70% in untreated hyperthyroidism. In the presence of fixed coronary lesions, blood flow may be inadequate to supply the increased metabolic need. In younger patients, thyrotoxicosis is associated with increased inotropic and chronotropic effects on the heart. Palpitations and occasionally atrial arrhythmias are the initial symptoms. Atrial fibrillation occurs in 33 to 47% of patients who are older than 60 years. Vascular resistance is decreased by peripheral vasodilation; the net effect is a marked increase in CO, which results in increased oxygen consumption. Peripheral edema is the most common symptom of overt heart failure in Graves' disease, although dyspnea on exertion can also be prominent.

Physical findings include a hyperdynamic precordium, accentuated heart sounds, and often a systolic murmur that can be heard over the precordium. Mitral valve prolapse may be present. Arrhythmias can range from sporadic premature beats to overt atrial fibrillation. Thyrotoxicosis is present in approximately 11% of patients with atrial fibrillation who are aged older than 60 years. Indeed, atrial fibrillation due to either hyper- or hypothyroidism is common enough that thyroid disease must be excluded at an early stage in the evaluation of this dysrhythmia. ECG findings are nonspecific. Heart failure in younger patients is generally reversible with adequate treatment. Whether a distinct thyrotoxic cardiomyopathy exists is debated; however, extensive cardiac remodeling occurs in some patients. This may also be aggravated by long-standing tachyarrhythmias. In elderly patients in whom underlying cardiac abnormalities exist, heart failure can be severe and may trigger atrial fibrillation. Acceleration of angina pectoris can be dramatic in the elderly, and overt myocardial infarction can occur in these patients if left untreated.

The diagnosis is established by elevated serum thyroxine in the presence of a suppressed TSH concentration. Early in the disease, triiodothyronine (T3) is elevated, which is usually followed by a T4 elevation.

Initial treatment with antithyroid drugs blocks thyroid hormone synthesis. Treatment of the thyroid disease does not always restore normal sinus rhythm. If patients fail to undergo remission in a reasonable period on antithyroid drugs,

Figure 54-2

The Hyperthyroid Heart

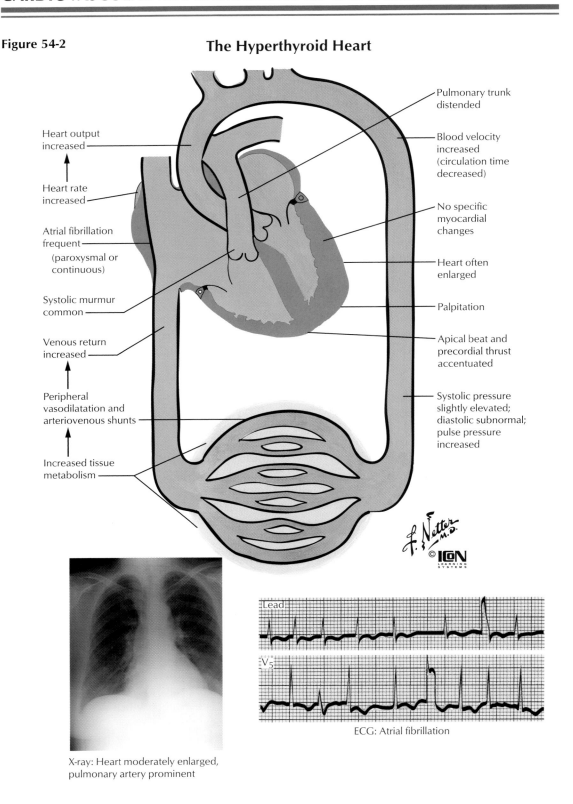

Heart output increased

Heart rate increased

Atrial fibrillation frequent (paroxysmal or continuous)

Systolic murmur common

Venous return increased

Peripheral vasodilatation and arteriovenous shunts

Increased tissue metabolism

Pulmonary trunk distended

Blood velocity increased (circulation time decreased)

No specific myocardial changes

Heart often enlarged

Palpitation

Apical beat and precordial thrust accentuated

Systolic pressure slightly elevated; diastolic subnormal; pulse pressure increased

X-ray: Heart moderately enlarged, pulmonary artery prominent

Lead

V₅

ECG: Atrial fibrillation

or if they do not tolerate these medications, they are generally treated with radioactive iodine. In elderly patients with multiple cardiac complications, initial therapy with radioactive iodine may be indicated. In younger patients, reversal of the thyrotoxic state generally restores the cardiac abnormalities to normal. With elderly patients, however, this may not always be the case. Both sets of patients may benefit initially from therapy with β-blockers, which limits most of the effects of catecholamines on the cardiovascular system that are accentuated in Graves' disease.

Hypothyroidism

Like hyperthyroidism, hypothyroidism is almost always caused by autoimmune thyroid disease. The most common cause of thyroid failure is Hashimoto's thyroiditis, which occurs in approximately 80% of women with hypothyroidism. In this disease, an autoantibody to the thyroid gland is produced that blocks thyroid function and thyroid hormone action. Eventually, this may result in destruction of the thyroid gland as a result of lymphocytic infiltration. However, it occurs over a period of several years, so the onset and the progression are usually insidious and unrecognized by the patient. Hypothyroidism also develops in a significant percentage of patients who receive radioactive iodine treatment for hyperthyroidism. Hypothyroidism can result from a pituitary tumor or other causes of anterior pituitary gland destruction, but these are rare compared to Hashimoto's disease.

Changes in the cardiovascular system are also common in patients with severe long-standing hypothyroidism (Fig. 54-3). These patients have an increase in peripheral vascular resistance, and a decrease in stroke volume causes decreased CO. As a result, mean arterial pressure is largely unaltered, although systolic pressure may decrease, and diastolic pressure may increase. The mechanism of increased vascular resistance is incompletely understood. The pre-ejection and isovolumetric contraction times are prolonged, and the ventricular relaxation rate during diastole is slower. The mechanism of reduced cardiac contractility is multifactorial. T3 stimulates the synthesis of calcium regulatory proteins that have been implicated in the cardiac manifestations of hypothyroidism. Blood

volume is decreased, and pericardial as well as pleural effusions are common. Echocardiographic evidence of pericardial effusion is present in approximately 40% of patients.

Physical examination reveals a slow pulse, diastolic hypertension, and soft first and second heart sounds. Cardiac enlargement, when present, is generally caused by a pericardial effusion. Peripheral edema may be present, but it is generally nonpitting and not caused by heart failure. The ECG may show bradycardia and low voltage with nonspecific ST or T-wave changes. First-degree heart block is also common. Silent myocardial ischemia does occur in patients with known coronary artery disease (CAD). Although symptomatic angina is not common, it can occur during thyroid hormone replacement therapy, particularly in patients with severe long-standing hypothyroidism. Therefore, any elderly patient with severe hypothyroidism should be given extremely low doses of thyroid hormone during the initial treatment phase. Hypothyroidism secondarily results in severe lipoprotein abnormalities, including hypercholesterolemia and low concentrations of high-density lipoprotein (HDL). Increased homocystine levels may also occur in hypothyroidism.

The treatment of hypothyroidism is thyroid hormone replacement therapy. Young patients can tolerate full replacement doses; however, elderly patients with angina need extremely low-dose therapy with gradual incremental increases as tolerated.

PARATHYROID DISORDERS

Hyperparathyroidism is an unusual cause of vascular pathogenesis. However, up to 69% of patients with primary hyperparathyroidism have systolic and diastolic hypertension. Generally, the degree of BP elevation is minimal. The cause of hyperparathyroidism in 85% of patients is a parathyroid hormone-producing tumor, generally leading to hypercalcemia, the most common presenting sign. The hypercalcemic state can cause increased BP, LV hypertrophy, increased heart muscle contractility, and arrhythmias. Calcium deposition in the myocardium, the heart valves, and the coronary arteries occurs in up to 69% of patients with hyperparathyroidism as compared to 17% of age-matched controls.

Figure 54-3

Myxedema Heart

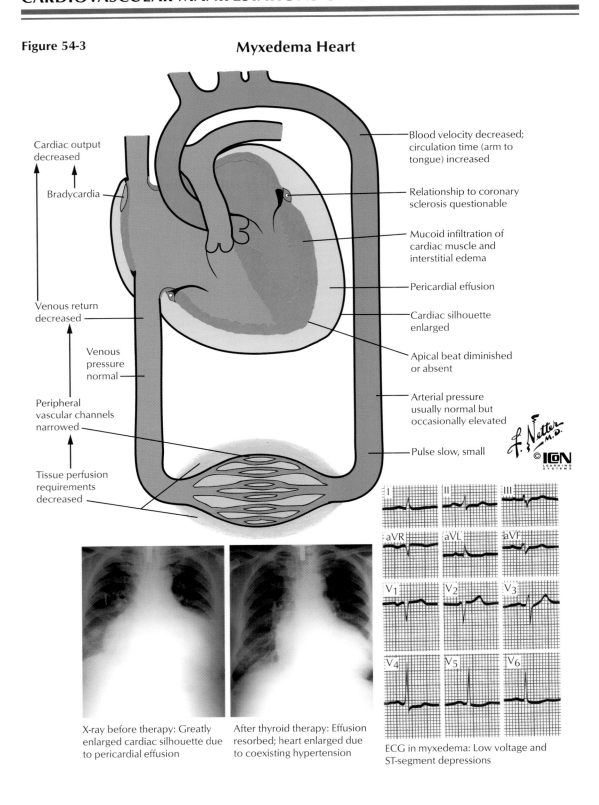

Cardiac output decreased

Bradycardia

Venous return decreased

Venous pressure normal

Peripheral vascular channels narrowed

Tissue perfusion requirements decreased

Blood velocity decreased; circulation time (arm to tongue) increased

Relationship to coronary sclerosis questionable

Mucoid infiltration of cardiac muscle and interstitial edema

Pericardial effusion

Cardiac silhouette enlarged

Apical beat diminished or absent

Arterial pressure usually normal but occasionally elevated

Pulse slow, small

X-ray before therapy: Greatly enlarged cardiac silhouette due to pericardial effusion

After thyroid therapy: Effusion resorbed; heart enlarged due to coexisting hypertension

ECG in myxedema: Low voltage and ST-segment depressions

Valvular calcifications are also noted in substantially more patients than controls. Usually, these changes occur with severe long-standing hyperparathyroidism; however, in recent years, the presentation and treatment of hyperparathyroidism have changed markedly, and probably a much lower percentage of patients have these abnormalities at the time of diagnosis because they are diagnosed and treated much earlier in the course of illness.

ADRENAL DISORDERS

Both glucocorticoid and mineralocorticoid excesses can lead to marked cardiovascular abnormalities.

Cushing's Disease and Syndrome

The most common cause of glucocorticoid excess is from pituitary tumors that overproduce ACTH, termed "pituitary Cushing's disease." Less common but equally deleterious to cardiovascular function are primary adrenal adenomas or ectopic tumors (tumors outside the pituitary) that overproduce ACTH.

Cushing's syndrome, or excess glucocorticoid production, often leads to severe skeletal muscle myopathy because glucocorticoids inhibit protein synthesis in muscle (Fig. 54-4). Because of its rapid onset, dramatic presentation, and severe deleterious effects, Cushing's syndrome is generally treated before a severe atrophic cardiomyopathy develops. Therefore, it is rare for patients to present with cardiomyopathic symptoms. Hypertension is common in Cushing's syndrome because of mineralocorticoid overproduction that leads to increased plasma volume and sodium retention. Severe hypokalemia can cause characteristic ECG changes. Whether atherosclerosis occurs independently of the changes in lipoprotein metabolism from Cushing's syndrome is not clear. However, marked increases in atherosclerosis in patients who receive long-term glucocorticoid therapy of pharmacologic doses have been reported.

Treatment involves removing the cause of the excess cortisol or ACTH. Generally, the cardiovascular abnormalities are easily ameliorated. Patients who receive pharmacologic doses of glucocorticoids for prolonged periods for underlying inflammatory disorders are just as suscepti-ble to cardiovascular complications. Glucocorticoid excess syndromes may precipitate CHF in susceptible patients because the resulting mineralocorticoids can cause salt retention.

Addison's Disease

Hypoadrenalism is most often caused by a primary autoimmune disorder, *Addison's disease*, in which the adrenal glands are progressively destroyed, leading to marked sodium loss with increased serum potassium. Orthostatic hypotension and decreased plasma volume are generally present. Decreased plasma volume can manifest as a reduction in the size of the cardiac silhouette on chest radiographs.

Occasionally, in patients with undiagnosed chronic adrenal insufficiency, acute adrenal insufficiency develops, usually in the setting of underlying physical stress, such as a car accident or a bacterial infection. During stress, healthy individuals secrete up to 10 times more cortisol than under normal conditions. Because this requirement cannot be met in patients with adrenal failure, symptoms of acute adrenal insufficiency develop: nausea or vomiting, hypotension, dizziness, and eventually vascular collapse and shock. The diagnosis should be suspected in patients with these findings and a low serum sodium concentration, a high potassium concentration, and evidence of low plasma volume. It is confirmed by administering 1.0 to 2.0 µg ACTH intravenously and measuring the plasma cortisol level after 30 or 60 minutes. A normal response to the ACTH challenge is a plasma cortisol level of 18 to 20 µg/dL. Treatment consists of fluid replacement and administration of hydrocortisone.

Several recently discovered hormones also have profound effects on salt and water balance and therefore on cardiovascular function. The most important of these are atrial natriuretic peptide (ANP), brain natriuretic peptide (BNP), and endothelin. *Atrial natriuretic peptide* is a 28–amino acid peptide produced by the left atrium. A circulating precursor form, 1-98, is believed to be biologically inactive. Normally, ANP-28 is made solely in the left atrium; however, in pathologic states such as LV hypertrophy or failure, ANP-28 can also be released from the left ventricle. Atrial wall tension is the primary factor that controls synthesis and secretion of

Figure 54-4

Cushing's Syndrome/Mineralocorticoid Hypertension

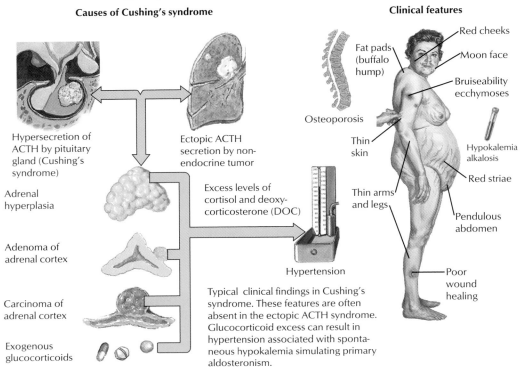

Causes of Cushing's syndrome

Hypersecretion of ACTH by pituitary gland (Cushing's syndrome)

Adrenal hyperplasia

Adenoma of adrenal cortex

Carcinoma of adrenal cortex

Exogenous glucocorticoids

Ectopic ACTH secretion by non-endocrine tumor

Excess levels of cortisol and deoxy-corticosterone (DOC)

Hypertension

Typical clinical findings in Cushing's syndrome. These features are often absent in the ectopic ACTH syndrome. Glucocorticoid excess can result in hypertension associated with spontaneous hypokalemia simulating primary aldosteronism.

Clinical features

Red cheeks

Moon face

Bruiseability ecchymoses

Fat pads (buffalo hump)

Osteoporosis

Thin skin

Thin arms and legs

Hypokalemia alkalosis

Red striae

Pendulous abdomen

Poor wound healing

Possible Mechanisms of Hypertension Associated With Glucocorticoid Excess

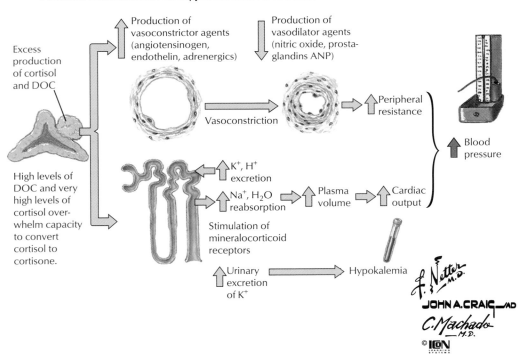

Excess production of cortisol and DOC

Production of vasoconstrictor agents (angiotensinogen, endothelin, adrenergics)

Production of vasodilator agents (nitric oxide, prosta-glandins ANP)

Vasoconstriction

Peripheral resistance

Blood pressure

High levels of DOC and very high levels of cortisol over-whelm capacity to convert cortisol to cortisone.

K^+, H^+ excretion

Na^+, H_2O reabsorption

Plasma volume

Cardiac output

Stimulation of mineralocorticoid receptors

Urinary excretion of K^+

Hypokalemia

F. Netter M.D.

JOHN A. CRAIG—MD

C. Machado—M.D.

© ICON LEARNING SYSTEMS

ANP-28. Therefore, ANP-28 is increased in acute and chronic volume expansion, CHF, and other conditions associated with elevated intra-atrial pressure. Negative feedback regulation of ANP-28 occurs, and volume contraction decreases its synthesis and secretion. ANP-28 binds to specific receptors in the kidney, where it increases capillary permeability, glomerular filtration rate, renal filtration fraction, urinary filtration, and excretion of sodium. This in turn lowers plasma volume and decreases BP. ANP is active in patients with acute renal failure, and its administration improves glomerular function.

A related peptide, *BNP*, is released by neural tissue. BNP is also stored in nerve endings in the atrium. This site of synthesis and release can be stimulated by many of the same stimuli that cause ANP-28 release. In general, BNP is released in response to more chronic changes in plasma volume. BNP acts on the same renal receptors that are activated by ANP and has similar effects on kidney function. Both peptides have direct effects on arterial smooth muscle cells and result in vasodilatation. Administration of ANP or BNP to patients with heart failure results in beneficial effects on plasma volume and CO and recent reports suggest that plasma BNP levels provide useful information in the longitudinal treatment of patients with congestive heart failure (see chapter 17).

Endothelin is a small peptide that is released by vascular endothelium and whose three isoforms are closely related. Endothelin receptors are present on vascular smooth muscle cells, cardiac myocytes, and renal glomerular endothelium. All three peptides are potent vasoconstrictors, an action that can be opposed by the release of nitric oxide. Endothelin is also a potent vascular mitogen. In addition to its effects on blood vessels and kidney function, endothelin also has direct inotropic and chronotropic effects on the heart; however, endothelin also decreases coronary blood flow because of its vasoconstrictive effects. It may act secondarily to decrease plasma volume by increasing ANP and BNP release. In vasculature, the major effect of endothelin seems to be the stimulation of smooth muscle cell contraction.

Mineralocorticoid Disorders

In addition to glucocorticoids, the adrenal gland synthesizes a group of steroids with sodium-retaining activity. Aldosterone is the principal steroid among this group. Unlike cortisol, which is regulated primarily by ACTH secretion, the primary stimulus for aldosterone synthesis is the renin–angiotensin system. In hypovolemic states, the afferent arterioles of the kidney contain specialized juxtaglomerular cells that sense low-flow or low-pressure states in these vessels. This triggers the release of the enzyme renin from the kidney, which is released directly into the blood. Renin acts on angiotensinogen, a peptide precursor that is synthesized in the liver, enzymatically converting angiotensinogen into angiotensin I. Angiotensin I passes through the pulmonary circulation and is cleaved by a second enzyme, termed *angiotensin-converting enzyme* (ACE), to angiotensin II. Angiotensin II is the most biologically active component of the renin–angiotensin system. This peptide, although labile, has direct vasoconstrictive effects on blood vessels and serves as a stimulus to maintain arteriolar tone. This stimulus is particularly important in maintaining normal BP when a person is assuming an upright posture. In addition to its acute effects on arteriolar tone, angiotensin II stimulates the adrenal gland to synthesize aldosterone. This is the principal mechanism for regulating aldosterone production.

Aldosterone acts on the distal convoluted tubule and collecting duct to increase sodium absorption (Fig. 54-5). This effect occurs via a sodium–potassium transporter. For each molecule of sodium that is reabsorbed, the tubular cells secrete a molecule of potassium. Under normal circumstances, this maintains a normal sodium–potassium balance and a normal plasma volume. Expansion of the plasma volume results in increased flow through the renal afferent arterioles, and this signals the system to increase renin, thus maintaining equilibrium.

Another important stimulus that controls the release of angiotensin II is potassium, which directly stimulates angiotensin II and aldosterone production. ACTH can also stimulate aldosterone secretion and is needed to maintain normal rates of aldosterone synthesis.

Figure 54-5

Primary Hyperaldosteronism/ Mineralocorticoid Hypertension

Mechanisms in Primary Aldosteronism

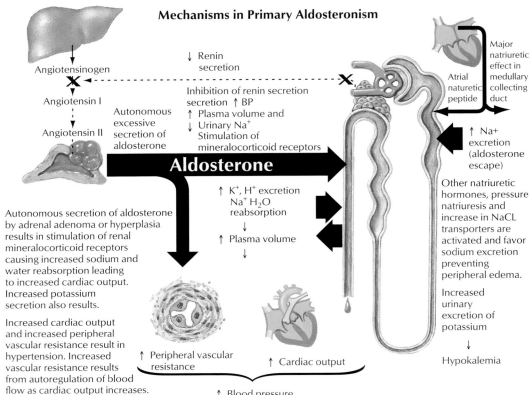

Angiotensinogen

↓ Renin secretion

Major natriuretic effect in medullary collecting duct

Atrial naturetic peptide

Angiotensin I

Angiotensin II

Autonomous excessive secretion of aldosterone

Inhibition of renin secretion ↑ BP
↑ Plasma volume and
↓ Urinary Na^+
Stimulation of mineralocorticoid receptors

Aldosterone

↑ Na^+ excretion (aldosterone escape)

↑ K^+, H^+ excretion Na^+ H_2O reabsorption
↓

↑ Plasma volume
↓

Autonomous secretion of aldosterone by adrenal adenoma or hyperplasia results in stimulation of renal mineralocorticoid receptors causing increased sodium and water reabsorption leading to increased cardiac output. Increased potassium secretion also results.

Increased cardiac output and increased peripheral vascular resistance result in hypertension. Increased vascular resistance results from autoregulation of blood flow as cardiac output increases. Aldosterone may also have direct effects on the vasculature.

Other natriuretic hormones, pressure natriuresis and increase in NaCL transporters are activated and favor sodium excretion preventing peripheral edema.

Increased urinary excretion of potassium
↓
Hypokalemia

↑ Peripheral vascular resistance

↑ Cardiac output

↑ Blood pressure

Clinical Features

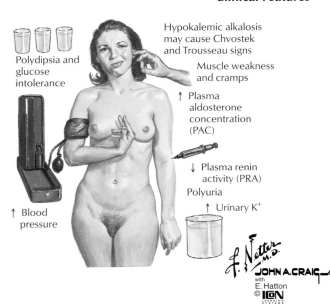

Polydipsia and glucose intolerance

Hypokalemic alkalosis may cause Chvostek and Trousseau signs

Muscle weakness and cramps

↑ Plasma aldosterone concentration (PAC)

↓ Plasma renin activity (PRA)

Polyuria

↑ Urinary K^+

↑ Blood pressure

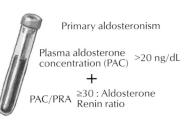

Primary aldosteronism

Plasma aldosterone concentration (PAC)   >20 ng/dL

+

PAC/PRA   ≥30 : Aldosterone Renin ratio

Purpose of serum screen is to distinguish between primary aldosteronism and low renin essential hypertension.

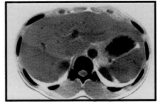

CT or MRI of adrenal glands used to select between surgically remedial APA and idiopathic hyperaldosteronism

f. Netter M.D.
JOHN A. CRAIG—AD
with
E. Hatton
© ICON

Disorders of this system are uncommon causes of hypertension and plasma volume expansion.

Primary tumors in which aldosterone is the principal secretory product are the most common disorder. Approximately 60% of patients with hyperaldosteronism have an aldosterone-producing adenoma. Another 34% have idiopathic bilateral enlargement of the zona glomerulosa in both adrenal glands and overproduce aldosterone, leading to increased sodium retention and potassium excretion. These patients usually present with mild hypertension, evidence of volume overload, and hypokalemia. Other than direct effects on the vasculature, hyperaldosteronism also leads to increased salt retention, which can precipitate CHF in elderly patients.

The diagnosis is usually established by obtaining the ratio of plasma aldosterone to renin. Because renin is suppressed by the increased plasma volume, this ratio is usually greater than 20:1, necessitating further investigation. Adrenal magnetic resonance imaging often confirms the diagnosis of an aldosterone-producing tumor.

Treatment for an adrenal adenoma consists of surgical removal, which cures hypertension in approximately 60% of patients. Patients with bilateral hyperplasia and no tumor respond well to diuretics that directly antagonize the effects of aldosterone, such as spironolactone. ACE inhibitors are effective for CHF in which secondary hyperaldosteronism is present.

Adrenal Medullary Tumors

Pheochromocytoma, while rare, is an important cause of acute changes in BP and cardiovascular function. These tumors are generally unilateral, but they can occur bilaterally and outside the adrenal medulla, for example: anywhere in the sympathetic ganglia chain (Fig. 54-6). The rapid release of norepinephrine or epinephrine from the tumor results in dramatic cardiovascular signs and symptoms.

Because catecholamines work directly on arterioles to cause severe vasoconstriction, the principle signs are rapid elevation of BP, palpitations, sweating, tremulousness, anxiety, and nervousness. Other symptoms can include headache, chest pain, extreme weakness, and fatigue. Acute symptoms occur in approximately 50% of patients and include severe headache, dyspnea, palpitations, sweating, and tremor. Signs that are notable on physical examination are hypertension, postural hypotension, tachycardia, weight loss, increased respiratory rate, and tremor. Postural hypotension occurs in approximately 90% of patients as a result of contraction of intravascular volume. Patients with underlying angina pectoris or heart failure may severely decompensate in the presence of an untreated pheochromocytoma. The diagnosis is established by measuring plasma catecholamines directly, urinary catecholamines, and the principal metabolites of epinephrine and norepinephrine, which include metanephrine.

Administration of β-blockers can precipitate a hypertensive crisis by leaving α activity unopposed. Other medications that can precipitate a crisis include monoamine oxidase inhibitors, tricyclic antidepressants, and catecholamine reuptake inhibitors. The hypertension responds well to α blockers, including dibenzyline. Management is usually surgical unless the tumor is malignant, in which case long-term therapy with α blockers is necessitated.

DIABETES

Both types of diabetes (type I from severe insulin deficiency and type II primarily from insulin resistance combined with insulin deficiency in the later stages) increase the incidence of atherosclerosis. Hypertension is also common in patients with long-standing diabetes, contributing to the high incidence of vascular disease in these patients. Patients in whom even moderate degrees of azotemia develop often become significantly hypertensive as a result of diabetic nephropathy.

In the majority of patients who have long-standing diabetes, significant lipoprotein abnormalities develop. These factors all contribute to extensive vascular disease, which occurs in 80% of patients with long-standing diabetes. As a factor that increases the relative risk for CAD, diabetes ranks second, behind only smoking.

It is difficult to separate the degree of risk conferred by diabetes from that conferred by hyperlipidemia. However, both are independent risk factors. It should be noted that the dyslipidemic syndrome that occurs in diabetes involves a profile that has been demonstrated to confer high risk

Figure 54-6

Pheochromocytoma

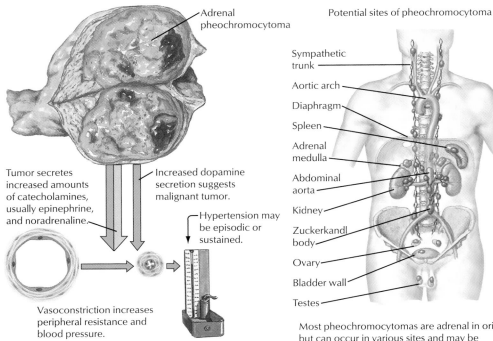

Adrenal pheochromocytoma

Potential sites of pheochromocytoma

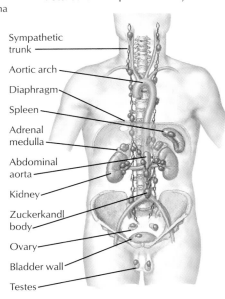

Sympathetic trunk

Aortic arch

Diaphragm

Spleen

Adrenal medulla

Abdominal aorta

Kidney

Zuckerkandl body

Ovary

Bladder wall

Testes

Tumor secretes increased amounts of catecholamines, usually epinephrine, and noradrenaline.

Increased dopamine secretion suggests malignant tumor.

Hypertension may be episodic or sustained.

Vasoconstriction increases peripheral resistance and blood pressure.

Pheochromocytoma is a chromaffin cell tumor secreting excessive catecholamines resulting in increased peripheral vascular resistance and hypertension.

Most pheochromocytomas are adrenal in origin, but can occur in various sites and may be associated with multiple endocrine neoplasia (MEN) syndromes. Most are sporadic, but some are hereditary.

Clinical features of pheochromocytoma

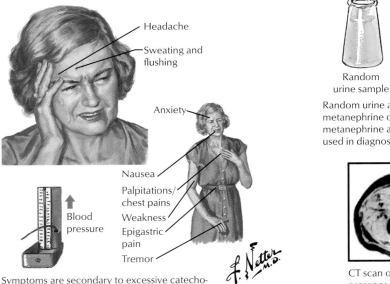

Headache

Sweating and flushing

Anxiety

Nausea

Palpitations/ chest pains

Blood pressure

Weakness

Epigastric pain

Tremor

Random urine sample

24-hour urine sample

Random urine assay for creatine and metanephrine or 24-hour urine assay of metanephrine and free catecholamines used in diagnosis

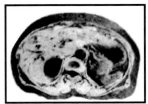

CT scan or MRI may reveal presence of tumor.

Symptoms are secondary to excessive catecholamine secretion and are usually paroxysmal. More than 90% of patients with pheochromocytoma have headaches, palpitations, and sweating alone or in combination.

for CAD. The lipoprotein phenotype common to patients with diabetes is overproduction of triglycerides and apolipoprotein B. Low-density lipoprotein cholesterol (LDL-C) levels are normal in approximately 65% of patients, but the small dense LDL fraction is often elevated, particularly in patients with extreme hypertriglyceridemia and low HDL levels. This is in part due to the activity of hepatic lipase, increased in type II diabetes, which results in processing of LDL to the small dense particles. Likewise, overproduction of triglycerides can lead to some suppression of HDL, particularly the most important subfraction, HDL_2C. This combination of abnormalities comprises the dyslipidemic syndrome that is common in patients with type II diabetes. The presence of nephropathy further aggravates the dyslipidemic syndrome in diabetes. Hypertriglyceridemia and a low HDL level are often accentuated, and dialysis can further worsen the profile.

A low HDL level is a strong predictor of CHD in patients with diabetes. Total triglycerides seem to have some predictive value, although the predictive value of total cholesterol in diabetic individuals is debated. In patients with diabetes, hypertriglyceridemia is much more predictive of CHD than in nondiabetic patients. Intimal–medial thickness is increased in patients with diabetes, suggesting the presence of a diffuse atherosclerotic process, even in those who have not had a myocardial infarction. Case fatality rates after an ischemic event are substantially higher among patients with diabetes.

The low HDL cholesterol (HDL-C) levels in persons with diabetes are associated with poor glycemic control. Improving glycemic control often lowers triglycerides. Treatment with oral hypoglycemic agents or insulin improves both triglyceride and HDL levels. Weight loss also improves both of these parameters.

Not surprisingly, peripheral vascular disease is also widespread in patients with diabetes. Many patients with coronary disease also have disease in the large peripheral arteries. Leg and foot amputations are far more frequent among patients with diabetes. Bilateral occlusive disease in medium-sized arteries below the knee is common in patients with long-standing disease. Medical treatment of peripheral vascular disease generally has limited success. Vascular surgery is the only option for many patients. Indications for Doppler ultrasonography followed by arteriography are pain at rest, ulcerations that fail to heal, and gangrene.

Cardiomyopathy

The possibility of a distinct diabetic cardiomyopathy has been debated. Postmortem examinations reveal cardiomegaly and myocardial fibrosis. Unexplained CHF occurs in a substantial number of patients with diabetes. Echocardiography of those patients with extensive microvascular disease shows compromised cardiac function. Impaired diastolic filling has been demonstrated in a substantial number of patients with type I diabetes with long-standing disease. A delayed increase in the ventricular ejection fraction during dynamic exercise is present in 29% of patients. The pathogenesis seems to be varied and multifactorial.

FUTURE DIRECTIONS

Several new drugs in the latter stages of development may be useful for cardiovascular manifestations of endocrine disorders. Studies of a GH receptor antagonist show that it significantly improves cardiomyopathy in acromegaly. Administration of this drug to patients with severe cardiomyopathy results in significant improvement in LV function. The GH receptor antagonist lowers IGF-I into the normal range and therefore results in ventricular remodeling. An aldosterone receptor antagonist functions similarly to spironolactone but is more potent and may provide patients with heart failure with another treatment option. This drug counteracts the effects of secondary hyperaldosteronism and lowers plasma volume, thus reducing manifestations of heart failure that are secondary to severe hyperaldosteronism.

Several drugs are in development for the treatment of hyperlipidemias. New medications that work to lower LDL-C levels by mechanisms other than the LDL receptor are in phase III development; it is presumed that their administration with a statin will further improve LDL-C levels in patients whose LDL-C level cannot be normalized on statin therapy. No primary drug therapy for low HDL levels has been developed; therefore, a drug that can be administered to patients who have only a low HDL level as a manifestation of their lipid disorder (e.g., most patients with diabetes) is needed. Such a drug would allow treatment of many patients who have no means other than exercise and alcohol ingestion to raise their HDL levels. One such drug is in late-stage development and has been shown to increases HDL levels significantly. Ongoing clinical studies will define the safety and efficacy of this approach and whether this approach will reduce mortality and morbidity rates in patients at risk.

Parathyroid hormone has been approved for treatment of severe osteoporosis. While PTH will be administered in relatively low doses, it will be important to determine whether cardiovascular manifestations of hyperparathyroidism such as hypertension and valvular calcification are exacerbated by this treatment. The role of estrogen replacement therapy in postmenopausal women for decreasing cardiovascular risk may also be resolved. While the combination of estrogen plus progesterone was found to increase cardiovascular risk, no increased risk was noted with estrogen alone. However, whether estrogen therapy alone confers a benefit both in terms of reducing high BP and in terms of atherosclerosis remains unproven. Epidemiologic studies, such as the ongoing Women's Health Study, should help to answer this question as well as the relative benefits of hormone replacement therapy for cardiovascular diseases versus the potential to increase the risk for ovarian and breast cancer.

REFERENCES

Bernstein R, Muller C, Midto K, et al. Silent myocardial ischemia in hypothyroidism. *Thyroid* 1995;5:443–447.

Bravo EL. Pheochromocytoma: New concepts and future trends. *Kidney Int* 1991;40:544–556.

Klein I, Ojamaa K. Thyrotoxicosis and the heart. *Endocrinol Metab Clin North Am* 1998;27:51–62.

Melmed S. Acromegaly. *N Engl J Med* 1990;322:966–977.

Rosen T, Bengtsson BA. Premature mortality due to cardiovascular disease in hypopituitarism. *Lancet* 1990;336:285–288.

Saruta T, Suzuki H, Handa M, et al. Multiple factors contribute to the pathogenesis of hypertension in Cushing's syndrome. *J Clin Endocrinol Metab* 1986;62:275–279.

Stefenelli T, Mayr H, Bergler-Klein J, et al. Primary hyperparathyroidism: Incidence of cardiac abnormalities and partial reversibility after successful parathyroidectomy. *Am J Med* 1993;95:197–202.

Turner RC, Millns H, Neil HA, et al. Risk factors for coronary artery disease in non-insulin dependent diabetes mellitus: United Kingdom Prospective Diabetes Study (UKPDS:23). *BMJ* 1998;316:823–828.

Chapter 55

Connective Tissue Diseases and the Heart

Yevgeniy Sheyn and Mary Anne Dooley

Connective tissue disorders commonly affect the cardiovascular system. The endocardium, myocardium, and pericardium all can be injured through different mechanisms by any rheumatologic disease, and the conducting system is affected by different mechanisms in many different connective tissue disorders. Each disease has a particular pattern of involvement; aortic root disease is more common in ankylosing spondylitis, whereas pericarditis is prevalent in systemic lupus erythematosus (SLE) and rheumatoid arthritis (RA). Direct inflammatory infiltration or fibrosis frequently causes conduction system damage, which often results in bundle branch blocks, AV blocks, and various electrophysiologic abnormalities; these can be associated with myocarditis, especially in polymyositis and scleroderma. In utero conduction damage may be associated with anti-Ro antibody passively transferred from the mother's circulation through placental blood flow. Valvular disease, coronary lesions, and pulmonary hypertension can lead to secondary bundle branch blocks, atrial fibrillation, and other arrhythmias. Autonomous nervous system abnormalities in RA, SLE, and ankylosing spondylitis decrease parasympathetic activity and variability.

Connective tissue abnormalities often correlate with disease severity and activity. However, in some cases, heart disease can be the first sign of rheumatic disease. The availability of sensitive and noninvasive cardiac tests and the recognition of increased cardiovascular mortality in patients with rheumatic disease has prompted cardiovascular injury to be considered frequent and of great clinical significance in rheumatic disorders.

ETIOLOGIES

With rare exception, the etiology of connective tissue diseases remains unclear, but is likely multifactorial. An individual with a susceptible genetic background may encounter an inciting factor such as infection, drugs, or environmental agents. Varying patterns of complement activation, T- and B-cell interactions, or tissue macrophage infiltration may produce inflammation and damage in rheumatic disorders but are also vital to normal blood vessel homeostasis. The factors promoting pathogenic rather than homeostatic effects are unknown and likely involve vascular, fibrotic, and immunologic features. Clinically significant heart disease may be caused by direct immunologic injury to the myocardium, endocardium, or pericardium or to the blood vessels supplying these tissues.

Certain antibodies are associated with cardiac involvement in rheumatologic diseases. Antiendothelial cell antibodies found in SLE, antiphospholipid syndrome (APS), scleroderma, and different forms of vasculitis may correlate with disease activity and severity of involvement. Antimyocardial antibodies are found in lupus and other connective tissue diseases; Ro/SSA and La/SSB antibodies are associated with cardiac involvement and are known to cause neonatal lupus with congenital heart block. Certain major histocompatibility complex haplotypes are associated with increased risk of particular rheumatologic diseases. Classic examples include the link between human leukocyte antigen (HLA) B27 and spondyloarthropathy, as well as HLA DR4 and rheumatoid arthritis. The interaction between inflammatory cells, endothelial injury response, and repair processes may influence clinical expression of vasculitides.

SYNDROMES
Rheumatoid Arthritis

Rheumatoid arthritis, characterized by a symmetric, additive, destructive synovitis, occurs in 1% of most populations. RA manifests with cellular infiltration, often with granulomas containing fibrinoid necrosis and predominantly

Table 55-1
Clinical Cardiac Manifestations in Rheumatologic Disorders

Disorder	Common	Less Common/Rare
Rheumatoid arthritis	Pericarditis Valvular lesions/endocardial involvement	Myocarditis Arrhythmia
SLE	Valvular lesions/endocardial involvement Pericarditis	Myocarditis Arrhythmia
Ankylosing spondylitis	Valvular lesions/endocardial involvement Aortitis Arrhythmia	Pericarditis Myocarditis (very uncommon)
Inflammatory myopathy	Myocarditis Arrhythmia	Valvular lesions Pericarditis
Scleroderma	Cardiomyopathy with microvascular dysfunction Arrhythmia	Pericarditis Valvular disease
APS	Valvular lesions/endocardial involvement CAD	

APS indicates antiphospholipid syndrome; SLE, systemic lupus erythematosus.

mononuclear inflammation. Its most frequent cardiac manifestations are pericarditis and valvular heart disease (Fig. 55-1). In nodular seropositive RA, valvular abnormalities and pericarditis are more common than in RA without extra-articular pathology. Pericarditis can present as thickening with or without a pericardial effusion in up to 60% of patients on echocardiography, though it is clinically evident in less than 5% (Tables 55-1 and 55-2). Pericardial fluid is exudative and typically serosanguinous or hemorrhagic with high acidity. Adhesions and loculations are common, often making pericardiocentesis ineffective. A significant proportion of patients with clinical pericarditis have constriction or tamponade with a grave prognosis. These patients, under some circumstances, may benefit from surgical pericardiectomy.

Despite frequent occurrence (up to 70%), valvular lesions are rarely symptomatic. Pathologically, endocardial lesions can be caused by fibrosis, nonspecific inflammation, or, rarely, by rheumatoid granulomas. Aortic or mitral insufficiency and aortic root dilation are the most common manifestations.

Myocarditis is rarely clinically evident but can be associated with various arrhythmias. Vasculitis of coronary vessels has been described, though the clinical significance is unknown.

Systemic Lupus Erythematosus

Lupus (SLE) is a multisystem autoimmune disorder characterized by the production of autoantibodies and a striking female predominance in the reproductive years (10:1 female:male). Autoantibodies and immunocomplexes with complement activation are the major factors in cardiovascular injury. In SLE, as in RA, the pericardium and endocardium are most commonly involved. Serositis in SLE is often associated with disease flare. Pericarditis is clinically evident in up to 20%, with prevalence on echocardiography or autopsy reaching 60%. Tamponade occurs in 1 to 2% of patients; constriction is even less common. Analysis of pericardial fluid is similar to that of RA, with high

Figure 55-1

Extra-articular Manifestations
in Rheumatoid Arthritis

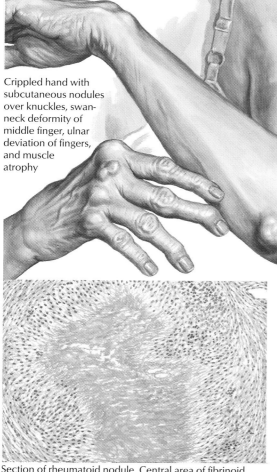

Crippled hand with subcutaneous nodules over knuckles, swan-neck deformity of middle finger, ulnar deviation of fingers, and muscle atrophy

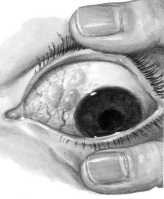

Nodular episcleritis with scleromalacia

Subcutaneous nodule just distal to olecranon process, and another in olecranon bursa

Section of rheumatoid nodule. Central area of fibrinoid necrosis surrounded by zone of palisading mesenchymal cells and peripheral fibrous tissue capsule containing chronic inflammatory cells.

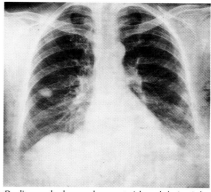

Radiograph shows rheumatoid nodule in right lung. Lesion may be misdiagnosed as carcinoma until identified by biopsy or postsurgical pathologic analysis.

acidity and increased polymorphonuclear cells.

Asymptomatic valvular involvement, usually mitral and aortic, is found in up to 70% of patients by transesophageal echocardiography (TEE). Libman and Sacks first described endocarditis in SLE. It consists of thrombotic–fibrinous clusters with proliferating endothelial cells, edema, and areas of necrosis. Immunoglobulins and complement deposits are often detected. The etiology of the lesions commonly found on the posterior mitral leaflet, advancing to the papillary muscles and chordae tendinae, is controversial. APS may influence valvular pathology of patients with SLE. Acute valvular insufficiency can lead to hemodynamic instability and require surgical correction. Libman-Sacks endocarditis

Table 55-2
Prevalence of Cardiac Involvement in Rheumatologic Disorders

Disorder	Noninvasive Tests	Autopsies
Rheumatoid arthritis	Pericarditis 20–60% (echo) Valvular lesions/endocardial involvement 30–40% (echo)	Pericarditis 20–60% Valvular lesions/endocardial involvement 30–50%
SLE	Pericarditis 20–60% (echo) Valvular lesions/endocardial involvement 30–40% (TTE), 53–73% (TEE)	Pericarditis 40–70% Valvular lesions/endocardial involvement 10–70% Myocarditis 8–81%
Ankylosing spondylitis	Aortic regurgitation 3–10% (echo) Conduction abnormalities 22–50% (ECG/Holter)	Aortic root thickening and dilation 20–60%
Inflammatory myopathy	Arrhythmias 30–50% (ECG/Holter) Pericarditis 10–25% (echo) Valvular lesions/endocardial involvement 8–20% (echo)	Myocarditis 30%
Scleroderma	Arrhythmias 50% (ECG) Pericarditis 30–50% (echo)	Cardiomyopathy 12–89% Pericarditis 30–70% (echo)

Echo indicates echocardiogram; SLE, systemic lupus erythematosus; TEE, transesophageal echocardiogram; TTE, transthoracic echocardiogram.

may predispose patients to infectious endocarditis. Lupus endocarditis also can cause various thromboembolic phenomena requiring anticoagulation, especially when associated with APS.

Conduction abnormalities, including AV block, bundle branch block, and dysautonomia, are found in up to 10% of patients with SLE; most are not clinically significant. In pregnant patients with SLE, screening for Ro/SSA/La/SSB antibodies is usually performed to estimate risk for neonatal lupus with congenital heart block. Only Ro/La antibodies are widely used in clinical practice to prevent and manage neonatal heart block. In mothers with positive antibodies, follow-up with fetal echocardiography between 17 and 24 weeks of gestation is recommended.

Another important manifestation of SLE, myocarditis, is clinically evident in less than 10% of patients but can cause severe systolic dysfunction. Myocarditis often develops with other organ involvement and may occur early in the course of SLE. Treatment with steroids or cytotoxic agents can be lifesaving.

New data suggest that homocysteine plays a significant role in the pathogenesis of coronary artery disease (CAD) in lupus and that folic acid supplementation should be considered in SLE patients with hyperhomocysteinemia.

Seronegative Spondyloarthropathies

Seronegative spondyloarthropathies (Spas) include ankylosing spondylitis, psoriatic arthritis, Reiter syndrome, and arthritis associated with inflammatory bowel disease. All of these conditions are associated with HLA B27, although the association is strongest in ankylosing spondylitis, which is considered the prototype Spa. The pathophysiology of cardiac lesions in Spa is characterized by mononuclear cellular inflammation with progressive fibrosis. Ankylosing spondylitis most commonly affects valvular structures and the aortic root and may present with aortic insufficiency (Fig. 55-2). Aortic thickening, dilation with some degree of aortic regurgitation, or both are found in 82% of patients with ankylosing spondylitis by means of TEE. Aortic insufficiency is associated with longstanding disease and older age. Aortic dissection may also occur. Progressive aortic dilation in ankylosing spondylitis may respond to corticosteroid and cytotoxic therapy. Mitral valve pathology is less common than aortic and is characterized by leaflet fibrosis or regurgitation. Diastolic dysfunction and left ventricular hypertrophy in ankylosing spondylitis are often consequences of valvular lesions. Conduction disturbances are usually caused by myocardial fibrosis. Bradyarrhythmias are associated with HLA B27 spondyloarthropathies.

Dermatomyositis and Polymyositis

Noninvasive tests show cardiac lesions in more than 70% of patients with dermatomyositis or polymyositis have inflammatory myopathies, but only 10% are symptomatic (Fig. 55-3). Dermatomyositis typically presents with vascular damage and microvasculopathy, whereas polymyositis shows significant T-cell muscle infiltration, and the initial presentation can be due to myocarditis. The pathology observed ranges from active inflammation to fibrosis and small vessel disease. Myocardial involvement can cause conduction abnormalities and life-threatening ventricular arrhythmias. Myocarditis often correlates with skeletal muscle disease. Pericarditis is usually asymptomatic but is detected by echocardiography in up to 25% of patients; valvular lesions are rare.

Scleroderma

Systemic sclerosis (SS) or *scleroderma* is a chronic connective tissue disorder characterized by inflammation, fibrosis, and degenerative changes in the skin, blood vessels, joints, skeletal muscle, and internal organs, such as the gastrointestinal tract, kidney, and lungs. SS is classified into limited scleroderma with skin changes prominently in distal extremites and diffuse scleroderma (Fig. 55-4). Scleroderma leads to immune-mediated endothelial injury with extensive fibrosis, producing a bland, intimal hyperplasia associated with tissue ischemia. It commonly involves the cardiovascular system. Mortality as a result of cardiopulmonary causes is more common than that from renal disease. The proposed mechanism for the myocardial injury in scleroderma is a myocardial Raynaud's phenomenon with microvascular dysfunction. Endomyocardial

biopsy shows myocardial fibrosis, contraction band necrosis, and myocytolysis in up to 80% of patients. Pericardial pathology is detected clinically in approximately 10% of patients, often being detected during life by echocardiography, or after death at autopsy. A high frequency of arrhythmias and electrophysiologic abnormalities is characteristic of scleroderma; life-threatening ventricular tachycardia and sudden cardiac death are described in patients with systemic sclerosis. Diastolic dysfunction often begins early in the disease and frequently precedes other cardiac abnormalities. Limited scleroderma less commonly affects the heart. Noninvasive methods in asymptomatic patients with limited SS detect approximately 10% each of arrhythmia, pericarditis, and cardiomyopathy. Pulmonary disease, particularly pulmonary hypertension, contributes significantly to cardiac abnormalities in limited and diffuse systemic sclerosis.

Vasculitis

The *vasculitides* are a heterogenous group of disorders characterized by destruction of blood vessels by several methods: direct antibody attack, immune complex formation, and cell-mediated and anticytoplasmic antibody-associated mediators. Systemic vasculitis embraces a range of relatively rare disorders, with an estimated incidence of 19.8 per million cases. When the inflammatory process compromises critical organ function, patients can experience severe symptoms or death. The prognosis for these disorders has improved, with more patients surviving for longer periods and a greater likelihood of remission. Treatment with corticosteroids and immunosuppressive drugs has proven to be beneficial.

Classification of these disorders is based on several features: the size of the blood vessels involved, the knowledge of disease pathophysiology, and the patterns of organ involvement. Large vessel arteritis includes giant cell arteritis (GCA) and Takayasu's vasculitis. They primarily affect the aorta and main branches but may also involve the coronary arteries. Medium vessel vasculitis includes polyarteritis nodosa (PAN) and Kawasaki disease that occurs predominantly in children. Although PAN typically spares the heart, Kawasaki disease causes coronary artery

Figure 55-2

Ankylosing Spondylitis

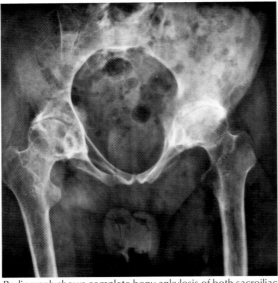

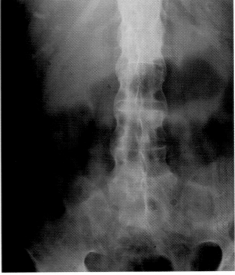

Radiograph shows complete bony ankylosis of both sacroiliac joints in late stage of disease.

"Bamboo spine." Bony ankylosis of joints of lumbar spine. Ossification exaggerates bulges of intervertebral discs.

Complications

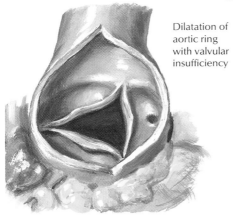

Dilatation of aortic ring with valvular insufficiency

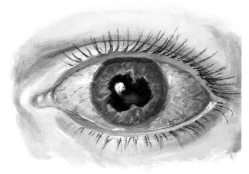

Iridocyclitis with irregular pupil due to synechiae

aneurysms in up to 25% of untreated patients and pericardial effusions in 30%, along with myocarditis and valvular regurgitation. Small vessel vasculitis adversely affects a variety of tissues and organs, including the skin, lungs, and kidneys. These diseases can be among the most devastating of rheumatic diseases.

SECONDARY CAUSES OF CARDIOVASCULAR DISEASE

Cardiac pathology in connective tissue disorders is common because the heart is often affected by the medications used to treat rheumatic disorders and by secondary or confounding conditions. Long-term steroid use increases

Figure 55-3

Polymyositis/Dermatomyositis

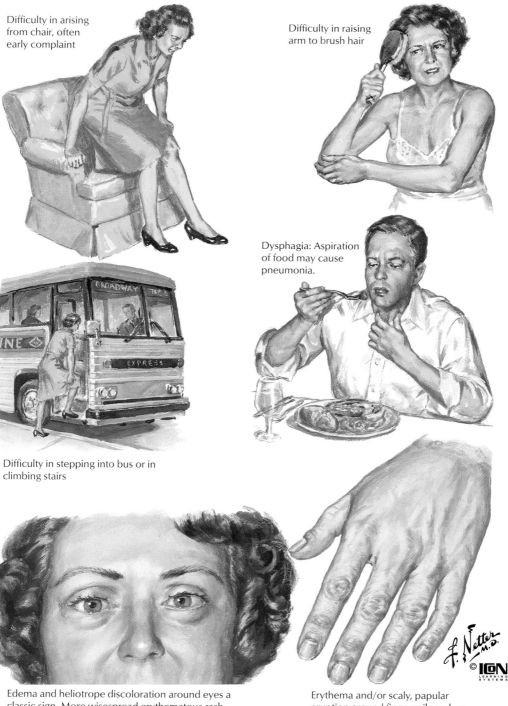

Difficulty in arising from chair, often early complaint

Difficulty in raising arm to brush hair

Dysphagia: Aspiration of food may cause pneumonia.

Difficulty in stepping into bus or in climbing stairs

Edema and heliotrope discoloration around eyes a classic sign. More wisespread erythematous rash may also be present.

Erythema and/or scaly, papular eruption around fingernails and on dorsum of interphalangeal joints

Figure 55-4

Progressive Systemic Sclerosis (PSS; Scleroderma); Lung Involvement

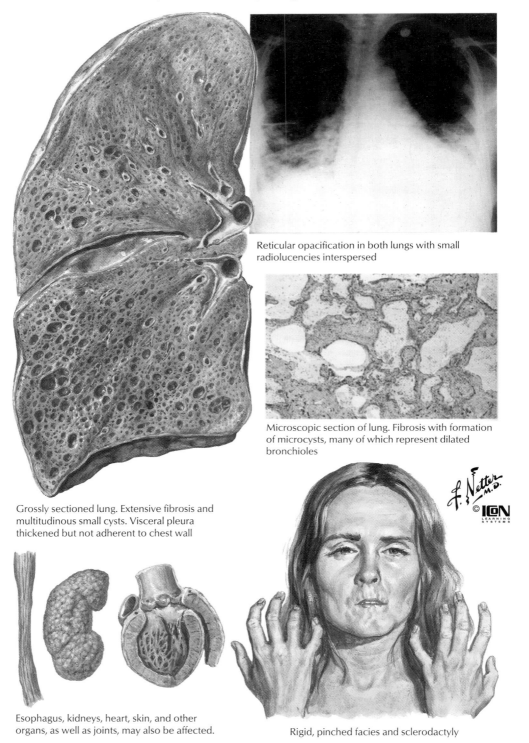

Reticular opacification in both lungs with small radiolucencies interspersed

Microscopic section of lung. Fibrosis with formation of microcysts, many of which represent dilated bronchioles

Grossly sectioned lung. Extensive fibrosis and multitudinous small cysts. Visceral pleura thickened but not adherent to chest wall

Esophagus, kidneys, heart, skin, and other organs, as well as joints, may also be affected.

Rigid, pinched facies and sclerodactyly

the risk of hypertension, diabetes, and advanced atherosclerosis, which are all associated with cardiovascular disease (see chapter 54). Methotrexate elevates homocysteine levels, an established risk factor for CAD.

Chronic inflammation with longstanding RA can lead to amyloidosis that may cause restrictive cardiomyopathy and conduction abnormalities. Felty's syndrome (splenomegaly with cytopenia in patients with RA) can cause severe immunodeficiency and theoretically can affect the pathogenesis of endocarditis on already damaged valves. Renal involvement in SLE is often associated with hypertension contributing to cardiomyopathy. Many patients with rheumatic disease have limited physical activity; sedentary lifestyle may contribute to CAD and increase the risk of thromboembolic complications. Chronic inflammation, one of the key features of rheumatologic diseases, can directly lead to accelerated atherosclerosis and CAD. Pulmonary fibrosis, common with dermatomyositis or scleroderma, may be complicated by pulmonary hypertension leading to right-sided heart failure. APS and pulmonary hypertension, commonly associated with many rheumatologic conditions, warrant additional discussion.

With or without coexistent rheumatic disease, APS is associated with recurrent arterial and venous thrombosis and fetal loss and may lead to significant morbidity and mortality. The two most common cardiac manifestations of APS are valvular lesions and coronary disease, including MI in 4% of patients. APS causes endothelial cell activation and atherosclerosis. It may play a significant role in the pathogenesis of CAD in patients without classic cardiac risk factors. Endocardial damage usually occurs in the mitral valve. The titer of anticardiolipin antibodies often correlates with the frequency and degree of valvular involvement.

Pulmonary hypertension is an important cause of morbidity and mortality in connective tissue disorders, especially in scleroderma and dermatomyositis as a result of arterial and myocardial effects of the disease process. Pulmonary hypertension can also occur as a result of pulmonary embolism secondary to a hypercoagulable state, most commonly in association with APS. Pulmonary hypertension decreases cardiac tolerance, with a significant increase in right ventricular pressures. This is probably why, in scleroderma, electrophysiologic abnormalities and arrhythmias originate mainly from the right side of the heart, in contrast to what happens in patients with CAD, in which left-sided arrhythmias predominate. Normalization of pulmonary pressure frequently improves cardiac function, especially if done early in the course of disease.

Coronary artery disease in connective tissue disorders causes significant cardiac mortality and morbidity in RA, SLE, and ankylosing spondylitis. The risk of premature CAD in SLE is dramatically increased. Rates of MI and death secondary to coronary disease in premenopausal women with lupus are 50 times higher than in controls. CAD is often silent, and, if it causes pain, patients tend to ignore it, overwhelmed with multiple musculoskeletal symptoms. For these reasons, patients with SLE, RA, and other rheumatologic disorders warrant aggressive diagnosis and treatment of CAD, even though at first glance these patients would seem to have a low risk based solely on their age (tending to be young) and in the absence of classic risk factors.

DIFFERENTIAL DIAGNOSIS

Underlying infection and malignancy should be excluded. Hepatitis B and C, possibly associated with cryoglobulinemia, can lead to medium or small vessel vasculitis. Subacute bacterial endocarditis, Lyme disease, and other chronic infections, such as tuberculosis and brucellosis, may complicate the diagnosis. Multiple myeloma may present similarly to polymyalgia rheumatica (PMR); however, the presence of paraproteins on serum and urine electrophoresis, as is found in multiple myeloma, can distinguish the two. Amyloidosis can mimic GCA, including jaw or arm claudication, and should be excluded. Other disorders, including cholesterol emboli, may mimic rheumatic disease.

Hypothyroidism, spondyloarthropathy, polymyositis, and, rarely, amyotrophic lateral sclerosis can present similarly to PMR. Polymyositis usually produces muscle weakness and, less commonly, muscle pain. Elevated creatine kinase (CK), electromyography, and muscle biopsy findings confirm the diagnosis. Temporal artery biopsy results are abnormal in up to 80 to 90% of GCA. As the lesions of GCA are patchy, this biopsy specimen should be 3 to 5 cm optimally, and, if results are negative, a contralateral biopsy should be considered to yield accurate results. The temporal artery biopsy shows fragmentation of the elastica lamina, luminal narrowing, intimal edema, granulomas with multinucleated giant cells, and monocellular infiltrate. Magnetic resonance angiography (MRA) and angiography can assess vessel involvement, particularly large vessel involvement in GCA. Noninvasive vascular studies identify only patients with pronounced luminal narrowing.

Drug-induced connective tissue disorders include vasculitis and lupus. Drug-induced lupus may be associated with a number of medications, most frequently procainamide or hydralazine. More recently, minocycline, alpha interferon, and tumor necrosis factor (TNF) α–blockers have been associated with antinuclear antibody (ANA) and anti-dsDNA antibody formation. Other agents such as propylthiouracil may induce lupus-like disorders or vasculitis.

Laboratory Abnormalities

There is no single diagnostic test for connective tissue diseases. The diagnosis relies on the history in combination with appropriate physical findings and laboratory and pathologic results. The American College of Rheumatology and other expert groups have established criteria that are useful clinically. ANA testing is a sensitive screening test because more than 95% of patients with lupus have positive test results when the test is performed using a substrate containing human nuclei such as HEP-2 cells. However, a positive test result for ANA is not specific for SLE. Positive ANA may occur in healthy individuals, especially in older adults; 15% of patients aged older than 65 years have an ANA, usually at a low titer. It is important to exclude other autoimmune diseases, particularly those associated with a positive ANA, such as RA, Sjögren's syndrome, scleroderma, isolated Raynaud's syndrome, or organ-specific autoimmune diseases, including idiopathic thrombocytopenic purpura, autoimmune thyroid disease, and hemolytic anemia. Family members of patients with SLE often manifest an ANA without development of clinical SLE features. Many autoimmune diseases have overlapping features, making strict classification difficult. The presence of antibodies to the Sm antigen, although found in only 30% of patients, is pathognomonic for SLE. Rheumatoid factor is elevated in most patients with RA, although it can be positive in various infectious, autoimmune, and oncologic disorders. Acute-phase reactants such as ESR and C-reactive protein (CRP) are often elevated in rheumatologic conditions and may correspond with flare of disease. An exception is the Spas, in which these test results may remain normal despite active disease.

DIAGNOSTIC APPROACH

The diagnosis of rheumatologic diseases relies on the history and physical examination. Antibody tests and acute-phase reactants should be considered in the context of clinical presentation, and diagnosis cannot rely on serologic tests alone. When evaluating cardiac involvement by rheumatologic condition, specific cardiac enzymes are used with some limitations; the MB fraction of CK can often be elevated from muscle injury and repair in myositis and may be less specific in these settings. CK and troponin levels are frequently normal in lupus cardiomyopathy, necessitating further investigation. Myocardial biopsy can help differentiate the pathologic process, particularly to distinguish active inflammation from fibrosis before instituting cytotoxic therapy with potentially serious side effects.

MANAGEMENT AND THERAPY

The choice of immunosuppressive medications to treat underlying rheumatologic disorders is often based on clinical experience, with few large randomized trials available. These medications include azathioprine, cyclophosphamide, methotrexate, mycophenolate, and mofetil, among others. Therapy of cardiac disease includes conservative or surgical management of heart failure, ischemia, arrhythmia, and valvular disease, as discussed in other chapters.

Symptomatic pericarditis is managed with nonsteroidal anti-inflammatory drugs and steroids; in cases of hemodynamic compromise, close monitoring is warranted. Pericardial tamponade occurs more commonly than previously recognized in rheumatic diseases. Pericardiocentesis can be life saving but is effective for only a short time and, although initial relief may result, pericardiocentesis rarely "cures" pericardial tamponade associated with collagen vascular diseases. Cardiothoracic surgery may be necessary for a pericardial window. Resistant pericardial effusions or constrictive pericarditis may necessitate pericardiectomy.

High-dose steroids and cytotoxic therapy are effective in SLE and inflammatory myocarditis. Myocardial biopsy often confirms inflammation and excludes other cardiomyopathy causes. Management of valvular lesions secondary to rheumatologic conditions is similar to other valve defects, except that inflammatory valvular lesions tend to progress more rapidly, necessitating close follow-up. Pulmonary hypertension therapy includes administration of calcium channel blockers, prostacyclin analogs, and endothelin antagonists.

Anticoagulation is used in most patients with significant pulmonary hypertension. Symptomatic APS often necessitates lifelong anticoagulation treatment.

FUTURE DIRECTIONS

The main cause of CAD in connective tissue disorders remains atherosclerosis. The role of coronary vasculitis is widely debated, and the precise molecular mechanisms remain to be elucidated. The role of immunocomplexes, APS, pro-oxidant environment, inflammation, and dyslipidemia are under investigation. Monoclonal antibodies to C5, TNF, and IL-1 are used more often in rheumatologic conditions; case reports showing the efficacy of biologic agents to treat endocarditis and myocarditis associated with connective tissue disorders have been published. Genetic and immunologic studies will continue and offer hope in earlier diagnosis and institution of appropriate therapy for these patients. New biomarkers of disease activity may arise; serum IL-6 levels may be more sensitive in detecting inflammation than are CRP or ESR.

REFERENCES

American College of Rheumatology. Available at: http://www.rheumatology.org/.

Classification Criteria for Rheumatic Diseases. Available at: http://www.rheumatology.org/research/classification/index.asp.

European League Against Rheumatism. Available at: http://www.eular.org/.

Klippel JH, ed. *Primer on the Rheumatic Diseases.* 12th ed. Atlanta: Arthritis Foundation; 2001.

Koopman WJ, ed. *Arthritis and Allied Conditions.* 14th ed. Philadelphia: Lippincott Williams & Wilkins; 2001.

National Institute of Arthritis and Musculoskeletal and Skin Diseases. Available at: http://www.niams.nih.gov/.

Rheuma 21st. Available at: http://www.rheuma21st.com/who_index.html.

Ruddy S, ed. *Kelley's Textbook of Rheumatology.* 6th ed. Philadelphia: WB Saunders; 2001.

Chapter 56

Cardiac Tumors

Hanna Kelly and Mark A. Socinski

Until the second half of the twentieth century, cardiac tumors were diagnosed almost exclusively at autopsy, and no treatment options existed for those rare instances of antemortem discovery. Advances in cardiac imaging—principally echocardiography—and the advent of cardiopulmonary bypass (CPB) made cardiac tumors treatable. Primary tumors of the heart are rare and typically benign. Because of their critical location, however, they are almost never clinically benign. Secondary tumors are more common, particularly in the setting of metastatic disease.

Data from autopsy series place the incidence of primary heart tumors around 0.02%, of which 75% are benign. Myxomas represent half of all benign primary tumors. Approximately 95% of primary malignant neoplasms are sarcomas.

Secondary malignant neoplasms have an autopsy incidence of 1%, commonly in the setting of widely disseminated metastatic disease. Of patients who die of metastatic cancer, 20% have some degree of cardiac involvement, frequently asymptomatic. The cancers most likely to involve the heart are lung, breast, lymphoma, and myeloid leukemia. Melanoma has a predilection for the heart—cardiac involvement is present in 50% of patients with advanced disease.

CLINICAL PRESENTATION

The clinical presentation of a cardiac tumor depends on its location. Tumors located on the endocardial surface, such as myxomas, usually present with various embolic phenomena or symptoms of valvular obstruction. Tumors that arise within the myocardium are more likely to produce arrhythmias and disruption of the conduction system. Diffuse myocardial infiltration can result in heart failure from systolic or diastolic dysfunction. Epicardial and pericardial involvement may manifest as pain, effusion, or heart failure in the form of constriction or tamponade. Myxomas also present with systemic illness: principally, constitutional symptoms and hematologic abnormalities.

DIFFERENTIAL DIAGNOSIS

Primary tumors of the heart should be considered in the differential diagnosis of embolic phe-

nomenon, valvular disease, heart failure, and arrhythmia. Infectious endocarditis may present in a manner virtually indistinguishable from that of a cardiac tumor—particularly myxomas that present with constitutional symptoms—and is a key component of the differential diagnosis. Other diagnostic considerations include atrial or ventricular thrombosis, endocrine derangements—particularly thyroid disease—and rheumatologic diseases such as lupus and systemic vasculitis.

Embolization

Emboli from cardiac tumors result from dislodgement of adherent thrombus or tumor fragments. The clinical picture from embolization of multiple small fragments may resemble small-vessel vasculitis or endocarditis. Larger emboli cause stroke and infarction of other viscera. Tumor emboli should always be included in the differential diagnosis of embolic phenomena. Hence, a pathologist should review all resected emboli.

Obstruction

Valvular obstruction by a tumor produces symptoms similar to valvular heart disease. Because atrial tumors are more common, obstruction of the AV valves mimicking mitral and tricuspid stenosis is typical. Classic symptoms caused by tumor obstruction can be distinguished from valvular disease by the paroxysmal and positional nature of obstruction by a mobile tumor.

Arrhythmia

Infiltration of the myocardium and irritation by an endocardial tumor can cause supraventricular and ventricular arrhythmias. Disruption of the conduction system may cause all degrees of AV nodal block. Sudden cardiac death is a risk; however, this presentation is unusual in patients with cardiac tumors.

DIAGNOSTIC APPROACH

Transthoracic echocardiography is the standard means by which many cardiac tumors are diagnosed. Echocardiography is most sensitive in the diagnosis of endocardial tumors and least well suited for diagnosing tumors originating from the pericardium. Transesophageal echocardiography allows further evaluation of right-sided tumors and better characterization of questionable masses seen on transthoracic cardiac imaging. MRI can further assess pericardial disease and the extent of cardiac involvement of a tumor.

PRIMARY BENIGN CARDIAC TUMORS

The majority of benign cardiac tumors are myxomas; however, a wide variety of tumors arise within the heart (Table 56-1).

Myxoma

Myxomas are the most common primary cardiac neoplasm, accounting for 50% of all benign cardiac tumors (Fig. 56-1). There is a female predominance of 2:1 to 3:1, and the median age of presentation is 50 years, though they do occur at all ages. Myxomas arise in the left atrium 75% of the time, usually on the interatrial septum near the fossa ovalis. Right atrial myxomas account for 20% of tumors (Fig. 56-2). The balance of myxomas occur in either ventricle and, in rare cases, on the cardiac valves. The majority of myxomas (>90%) is solitary.

There is, however, an autosomal dominant, familial myxoma syndrome: the Carney complex. Affected individuals demonstrate variable phenotypic expression but have in some form at least two of the main features: heavy facial freckling, endocrine hyperactivity (i.e., Cushing syndrome), both myxomatous and nonmyxomatous endocrine neoplasia, noncardiac myxomas (typically breast and skin), and cardiac myxomas. Cardiac myxomas associated with the Carney complex have an equal male to female ratio, occur at a younger age (mean age of diagnosis, 25 years), and are more likely to be multiple or

Table 56-1
Histologic Distribution of Primary Benign Cardiac Neoplasms

	Percentage of Tumors	
Benign Tumor	Adults	Children
Myxoma	45	15
Lipoma	21	0
Papillary fibroelastoma	16	0
Rhabdomyoma	2	45
Fibroma	3	15
Hemangioma	5	5
Teratoma	1	13
Other	6	6

With permission from Allard MF, et al. Primary cardiac tumors. In: Goldhauber, S, Braunwald, E, eds. *Atlas of Heart Diseases.* Philadelphia: Current Medicine; 1995:15.1–15.22.

ventricular and to recur after resection. Linkage analysis has mapped gene loci to both 17q22-17q24 and 2p16. Analysis of four unrelated kindred has implicated mutations in the protein kinase A type I-α regulatory subunit as a causative factor in the Carney complex tumors in these families.

Myxomas originate from multipotent mesenchymal cells. Grossly, they are gelatinous, pedunculated tumors with an average size of 4 to 8 cm. The tumor surface may be friable or smooth. A smooth surface is associated with systemic signs and symptoms. Friable tumors are more likely to present with embolization.

Clinical Presentation

Myxomas typically present with embolization, obstruction, and arrhythmia but may also cause systemic signs and symptoms similar to those of collagen vascular disease, endocarditis, vasculitis, and malignant neoplasms. Typical signs and symptoms are fever, anorexia and weight loss, malaise, arthralgia, increased ESR and C-reactive protein, leukocytosis, thrombocytopenia, hypergammaglobulinemia, and anemia. The mechanism by which myxomas cause systemic manifestations is not fully understood; however, many myxomas produce IL-6, which leads to hepatic synthesis of acute-phase reactants and

Figure 56-1

Heart Tumors

Myxoma. Characteristically originating from interatrial septum and almost filling L. atrium; R. ventricular hypertrophy

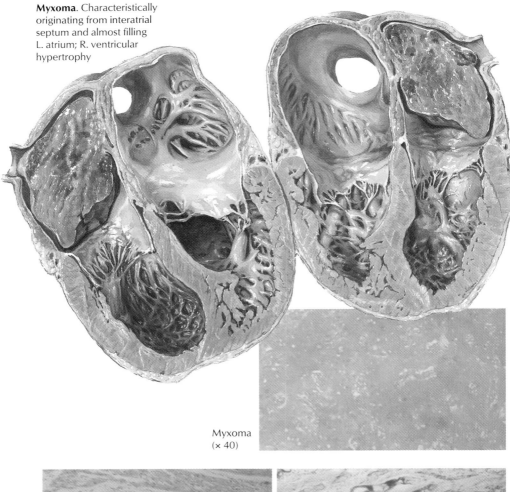

Myxoma
(× 40)

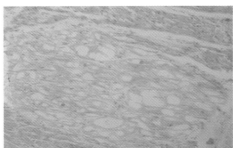

Rhabdomyoma (× 40)

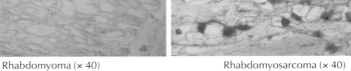

Rhabdomyosarcoma (× 40)

Figure 56-2
Echocardiographic Image of a Right Atrial Myxoma

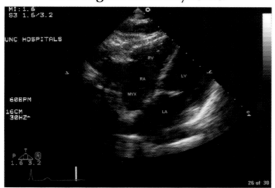

Image courtesy of Dr. Alan Hinderliter

Echocardiographic image of a right atrial tumor. At the time of resection, the tumor was found to be a myxoma.

subsequent systemic illness. These constitutional symptoms usually resolve with resection of the tumor. In addition, antimyocardial and antineutrophil antibodies may be found at presentation, and then resolve with removal of the myxoma. It is unclear whether these antibodies play a pathologic role or are an incidental finding. Of these presentations, cardiac symptoms are the most common, followed equally by embolization and constitutional symptoms.

The physical examination may direct the differential diagnosis toward myxoma. In the setting of left atrial tumors, auscultation may reveal a tumor plop that occurs in early diastole and is often confused with an S_3 gallop. Mitral diastolic rumbles and mitral systolic murmurs may be present.

Management and Therapy

Given the propensity of myxomas to cause serious, life-threatening complications, resection using CPB should be performed on an urgent or semiemergent basis. Only in rare instances should myxomas be managed nonoperatively, principally in persons with a short life expectancy and serious comorbid conditions. In these instances, it is prudent to initiate life-long anticoagulation. With thorough resection of the tumor, including a wide resection of the myocardium at the base of the tumor stalk, recurrence is rare. Patients with sporadic myxomas have a recurrence rate of 1%, whereas patients with familial myxoma syndrome have a 7 to 22% rate of

recurrence or second myxoma. Recurrence is usually within the first 4 years after resection. Follow-up echocardiography is recommended for patients with Carney complex, but may not be necessary following surgical resection of a sporadic myxoma, given the high cure rate.

Lipoma

Lipomas are the second most common benign primary cardiac tumor. Lipomas can occur at any age and have no gender predeliction. They are encapsulated tumors usually located in the epicardium or the myocardium, though endocardial tumors do occur. Most are small and asymptomatic, but they occasionally grow to massive proportions. Symptoms, when present, are usually referable to effusion or infiltration of the myocardium, with subsequent arrhythmia or conduction defect. Large, asymptomatic lipomas are sometimes found incidentally on the chest radiograph or during echocardiography. Similar to all cardiac tumors, symptomatic lipomas may necessitate at least partial resection.

Lipomatous hypertrophy warrants consideration because the treatment is drastically different than that for the presence of a circumscribed lipoma. Lipomatous hypertrophy of the atrial septum is a relatively common nonneoplastic condition characterized by massive fatty infiltration of the interatrial septum. This condition is found in obese persons 50 years or older—typically older than 65 years. Septal thickening may be marked: up to 7 cm. Atrial tachyarrhythmias are common. The only effective therapy for lipomatous hypertrophy is weight loss.

Fibroma

Fibromas are tumors of childhood, occurring in the ventricular myocardium, often located in, or extending to, the intraventricular septum. Symptoms result from involvement of the conduction system, which may lead to sudden death. Because they are located in a crucial part of the myocardium, resection is usually not feasible. Cardiac transplantation may be the only treatment option.

Rhabdomyoma

Rhabdomyoma is the most common benign cardiac tumor type of infancy and childhood. Multiple tumors usually occur and appear within the ventricular myocardium, though some project into the ventricular cavity. One third of rhabdomyomas are associated with tuberous sclerosis. It is not uncommon for tumors to regress spontaneously; as a result, conservative management is generally recommended.

Papillary Fibroelastoma

Papillary fibroelastomas are the most common "tumors" of the cardiac valves. These are not truly neoplasms, but avascular growths resembling a sea anemone because of their frondlike arms around a central base of attachment. The pathogenesis of fibroelastomas is unknown. They may originate from endocardial trauma and organization of thrombus. Previously diagnosed only at autopsy, they are seen frequently during echocardiography and may be confused with valvular vegetations. Fibroelastomas occur most commonly on the ventricular surface of the aortic valve or on the atrial surface of the mitral valve. They are usually small (measured in millimeters), solitary, and mobile. Fibroelastomas usually do not cause valvular dysfunction, but can be a source of embolization to the coronary or cerebral vasculature; therefore, management focuses on preventing emboli via anticoagulation or removal.

Pericardial Cysts

Also known as Springwater cysts, these benign, non-neoplastic, congenital cysts are usually located in the right costophrenic angle outside the pericardial cavity. The diagnosis is usually made by an incidental finding of a mass on chest radiograph or echocardiograph. No intervention is recommended except in the rare case of symptomatic cysts that cause chest pains, dyspnea, cough, or tachycardia.

PRIMARY MALIGNANT CARDIAC TUMORS

Approximately 25% of primary cardiac neoplasms are malignant. A majority (95%) are sarcomas (Table 56-2). Lymphomas, although rare, represent most of the remaining primary tumors of the heart. The incidence of primary lymphoma may be increasing given the number of people with impaired cellular immunity from AIDS and organ transplantation.

Table 56-2
Histologic Distribution of Primary Malignant Cardiac Tumors

	Percentage of All Tumors	
Malignant Tumor	Adults	Children
Angiosarcoma	33	0
Rhabdomyosarcoma	21	33
Mesothelioma	16	0
Fibrosarcoma	11	11
Lymphoma	6	0
Osteosarcoma	4	0
Thymoma	3	0
Neurogenic sarcoma	3	11
Leiomyosarcoma	1	0
Liposarcoma	1	0
Synovial sarcoma	1	0
Malignant teratoma	0	44

With permission from Allard MF, et al. Primary cardiac tumors. In: Goldhaber, S, Braunwald, E, eds. *Atlas of Heart Diseases.* Philadelphia: Current Medicine; 1995: 15.1–15.22.

Sarcoma

Sarcomas are aggressive tumors that present most commonly in the third to fifth decades of life with signs and symptoms of cardiac dysfunction from obstruction or myocardial infiltration. The most common sites of involvement, in descending order, are the right atrium, the left atrium, the right ventricle, the left ventricle, and the interventricular septum. Sarcomas grow quickly, and affected individuals usually have a rapidly downhill course. Death within a few weeks or months is typical; rarely do patients survive for a few years after diagnosis. Death is a result of heart failure from myocardial replacement by tumor, tumor obstruction, or distant metastasis. At the time of death, 75% of individuals have distant metastases; the lungs, thoracic lymph nodes, mediastinal structures, and vertebral column are the sites most commonly affected. Sarcomas derive from mesenchymal cells and, therefore, may present as subtypes. The two most common sarcomas are angiosarcoma and rhabdomyosarcoma.

Angiosarcoma, including Kaposi sarcoma, is the more common subtype. There is a 2:1 male predominance. Angiosarcomas typically arise in the right atrium. Malignant cells form vascular channels and a continuous precordial murmur may be present. Death is a result of obstruction of the right side of the heart, either by tumor or thrombus, or from rupture of the sarcoma with hemopericardium and subsequent hemorrhagic tamponade. Rhabdomyosarcomas have no chamber predilection and often involve multiple sites. Death is a result of obstruction or infiltration of the myocardium.

The prognosis for all morphologic subtypes of cardiac sarcoma is poor. Resection with adjuvant chemotherapy is usually not an option because the degree of cardiac involvement precludes adequate operative resection. The role of preoperative chemotherapy is not defined.

Lymphoma

Primary cardiac lymphoma is almost exclusively non-Hodgkin and is usually a diffuse B-cell lymphoma. It comprises about 1% of all cardiac tumors and 0.5% of extranodal non-Hodgkin lymphomas. It usually presents with effusion, heart failure, or arrhythmia. Because typically it is rapidly progressive, most patients die before initiation of chemotherapy. Patients who survived to undergo standard therapy with CHOP (cyclophosphamide, doxorubicin, vincristine, prednisone) or an equivalent regimen still had a median survival of only 7 months in recent studies. In addition, immediately after initiation of chemotherapy, tumor necrosis may cause death as a result of refractory heart failure and refractory ventricular tachycardia.

Pericardial Mesothelioma

Pericardial Mesothelioma is a rare tumor that occurs in young people, presenting as constriction or pericardial effusion with or without tamponade. Primary cardiac mesotheliomas typically involve the parietal and the visceral pericardium, but usually do not invade the myocardium. Suspected links to asbestos exposure are insufficiently substantiated. Chemotherapy and radiation therapy may give temporary improvement in a palliative setting, but the disease is uniformly and rapidly fatal.

SECONDARY MALIGNANT CARDIAC TUMORS

Metastatic disease to the heart is much more common than primary neoplasia. At autopsy, 1% of unselected persons had secondary tumors of the heart. In comparison with primary cardiac neoplasms, which are rare but never clinically silent, only 10% of secondary tumors are symptomatic. The majority of symptomatic individuals have pericardial metastases. A diagnosis of cardiac metastasis should be considered when patients with known malignant neoplasms have any new onset of cardiac dysfunction (heart failure, arrhythmia, cardiomegaly, among others). Rarely, cardiac involvement, in the form of a large pericardial effusion, is the initial presentation of a malignant process.

Cancers that most commonly metastasize to the heart are lung, breast, lymphoma, and leukemia (Fig. 56-3). Lung and breast cancers involve the heart via local spread and subsequent infiltration of the pericardium, causing effusion and constriction. Lung cancer can invade the left side of the heart through the pulmonary artery, and its adrenal metastases can invade the right side of the heart via the inferior vena cava. In myeloid leukemias, leukemic cells are seen on light microscopy infiltrating between myocytes. As a result, thrombocytopenic patients may experience fatal hemorrhages into the myocardium or the pericardial space. Non-Hodgkin lymphomas have a high rate of cardiac involvement—up to 25% of patients may have grossly visible epicardial or myocardial disease—but it is often clinically silent. Melanomas are rare and comprise a small portion of secondary cardiac tumors. However, for unknown reasons, melanoma has the highest rate (approximately 50%) of cardiac metastasis. It may involve any site and is often present in all four chambers of the heart. Most cancers, with the exception of primary central nervous system malignant neoplasms, can metastasize to the heart; therefore, cardiac involvement should be considered if consistent symptoms arise.

MANAGEMENT AND THERAPY

Echocardiography and surgical technique allow for prompt diagnosis and safe, curative operative intervention for most benign tumors.

Figure 56-3

Metastic Tumors of the Heart

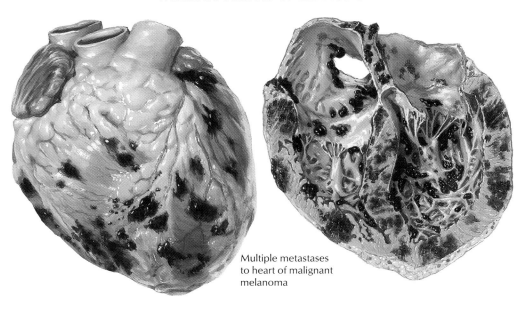

Multiple metastases
to heart of malignant
melanoma

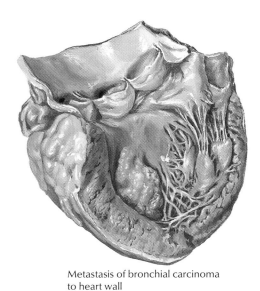

Metastasis of bronchial carcinoma
to heart wall

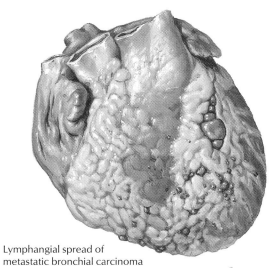

Lymphangial spread of
metastatic bronchial carcinoma

Unfortunately, malignant disease of the heart is uniformly fatal; resection for cure is impossible and, with the exception of lymphoma, these tumors are not sensitive to chemotherapy or radiotherapy. Cardiac transplantation has been suggested as an alternative curative method for benign tumors in critical locations that preclude resection and for unresectable malignant disease without evidence of metastasis. Micrometatstatic disease is a valid concern, however, given the suppression of cell-mediated immunity that must follow cardiac transplantation. In children with inoperable benign tumors, transplantation is likely the only option.

FUTURE DIRECTIONS

Successes in the treatment of cardiac tumors have stemmed from modern imaging and surgical techniques. Cardiac transplantation is a compelling treatment method in the young and healthy. Demand already significantly outstrips the supply of organs, however, and transplantation is unlikely to become a prevalent solution.

Future progress in the realm of cardiac tumors will likely come from our increasing knowledge about the molecular and genetic pathology of this diverse group of neoplasms. Recent identification of gene loci implicated as causative in the Carney complex may lead to genetic testing. Affected family members could be identified early and receive targeted surveillance and treatment before complications arise. Drugs designed to target specific cell-surface markers and proteins within tumors have had excellent early success in other neoplasms—most notably the tyrosine kinase inhibitor imatinib used to treat chronic myelogenous leukemia. As researchers develop a better understanding of the molecular derangements of these tumors, similar targeted, tumor-specific therapy may become available.

REFERENCES

Aisner J, Antman K, Belani C. Pleura and mediastinum. In: Abeloff MD, ed. *Clinical Oncology.* 2nd ed. New York: Churchill Livingstone; 2000:1478–1516.

Burke A, Virmani R. *Atlas of Tumor Pathology. Tumors of the Heart and Great Vessels.* Washington, DC: Armed Forces Institute of Pathology; 1996:231.

Lam KY, Dickens P, Chan ACL. Tumors of the heart. A 20-year experience with review of 12485 consecutive autopsies. *Arch Pathol Med* 1993;117:1027–1031.

Pinede L, Duhaut P, Loire R. Clinical presentation of left atrial cardiac myxoma. A series of 112 consecutive cases. *Medicine* 2001;80:159–172.

Roberts WC. Primary and secondary neoplasms of the heart. *Am J Cardiol* 1997;80:671–682.

Rolla G, Bertero MT, Pastena G, et al. Primary lymphoma of the heart. A case report and review of the literature. *Leukemia* Res 2002;26:117–120.

Salcedo EE. Cardic tumors: Diagnosis and management. *Curr Prob Cardiol* 1992;17:73–129.

Shapiro LM. Cardiac tumors: Diagnosis and management. *Heart* 2001;85:218–222.

Chapter 57

Pulmonary Hypertension and Thromboembolic Disease

Timothy C. Nichols and Thomas R. Griggs

By definition, pulmonary blood flow equals peripheral blood flow under normal conditions, but at much lower driving hemostatic pressures. This reflects, to a major degree, the large cross-sectional area of the pulmonary capillary bed and the ability of small pulmonary vessels to respond to numerous vasodilatory and vasoconstrictive influences. This system has enormous reserve, so major challenges, such as surgical excision of lung tissue or advanced pulmonary disease, are usually tolerated with minimal symptoms. However, when the pulmonary circuit is suddenly occluded, as with massive pulmonary thromboembolism, or when chronic disease overwhelms the anatomic and physiologic reserve, the result can be severe disability and/or death.

ETIOLOGY AND PATHOGENESIS

Pulmonary artery pressure (PAP), the pressure that must be sustained by the right ventricle, is equal to pulmonary flow (PF) times pulmonary vascular resistance (PVR) plus pulmonary venous pressure (PVP) [PAP = (PF × PVR) + PVP]. Normal PAP in systole is 18 to 25 mm Hg and mean PAP is 12 to 16 mm Hg. The normal pulmonary venous pressure is about 6 to 10 mm Hg, giving a total pressure gradient that averages about 5 mm Hg. Pulmonary hypertension, defined as systolic pressures above 30 mm Hg and mean pressures above 20 mm Hg, can occur as a result of reduced pulmonary arterial flow, increased pulmonary arterial resistance, or increased pulmonary venous pressure.

Table 57-1 shows the physiologic and pathologic influences that can affect PAP. Chronically increased blood flow as a cause of symptomatic pulmonary hypertension was classically seen in patients with congenital heart disease and left-to-right shunting of blood before the development of techniques to repair these lesions surgically. This is less common today because these shunts have been routinely treated surgically, early in life, for more than three decades.

The various disease processes that cause pulmonary hypertension by increasing pulmonary vascular resistance can be divided into four categories. First, pulmonary artery resistance increases when the arteries are occluded, as with massive pulmonary embolism, or when the vascular tree is decreased in area by virtually any process that destroys lung parenchyma. Second, there are processes that can constrict or obliterate the resistance vessels of the lung. Long-term high-flow states, chronic hypoxia, as with altitude or sleep apnea, certain toxins, and chronic thromboembolism and in-situ thrombosis, are commonly implicated in pulmonary hypertension. Portal hypertension and HIV infection also cause obliterative pulmonary microvascular disease. Primary pulmonary hypertension (PPH), a devastating disease with a genetically determined etiology in a proportion of patients, is characterized by proliferative and necrotic obliteration of the pulmonary microvasculature. Third are diseases that cause increased blood viscosity. The fourth are processes that increase intrathoracic pressures, such as COPD and positive-pressure ventilation. Finally, any process that obstructs blood flow in the pulmonary veins or at the level of the left atrium will necessitate increased upstream pressures. The most common of these include left ventricular (LV) dysfunction from any cause and mitral valve disease (either mitral regurgitation or mitral stenosis).

Pulmonary thromboembolism occurs when thrombi migrate from the deep veins of the legs through the right side of the heart into the pulmonary arteries. The fundamental pathophysiology, therefore, is that promoting thrombosis in the peripheral veins. This may involve one or a

Table 57-1
Factors That Can Increase PAP

Factor	Cause
Increased pulmonary blood flow	Left-to-right shunts Exercise Severe anemia
Increased pulmonary vascular resistance Pulmonary artery disease	Pulmonary embolism Loss of pulmonary parenchyma COPD Fibrosis Sarcoidosis Scleroderma Surgery Neoplastic infiltration Inflammatory infiltration Kyphoscoliosis
Arteriolar vasoconstriction or obliteration	Alveolar hypoxia Altitude COPD Hypoventilation/sleep apnea Acidosis Response to chronic high flow (congenital heart disease) Response to chronic left atrial hypertension (mitral stenosis) Toxic substances (weight loss drugs) HIV infection Cocaine Portal hypertension PPH
Increased blood viscosity	Polycythemia vera Leukemias
Increased intrathoracic pressure	COPD Positive end-expiratory pressure
Pulmonary venous hypertension or obstruction	Left atrial hypertension Mitral stenosis LV failure, systolic and diastolic Pulmonary venous thrombosis Pulmonary venoocclusive disease (sickle cell syndrome and others) Cor triatriatum Left atrial myxoma

PAP = (pulmonary flow × pulmonary vascular resistance) + pulmonary venous pressure.
PAP indicates pulmonary artery pressure; PPH, primary pulmonary hypertension; LV, left ventricular.

combination of factors, including venous stasis, hypercoagulability, and injury to the vessel wall. These three factors are termed *Virchow's triad*. Stasis and turbulence around venous valves promote platelet deposition, platelet aggregation, and formation of a fibrin thrombus. The thrombi formed include entrapped red blood cells, giving the thrombus a deep red color. Pulmonary thrombi, when recovered intact from the lungs at autopsy, most often are a "cast" of the peripheral vein complete with the impressions formed by the venous valves (Fig. 57-1).

CLINICAL PRESENTATION

The symptoms of pulmonary hypertension are common to multiple etiologies. Most patients with mild or moderate pulmonary hypertension are asymptomatic. Initial symptoms may be dyspnea with exertion, fatigue, and exertional intolerance. Many patients experience chest pain. Syncope suggests severe pulmonary hypertension with marked limitation of flow reserve. Hemoptysis is not common, but in some patients, it is dramatic and fatal. The clinical presentation depends in part on the chronicity of the process. Adaptive changes in the right ventricle allow patients with chronic pulmonary hypertension to sustain near-systemic levels of pressures with minimal symptomatic effects. However, acute increases in pulmonary pressure, as with massive pulmonary thromboembolism, cause immediate overt distress and, in many cases, collapse and death (Fig. 57-2).

Two keys to the diagnosis of pulmonary hypertension are a high degree of suspicion raised by the clinical history and physical findings that suggest RV failure and systemic congestion (see also chapter 1). Increased PAPs are reflected in elevated RV systolic and, later, diastolic pressures. As a result of chronically elevated RV systolic and diastolic pressure, the geometry of the right ventricle is altered, usually sufficiently to render the tricuspid valve incompetent. Inspection of the jugular veins, in this case, demonstrates a visible "meniscus" at a level of more than 10 cm above the right atrium. As a rule, this means filling of the deep neck veins above the clavicle is visible with the patient sitting upright. Tricuspid regurgitation creates a prominent *v* wave in the jugular venous pulse. Significant tricuspid regurgitation can also often be appreciated as pulsation of the liver. Less common and subtler physical findings with pulmonary hypertension are a right ventricular (RV) precordial heave, an RV third heart sound, and increased intensity of the pulmonic component of the second heart sound.

Pulmonary thromboembolism should be suspected in patients with acute dyspnea, chest pain, syncope, or hemoptysis. Risk factors that reinforce clinical evidence of pulmonary thromboembolism include advanced age, immobilization, and history of recent surgery, malignant neoplasms, and thromboembolic disease. Recent travel, obesity, pregnancy, or a family history of thrombosis are also clues. In some seriously ill or debilitated patients, the presentation may be subtle, with events such as mental status changes, fever, or otherwise unexplained hypoxemia leading ultimately to the diagnosis.

DIFFERENTIAL DIAGNOSIS

Table 57-1 lists the numerous causes of pulmonary hypertension. The most common are chronic LV dysfunction with or without valve disease and chronic lung diseases. These are usually recognized by history, and treatment is focused on the primary disease. It is only after all potential causes of secondary pulmonary hypertension are excluded that the diagnosis of PPH is considered. A major diagnostic challenge is to identify acute or recurrent pulmonary thromboembolism, because antithrombotic treatment can be lifesaving.

The diseases of the pulmonary circulation are divided into acute and chronic classifications. Chronic illnesses are rarely an immediate danger to the patient, except at the end-stage of the disease process. Pulmonary thromboembolism is the most common and immediately life-threatening acute process. Therefore, the physician must remain vigilant for this diagnosis in patients with evidence of impairment of the pulmonary circulation.

PULMONARY THROMBOEMBOLISM
Diagnostic Approach

In the acute setting, the traditional initial diagnostic tests are ECG and chest radiography. While neither is diagnostic of acute pulmonary thromboembolism, both can yield clues to the

Figure 57-1

Deep Venous Thrombosis

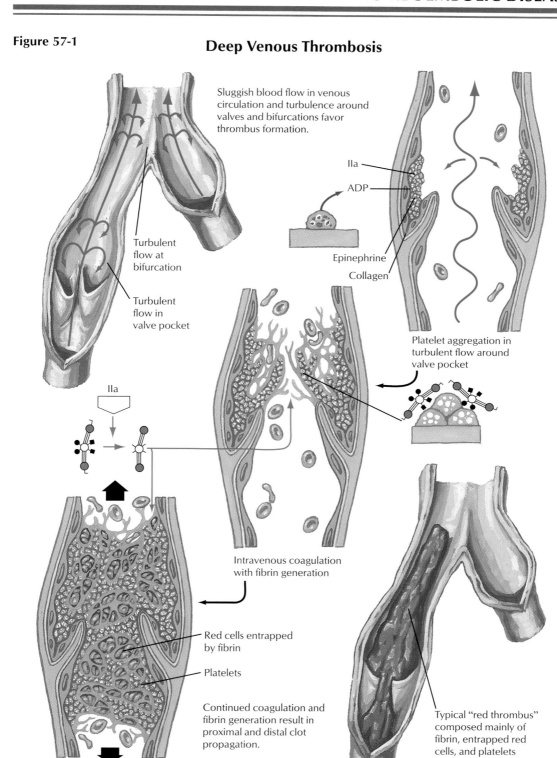

Sluggish blood flow in venous circulation and turbulence around valves and bifurcations favor thrombus formation.

IIa

ADP

Epinephrine

Collagen

Turbulent flow at bifurcation

Turbulent flow in valve pocket

Platelet aggregation in turbulent flow around valve pocket

IIa

Intravenous coagulation with fibrin generation

Red cells entrapped by fibrin

Platelets

Continued coagulation and fibrin generation result in proximal and distal clot propagation.

Typical "red thrombus" composed mainly of fibrin, entrapped red cells, and platelets

JOHN A.CRAIG—AD
©ICON

Figure 57-2

Massive Embolization

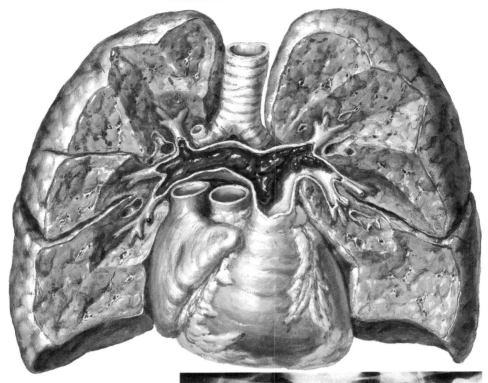

Saddle embolus completely occluding R. pulmonary artery and partially obstructing main and left arteries

X-ray film showing dense shadow of R. pulmonary artery with increased luminescence of peripheral lung fields

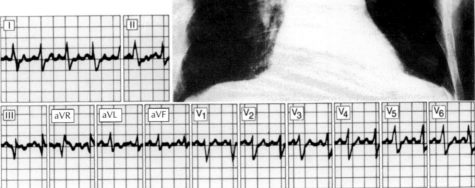

Characteristic electrocardiographic findings in acute pulmonary embolism. Deep S_1; prominent Q_3 with inversion of T_3; depression of ST segment in lead II (often also in lead I) with staircase ascent of ST_2; T_2 diphasic or inverted; R. axis deviation; tachycardia

astute clinician. Classic changes of acute massive pulmonary embolism (PE) on ECG are sinus tachycardia, right axis deviation and new incomplete right bundle branch block, producing a pattern sometimes described as "S1-Q3-T3" (Fig. 57-2, lower). Unfortunately, this pattern is noted in a minority of patients with documented pulmonary embolism. More commonly, the ECG shows only nonspecific ST and T wave changes or is normal.

Chest films in patients with acute pulmonary thromboembolism may be normal or show atelectatic segments and patchy infiltrates. Rarely, pleural-based infiltrates associated with pulmonary infarction are documented.

Transthoracic echocardiography can demonstrate RV hypokinesis and dilation. Doppler measures of tricuspid regurgitant velocity are reliable estimates of pulmonary systolic pressure (see also chapter 31). These data help establish the hemodynamic effects of acute PE. Rarely a thrombus in transit in the right ventricle can be imaged. However, there are many causes of RV dysfunction and tricuspid regurgitation other than PE and, conversely, echocardiograms may be normal in patients with small emboli.

Recently, transesophageal echocardiography has been used to visualize large pulmonary artery thromboemboli. However, this technique is insensitive for visualization of distal emboli, and technical challenges exist with imaging certain parts of the pulmonary arteries. ECG, chest radiography, and echocardiography are, therefore, too insensitive and nonspecific to reliably diagnose or exclude acute pulmonary thromboembolism. Despite a remarkable evolution in the technology of diagnosis of PE, the importance of clinical judgment continues.

The most venerable diagnostic procedure for suspected PE is ventilation/perfusion (V/Q) lung scanning. The consensus in most of the literature is that normal lung scan results essentially exclude the diagnosis of PE. Unfortunately, PE is commonly a complication of other disease processes affecting the lungs, meaning that few ventilation scans are normal in those patients evaluated. Therefore, in only a minority of patients with suspicious clinical presentation but no PE is the V/Q scan normal. Scans that show multiple segmental or lobar defects in

flow with normal ventilation, on the other hand, reflect PE in 85 to 90% of cases (with PE documented subsequently by pulmonary angiography). However, scans of many patients with suspected PE are neither normal nor high probability. These intermediate, or indeterminate, probability scans are not diagnostic and must be supplemented to confirm or exclude PE. A highly specific diagnosis is necessary because the only alternative is empiric treatment with full anticoagulation, a treatment that carries the risk of serious complications.

Recently, the place for V/Q scanning in evaluation of suspected PE has been challenged by contrast-enhanced spiral CT of the chest. Spiral CT is highly sensitive for emboli in the proximal pulmonary arteries and large branches; however, emboli in small, distal arteries are not reliably detected. Hence, the sensitivity of CT varies. Nonetheless, CT has gained widespread acceptance because it has a much higher degree of specificity than V/Q scanning, reliably demonstrates the large emboli that are probably the most clinically important, and can document an array of alternate diagnostic possibilities. Moreover, CT scans are generally available more quickly and more easily interpreted than V/Q scans.

The gold standard for PE diagnosis is pulmonary arteriography. This invasive procedure involves placement of a catheter into the pulmonary artery and injection of contrast media (Fig. 57-3). Although it is recommended as the initial follow-up test for patients with intermediate-probability lung scans, the technical challenge and perceived risk of the procedure have prevented its wide application for this purpose.

Another alternative that has gained consideration is the use of venous ultrasound imaging of the leg. This approach is based on the knowledge that virtually all large pulmonary emboli originate in the deep veins of the legs. In patients with PE documented by high-probability lung scans or pulmonary angiography, only a small proportion has deep vein thrombosis identified by venous ultrasound techniques, justifying the argument that these venous clots have migrated out of the legs. However, when lung scans or spiral CT suggest low probability of PE and ultrasound studies repeated serially over a 2-week period remain negative, the risk of recur-

Figure 57-3

Embolism of Lesser Degree Without Infarction

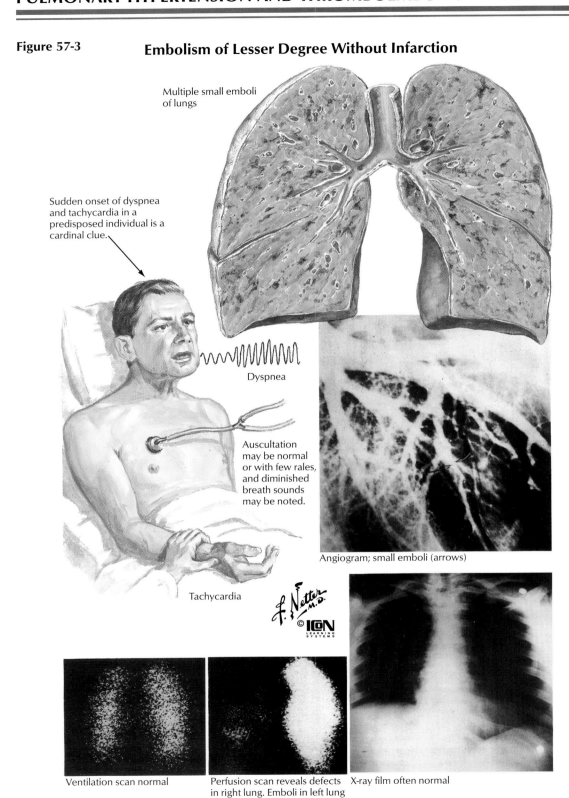

Multiple small emboli of lungs

Sudden onset of dyspnea and tachycardia in a predisposed individual is a cardinal clue.

Dyspnea

Auscultation may be normal or with few rales, and diminished breath sounds may be noted.

Tachycardia

Angiogram; small emboli (arrows)

Ventilation scan normal

Perfusion scan reveals defects in right lung. Emboli in left lung not visualized

X-ray film often normal

rent PE is so low as to justify withholding anticoagulation. Unfortunately, this approach is inconvenient and costly, and for this reason is used routinely in only a few centers.

D-dimer, a degradation product of cross-linked fibrin measured in blood, is a sensitive marker for thrombosis. However, the test also represents "acute phase reactivity," as is found in many disease states other than PE. A negative D-dimer assay result is useful in clinically low-risk patients who have a low pretest probability—reliably predicting the absence of PE. However, in patients with a high pretest probability, a negative D-dimer test result has only a 64% negative predictive value. Because the sensitivity and specificity of each of these tests are imperfect, the concept of pretest probability is critical (see also chapter 1). A validated algorithm that differentiates low-, moderate-, and high-risk groups with 3, 28, and 78% prevalence of PE, respectively, is shown in Table 57-2.

The use of pretest probability can be coupled with known sensitivity and specificity of the diagnostic tests to design a logical treatment strategy. For example, patients with a moderate or high pretest probability and a high-probability lung scan have adequate indication for anticoagulation. Conversely, patients with low pretest probability of PE and a high-probability lung scan would be candidates for further evaluation.

Management and Therapy

The goals in treating PE are to stabilize critically affected patients and then prevent recurrence of emboli by treating the underlying venous thrombosis. Patients with hypotension, shock, cardiac arrest, or refractory hypoxemia may require inotropic support and mechanical ventilation. In this subset of unstable patients, thrombolysis may be lifesaving. Although multicenter studies have shown a mortality benefit for thrombolytic therapy in unstable patients, no such benefit is seen (in comparison with conventional therapy using heparin—see below) in stable patients with PE. Patients with refractory shock or hypoxemia who do not respond to thrombolysis, or who have contraindications to thrombolytic therapy but not surgery, are candidates for surgical thrombectomy. Because mortality rate is high, surgical thrombectomy is a

Table 57-2
Variables Used to Determine Patient Pretest Probability for PE

Variable	Value
Clinical signs and symptoms of DVT	3.0 points
PE as or more likely than an alternate diagnosis	3.0 points
Heart rate greater than 100 beats/min	1.5 points
Immobilization or history of surgery in the previous 4 weeks	1.5 points
Previous DVT or PE	1.5 points
Hemoptysis	1.0 points
Malignant neoplasm (at treatment, treated in the last 6 months, or palliative)	1.0 points

Low probability <2.0; moderate probability 2.0– 6.0; high probability >6.0. DVT indicates deep vein thrombosis; PE, pulmonary embolism. With permission from Rodger M, Wells PS. Pulmonary embolism. *Thromb Res* 2001;103:V225–238.

consideration for only the highest risk patients. Percutaneous catheter suction or dislodgement of massive proximal emboli may be other options, although no randomized studies using these approaches have been conducted.

Fortunately, most patients who survive the first few minutes after PE are relatively stable and can be evaluated and managed in a deliberate manner. The accepted treatment initially or after thrombolysis is heparin. Unfractionated heparin (UFH) or low-molecular-weight heparin (LMWH) should be started when the diagnosis is considered, assuming there are no serious contraindications, such as active bleeding; history of recent surgery, stroke, intracranial malignancy, among others; or documented heparin-associated thrombocytopenia. Contraindications to thrombolytic therapy for patients with PE are the same as those for acute MI (see chapter 9). The dose of UFH should be adjusted for weight with an initial bolus of 80 U/kg followed by an infusion of 18 U · kg^{-1} · h^{-1} by intravenous infusion. Subsequent adjustments should be made to achieve an activated partial thromboplastin time of 1.5 to 2.5 times control. Use of a LMWH is increasingly popular because of its ease of administration, reduced laboratory costs, and reduced propensity to precipitate thrombocytopenia. Regardless of the heparin used, the administration should be aggressively managed because inadequate doses are associated with increased recurrence of PE. Heparin-associated thrombocytopenia is a potentially serious complication of heparin therapy. Platelet counts of all patients on heparin should be monitored daily. Direct inhibitors of thrombin, such as recombinant hirudin can be substituted for heparin in patients in whom thrombocytopenia develops.

Heparin administration should continue for a minimum of 5 days after the initiation of warfarin therapy. This allows time for adequate reduction of the plasma procoagulant factors II, VII, IX, and X and prevents the state of thrombophilia that occurs early after initiation of warfarin therapy when the anticoagulant factors S and C are reduced more quickly than the procoagulant factors. The intensity of warfarin therapy should be sufficient to prolong the prothrombin time international normalization ratio to 2 to 3. Treatment duration is individualized but should continue for a minimum of 3 months in all patients until possible precipitating issues have resolved.

Placement of an inferior vena cava filter device should be considered in several settings. These devices can be used in patients with absolute contraindications to anticoagulation, either at the time of initial therapy or thereafter. In addition, inferior vena cava filters will reduce the likelihood of recurrent PE in patients with recurrence who are undergoing adequate anticoagulation or who have had multiple PEs over time.

PULMONARY HYPERTENSION
Diagnostic Approach

Table 57-3 describes the diagnostic approach to pulmonary hypertension. This approach distinguishes secondary forms of pulmonary hypertension from PPH (defined as sustained elevation of PAPs without a demonstrable cause), thereby guiding appropriate therapy.

Critical information on the degree and possible cause of pulmonary hypertension can be

Table 57-3
Evaluation of Patients With Suspected Pulmonary Hypertension

Diagnostic Test	Potential Findings
Electrocardiography	P pulmonale (P wave in lead II greater than 3 mV)
	Right-axis deviation
	R wave greater than S wave in V^1
Chest radiography	Enlarged pulmonary arteries
	RV enlargement
	Parenchymal lung disease
	Skeletal abnormalities
Echocardiography	PAP estimated by TR velocity
	RV hypertrophy
	RV enlargement
	LV function/LA size
	Valvular disease
	Imaging to detect ASD or VSD
Pulmonary function testing with ABG	COPD
	Restrictive lung disease
	Hypoventilation
Ventilation/perfusion lung scan	To diagnose or exclude pulmonary embolism
PA angiography	For further evaluation of indeterminate lung scan to exclude thromboembolism
Cardiac catheterization	Pressure determinations at rest and after inhalation of 100% oxygen
	Pulmonary wedge pressure
	Response to vasodilators

ABG indicates arterial blood gas; PA, pulmonary artery; PAP, pulmonary artery pressure; LA, left atrial; LV, left ventricular; RV, right ventricular; TR, tricuspid regurgitation.

gained from a transthoracic echocardiogram. PAP can be estimated from the Doppler-derived velocity of tricuspid regurgitation and from the degree of RV dilation and hypertrophy. These data provide diagnostic and prognostic information. The echocardiogram also provides data on LV function, mitral valve structure and function, and the existence of an intracardiac shunt, all key clues to the possibility that the pulmonary hypertension is an effect of cardiac disease.

Information about primary pulmonary disease must also be pursued. Pulmonary function testing provides information on parenchymal and functional lung disease. V/Q scans are useful in excluding chronic pulmonary thromboembolism as the underlying etiology for pulmonary hypertension. The need to document thromboembolism is so critical to treatment and survival that pulmonary angiography must be considered for every patient with otherwise undiagnosed pulmonary hypertension. However, particularly in patients with severe pulmonary hypertension, pulmonary angiography presents increased risk of morbidity and death. For this reason, pulmonary angiography in this setting should be performed in a center and by an operator with experience in dealing with these patients.

Evaluation by teams experienced with pulmonary hypertension should always be considered for patients who have disease that evades diagnosis by noninvasive means. For most of these patients diagnosed as having PPH, the prognosis is grave and survival depends on sophisticated evaluation and management. Key to this evaluation are the levels of pulmonary hypertension and pulmonary vascular resistance, and documentation of the effects of vasodilators on the pulmonary vascular resistance and pressure. Testing the effect of vasodilators on pulmonary vascular resistance is accomplished in part by right-sided heart catheterization. Response to acute vasodilators such as nitric oxide, adenosine, and epoprostenol is associated with subsequent response to long-term therapy with vasodilators such as calcium channel blockers and epoprostenol. The desired response to a vasodilator challenge is a reduction of PAP, with associated increases in cardiac output but without systemic hypotension or hypoxemia.

Management and Therapy

The severity of pulmonary hypertension and the patient degree of functional limitation are accurate predictors of prognosis. However, the disease is progressive; PPH virtually always leads to death. The average survival time in a national registry was 2.5 years after diagnosis. Experience with vasodilator and anticoagulation therapy has improved that prognosis considerably. Warfarin anticoagulation is recommended for all patients without contraindications because it doubles survival time. Patients who respond to calcium channel blockers have a 95% survival rate at 5 years. Recent studies have demonstrated that continuous intravenous infusion of epoprostenol improves survival in patients with severe pulmonary hypertension. Because the response to epoprostenol is more predictable and more easily than the response to calcium channel blockers, increasing numbers of patients with severe pulmonary hypertension are being treated with epoprostenol.

Despite improved survival rates with anticoagulation and vasodilator therapies, a large subset of patients have no improvement in hemodynamic parameters or symptoms. These patients are candidates for lung or heart–lung transplantation. The posttransplantation mortality rates for patients with severe pulmonary hypertension are higher than the rates for patients who undergo organ transplantation for other reasons. The 1-year survival rate for those with pulmonary hypertension is about 65%.

Individuals with pulmonary hypertension caused by chronic pulmonary thromboembolism constitute an important subset of patients. These patients benefit from pulmonary thromboendarterectomy followed by long-term anticoagulant therapy.

FUTURE DIRECTIONS

For thromboembolism, the challenge is improvement of prevention and detection of deep vein thrombosis in populations at increased risk. Diagnostic testing for pulmonary thromboembolism will improve as experience with high-definition imaging evolves. New antithrombotic agents are being developed that are easier to manage than warfarin and that have a reduced risk of heparin-associated thrombocytopenia.

The discovery that a mutation in the gene for bone morphogenetic protein receptor II is associated with PPH may increase understanding of the familial transmission of the disease. It is likely that understanding the role of this protein in PPH will also provide clues to the pathophysiologic processes involved in pulmonary hypertension associated with HIV infection, cocaine use, portal hypertension, and use of weight-loss drugs.

New information from basic studies of vascular biology will bring new therapies for safer and more convenient treatment of pulmonary hypertension. Examples of new and promising agents include sildenafil and bosentan.

REFERENCES

Fedullo PF, Auger WR, Kerr KM, Rubin LJ. Chronic thromboembolic pulmonary hypertension. 2001;345:1465–1472.

Ginsberg JS, Wells PS, Kearon C, et al. Sensitivity and specificity of a rapid whole-blood assay for D-dimer in the diagnosis of pulmonary embolism. *Ann Intern Med* 1998;129:1006–1011.

Newman JH, Wheeler L, Lane KB, et al. Mutation in the gene for bone morphogenic protein receptor II as a cause of primary pulmonary hypertension in a large kindred. *N Engl J Med* 2001;345:319–324.

Riedel M. Venous thromboembolic disease. Acute pulmonary embolism: Pathophysiology, clinical presentation, and diagnosis. *Heart* 2001;85(pt 1):229–240.

Riedel M. Venous thromboembolic disease. Acute pulmonary embolism: Treatment. *Heart* 2001;85(pt 2):351–360.

Rodger M, Wells PS. Pulmonary embolism. *Thromb Res* 2001;103:V225–V238.

Rubin LJ. Current concepts: Primary pulmonary hypertension. *New Engl J Med* 1997;336:111–117.

Chapter 58

Substance Abuse and the Heart

David A. Tate

Substance abuse has enormous social, economic, and medical consequences. Although the effect of illegal abused substances on the cardiovascular system is important, two legal substances—tobacco and alcohol—have a far greater impact on the cardiovascular health of citizens of the United States and other industrialized countries (Fig. 58-1).

TOBACCO

From a cardiologic perspective, given the impact of smoking on coronary artery disease, tobacco is by far the most lethal of abused substances. Although the adverse effects of smoking on atherosclerotic disease have been known for years, studies continue to emphasize the striking magnitude of the effect. The incidence of coronary disease in smokers is approximately twice the incidence in nonsmokers. Indeed, the deleterious effects of smoking were recently demonstrated in the Women's Health Study, which suggested that half of all coronary deaths in women could be attributed to smoking. In primary prevention trials of the use of statins for hypercholesterolemia, coronary event rates were 74 to 86% higher in smokers than in nonsmokers. Following myocardial infarction (MI), recurrent MI is twice as frequent among those who continue to smoke than among those who quit. It can therefore be argued that smoking cessation is likely to be more effective than statins for primary prevention of cardiovascular disease and more effective than aspirin, β-blockers, or angiotensin-converting enzyme inhibitors for secondary prevention. Despite a decline in smoking in recent decades, approximately 20 to 25% of adult Americans remain addicted to tobacco. Moreover, smoking among adolescents continues to increase, particularly among young women.

The medical and lay communities share a pessimistic view of smoking cessation, which may not be fully justified. It is true, and caregivers must recognize, that tobacco is a genuinely addictive substance, recognized as such by the US Surgeon General's Office. It must also be acknowledged that smokers who want to quit often fail in their attempts to stop smoking. Nevertheless, many smokers do ultimately succeed, and by facilitating smoking cessation, the healthcare provider is likely to have a more salutary effect on a patient's health than is almost any other medical intervention. Counseling by physicians makes a difference. The efficacy of counseling is directly related to the intensity of the counseling program, and that efficacy can be greatly increased by the use of questionnaires, written materials, and follow-up. Smoking cessation rates are greatly increased when a cardiovascular event has heightened patient concern. In a group of smokers with MI, cessation rates of 24.5% with standard advice and 63.2% with intensive advice were achieved.

Several pharmacologic adjunctive agents for smoking cessation are available and may increase success rates. In a standard outpatient setting, modest but significant success has been achieved with nicotine replacement therapy, with abstinence rates of approximately 20% at 1 year. Considerable success has also been achieved with the non-nicotine therapy bupropion. Most promising, however, are programs that combine non-nicotine medications with nicotine replacement therapy. Long-term smoking cessation rates of 36% have been demonstrated for the combination of bupropion and the nicotine patch as compared to 16% quit rates with double placebo. Given the remarkable efficacy of smoking cessation in reducing cardiovascular morbidity and mortality, aggressive efforts at helping patients to stop smoking are warranted.

ALCOHOL

Alcohol abuse takes an enormous toll, with the strictly medical effects (liver disease, pancre-

Figure 58-1

Substance Abuse and the Heart

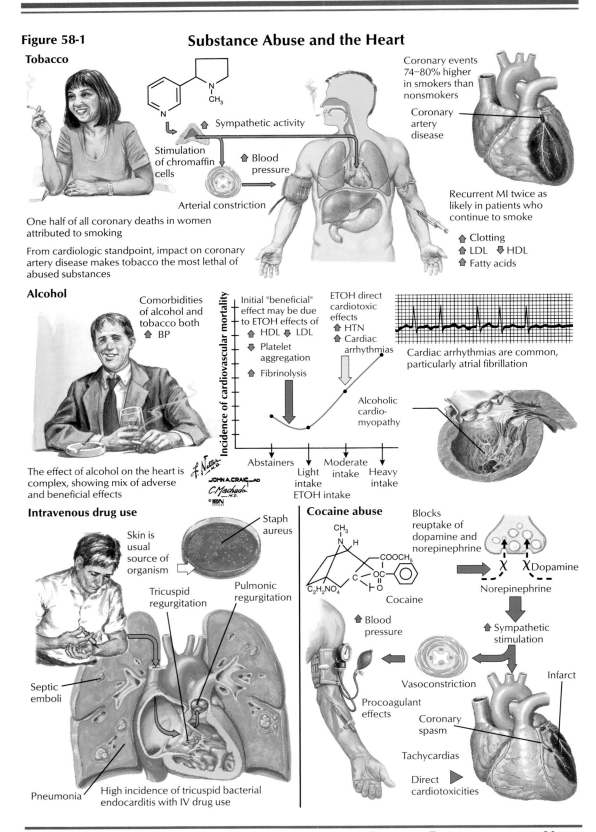

Tobacco

Coronary events 74–80% higher in smokers than nonsmokers

Coronary artery disease

Sympathetic activity

Stimulation of chromaffin cells

⬆ Blood pressure

Arterial constriction

Recurrent MI twice as likely in patients who continue to smoke

⬆ Clotting
⬆ LDL ⬇ HDL
⬆ Fatty acids

One half of all coronary deaths in women attributed to smoking

From cardiologic standpoint, impact on coronary artery disease makes tobacco the most lethal of abused substances

Alcohol

Comorbidities of alcohol and tobacco both ⬆ BP

Initial "beneficial" effect may be due to ETOH effects of
⬆ HDL ⬇ LDL
⬇ Platelet aggregation
⬆ Fibrinolysis

ETOH direct cardiotoxic effects
⬆ HTN
⬆ Cardiac arrhythmias

Cardiac arrhythmias are common, particularly atrial fibrillation

Alcoholic cardiomyopathy

Incidence of cardiovascular mortality

Abstainers | Light intake | Moderate intake | Heavy intake

ETOH intake

The effect of alcohol on the heart is complex, showing mix of adverse and beneficial effects

Intravenous drug use

Staph aureus

Skin is usual source of organism

Tricuspid regurgitation

Pulmonic regurgitation

Septic emboli

Pneumonia

High incidence of tricuspid bacterial endocarditis with IV drug use

Cocaine abuse

Blocks reuptake of dopamine and norepinephrine

Dopamine

Norepinephrine

Cocaine

⬆ Blood pressure

⬆ Sympathetic stimulation

Vasoconstriction

Procoagulant effects

Coronary spasm

Infarct

Tachycardias

Direct cardiotoxicities

atitis, etc.) compounded by the sociobehavioral health effects (suicide, homicide, trauma, domestic abuse, etc.). The effect of alcohol on the heart, however, is complex, with a mix of adverse and probably beneficial effects.

The apparent beneficial effect of modest alcohol intake was first noted in France, where a surprisingly low coronary disease mortality rate was observed despite a high intake of dietary fat. This observation came to be called the "French paradox." There appears to be a J-shaped relationship between alcohol intake and total mortality. The initial descending portion of the curve derives from the reduced cardiovascular mortality associated with modest alcohol intake (1–3 drinks a day). Although the effect may be somewhat more apparent with red wine, most evidence suggests that the effect is from alcohol per se. The mechanism may relate to a variety of factors, including increased high-density lipoprotein cholesterol, decreased low-density lipoprotein cholesterol, antioxidant effects, decreased platelet aggregation, and enhanced fibrinolysis.

It is important to note that despite this finding, there are no controlled trials that suggest a benefit from advising or instigating modest alcohol intake. The potential beneficial effect must be weighed against the catastrophic effect of immoderate consumption or even of moderate consumption in at-risk segments of the population (genetic risk for alcoholism, women of childbearing age, drivers, etc.). Thus, it is likely that an intervention trial would demonstrate both positive and negative effects, and randomized studies have not yet been performed.

Alcohol has numerous deleterious effects on the cardiovascular system, particularly in high doses. The most commonly encountered of these effects are alcoholic cardiomyopathy, alcohol-associated arrhythmias, and aggravation of hypertension. Ethanol and its metabolites have direct cardiotoxic effects on systolic and diastolic function. When severe, these direct cardiotoxic effects produce a clinical syndrome identical to idiopathic dilated cardiomyopathy. In general, therapy for alcoholic cardiomyopathy is similar to that used for other forms of heart failure (see chapters 12 and 17). However, of paramount importance is the cessation of alcohol intake. In patients who abstain from alcohol consumption, the disease is reversible in a large number of patients. In patients who continue to consume alcohol, the disease is usually persistent and often progressive and fatal.

Alcohol use may trigger a wide range of cardiac arrhythmias, from premature atrial and ventricular contractions to ventricular fibrillation and sudden cardiac death. By far the most common arrhythmia associated with alcohol use, however, is atrial fibrillation. Indeed, this symptom has been noted commonly enough after weekends and holidays to be labeled "holiday heart." The mechanisms may include heterogeneous delayed cardiac conduction, QT prolongation, electrolyte imbalance, or excess catecholamine activity.

The deleterious cardiovascular effect of alcohol that affects the most individuals is its contribution to hypertension. Even low levels of alcohol intake cause a mild increase in systolic blood pressure. This finding is probably of great significance given the high prevalence of both hypertension and moderate alcohol intake. At high doses, alcohol exerts a significant pressor effect and is a leading cause of reversible hypertension.

INTRAVENOUS DRUG USE

Regardless of the substance involved, IV drug use may cause endocarditis. Whereas other patients in whom endocarditis develops generally have a predisposing valvular lesion, the vast majority of IV drug users with endocarditis do not have such a lesion. In addition, there is some evidence from echocardiographic studies that chronic IV drug use may cause a mild degree of tricuspid and pulmonic regurgitation, even in the absence of endocarditis.

Endocarditis associated with IV drug use is usually right-sided, involving the tricuspid valve. Not surprisingly, therefore, IV drug–related endocarditis is often associated with pneumonia or septic pulmonary emboli. The infectious agent that causes the endocarditis is most commonly a skin organism, rather than a contaminated agent itself. Staphylococcus aureus is the most common organism causing endocarditis in IV drug users, comprising approximately 60% of cases. Interestingly, cocaine use is also a predisposing factor for development of left-sided endocarditis, perhaps a result of valvular trauma from cocaine-induced extreme hemodynamic stress (as discussed in the next section), creating a nidus for bacterial infection.

COCAINE

Cocaine inhibits the reuptake of norepinephrine and dopamine at sympathetic nerve terminals. It thereby produces intense activation of the sympathetic nervous system, leading to severe hypertension and tachycardia. Cocaine also has complex interactions with cellular ion transport (sodium, potassium, and calcium), and these interactions likely contribute to the vasospastic and arrhythmogenic effects of cocaine. Finally, cocaine has procoagulant, atherosclerotic, and direct myocardial toxic effects.

Cocaine-induced MI can occur via several mechanisms. In individuals with preexisting coronary disease, the severe tachycardia and hypertension associated with cocaine use may lead to a supply–demand imbalance. Even in the absence of underlying coronary disease, focal or diffuse coronary vasospasm may occur. Thrombosis may develop in some subjects because of endothelial disruption caused by the mechanisms just mentioned or because of direct procoagulant effects. Cocaine-induced MI may occur up to 15 hours after use of the drug. It is important to note that individuals who use cocaine over prolonged periods of time are often found to have advanced coronary atherosclerosis, out of proportion to their underlying risk factor profile. Thus, in a young individual with chest pain and a history of cocaine abuse, coronary atherosclerosis must be considered. This creates a diagnostic dilemma since many cocaine users also present with chest pain unrelated to myocardial ischemia.

Appropriate therapy for cocaine-associated cardiac toxicity must consider the many complex pharmacologic actions of cocaine. An understandable but potentially catastrophic mistake with these patients, whose sympathetic nervous systems are stimulated by the cocaine, is the use of β-blockers. β-Blockade produces unopposed α-receptor stimulation, which may lead to severe hypertension and coronary vasoconstriction. Calcium channel blockers should also be avoided because the effect of cocaine on calcium transport leads to an unpredictable clinical response. α-Blockers, such as phentolamine, or direct-acting vasodilators, such as nitroglycerin, nitroprusside, and hydralazine, are the preferred therapeutic options.

Antiarrhythmic drugs should be avoided if possible in patients with cocaine intoxication because drug interactions involving electrolyte transport may lead to proarrhythmic effects or hemodynamic instability. Given the relatively short half-life of cocaine (30–60 minutes), it is generally best to simply monitor the patient until the cocaine-induced arrhythmias subside. DC cardioversion may be necessary for treatment of hemodynamically unstable rhythms, and adenosine is probably safe for termination of sustained supraventricular arrhythmias.

Amphetamine, LSD, and psilocybin intoxication are often associated with marked tachycardia, hypertension, and arrhythmia and are managed in much the same way as cocaine intoxication.

NARCOTICS

Depressant effects on the respiratory and central nervous systems dominate the clinical picture of narcotic intoxication. However, narcotic agents such as heroin and morphine also have potentially life-threatening cardiovascular effects. These agents act directly on the vasomotor center to reduce sympathetic activity and enhance parasympathetic activity. These agents also stimulate histamine release from mast cells and increase electrophysiologic automaticity. Narcotic intoxication may therefore be associated with profound bradycardia and hypotension as well as with supraventricular and ventricular arrhythmias. In addition, narcotic use may precipitate noncardiogenic pulmonary edema, which can mimic and complicate true cardiovascular effects.

Therapy for narcotic overdose is predominantly supportive. Severe hemodynamic instability is treated with naloxone, a narcotic-receptor antagonist. Experience with antiarrhythmic drugs is limited in the setting of narcotic overdose, and as with cocaine, it is best to avoid pharmacologic agents if possible and allow the narcotic to be metabolized. DC cardioversion is appropriate for hemodynamically unstable rhythms. If necessary, supraventricular arrhythmias may be treated with adenosine, β-blockers, verapamil, or digoxin.

SUBSTANCE ABUSE AMONG ATHLETES

Competitive athletes and bodybuilders often abuse substances, with a goal of enhancing performance or building muscle mass. The primary ingredients of most cardiac stimulant products used by this population are ephedrine, often called by its Chinese name, "ma huang," and caffeine. Ephedrine and caffeine may cause or exacerbate hypertension and rarely can be associated with a catecholamine cardiomyopathy. In addition, the effects of ephedrine and caffeine on myocardial contractility, myocardial irritability, and coronary vasoconstriction may sometimes be hazardous, particularly in the occasional subject with hypertrophic cardiomyopathy or a preexcitation syndrome.

Anabolic steroids are widely used and have multiple adverse effects on the cardiovascular system. Anabolic steroids promote atherogenesis by dramatically increasing low-density lipoprotein cholesterol and decreasing high-density lipoprotein cholesterol. Anabolic steroids appear to promote left ventricular hypertrophy secondarily by causing hypertension but possibly also by a direct anabolic effect on the myocardium. Finally, anabolic steroids may have effects on platelet aggregation and cardiac conduction. Sporadic cases of MI and sudden cardiac death have been reported among anabolic steroid users.

FUTURE DIRECTIONS

Substance abuse is epidemic in Western societies and is likely to remain so. Primary prevention in this area relies on public education. The legal substances tobacco and alcohol exacerbate two of the major killers in cardiovascular medicine, coronary artery disease and hypertension. The use of illegal substances takes a disproportionate toll on youth, who otherwise would be expected to be free of cardiovascular disease. Physician awareness of and attention to these issues can highlight their importance for the general public.

REFERENCES

Burt A, Illingworth D, Shaw PR, et al. Stopping smoking after myocardial infarction. *Lancet* 1974;1:304–306.

Fiore MC, Smith SS, Jorenby DE, et al. The effectiveness of nicotine patch for smoking cessation: A meta-analysis. *JAMA* 1994;263:2760–2765.

Hurt RD, Sachs DL, Glover ED, et al. A comparison of sustained-release bupropion and placebo for smoking cessation. *N Engl J Med* 1997;337:1195–1202.

Jorenby DE, Leischow SJ, Nides MA, et al. A controlled trial of sustained-release bupropion, nicotine patch, or both for smoking cessation. *N Engl J Med* 1999;340:658–691.

Milionis HJ, Rizos E, Mikhailidis DP. Smoking diminishes the beneficial effect of statins: Observations from the landmark trials. *Angiology* 2001;52:575–587.

Mouhaffel, AH, Madu EC, Satmary WA, Fraker TD. Cardiovascular complications of cocaine. *Chest* 1995;107: 1426–1434.

Ronnevik PK, Gunderson T, Abrahamsen AM. Effect of smoking habits and timolol treatment on mortality and reinfarction in patients surviving acute myocardial infarction. *Br Heart J* 1985;54:134.

Russell MA, Wilson C, Taylor C, Baker CD. Effect of general practitioners' advice against smoking. *Br Med J* 1979;2: 231–235.

Willet WC, Green A, Stampfer MJ, et al. Relative and absolute excess risks of coronary heart disease among women who smoke cigarettes. *N Engl J Med* 1987;317: 1303–1309.

Chapter 59

HIV and the Heart

Kristine B. Patterson and Joseph J. Eron

Human immunodeficiency virus (HIV) and acquired immunodeficiency syndrome (AIDS) affect more than 45 million people worldwide. *AIDS*—defined immunologically as a CD4[+] T-cell count of 200/μL or less, or by the occurrence of an opportunistic illness—is the most advanced manifestation of HIV infection. The spectrum of disease, however, is diverse and the period between HIV acquisition and the development of AIDS can be many years. Advances in the knowledge and treatment of HIV infection have resulted in longer survival for patients. Because of the increased longevity, HIV-related cardiac diseases are becoming more prevalent. Common cardiac manifestations of HIV include dilated cardiomyopathy, myocarditis, pericardial effusions, endocarditis, pulmonary hypertension, malignant neoplasms, and complications from combined antiretroviral therapy, including alterations in lipid metabolism. The HIV-infected individual is also subject to the development of traditional cardiovascular diseases, some of which may be accelerated by antiretroviral therapy or by the virus itself. This chapter explores the most common cardiac diseases in HIV-infected individuals and the ways in which the etiologies of these diseases are different in these patients (Fig. 59-1). Special considerations in treating lipid abnormalities and evaluating atherosclerosis are also discussed.

CARDIAC MANIFESTATIONS OF AIDS

Cardiac involvement is commonly reported in HIV-infected patients, especially in the late stage of the disease. Important differences exist in the type and frequency of abnormalities found in HIV-related cardiac involvement versus that in the general population. Among individuals who are HIV-infected, pericarditis and pericardial effusions are the most frequently seen cardiovascular abnormalities. However, with the exception of evaluation for opportunistic infections, the evaluation of cardiac disease in HIV patients does not differ from the evaluation of cardiac disease in the general population. Because AIDS patients are subject to opportunistic bacterial, viral, mycotic, and protozoal infections, cardiac disease in HIV-infected individuals commonly arises from opportunistic pathogens. In all cases, treatment is directed at the underlying etiology when possible.

MYOCARDIAL INVOLVEMENT
Dilated Cardiomyopathy

AIDS is an increasingly recognized etiologic factor in dilated cardiomyopathy. Echocardiographic findings consistent with dilated cardiomyopathy are found in 20 to 40% of patients with AIDS and also in long-standing HIV infec-

tion in the absence of an AIDS-defining diagnosis or a CD4 cell count ($\leq$200 cells/mm[3]). The most common echocardiographic findings are four-chamber enlargement, diffuse left ventricular hypokinesis, and decreased fractional shortening. Dilated cardiomyopathy typically occurs late in the course of HIV infection and is usually associated with a reduced CD4 count.

The pathogenesis of the AIDS- or HIV-related cardiomyopathy is a matter of controversy. Hypotheses include ventricular dysfunction resulting from myocarditis, myocarditis resulting from opportunistic infections, impaired immune function, and nutritional and drug-induced cardiomyopathies. The development of ventricular dysfunction resulting from myocarditis may be the most logical hypothesis, because HIV has been cultured from cardiac muscle biopsy specimens. However, there is little theoretical reason, or in vitro evidence, to support HIV infection of myocardial cells, which lack CD4 receptors. Histologically, there are three features: lymphocytic infiltrates with necrosis of the myocardial fibers, lymphocytic infiltrates without necrosis, and focal and mild myocarditis with a mononuclear infiltrate. Mononuclear infiltrates tend to be more common, but are not found exclusively, in individuals coinfected with an opportunistic infection.

Figure 59-1

Cardiac Manifestations of AIDS

Ischemic cardiovascular disease in HIV-positive patients

Protease inhibitors (PI) may be associated with the development of accelerated atherosclerosis by inducing insulin resistance, hypertension, and dyslipidemia in HIV-infected patients.

Dilated cardiomyopathy

This condition typically occurs late in the course of HIV infection, with associated low CD4 count, and may be associated with nucleoside reverse transcriptase inhibitor usage. The most common findings are four-chamber enlargement, left ventricular hypokinesis, and decreased fractional shortening.

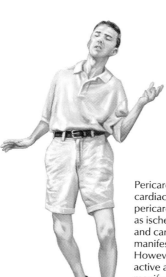

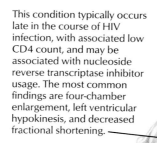

Pericarditis, pericardial effusion, cardiac neoplasms, infective pericarditis and endocarditis, as well as ischemic cardiovascular disease and cardiomyopathies, are common manifestations of HIV disease. However, in the presence of highly active antiretroviral therapy, these manifestations are relatively rare.

Pulmonary hypertension, which is more commonly seen in the younger population, is usually caused by left ventricular dysfunction.

C. Machado
—M.D.

©**ICON**
LEARNING
SYSTEMS

It seems unlikely in most cases that opportunistic infections lead to myocarditis, because in 80% of patients with myocarditis found on biopsy, no specific etiologic factor can be found. Myocardial opportunistic pathogens found in the remaining 20% include viral (cytomegalovirus, herpes simplex), protozoal (*Toxoplasma gondii*), bacterial (*Mycobacterium tuberculosis*, *Mycobacterium avium-intracellulare*), and fungal (*Cryptococcus neoformans*, *Aspergillus fumigatus*, *Candida albicans*, *Histoplasma capsulatum*, and *Coccidioides immitis*).

Impaired immune response is another possible etiology. Patients with AIDS have an abnormality of T-helper cell function frequently resulting in uncontrolled hypergammaglobulinemia and high concentration of serum immune complexes that may cause inflammatory lesions within the myocardium. The HIV gene products may either attach to or modify myocardial cell surface proteins, resulting in the induction of circulated cardiac autoantibodies, which can trigger a progressively destructive autoimmune reaction.

Nutrient deficiencies have also been postulated to play a role in AIDS- or HIV-related cardiomyopathy. Various studies have implicated deficiencies of specific micronutrients, including selenium, l-carnitine and vitamin B_1, have been implicated. Illicit drugs (cocaine and alcohol) and therapeutic medications (zidovudine and other nucleoside analogues such as didanosine) both have also been implicated, leaving open the possibility that multiple etiologies contribute to this cardiomyopathy, as is the case with other synergistic contributors to dilated cardiomyopathy (see chapter 12).

Clinical manifestations of dilated cardiomyopathy in HIV-positive patients are similar to those in uninfected patients. Reversible etiologies, such as infections and nutritional deficiencies that could contribute to the cardiomyopathy, should be considered during evaluation. Consultation with an infectious disease specialist may be helpful. Standard management, including diuretics, angiotensin-converting enzyme inhibitors or angiotensin antagonists (and/or other vasodilators) and β-blockers is advisable. Inotropic agents are useful in short-term treatment of hemodynamic compromise as in other cardiomyopathy patients. If a specific opportunistic pathogen is contributing to the cardiomyopathy, directed therapy is appropriate. Anticoagulants should be used cautiously because HIV-infected patients, especially those with AIDS, appear to be at higher risk for vasculopathy and intracranial lesions that may lead to intracerebral bleeding.

Pulmonary Hypertension

The incidence of HIV-associated pulmonary hypertension is 1 in 200 compared with 1 in 200,000 in the general population. This condition is more common in young male patients. Common risk factors are intravenous drug use, homosexual encounters, and hemophilia. No correlation exists between a history of opportunistic infections or the CD4 count and pulmonary hypertension. Possible etiologies of secondary pulmonary hypertension include recurrent viral, bacterial, parasitic, and fungal pulmonary infections; necrotizing angiitis secondary to injection drug use; thromboembolic events; and left ventricular dysfunction. Symptoms reflect the degree of pulmonary hypertension and cor pulmonale.

Cardiac Neoplasm

The two most common malignant neoplasms associated with HIV disease, Kaposi's sarcoma (KS) and non-Hodgkin's lymphoma, may involve the heart.

Cardiac involvement with KS is usually part of disseminated KS. AIDS-related metastatic KS involves either the visceral layer of serous pericardium or the subepicardial fat, especially the tissue adjacent to a major coronary artery. Clinical cardiac findings are usually obscure; most cases are found at autopsy. Fatal cardiac tamponade and pericardial constriction may occur. Pericardiocentesis does not have a diagnostic role in these patients; it is considered a high-risk procedure because of the vascular nature of KS lesions. When a pericardial effusion due to KS is suspected, a pericardial window is the procedure of choice for providing decompression in addition to establishing the diagnosis.

Non-Hodgkin's lymphoma, usually of B-cell origin, is typically high grade and disseminates early in HIV-infected patients, particularly in those with AIDS, and results in cardiac involvement in a small fraction of patients. Patients may present with intractable heart failure, pericardial effusion, cardiac tamponade, or arrhythmias. Patients with mechanical obstruction may benefit from surgical resection. The prognosis is generally poor, although clinical remission has been observed with combination chemotherapy, an outcome that may be more frequent in the era of highly active antiretroviral therapy (HAART).

PERICARDIAL INVOLVEMENT
Pericardial Effusions and Pericarditis

Pericardial effusion is the most common form of cardiac involvement in HIV-infected individuals and typically arises with more advanced HIV disease. Clinical manifestations include asymptomatic effusions detected on echocardiography, pericarditis with or without constriction, and fatal tamponade. The clinical presentation of pericarditis alone is no different in HIV-positive patients and uninfected individuals. Pericarditis can occur with or without an effusion. The etiology of pericarditis in HIV infection is most often not determined, as is the case in uninfected individuals. Specific causes of the pericardial effusion, when found, often relate to opportunistic infections, including mycobacterial and fungal pathogens, and malignancies such as KS and non-Hodgkin's lymphoma as described above. A pericardial effusion may also appear with HIV-associated nephropathy and renal failure.

Pericardiocentesis is currently recommended only for large or poorly tolerated effusions (including cardiac tamponade; see chapters 35 and 36), for evaluation of a disseminated opportunistic infection or a systemic illness in addition to HIV infection. HIV/AIDS patients with pericardial effusions have a 9% annual incidence of cardiac tamponade. The size of the effusion does not correlate with shortened survival; the presence of an effusion is solely predictive of high mortality. This high mortality is likely related to lower CD4 counts in those patients and, therefore, to more advanced disease.

ENDOCARDIAL INVOLVEMENT
Nonbacterial Thrombotic Endocarditis

In AIDS, the most common endocardial lesion reported is nonbacterial thrombotic endocarditis (NBTE). These friable vegetations can occur on any of the four valves, but left-sided lesions are the most common. Systemic embolization from NBTE is a rare cause of death in AIDS patients. Overall, NBTE is estimated to occur in 3 to 5% of AIDS patients, typically in those older than 50 years and most commonly in patients with HIV wasting syndrome.

Infective endocarditis

Infective endocarditis (IE) in patients with AIDS typically occurs in parenteral drug users. *Staphylococcus aureus* and *Streptococcus viridans* are the major responsible organisms. HIV-infected patients have a higher risk of developing *Salmonella* endocarditis than do immunocompetent patients because they are more likely to develop bacteremia during *Salmonella* infections. Fungal endocarditis, including *C. albicans*, *A. fumigatus*, *H. capsulatum*, and *C. neoformans*, is also more common. The tricuspid valve is most commonly affected. There is generally no difference in presentation and survival of IE in patients with and without HIV infection. However, patients with late-stage HIV disease have higher mortality than patients who are earlier in the disease course.

DYSLIPIDEMIA IN AIDS PATIENTS

Dyslipidemia and the potential for accelerated atherosclerosis have become important issues for physicians treating patients with AIDS or HIV infection. It is important to note, however, that HIV-infected patients had perturbations in lipid metabolism even before the institution of HAART therapy. Increased serum triglyceride levels, lower levels of high-density lipoprotein (HDL) and low-density lipoprotein (LDL), and decreased total cholesterol levels are all associated with progression toward AIDS. However, the more common problem of dyslipidemia affects HIV-infected patients who are receiving HAART. The clinical implications of antiretroviral therapy–associated dyslipidemia are not fully known. Treatment-related elevations in LDL (or non-HDL) cholesterol and, to a lesser extent, triglycerides might be expected to increase cardiovascular mortality, especially when combined with other HIV-associated conditions and treatment-associated metabolic abnormalities, such as insulin resistance and visceral adiposity.

Protease inhibitors (PIs) increase total serum cholesterol on average by 20 to 30 mg/dL within weeks of institution, although the extent of cholesterol elevations varies markedly among patients. These increases in total cholesterol are typically from increases in LDL cholesterol and, to a more variable extent, increases in HDL. Total cholesterol to HDL ratios therefore may or may not increase. Hypertriglyceridemia is also associated with PIs, although increases are not consistently seen with all PIs. Elevations in triglycerides may be extreme, with elevations of more than 1000 mg/dL, particularly with ritonavir or ritonavir-containing PI combinations. The non-nucleoside reverse transcriptase inhibitor (NNRTI) efavirenz is also associated with increases in lipids. Total cholesterol rises in individuals treated with efavirenz, but HDL increases, as well as LDL cholesterol, in these individuals. When efavirenz is used in combination with ritonavir, lipid elevations, including increases in triglyceride levels, may be more marked. Conversely, the NNRTI nevirapine may be associated with improvements in lipid profiles.

A fasting lipid profile should be obtained before initiation of HAART and 3 to 6 months after initiation. Patients should be screened for other cardiovascular risk factors as though they were uninfected individuals with elevated lipids. Smoking, hypertension, and diabetes are common comorbid diseases in HIV-infected individuals. Also, at least some of the inhibitors of HIV protease (e.g., indinavir) are associated with decreases in insulin sensitivity; these decreases may precipitate manifestation of underlying glucose intolerance with possible attendant cardiovascular risk, despite continued blood sugar control. Perhaps compounding the problem, individuals receiving certain antiretroviral agents were instructed to take their medication with a high-fat meal. Nondrug therapies including diet modification and exercise should be attempted first, except when urgent intervention is needed, such as in patients with established coronary artery disease.

Therapy should follow the National Cholesterol Education Program Treatment Guidelines. Drug treatment of HIV-infected patients with dyslipidemia is problematic because of potential drug interactions. Many of the 3-hydroxy-3-methylglutaryl coenzyme A reductase inhibitors, or statins, are primarily metabolized via cytochrome P450 3A4. Therefore, interactions between these drugs and the HIV PIs, which inhibit CYP3A4, are likely. Potential problems include an increased propensity toward skeletal muscle toxicity (myalgias) or liver toxicity from increased levels of statins. Similarly, interactions between the statins and the NNRTIs nevirapine and efavirenz, which induce CYP3A4, may result in lower serum concentrations of the statins. Because lovastatin and simvastatin are extensively metabolized by CYP3A4, a high likelihood of toxicity is present when these agents are administered with PIs; their use should be avoided in these patients. Fluvastatin, however, is metabolized by CYP2C9 and, therefore, more likely to interact with nelfinavir. Atorvastatin metabolism is less dependent on CYP3A4; therefore, more modest increases in atorvastatin concentrations may be expected when it is coadministered with ritonavir, saquinavir, or both. Pravastatin has no significant P450 interactions, although its levels may be lower when administered with inducers of hepatic metabolism such as ritonavir, nevirapine, or efavirenz.

Fibrates may be effective alternatives for patients with both hypercholesterolemia and hypertriglyceridemia. Lipoprotein lipase (LPL) activity is decreased in hyperlipidemic HIV-infected patients treated with PIs, causing a shift to the more atherogenic dense LDL. Fibrates augment LPL activity and induce a reduction of dense LDL, reducing both LDL and triglycerides. Fibrates are predominantly metabolized by hepatic P450 enzymes, primarily affecting only CYP4A; hence clinically significant drug interactions with PIs are unlikely. With refractory hypertriglyceridemia and hypercholesterolemia, both a fibrate and a statin may be necessary, although toxicity risk may be compounded. Niacin lowers LDL but potentially worsens insulin resistance and should be avoided in patients taking PIs. However, niacin may have a role in isolated hypertryglyceridemia. Bile-sequestering resins are discouraged because their use can be associated with increased triglyceride levels and their effects on antiviral drug absorption are unknown. Switching patients from PIs to potent agents that have a lesser impact on lipids, such as nevirapine or abacavir, or one of the newest

PIs, atazanavir, which does not have any effect on lipis, may be an option.

ISCHEMIC CARDIOVASCULAR DISEASE IN AIDS PATIENTS

Ischemic cardiovascular disease is increasingly reported in association with HIV infection and HAART. Ischemic cardiovascular events are most common in HIV-infected individuals with traditional risk factors, including cigarette smoking, hypertension, family history of premature coronary disease, and hypercholesterolemia. The contribution of HIV infection to the process is complex. Lower CD4 lymphocyte counts and longer duration of HIV infection may be additional risk factors. When compared with age-matched HIV-uninfected individuals, HIV-infected persons in one study had nearly twice the incidence of coronary disease and coronary events, such as myocardial infarctions. This potential for accelerated atherosclerosis in HIV-infected patients may be related to the use of PIs, which may indirectly contribute to the development of cardiovascular disease through the induction of insulin resistance, hypertension, premature menopause, and dyslipidemia, or may be related to the HIV itself. Since the institution of HAART, the overall mortality of HIV-infected individuals has decreased. However, nearly 7% of deaths are related to cardiovascular disease. Clinicians must aggressively treat traditional risk factors and be aware of the potential for accelerated atherosclerosis.

FUTURE DIRECTIONS

The incidence of cardiac disease is higher in HIV-infected individuals than in age-matched individuals in the general population. Since the introduction of HAART, however, the overall incidence has significantly decreased, especially the incidence of pericarditis and dilated cardiomyopathy. This reduction most likely reflects a decrease in opportunistic infections, increased control of HIV replication, improved immune function, and increased overall well-being seen in these patients. Unfortunately, dyslipidemia and potentially accelerated atherosclerosis will likely occur more frequently as more patients are treated with combination antiretroviral regimens of PIs and possibly other antiretroviral agents associated with increases in cholesterol and triglycerides.

REFERENCES

Barbaro G, Di Lorenzo G, Grisorio B, et al. Incidence of dilated cardiomyopathy and detection of HIV in myocardial cells of HIV-positive patients. Gruppo Italiano per lo Studio Cardiologico dei Pazienti Affetti da AIDS. N Engl J Med 1998;339:1093–1099.

David M, Hornung R, Fichtenbaum CJ. Ischemic cardiovascular disease in persons with human immunodeficiency virus infection. Clin Infect Dis 2002;34:98–102.

Dubé, MP, Sprecher D, Henry WK, et al. Preliminary guidelines for the evaluation and management of dyslipidemia in adults infected with human immunodeficiency virus and receiving antiretroviral therapy: Recommendations of the Adult AIDS Clinical Trial Group Cardiovascular Disease Focus Group. Clin Infect Dis 2000;31:1216–1224.

Lewis, W. Cardiomyopathy in AIDS: A pathophysiological perspective. Prog Cardiovasc Dis 2000;43:151–170.

Merigan TC Jr, Bartlett JG, Bolognesi D, eds. Textbook of AIDS Medicine. 2nd ed. Baltimore: Williams & Wilkins, 1999.

National Institutes of Health. Cholesterol lowering in the patient with coronary artery disease: Physician monograph—National Cholesterol Education Program. September 1997 (NIH Publication 97-3794).

Pugliese A, Isnardi D, Saini A, et al. Impact of highly active antiretroviral therapy in HIV-positive patients with cardiac involvement. J Infect 2000;40:282–284.

Yunis NA, Stone VE. Cardiac manifestations of HIV/AIDS: A review of disease spectrum and clinical management. J Acquir Immune Defic Syndr Hum Retrovirol 1998;18:145–154.

Section X

AFFECTING HEART DISEASE— FUTURE DIRECTIONS

Chapter 60

Cardiovascular Epidemiology

Georgeta D. Vaidean

Cardiovascular epidemiology originated from the necessity to quantify the likelihood of developing a coronary event; it emerged as a bridge between the basic sciences, population, and clinical research, and triggered interdisciplinary research in pharmacogenetics, proteomics, biomarkers, bioinformatics, and functional imaging. This explosive growth of information is illustrated by MEDLINE searches for "cardiovascular risk factors": one restricted to the years 1960–1990 retrieves 845 articles, whereas a similar search for the years 1991–2002 retrieves 6883 articles. A better understanding of the pathogenesis, etiology, natural history, underlying mechanisms, and molecular basis of CVD, and a better approach to the design and interpretation of interventional studies have revealed multiple applications for cardiovascular epidemiology research.

CARDIOVASCULAR RISK FACTORS

Cardiovascular epidemiology and evidence-based preventive cardiology evolved around the concept of cardiovascular risk factors, which became an integral part of clinical assessment and decision-making. A cardiovascular risk factor is a personal or environmental (natural or social) characteristic whose presence is associated with an increased likelihood that a particular cardiovascular outcome will develop at a later time in the short or long term. Characteristics of these factors include the following: their distribution and influence are different in different populations; they are not always necessary and/or sufficient for development of clinically apparent coronary heart disease; they have a probabilistic character because their importance resides in their statistical associations in populations; and they are not necessarily elastic. The magnitude of risk reduction achieved by therapy may not be equivalent to the increment in risk .

Categories of Risk Factors

Coronary heart disease (CHD) is a multifactorial disease with multilayered and overlapping "causes" (Table 60-1). More than 300 factors are described as "associated" with CHD. A National Heart, Lung, and Blood Institute (NHLBI) workshop on cardiovascular risk assessment classified factors implicated in the pathogenesis of a major coronary event into several levels: major atherogenic, plaque burden, conditional, underlying, susceptibility, undetermined, and protective. The

multilayered–overlapping paradigm has a variety of mechanisms of action and interactions between levels.

CARDIOVASCULAR RISK PREDICTION: APPROACHES TO GLOBAL RISK ASSESSMENT

Clinical Importance of Global Estimates for CHD Risk

Assessment of global cardiovascular risk based on all major cardiovascular risk factors has three purposes of clinical interest: identification of high-risk patients who should have immediate attention and undergo immediate intervention, motivation of patients to adhere to risk-reduction therapies, and modification of the intensity of risk-reduction efforts based on the total risk estimate (Fig. 60-1). Therapeutic decisions based on quantifiable measurements improve clinical decision-making, increase motivation and compliance of patients, and can be evaluated for economic planning. Guidelines for the management of individual risk factors recommend matching the intensity of preventive therapy to the absolute global cardiovascular risk. Cardiovascular epidemiologic research strives to quantify this global risk via predictive models.

The most common predicted event is the incidence of CHD. This can be defined as including angina pectoris, unstable angina, unrecognized myocardial infarction (MI), recognized MI, and CHD death. When risk cut points are defined to select patients for specific therapies, definitions

Table 60-1
Categories of Risk Factors

Plaque Burden as Risk Factor

· Age (relating to the length of time an individual is exposed to risk factors)

Major Risk Factors

· Smoking
· Increased blood pressure
· Increased serum total and LDL cholesterol concentration
· Low serum concentrations of HDL-C
· History of diabetes mellitus

Conditional Risk Factors

· Increased serum triglyceride concentration
· Small LDL particles
· Increased serum lipoprotein (a) concentration
· Increased serum homocysteine concentration
· Prothrombotic factors: PAI-1, fibrinogen
· Inflammatory markers (e.g., CRP)

Underlying Risk Factors

· Overweight, obesity (especially abdominal obesity)
· Lack of physical activity
· Male gender
· Family history of premature CHD death
· Insulin resistance
· Socioeconomic factors
· Psychological and behavioral factors related to inadequate reaction to stress

Other Risk Factors With Value to Be Established

· Uric acid
· Hematocrit
· Heart rate at rest
· Infectious agents
· Environmental factors: air pollution

CHD indicates coronary heart disease; CRP, C-reactive protein; HDL-C, high-density lipoprotein cholesterol; LDL, low-density lipoprotein; PAI-1, plasminogen activator receptor 1.
With permission from Smith SC Jr, Greenland P, Grundy SM. AHA Conference Proceedings. Prevention conference V: Beyond secondary prevention: Identifying the high-risk patient for primary prevention: Executive summary. American Heart Association. *Circulation* 2000;101:111–116.

of coronary end points have critical importance. However, of an increased interest are symptomatic heart failure, hospital admission for unstable angina, need for revascularization procedures, and changes in functional capacity and quality of life.

Relative Versus Absolute Risk

Absolute global risk is defined as the likelihood that CHD will develop in a person over a specified period, given the presence of cardiovascular risk factors. Absolute risk is considered the crucial determinant of whether and when to initiate pharmacologic therapy. Absolute risk can be calculated as short-term, usually 10 years, long-term, or lifetime risk. *Relative risk* is the ratio of the likelihood of CHD developing in persons with and without given risk factors or at a given intensity of a risk factor. The difference between relative and absolute risk can be explained with an example of serum cholesterol concentration.

Figure 60-1

Cardiovascular Risk Prediction

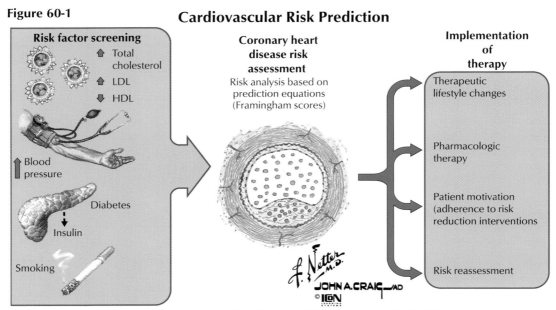

Risk factor screening

⬆ Total cholesterol

⬆ LDL

⬇ HDL

⬆ Blood pressure

Diabetes

↓ Insulin

Smoking

Coronary heart disease risk assessment

Risk analysis based on prediction equations (Framingham scores)

Implementation of therapy

Therapeutic lifestyle changes

Pharmacologic therapy

Patient motivation (adherence to risk reduction interventions

Risk reassessment

In clinical setting CHD risk analysis is important in identification of high risk patients, who should have immediate intervention, motivation of patients to adhere to risk reduction therapy, and modification of risk reduction efforts based on total risk estimate.

Screening to detect subclinical atherosclerosis

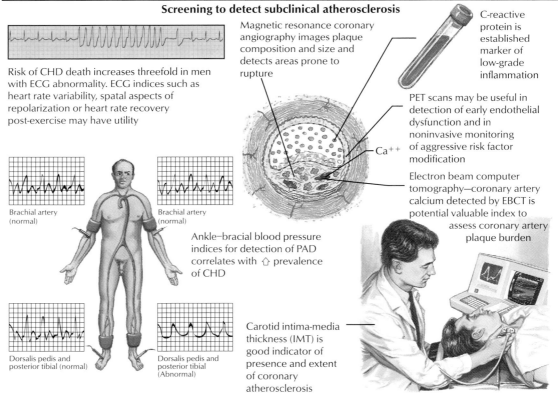

Risk of CHD death increases threefold in men with ECG abnormality. ECG indices such as heart rate variability, spatal aspects of repolarization or heart rate recovery post-exercise may have utility

Magnetic resonance coronary angiography images plaque composition and size and detects areas prone to rupture

C-reactive protein is established marker of low-grade inflammation

PET scans may be useful in detection of early endothelial dysfunction and in noninvasive monitoring of aggressive risk factor modification

Ca++

Electron beam computer tomography—coronary artery calcium detected by EBCT is potential valuable index to assess coronary artery plaque burden

Brachial artery (normal)

Brachial artery (normal)

Ankle–bracial blood pressure indices for detection of PAD correlates with ⬆ prevalence of CHD

Dorsalis pedis and posterior tibial (normal)

Dorsalis pedis and posterior tibial (Abnormal)

Carotid intima-media thickness (IMT) is good indicator of presence and extent of coronary atherosclerosis

A major objective of preventive cardiology is to measure and monitor atherosclerosis in asymptomatic individuals and identify appropriate candidates for aggressive primary prevention

A young adult with a very high serum cholesterol concentration is at a low absolute risk for CHD but is at a high relative risk compared with a young adult with a low serum cholesterol concentration. CHD is unlikely to develop in the hypercholesterolemic young adult in the next 10 years, but the individual's chances of experiencing premature CHD in the long term (e.g., before age 65) are high.

The goal for reducing elevated serum cholesterol concentration in young adults, therefore, is to retard atherogenesis throughout life, not only to prevent MI in the next decade.

Methods of Risk Assessment

Cardiovascular risk assessment uses two major approaches: simple counting and mathematical models.

Counting

Simple counting of the major cardiovascular risk factors can grossly rank asymptomatic subjects by the likelihood of a coronary event developing. It is a rapid approach of limited complexity for daily practice and easy to implement. However, it does not apply the intensity of risk factors nor their synergistic impact on the global cardiovascular risk. Hence, simple counting has a reduced predictive ability.

Risk Scores Based on Mathematical Models

A more refined approach is the use of predictive equations, which offer quantification of the absolute risk. Predictive equations have been generated by several cohort studies, the most well-known being the Framingham risk equations.

Estimating Risk Using the Framingham Risk Scores

The Framingham Heart Study has generated prediction equations based on multivariate regression models to estimate CHD risk. The outcomes predicted are total CHD and "hard CHD." In the Framingham study, total cholesterol (TC)— and LDL-C—based approaches, whether as continuous or categorical variables, are similar in their ability to predict initial CHD events. However, extensive clinical data and clinical trial results suggest that LDL-C is the major atherogenic lipoprotein. Therefore, the use of LDL-C concentrations in the clinical set-

ting is important whenever fasting samples are available. Despite studies advocating the use of the total cholesterol:HDL-C ratio, it was not used in Framingham predictions for two reasons. At the extremes of the TC or LDL-C distribution, equal ratios may not signify the same CHD risk, and, as importantly, the use of a ratio may make it more difficult for the physician to focus on the separate values.

The BP value used in the Framingham Risk Score is obtained at the time of assessment, regardless of whether the patient is taking antihypertensive drugs. The average of several BP measurements is needed for an accurate determination of the baseline concentration. Diabetes is defined as a fasting plasma glucose concentration greater than 126 mg/dL. The designation of "smoker" indicates any use of cigarettes within the past month.

Framingham risk scores provide two ways to estimate cardiovascular risk: (1) Comparison of a an individual's estimated risk with the absolute risk of an individual at low risk, that is, a person who is largely without risk factors. This is the best way to assess the full potential for risk reduction, when introduced relatively early in life (Table 60-2). Total excess risk for an individual patient can be estimated by subtracting the absolute risk of a person of the same age and sex who is at low risk from that of the individual in question. (2) Comparison of an individual's estimated risk with the risk of an average person of the same age and sex. This approach is commonly used, though it tends to underestimate the preventable component of coronary risk because of the high prevalence of coronary atherosclerosis in the United States and most developed countries. To facilitate the use of risk prediction in clinical practice, based on these equations, simple risk score sheets are widely distributed and available for public use (see Resources at the end of this chapter).

These risk prediction equations can be confidently extrapolated to other settings. Recent comparisons show that within sampling fluctuations, the Framingham equations discriminate reasonably well between subjects in whom clinical CHD developed and in those whom it did not in other (non-Framingham) populations. However, when applied to Japanese American,

Table 60-2
Low Risk

Definition

The Framingham Heart Study defines low risk as the risk for CHD at an age that is conferred by a combination of all of the parameters listed below.

Parameters

· Serum total cholesterol 160–199 mg/dL or LDL-C 100–129 mg/dL

· HDL-C ≥45 mg/dL in men and ≥55mg/dL in women

· SBP <120 mm Hg systolic and DBP < 80 mm Hg

· Nonsmoker

· No history of diabetes mellitus

CHD indicates coronary heart disease; HDL-C, high-density lipoprotein cholesterol; LDL-C, low-density lipoprotein cholesterol.
With permission from Grundy SM, Pasternak R, Greenland P, et al. Assessment of cardiovascular risk by use of multiple-risk-factor assessment equations: A statement for healthcare professionals from the American Heart Association and the American College of Cardiology. *Circulation* 1999;100:1481–1492. Available at: http://circ.ahajournals.org/cgi/reprint/100/13/1481.pdf

Hispanic, and Native American men and women, some recalibration is needed by future work using data on prevalence and CHD event rates specific to the population of interest.

IMPLEMENTATION: THE FINAL FRONTIER OF PREVENTIVE CARDIOLOGY

A large body of evidence supports the efficacy of risk factor modification in subjects with atherosclerosis. Cardiovascular risk factors are seen interventionally through their amenability to be changed, from proven effective interventions to those that are unlikely to be effective (Table 60-3).

Guidelines for risk factor management have been developed based on convincing results of pathophysiology, molecular biology, epidemiologic studies, and randomized clinical trials, in primary and secondary prevention. However, guidelines often fall short of implementation and fail to influence clinical practice, despite the wide dissemination of algorithms for the screening for cardiovascular risk factors and management of hypertension and lipid disorders.

Table 60-3
Classification of Cardiovascular Risk Factors From the Intervention Point of View

Factors for which intervention has been proven to lower coronary CAD risk

· Diet
· TC and LDL-C
· Antithrombotic therapy
· Smoking
· Hypertension
· Multifactorial risk modification

Factors for which interventions are likely to lower CAD risk

· History of diabetes
· Physical inactivity/exercise
· Obesity
· HDL-C
· TG and small, dense LDL-C
· Hormone replacement therapy

Factors that if modified, might lower CAD risk

· Psychoscial factors
· Oxidative stress
· Lipoprotein(a)
· Hyperhomocysteinemia

Factors that cannot be modified or for which modification would be unlikely to lower CAD risk

· Family history and genetics
· Age

CAD indicates coronary artery disease; HDL-C, high density lipoprotein cholesterol; LDL-C, low-density lipoprotein cholesterol.
Data from Forrester JS, Merz CN, Bush TL, et al. 27th Bethesda Conference: Matching the intensity of risk factor management with the hazard for coronary disease events. Task Force 4. Efficacy of risk factor management. *J Am Coll Cardiol* 1996;27:991–1006.

Screening and Management of Cardiovascular Risk Factors in Medical Practice

It is often claimed that approximately 50% of MIs occur in patients without prior manifestations of risk factors. Recently, some investigators have argued that this number is less than 50%; it nonetheless remains significant and has stimulated efforts in the research community to search for new risk factors that could aid early identification and treatment, and could prevent future events. Of equal importance, however, is the question of whether adequate preventative strategies were used for the other 50%, in whom traditional cardiovascular risk factors were present at the time of symptoms. In a random sample of retrospective chart reviews of patients admitted to coronary care units, rates of physician screening for CHD risk factors; rates of counseling for cigarette cessation, diet, and exercise; and extent of use of National Cholesterol Education Program (NCEP) algorithms were disappointing. Approximately 50% of smokers report that their physician has never advised them to quit. Even in secondary prevention, the management of risk factors is less than satisfactory.

Blood pressure control rates are poor. Data from The National Health and Nutrition Examination Survey—the barometer of hypertension awareness, treatment, and control—show that the initial improvements since the publication of the recommendations of the Fifth Joint National Committee on the Prevention, Detection, Evaluation, and Treatment of High Blood Pressure (JNC V) in 1993 have begun to deteriorate.

Aggressive lipid-lowering therapy prevents recurrent cardiac events and lowers total mortality rate in patients with known CHD, as well as in asymptomatic individuals. Despite strong evidence of benefits, patients continue to be underscreened and undertreated for hyperlipidemia. For instance, in numerous studies performed in varying clinical settings (such as coronary care units, VA hospitals or medical practices), 33% of patients with CVD were not screened using lipid panels and only approximately 35% of those in whom medical therapy was indicated—according to National Cholesterol Education Program guidelines—actually received lipid-lowering medications in primary prevention and only about 67% received medications in secondary prevention. Furthermore, among patients being prescribed lipid-lowering medications, only a fraction achieve acceptable LDL-C reduction. In the Lipid Treatment Assessment Project, overall, target LDL-C concentrations or values lower than the goal were attained in only 38% of the patients. Moreover, the greater the number of risk factors, the lower the proportion of target concentrations achieved in patients.

Table 60-4
Barriers to Implementation of Preventive Services

Patient

· Lack of knowledge and motivation
· Lack of access to care
· Cultural and social factors

Physician

· Problem-based focus
· Feedback on prevention is negative or neutral
· Time constraints
· Lack of incentives
· Lack of training
· Lack of specialist–generalist communication
· Lack of perceived legitimacy

Healthcare Settings

· Acute care priority
· Lack of resources and facilities
· Lack of systems for preventive services
· Time and economic constraints
· Poor communication specialists and primary care providers
· Lack of policies and standards

Community/Society

· Lack of policies and standards
· Lack of reimbursement

Reprinted from the *Journal of the American College of Cardiology* 27(5), Pearson TA, McBride PE, Miller NH, et al. 27th Bethesda Conference: Matching the intensity of risk factor management with the hazard for coronary disease events. Task Force 8. Organization of preventive cardiology service, 1039–47, 1996, with permission from the American College of Cardiology Foundation.

Barriers to Implementation of Preventive Services and Strategies to Improve Guideline Adherence

It is inevitable that there are delays before research results are accepted by the medical community and adopted into routine clinical practice. However, it is important that validated guidelines and new findings be adopted as widely and quickly as possible. Potential barriers to the adoption of new approaches comprise three areas: those relating to the patient, those relating to the healthcare system and society as a whole, and those affecting physician behavior (Table 60-4).

FUTURE DIRECTIONS

A major objective of preventive cardiology is to measure and monitor atherosclerosis in asymptomatic individuals and to identify appropriate candidates for aggressive primary prevention. Although noninvasive imaging of atherosclerosis and identification of serum markers hold great promise to quantify atherosclerotic burden and predict coronary events, they should not be considered substitutes for traditional risk factor screening, but should have instead a complementary role. In evaluating their potential as screening and predictive tools, these novel tests should answer whether screening with a new tool has incremental value in assessing cardiovascular risk and whether such a screening test would further improve outcomes over currently advocated guidelines for risk reduction. Tests with promise include recently appreciated ECG findings, electron beam CT, magnetic resonance coronary angiography, PET, ankle–brachial BP index, carotid intima– media thickness on ultrasound, C-reactive protein, and possibly evidence of exposure to certain infectious agents.

In the Multiple Risk Factors Intervention Trial (MRFIT) study, the risk of CHD death for men with any ECG abnormality was three times the risk of those without abnormalities. Novel ECG indexes, such as heart rate variability, spatial aspects of repolarization, or heart rate recovery after the exercise test, may add clinical and epidemiologic utility.

Because coronary calcification increases with age, the highly sensitive electron beam CT score might be able to replace age as a surrogate for coronary plaque burden. However, because it lacks the ability to detect noncalcified atheroma electron beam CT may offer an improvement over conventional risk factors in predicting the angiographic burden of atherosclerosis, but not in predicting coronary events.

Magnetic resonance coronary angiography is a research tool intended to image plaque composition and size and detect areas vulnerable to rupture. Although it cannot accurately detect small stenoses, it is a potential source of information on anatomic and functional significance of atherosclerotic plaques, by allowing three-dimensional visualization of coronary arteries and evaluation of perfusion, coronary flow and

flow reserve, contractility, stress-induced wall-motion abnormalities, and cardiac metabolism. PET, as used today, has limited applicability as a screening test. It lacks the ability to detect coronary stenoses less than 50%. PET may have a future role in the detection of early endothelial dysfunction and in noninvasive monitoring of aggressive risk factor modification in asymptomatic individuals.

Ankle–brachial BP index (ABI) detection of peripheral artery disease (PAD) correlates with a higher prevalence of CHD, demonstrates the atherosclerotic involvement of multiple vascular beds, and is a simple and inexpensive test. An ABI less than 0.90 in either leg indicates peripheral artery disease; the lower the value of the index, the more severe the obstruction. An abnormal ABI elevates asymptomatic individuals to a higher risk category.

A correlation between carotid intima–media thickness and cardiac risk has been demonstrated within populations, but this less clearly predicts CHD risk in individuals. Carotid intima–media thickness is a good indicator of the presence and extent of coronary atherosclerosis; a direct relation exists between intima–media thickening and the likelihood of coexistent significant CHD.

C-reactive protein, especially measured by highly sensitive assays (hs-CRP), is an established marker of low-grade systemic inflammation, and its association with cardiovascular disease is well-documented. CRP advantages include its sensitivity, safety, convenience, and cost-effectiveness; standardized assays are available to provide good validity and repeatability.

Several large-scale clinical trials are studying certain infectious agents (*Helicobacter pylori*, Cytomegalovirus, *Chlamydia pneumoniae*) and their role in atherogenesis and CHD end points, but it is not yet clear whether evidence of these infectious agents represents causation or whether these are, in effect, "innocent bystanders."

Research in cardiovascular epidemiology has contributed to understanding the atherosclerosis process and shaped the development of intervention tools in individuals and communities. The answers obtained have prompted new questions and generated new hypotheses. Future avenues for research will likely seek a better understanding of how the identified cardiovascular risk factors modify genetic predispositions and of the interplay between behavioral and environmental factors, and the development of more accurate risk prediction tools and more targeted prevention strategies.

REFERENCES

D'Agostino RB, Grundy S, Sillva LM, Wilson P, for the CHD Risk Prediction Group. Validation of the Framingham Coronary Heart Disease Prediction Scores results of a multiple ethnic groups investigation *JAMA* 2001;286:180-187.

Expert Panel on Detection, Evaluation, and Treatment of High Blood Cholesterol in Adults. Summary of the third report of the National Cholesterol Education Program (NCEP) Expert Panel on Detection, Evaluation, and Treatment of High Blood Cholesterol in Adults (Adult Treatment Panel III). *JAMA* 2001; 285:2486-2497.

Forrester JS, Merz CN, Bush TL, et al. 27th Bethesda Conference: Matching the intensity of risk factor management with the hazard for coronary disease events. Task Force 4. Efficacy of risk factor management. *J Am Coll Cardiol* 1996;27:991-1006.

Greenland P, Abrams J, Aurigemma GP, et al. Beyond secondary prevention: Identifying the high-risk patient for primary prevention: Noninvasive tests of atherosclerotic burden: Writing Group III. *Circulation* 2000;101:E16-22.

Grundy SM. D'Agostino RB Sr, Mosca L, et al. Cardiovascular risk assessment based on US cohort studies: Findings from a National Heart, Lung, and Blood Institute workshop. *Circulation* 2001;104:491-496.

Pearson TA. New tools for coronary risk assessment. What are their advantages and limitations? *Circulation* 2002;105:886-892.

Pearson TA, McBride PE, Miller NH, Smith SC. 27th Bethesda Conference: Matching the intensity of risk factor management with the hazard for coronary disease events. Task Force 8. Organization of preventive cardiology service. *J Am Coll Cardiol* 1996;27:1039-1047.

Smith SC Jr, Greenland P, Grundy SM. AHA Conference Proceedings. Prevention conference V: Beyond secondary prevention: Identifying the high-risk patient for primary prevention: Executive summary. American Heart Association. *Circulation.* 2000;101:111-116.

RESOURCES

An Online Risk Assessment Tool for Estimating 10-Year Risk of Developing Hard CHD (Myocardial Infarction and Coronary Death) [NCEP-NIH-NHLBI Web site]. Available at: http://hin.nhlbi.nih.gov/atpiii/calculator.asp?usertype=prof

A Risk Assessment Tool for Estimating 10-Year Risk of Developing Hard CHD (Myocardial Infarction and Coronary Death) [NIH, NHLBI, NCEP ATPIII Web site]. Available at: http://www.nhlbi.nih.gov/guidelines/cholesterol/. Online assessment available at: http://hin.nhlbi.nih.gov/atpiii/calculator.asp?usertype=prof. Download on Palm OS available at: http://hin.nhlbi.nih.gov/atpiii/atp3palm.htm

CHD Risk score sheets. [NIH-NHLBI Web site]. Available at: http://www.nhlbi.nih.gov/about/framingham/riskabs.htm

Chapter 61

Cardiovascular Disease in Women and Special Populations

Eileen A. Kelly and Sidney C. Smith, Jr

Changes in the US ethnic mix coupled with an aging population and an increasing prevalence of cardiovascular risk factors, and the notable increase in obesity, necessitate a broader understanding of cardiovascular disease (CVD) in special populations. The aging of the population has resulted in an increased prevalence of CVD among women, in whom the onset of clinical events is generally approximately 10 years later than it is in men. By 2050, it is projected that more than 45% of the US population will have a BMI above 30: a marker of obesity and a risk factor for both coronary heart disease (CHD) and diabetes. Finally, increases in black, Latino, Asian Pacific, and Southeast Asian groups in the US population will result in major shifts in the demographic patterns of CVD.

DIABETES

The prevalence and incidence of diabetes in the United States have increased significantly (see also chapter 54). Almost 35 million Americans and 35% of elderly Americans have some degree of glucose intolerance. The rates of morbidity and mortality from cardiovascular disease and from atherosclerotic disease involving the cerebral and peripheral vessels is two to eight times higher among individuals with diabetes (Fig. 61-1). Diabetes is more common among Hispanic individuals, black individuals, and Native Americans than among white individuals. The increase in type 2 diabetes among children and adolescents is likely to result in further increases in the incidence of premature CHD. The National Cholesterol Education Program Adult Treatment Panel III identifies diabetes as a CHD equivalent and recommends the same aggressive risk factor modification and preventive therapy for patients with diabetes as for patients with known CHD.

The evaluation of the patient with diabetes begins with a careful medical history (see also chapter 1). Symptoms of atherosclerotic vascular disease, such as claudication and angina, deserve special attention. Patients with diabetes should be evaluated for signs and symptoms of congestive heart failure, although it must be appreciated that diabetic individuals often have atypical symptoms or no symptoms at all in the presence of significant CHD. The resting ECG should be evaluated for evidence of left ventricular hypertrophy, a marker for increased cardiovascular risk. The value of screening tests such as exercise treadmill electrocardiography, ankle–brachial index, and electron beam CT is not well established. The use of medical therapies such as lipid-lowering treatment should be based on the presence of diabetes, a CHD equivalent, rather than on symptoms or on the identification of an abnormality on noninvasive testing. The Adult Treatment Panel III recommends a target low-density lipoprotein (LDL) cholesterol below 100 mg/dL for patients with diabetes. The American Heart Association/American College of Cardiology secondary prevention statement recommends that blood pressure be kept below 130/80 and hemoglobin A_{1c} below 7.0 as treatment goals for patients with diabetes. For patients who have triglyceride levels above 200 mg/dL in spite of appropriate diet and exercise and who have received statin therapy, treatment with a fibrate is recommended. Because a prothrombotic state accompanies diabetes, patients with diabetes should be treated with daily aspirin even in the absence of clinical CHD. Physical activity and maintenance of BMI below 25 will also improve diabetic control and reduce the risk of CHD-related events in diabetic individuals.

The hospitalization and long-term mortality rates following acute myocardial infarction (MI) are twice as high among individuals with diabetes than they are among individuals without dia-

Figure 61-1

Cardiovascular Disease in Diabetes

Diabetes mellitus

High BMI
(⬆ insulin resistance)

Smoking

Elevated
blood
pressure

⬆ Clotting
factors

⬆ HGB A$_{1c}$

⬆ LDL and
triglycerides
⬇ HDL

Microalbuminuria
(⬆ risk of loss of
renal function
and CHD)

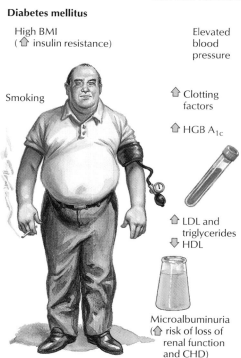

Diabetic patient with high-risk
factors for cardiovascular disease

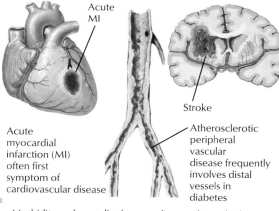

Acute
MI

Stroke

Acute
myocardial
infarction (MI)
often first
symptom of
cardiovascular disease

Atherosclerotic
peripheral
vascular
disease frequently
involves distal
vessels in
diabetes

Morbidity and mortality from cardiovascular and other
atherosclerotic disease involving cerebral and peripheral
vessels 2–3 times higher among persons with diabetes

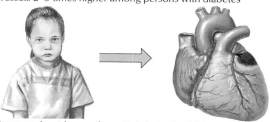

Increased incidence of type II diabetes in children and
adolescents raises likelihood premature coronary heart
disease (CHD) will develop

Management goals

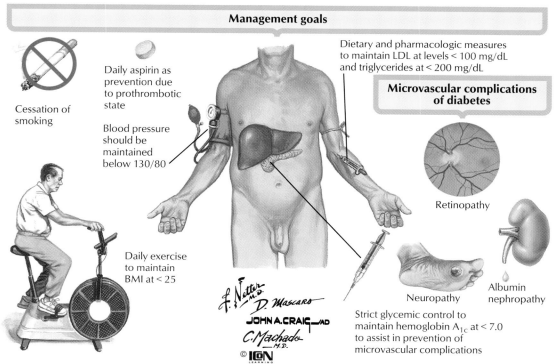

Cessation of
smoking

Daily aspirin as
prevention due
to prothrombotic
state

Blood pressure
should be
maintained
below 130/80

Daily exercise
to maintain
BMI at < 25

Dietary and pharmacologic measures
to maintain LDL at levels < 100 mg/dL
and triglycerides at < 200 mg/dL

**Microvascular complications
of diabetes**

Retinopathy

Neuropathy

Albumin
nephropathy

Strict glycemic control to
maintain hemoglobin A$_{1c}$ at < 7.0
to assist in prevention of
microvascular complications

betes. Diabetes is a major risk factor for adverse outcomes in patients with unstable angina. Although the prevalence of diabetes is about 8% among the general population, it is about 30% among patients with acute MI. Often, acute MI is the first symptom of CVD in a patient with diabetes. Because symptoms may be atypical, due in part to the presence of autonomic neuropathy, late recognition by the patient may delay implementation of reperfusion therapies, thus leading to a poorer prognosis. The ventricle in patients with diabetes often has undergone maladaptive remodeling, which contributes to heart failure and cardiogenic shock. Among diabetic individuals presenting with acute MI who are undergoing primary coronary intervention, the use of a IIb/IIIa receptor antagonist results in better outcomes. Similar benefits have been observed with IIb/IIIa receptor antagonists in patients with diabetes who have unstable angina or non–ST-segment elevation MI. For patients with diabetes, the use of β-blockers results in early and late survival benefits compared to patients without diabetes. The admission glucose level is an independent predictor of early and late mortality after MI in patients with diabetes. Strict glycemic control reduces cardiovascular risk. Studies of MI survivors with diabetes have demonstrated a significant survival benefit in those with tight glycemic control for up to 3 years following their MI.

The control of cardiovascular risk factors in patients with diabetes must be a high priority. In patients with diabetes who smoke cigarettes, cardiovascular risk is doubled. In addition to the benefits of glycemic control in terms of blood pressure and lipid abnormalities, the control of hyperglycemia assists in the prevention of the microvascular complications of diabetes (nephropathy, neuropathy, and retinopathy). Diabetes is the leading cause of end-stage renal disease in the United States, with a 5-year survival of only 20% for patients with diabetes in this category. Microalbuminuria is a major predictor of renal function loss and CHD. The early use of angiotensin-converting enzyme inhibitors among patients with diabetes even in the absence of hypertension reduces the rates of cardiovascular morbidity and mortality.

Of the nearly 1.5 million percutaneous and surgical revascularization procedures carried out annually in the United States, roughly 25% are performed on patients with diabetes. In this group, comorbidities such as hypertension, dyslipidemia, systolic and diastolic heart failure, nephropathy, and peripheral vascular, cerebrovascular, and microvascular diseases contribute to poorer outcomes compared to patients without diabetes. In addition to the extent of coronary artery disease, the presence of diabetes alone may govern the revascularization approach chosen. For instance, significant differences in survival, in favor of CABG, exist for patients with diabetes and two- or three-vessel CAD randomized to CABG surgery compared with PTCA. The benefits of CABG surgery are seen only when at least one arterial conduit is utilized. The increased use of stents and IIb/IIIa receptor antagonists in percutaneous revascularization procedures has improved outcomes and further studies will help define the relative benefits of coronary artery stenting versus CABG in diabetic individuals.

THE ELDERLY

Although cardiovascular events can occur at any age, the absolute risk increases incrementally as the population ages and is greatest in the elderly population (≥65 years). Approximately 85% of cardiovascular deaths occur after age 65. In the United States alone there are more than 25 million people 65 years or older. In 2000, elderly individuals represented 12.6% of the population. By 2020, the elderly population will increase to 16.5%. The 31% increase in this group of individuals with a high prevalence of CVD will further increase the demands on the health care system and underscores the importance of treatment strategies for elderly individuals (Fig. 61-2, upper).

Clinically, CHD in elderly individuals often presents in an atypical manner, with dyspnea or heart failure as the initial symptom. Although not always the case, CHD in elderly individuals is often essentially asymptomatic. The atypical nature of symptoms often delays diagnosis and treatment. This delay combined with an increase in comorbidities and the underuse of proven beneficial therapies (pharmacologic and interventional) contributes to the increased rates of mor-

Figure 61-2

Cardiovascular Disease in Women and the Elderly
Cardiovascular disease in the elderly

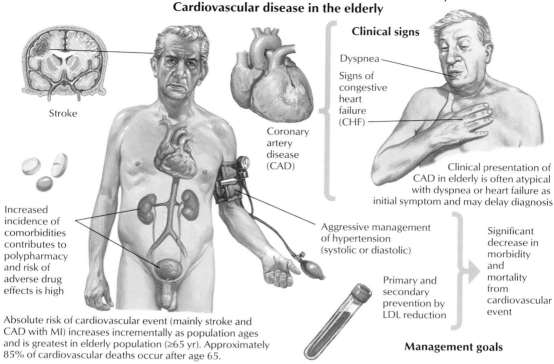

Stroke

Coronary artery disease (CAD)

Clinical signs

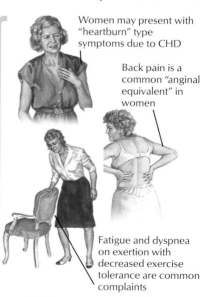

Dyspnea

Signs of congestive heart failure (CHF)

Clinical presentation of CAD in elderly is often atypical with dyspnea or heart failure as initial symptom and may delay diagnosis

Increased incidence of comorbidities contributes to polypharmacy and risk of adverse drug effects is high

Aggressive management of hypertension (systolic or diastolic)

Significant decrease in morbidity and mortality from cardiovascular event

Primary and secondary prevention by LDL reduction

Absolute risk of cardiovascular event (mainly stroke and CAD with MI) increases incrementally as population ages and is greatest in elderly population (≥65 yr). Approximately 85% of cardiovascular deaths occur after age 65.

Management goals

Cardiovascular disease in women

Risk factors

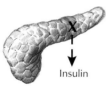

Insulin

Diabetes in women more powerful risk factor than in men, associated with 3–7 times increase in CHD development

Smoking stronger risk factor for MI in middle aged women than men

Hormone replacement contraindicated as cardio-protection in post-menopausal women

Treatment of dyslipidemias (⬆ LDL, ⬇ HDL, ⬆ triglycerides) offers reduction in cardiovascular event risk

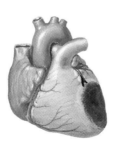

Cardiovascular disease is leading cause of death in both men and women. More women die of cardiovascular disease than of breast cancer.

f. Netter M.D.

JOHN A. CRAIG —MD

C. Machado M.D.

©ICN

Clinical presentation

Women may present with "heartburn" type symptoms due to CHD

Back pain is a common "anginal equivalent" in women

Fatigue and dyspnea on exertion with decreased exercise tolerance are common complaints

CHD symptoms reported by women often differ from those reported by men. These vague or confusing symptoms may contribute to a delayed or missed diagnosis.

bidity and mortality among post-MI elderly patients. The increased incidence of comorbid conditions contributes to polypharmacy in elderly patients—with the attendant risk of adverse effects—and prevents the addition of medications that would likely lower cardiac risk. Despite the need for multiple medical therapies among elderly patients, risk factor modification in this group translates into decreased cardiovascular events.

Elevated LDL plays an important role in the pathogenesis of CHD, and reduction of LDL cholesterol levels decreases the risk of cardiovascular events. Despite widespread information indicating a therapeutic benefit, underdiagnosis and undertreatment of dyslipidemia continue among elderly individuals. In fact, preventive therapies (pharmacological and non-pharmacological) in elderly individuals decrease in cardiovascular endpoints even more dramatically than in younger cohorts, probably because of the increased incidence of CHD in elderly individuals. Age should not exclude patients from treatment for LDL-lowering in the secondary prevention setting. In primary prevention, treatment of elevated LDL has been more controversial. However, the benefits of preventive treatment in this population are substantiated by several smaller trials and by the Heart Protection Study, which included patients up to the age of 80. The Adult Treatment Panel III recommends therapeutic lifestyle changes as first-line therapy.

Hypertension (blood pressure ≥140/90) occurs in more than 50% of the population aged 65 years and older. It is a major risk factor for stroke, heart failure, and CHD. Although hypertension was once considered part of "normal aging," the benefit of treating elderly patients with elevated systolic and/or diastolic blood pressure is clear. Aggressive treatment of isolated systolic hypertension can provide a 30% reduction in rate of combined fatal and nonfatal stroke, a 26% reduction in the rates of fatal and nonfatal cardiovascular events, and a 13% reduction in the total mortality rate.

WOMEN

Cardiovascular disease is the leading cause of death in men and women. In the United States in 2001, CVD claimed the lives of 498,863 women and 432,245 men. Unfortunately,

although the cardiovascular mortality rate has declined steadily for men, it has remained virtually unchanged for women. It is uncertain whether this difference reflects a gap in awareness and education, undertreatment of women, or an increase in the prevalence of CHD in women. Among respondents to an American Heart Association survey, most women believed that cancer was their biggest health threat. However, in 2001, the death rate for women from cardiovascular disease was 281.7 (per 100,000) compared to 26.0 for breast cancer.

In addition to receiving information on disease prevalence, women must be educated that their CHD symptoms can differ from the symptoms that men commonly report. Women often have dyspnea on exertion, "heartburn," fatigue, decreased exercise tolerance, or back pain as their "anginal equivalent." These somewhat vague or confusing symptoms often contribute to delayed or missed diagnoses of CHD (Fig. 61-2, lower).

Most CHD risk factors and strategies for preventing disease applicable to men also apply to women. However, the magnitude of the effects of these risk factors and prevention strategies may be different. For example, diabetes is an even more powerful risk factor for CHD in women. It is associated with a three- to sevenfold increase in the frequency of CHD development. A woman with diabetes is twice as likely to have a recurrent MI compared to the likelihood of recurrent MI in a man with equal risk factors. Smoking is also a stronger risk factor for MI in middle-aged women than it is in men, a concern because smoking rates are declining at a slower rate among women than among men. Dyslipidemias, especially elevated triglycerides and low high-density lipoprotein cholesterol, are more commonly seen with CHD in women and are most commonly seen in postmenopausal women. Cholesterol reduction strategies with statins have shown at least an equivalent reduction in risk in women compared with men. In fact, in some studies the risk of primary or secondary cardiovascular events was more favorably influenced by statin therapy in women than in men. Risk factors unique to women include menopause, with its associated estrogen loss and effect on the lipid profile, and hormone replacement therapy (HRT). Historically, a cardioprotective effect of HRT in women was inferred, based largely on observational data, regardless of the women's cardiovascular disease status. However, no benefit in the rates of nonfatal MI or death from CHD in women with known heart disease receiving combined HRT was found in the largest randomized clinical trial conducted to date. Indeed, an increase in CHD events was observed during the first year of HRT use in that trial. Consequently, the American Heart Association has released a statement for health care professionals recommending that HRT *not* be initiated for the prevention of heart attack or stroke in women with CVD. Furthermore, a large-scale trial investigating the primary prevention benefits of combined HRT was stopped early primarily because of the risk of associated invasive breast cancer. However, a significant increase in cardiovascular events was also observed. Taken together, clinical trials do not support the use of combined HRT in the primary or secondary prevention of cardiovascular events.

RACIAL AND ETHNIC CONSIDERATIONS

The prevalence and incidence of CVD varies among the major ethnic and racial groups in the United States. These variations are increasingly important in developing strategies for prevention and treatment as minority populations increase in number. For instance, in California it is estimated that over the next decade, the Hispanic and African American populations will constitute more than 50% of residents.

Cardiovascular disease mortality rate varies significantly by US region, with a greater than twofold difference between the states with the lowest and the highest rates. In part, these differences in mortality rates reflect variations in the ethnic composition of a given region. Black individuals have the highest mortality rates for CHD and stroke; the mortality rate from CHD is lower among the Hispanic, Asian, and Native American populations. Among Asians, probably because of the high prevalence of hypertension, the mortality rate from stroke is nearly equal that among non-Hispanic whites but it is still less than that seen among black individuals. The highest

mortality rates from CHD are seen in the Mississippi Delta, Appalachia, and the Ohio River Valley. A high mortality rate from stroke continues to exist in the southeastern United States, but stroke rates have increased in the northwestern United States, possibly because of an increase in the Asian population of those states. The areas with the highest CVD mortality in the United States are frequently poor and rural.

Racial differences in health care outcomes are well documented in the United States. Members of minority populations, especially black individuals, are less likely to receive invasive cardiovascular procedures shown to improve outcomes. The reasons for this disparity may include racial differences in access to care, patient preferences, and provider bias. Although the preponderance of literature on racial differences in the use of cardiovascular procedures reflects comparisons between black and white patients, similar findings are described for Hispanic and Asian patients.

LOWER SOCIOECONOMIC GROUPS

Socioeconomic differences in CVD mortality rates are reported for many countries, including the United States. In most reports, a clear gradient in mortality rates exists; the CVD mortality rate is higher in individuals with lower education levels or in lower occupational classes. In Western Europe, a north–south gradient exists for CHD, with a higher mortality rate in the north. These differences may reflect differences in risk factors, such as diet, cigarette smoking, and obesity. Unfortunately, reports suggest that the gap in the CVD mortality rates between the poor and undereducated and the wealthy and well educated has not narrowed and may even be widening.

FUTURE DIRECTIONS

Future directions for prevention of CHD in special populations must target the special needs of each population. Clinical trials testing new strategies need to establish appropriate guidelines for revascularization strategies in patients with diabetes. The Bypass Angioplasty Revascularization Investigation 2 Diabetes trial, which will compare tight diabetic control with and without various revascularization procedures, should contribute significantly to the understanding of appropriate strategies for managing patients with diabetes.

Cardiovascular disease in elderly individuals, the most rapidly expanding subgroup in the United States, is an important public health issue. Prevention efforts should be undertaken. Elderly individuals must be included in clinical trials, and aggressive risk factor identification and modification must be pursued. Because of the potentially debilitating nature of cardiovascular events, primary and secondary prevention in elderly individuals are crucial.

Coronary heart disease is largely preventable in women through diet and lifestyle modification. Education, lifestyle changes, and prevention efforts will make a difference in this patient population.

Major federal initiatives have been launched to eliminate the racial and ethnic differences in cardiovascular outcomes. The challenges of changing behavior and CVD risk are magnified among those of lesser educational background and lower economic income where resources may be lacking to understand and afford necessary measures. Developing effective interventions for risk factor reduction among lower socioeconomic groups must be a priority.

REFERENCES

American Heart Association. 2003 Heart and Stroke Statistical Update. Dallas: American Heart Association; 2002.

American Heart Association. Women and Heart Disease: A Study Tracking Women's Awareness of and Attitudes Toward Heart Disease and Stroke. Dallas: American Heart Association; 2000.

Benjamin EJ, Smith SC, Cooper RS, et al. Magnitude of the prevention problem: Opportunities and challenges. 33rd Bethesda Conference. *J Am Coll Cardiol* 2002;40:588–603.

Cooper R, Cutler J, Desvigne-Nickens P, et al. Trends and disparities in coronary heart disease, stroke, and other cardiovascular diseases in the United States. *Circulation* 2000;102:3137–3147.

Executive Summary of the third report of the National Cholesterol Education Program (NCEP) Expert Panel on Detection, Evaluation, and Treatment of High Blood Cholesterol in Adults (Adult Treatment Panel III). *JAMA* 2001;285:2486–2497.

Grundy SM, Howard B, Smith S Jr, Eckel R, Redberg R, Bonow RO. Prevention Conference VI: Diabetes and Cardiovascular Disease: Executive Summary: Conference proceeding for healthcare professionals from a special writing group of the American Heart Association. *Circulation* 2002;105:2231–2239.

Mosca L, Collins P, Herrington DM, et al. Hormone replacement therapy and cardiovascular disease: A statement for healthcare professionals from the American Heart Association. *Circulation* 2001;104:499–503.

Smith SC, Blair SN, Bonow RO, et al. Guidelines for preventing heart attack and death in patients with atherosclerotic cardiovascular disease: 2001 update. *Circulation* 2001;104:1577–1579.

Chapter 62

Genetics in Cardiovascular Disease

Marschall S. Runge

In the 50 years since Watson and Crick published their landmark manuscript on the molecular structure of nucleic acids, genetics has changed profoundly. The human genome (and the genomes of many other species) has been sequenced, and the search to identify and characterize the estimated 30,000 genes in the human genome continues.

A major challenge for physicians and health care providers will be fluency in the language of genetics as decisions on who should be screened for genetic causes of disease, how to best approach families with heritable diseases, and, ultimately, selection of patients for genetic-based therapies become more common. This information will be particularly important for caregivers of patients with cardiovascular diseases, a field dominated by common diseases with complicated genetics.

This chapter on genetics is not comprehensive. Many excellent texts describe all aspects of genetics, from the genetic basis of disease to gene therapy. Rather, the goal of this chapter is to introduce the clinically important principles of genetics and the application of these principles to clinical medicine, with particular emphasis on the genetics of cardiovascular diseases (Fig. 62-1).

TERMINOLOGY

The following is a brief glossary of the clinically important terms in this chapter:

Genotype. The genetic makeup of an individual. Genotype can refer to specific genes or to the overall genetic profile.

Alleles. Copies of a specific gene. Humans have two alleles for each gene (one each from the biological father and mother). Alleles may have functional differences in their DNA sequence. A person with two identical copies of an allele is termed homozygous; a person with two different copies of an allele is called heterozygous.

Phenotype. The functional effects of genetic changes together with environmental influences. For instance, a person's appearance (body build, muscularity, hair color), the pres-

ence of measurable abnormalities that may reflect underlying disease processes, or other physical features demonstrate phenotypes. The list of measurable abnormalities is almost infinite, from blood pressure abnormalities to abnormal biochemical measurements (e.g., serum glucose levels) to ECG abnormalities reflecting ion channel abnormalities (as occur in the long QT syndrome [LQTS]) to coronary heart disease measured by angiography or endothelial dysfunction measured by forearm blood flow variability.

Mutation. Changes in the DNA sequence of a gene that result in a gene product (protein) that has an altered sequence. For this chapter, mutations are considered to be changes in the DNA sequence of a gene that result in either loss of function or severely altered function.

Dominant mutation. A mutation in one allele of a gene that is sufficient to cause disease. More severe disease or lethality may result from a dominant mutation in both alleles of a gene.

Recessive mutation. A mutation that requires alterations in both alleles of a gene to cause disease (except in the case of mutations in the X and Y chromosomes).

Polymorphism. An inherited variation in the DNA sequence of a gene that occurs at a greater frequency than would be expected of a mutation. Humans have thousands of polymorphisms, none of which are thought to be solely responsible for disease. Technically no different from mutations (a change in DNA sequence from "normal"), polymorphisms typically alter the gene product more subtly than mutations. It is thought that many human phenotypes result from the interplay between an individual's mix of polymorphisms and the environment.

Genetics in Cardiovascular Medicine

Figure 62-1

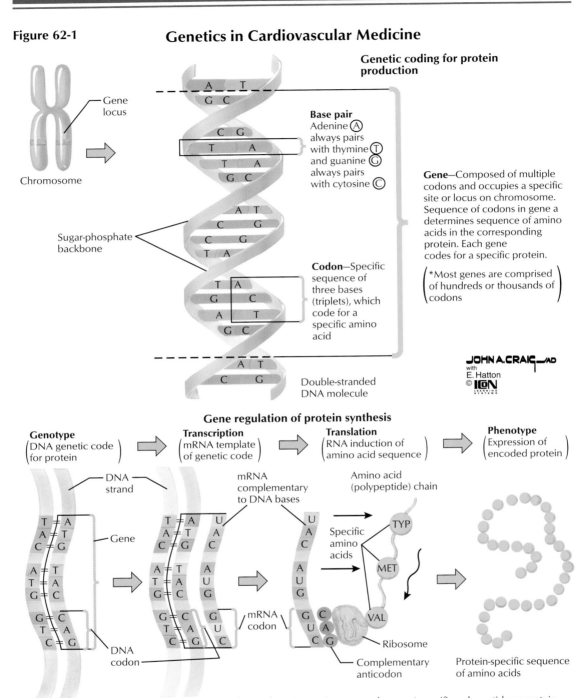

A gene is a segment of DNA that directs the synthesis of one (sometimes more than one) specific polypeptide or protein. Synthesis of a polypeptide occurs in a stepwise sequence in which the DNA base triplets (codons) are translated into a complementary set of mRNA codons, which then induce formation of anticodons, identical in sequence to the DNA codons (except "U" replaces "T" in mRNA sequences). The three-base genetic code then directs the sequential synthesis of amino acids into a polypeptide chain. Of note, on any particular segment of a chromosome, DNA sequences are considered to fall into two general categories: (1) **exons**, which are nucleotide sequences that code information for protein synthesis that is copied and spliced together with other sequences to form mRNA, and (2) **introns**, which are nucleotide sequences that do not code information for protein synthesis and are removed before translation of mRNA. For simplicity, a single exon is shown in diagram.

Environmental effects. For this chapter, any potentially controllable influence on an individual. Examples are diet, exercise, air quality, a response to a prescribed or an over-the-counter medication, cigarette smoking, and alcohol use.

MODERN HUMAN GENETICS IN THE ETIOLOGY OF DISEASE

Before Mendel described the principles of genetics on the basis of his plant studies, it was recognized that a wide variety of diseases were familial. Although not the first, Sir William Osler is the most recognized modern physician to propose that familial clusterings of diseases were linked to specific gene abnormalities. Medical genetics became a specialty with the recognition that a detailed pedigree made it possible to understand the genetic basis of a given familial disease. However, in the mid-20th century, genetic screening was only a concept and no quantitative tools existed for genetic screening. Biochemical screening tests, reflecting the downstream effects of a genetic abnormality, were the first "genetic tests" developed. Population-wide screening for Tay-Sachs disease, a disease with autosomal recessive inheritance found predominantly in Ashkenazi Jews, was one of the first successful applications of such a test. A combination of biochemical screening and genetic counseling has resulted in a greater than 90% decrease in the occurrence of the disease over the past 2 decades, underlining the importance of this type of screening.

In the late 20th century, with the advent of reliable DNA sequencing, it became possible to demonstrate that diseases could be assigned to a single nucleotide change in a specific, important gene. This development led to the idea that single mutations "caused" disease, extending the principles of Osler: one abnormality, one disease.

With the advent of high-speed DNA sequencing, it has become clear the genetic basis of human disease is much more complex than was previously recognized. There are several reasons for this greater complexity. First, mutations in specific genes are rarely unique; the same phenotype can result from any of a number of mutations in the same gene. Second, nearly identical phenotypes can result from a mutation in more than one gene. Third, just as genes do not act in isola-

tion, mutations often do not have a strict cause-and-effect relationship with disease (Fig. 62-2). Often, an interaction of a mutation with a broad array of environmental factors leads to a given phenotype. Finally, humans are not a product of changes in single genes in isolation, but of many, perhaps hundreds of, polymorphisms (Fig. 62-3, upper). Commonly, susceptibility to environmental effects depends not on a single gene but on the interactions of many genes, often genes for nuclear factors that regulate the expression of entire classes of genes. Practical examples follow.

GENETIC EVALUATION: SELECTED EXAMPLES
Hypertrophic Cardiomyopathy

Hypertrophic cardiomyopathy (HCM) was first described as a myocardial abnormality that clinically mimicked aortic stenosis, often resulted in sudden cardiac death, and pathologically was characterized by asymmetric septal hypertrophy and myocardial fiber disarray (see chapter 13). The genetic characterization of HCM was first reported in the late 1980s in a study that implicated an abnormality on chromosome 14. Subsequently, it was found, on the basis of studies of a large family, that a single mutation in the *β-myosin heavy chain* was responsible for HCM. However, in less than a decade, more than 100 mutations in 10 genes (ranging from *myosins* to *troponins* and including other proteins of the contractile apparatus) have been reported to produce the phenotype of HCM (Fig. 62-3, middle). Specific mutations in certain genes are associated with more or less severe phenotypes and outcomes. Further complicating the genetic analysis of HCM is the status of HCM as an autosomal dominant disorder characterized by incomplete penetrance. Thus, even though siblings may all carry a mutation, the severity of the phenotype varies on the basis of factors yet to be elucidated.

For these reasons, HCM is an excellent example of the types of genetic diseases that cardiovascular specialists see. HCM cannot be attributed to a single mutation, nor does the precise mutation entirely predict the outcome of the disease. The genetics for other cardiovascular diseases is likely to be even more complicated. Given these issues, there has been much debate

Figure 62-2

Normal, Mutant, and Polymorphic Gene Expression

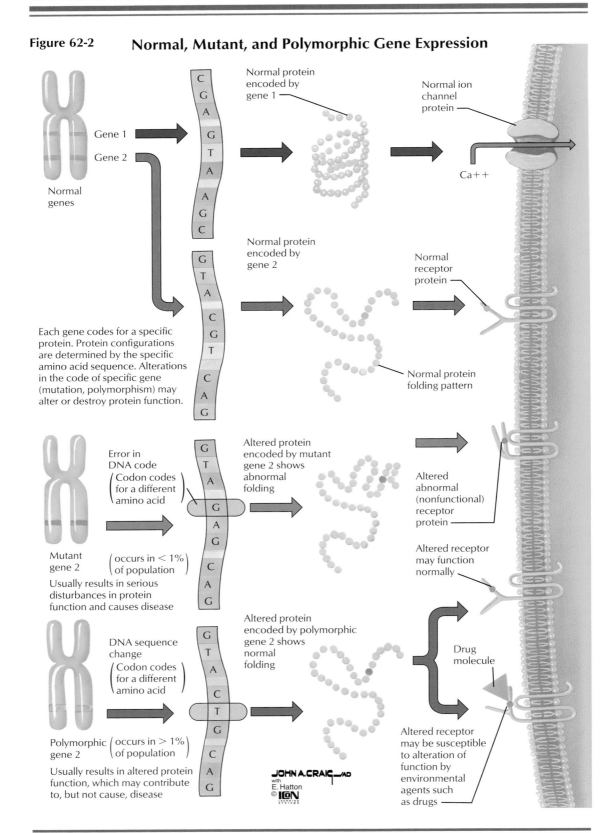

Gene 1

Gene 2

Normal genes

Each gene codes for a specific protein. Protein configurations are determined by the specific amino acid sequence. Alterations in the code of specific gene (mutation, polymorphism) may alter or destroy protein function.

Normal protein encoded by gene 1

Normal ion channel protein

Ca++

Normal protein encoded by gene 2

Normal receptor protein

Normal protein folding pattern

Error in DNA code
(Codon codes for a different amino acid)

Mutant gene 2 (occurs in < 1% of population)

Usually results in serious disturbances in protein function and causes disease

Altered protein encoded by mutant gene 2 shows abnormal folding

Altered abnormal (nonfunctional) receptor protein

Altered receptor may function normally

DNA sequence change
(Codon codes for a different amino acid)

Polymorphic gene 2 (occurs in > 1% of population)

Usually results in altered protein function, which may contribute to, but not cause, disease

Altered protein encoded by polymorphic gene 2 shows normal folding

Drug molecule

Altered receptor may be susceptible to alteration of function by environmental agents such as drugs

JOHN A. CRAIG—AD
with
E. Hatton
© ICON

Figure 62-3

Genetic and Environmental Factors in Cardiovascular Disease

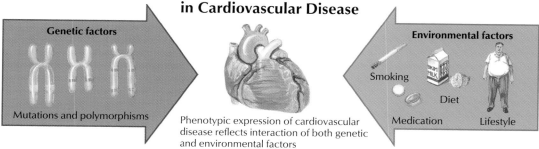

Genetic factors

Mutations and polymorphisms

Phenotypic expression of cardiovascular disease reflects interaction of both genetic and environmental factors

Environmental factors

Smoking

Diet

Medication

Lifestyle

Hypertrophic cardiomyopathy (HCM)

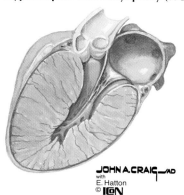

JOHN A. CRAIG—AD
with
E. Hatton
© ICN

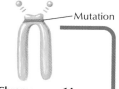

—Mutation

Chromosome 14

Original genetic studies revealed mutation in gene encoding β-myosin heavy chain. Subsequently, 200 mutations in 10 genes coding for contractile proteins have been identified.

Inheritance pattern of familial-type hypertrophic cardiomyopathy is autosomal dominant with incomplete penetrance

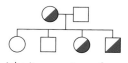

Tropomyosin — Troponins (F, T, C)
— Actin

Thin filament {

Myocardial abnormality marked by asymmetric septal hypertrophy and myocardial fiber disarray. Clinically, it mimics aortic stenosis and often results in sudden cardiac death, particularly in young athletes. Causes are multifactorial but genetic predisposition is a strong factor.

Myosin head
β-myosin heavy chain

Thick filament {

Myocardial sarcomere

Long QT syndrome (LQTS)

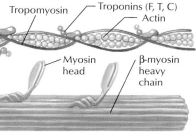

Rate = 71/min

QT
0.42 s

Abnormal prolongation of QT interval on ECG is phenotypic expression of all causes of LQTS. QT prolongation is associated with sudden cardiac death.

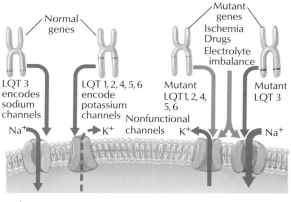

Normal genes

Mutant genes
Ischemia
Drugs
Electrolyte imbalance

LQT 3 encodes sodium channels

Na⁺

LQT 1, 2, 4, 5, 6 encode potassium channels

K⁺

Mutant LQT1, 2, 4, 5, 6 Nonfunctional channels

K⁺

Mutant LQT 3

Na⁺

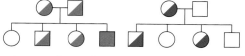

Autosomal recessive   **Autosomal dominant**

LQTS exhibits either an autosomal dominant or a recessive inheritance pattern, depending on specific gene involved

The genetic factors that underlie the LQTS involve the genes that encode for sodium and potassium ion channel proteins. To date, six genes (LQT1–LQT6) on five chromosomes have been identified. Mutations in these genes alter ion channel function and repolarization. Some forms of LQTS become manifest only when a secondary cause of QT prolongation (electrolyte disturbance, drugs, myocardial ischemia) is present.

on the value of genetic screening for HCM. The genetic analysis may not entirely predict the phenotype, and there is little to be done, at present, even if the genotype is known. The situation with HCM is in contrast with that of Tay-Sachs disease, or even with that of cystic fibrosis, both of which diseases result predominantly from a single mutation and the mutation itself is entirely sufficient to cause the disease. However, HCM is the most common cause of sudden cardiac death in young athletes, and often this is the initial presentation of the disease. Because the disease can usually be detected by physical examination, particularly in combination with noninvasive testing (ECG is helpful, and echocardiography is diagnostic), the best advice for clinicians is to screen individuals on the basis of medical criteria. In families with a known history of HCM, genetic screening can add prognostic information. When genetic screening becomes more rapid and less expensive, it will become increasingly useful to clinicians.

Long QT Syndrome

The LQTS describes a group of patients whose most common phenotype is an abnormal QT interval on the ECG, usually patients with a corrected QT interval greater than 440 ms. QT prolongation is associated with sudden cardiac death, presumably because of the propensity for polymorphic ventricular tachycardia when a premature ventricular contraction occurs in the refractory period (prolonged in these cases; see chapter 23). More than 200 mutations in five different genes (all coding for sodium or potassium channel proteins) have been reported to cause LQTS (Fig 62-3, lower). Unlike in families with HCM, both autosomal dominant and autosomal recessive inheritance are described for LQTS, the inheritance depending on the gene involved. Some forms of LQTS manifest only when a secondary cause of QT prolongation is present, such as electrolyte abnormalities, medications, or myocardial ischemia. As with HCM, the diagnosis of LQTS can be made by noninvasive (ECG) testing in most cases (except in the case of LQTS provoked by a secondary cause). For individuals from families with a history of sudden cardiac death, careful analysis of the ECG is necessary and provocative testing may

be indicated in some circumstances. LQTS also represents a spectrum of diseases that could benefit from *pharmacogenomics*, the use of specific medications based on genotype.

Atherosclerosis in Individuals With Metabolic Syndrome or Diabetes Mellitus

Atherosclerosis is the most common polygenic disorder seen by cardiovascular specialists. The genetics of atherosclerosis ranges from individuals with defects in the low-density lipoprotein receptor (familial hypercholesterolemia), who almost all die prematurely of heart attack or stroke regardless of therapy, to the much larger group whose disease progression is highly dependent on environmental factors, such as diet, exercise, and cigarette smoking. The genetics of this latter group, even with what we have learned thus far, remains largely unknown.

With regard to the large group of individuals at risk for heart attack, some advances have been made in understanding the interplay of obesity, diabetes, and atherosclerosis. Although much progress has been made in reducing the prevalence of most cardiac risk factors (including hypertension, hypercholesterolemia, and cigarette smoking), this favorable trend has been counterbalanced by increases in obesity and diabetes. As discussed in chapters 2 and 54, there is a powerful relationship between diabetes mellitus and atherosclerosis. According to the Framingham risk calculator, the presence of diabetes is equivalent to the presence of some degree of coronary heart disease.

Analogous to the genetics of familial hypercholesterolemia, some individuals with diabetes mellitus have well-described mutations, whereas the vast majority of individuals with diabetes mellitus likely have a spectrum of polymorphisms that makes them particularly susceptible to environmental influences. This susceptibility can often be most easily detected in genetically homogeneous populations. One of the best characterized groups with a genetic susceptibility to diabetes is the Pima Indians. In a manner analogous to studies of Amish families, or more recently described studies of colon cancer in Mormon families, Pima families from the Gila River Indian Community in Arizona are being intensively studied in the search for genes and polymorphisms important in obesity, diabetes, and even the propensity for the metabolic syndrome. Interestingly, in the early 1900s, these individuals were lean and the incidence of diabetes was low. By the year 2000, nearly all of these individuals were morbidly obese and had diabetes. During the intervening 100 years, there was little genetic change, but major environmental changes occurred, as the members of these families became more sedentary and their diets became richer in animal fats. Insulin resistance (uniformly present in patients with the metabolic syndrome) seems to underlie the propensity for diabetes in these individuals. At least two different groups of genes, fatty acid–binding proteins, such as FABP2, and protein phosphatases, such as protein phosphatase 1, are being studied. It is likely that polymorphisms are present in this population (either in the target genes being studied or in nuclear factors that regulate the expression of those genes) that were benign under the environmental conditions of the 19th century but that cause significant morbidity today. Studies such as these will lead to a better understanding of atherosclerosis risk mechanisms and diagnostic and therapeutic approaches for intervention.

Molecular Signatures

It has become possible to assess gene regulation simultaneously for hundreds to thousands of genes using technology commonly referred to as "microarray" analysis. A microarray consists of samples of DNA for particular genes or antibodies specific for certain proteins robotically placed on a microscope slide. A single slide may hold thousands of individual samples of known DNAs or antibodies. Blood or tissue samples are then processed, and the messenger RNA samples or proteins are hybridized to microarrays containing DNA or antibodies. The relative signal for a specific gene or protein from the patient can be quantified, comparing expression in "normal" and "abnormal" tissue or blood samples. The goal is to use the assessment of these complex, multivariate patterns of gene expression to predict the likelihood of disease, disease progression, and response to therapy.

The results obtained from microarray analysis suggest that by analyzing the response of large classes of genes, it will be possible to account for the intrinsic variation resulting from the interplay of polymorphisms with the environment. Much of what is known is based on analysis of gene expression at the mRNA level. It is likely that the analysis of gene expression at the protein level will provide even more meaningful data.

Molecular signatures are still under investigation for patients with cardiovascular disease, but molecular signatures have been used in patients with cancer. One of the best examples is in women with breast cancer. Gene expression patterns in breast cancer tumor biopsy samples have been examined with regard to disease progression and the efficacy of chemotherapy. Several studies have shown that gene expression patterns can accurately predict high-risk versus low-risk status.

Many studies are under way to determine whether molecular signatures will enable clinicians to predict the presence of disease and the response to therapy for atherosclerosis, hypertension, diabetes, and other cardiovascular diseases.

FUTURE DIRECTIONS

As our knowledge of the genetics of cardiovascular diseases increases, tools for the treatment of cardiovascular diseases will emerge. Many of the approaches described here will become clinically useful in coming years. We must be circumspect in speculating on when use of these technologies will become commonplace; in cardiovascular diseases, optimal clinical outcomes often lag decades behind the development of new technologies. Two areas of common interest not addressed in this chapter are gene therapy for cardiovascular diseases and individualized pharmacotherapy for patients with cardiovascular diseases.

Gene therapy, the replacement of defective genes with normally functioning genes or the use of exogenously administered genes to alter function at the cellular level, has been performed for several single-gene diseases, with variable efficacy. In the field of cardiovascular diseases, several studies have reported the use of angiogenic factors or genes for the treatment of severe angina or severe peripheral vascular disease. The results are minimally positive, sufficient to continue studies but not sufficient to indicate clinical utility. A more promising approach than single-gene replacement is the use of stem cells to replace entire classes of genes and even to effect tissue repair. The use of stem cells is an area of active investigation, considered more promising than single-gene therapy by many, which is also being tested in clinical trials. It is hoped that it will become possible to individualize therapeutic choices. It is also hoped that it will even be possible to develop entire new portfolios of pharmacologic approaches that are customized to particular genetic backgrounds.

REFERENCES

Arad M, Seidman JG, Seidman CE. Phenotypic diversity in hypertrophic cardiomyopathy. *Hum Mol Genet* 2002;11: 2499–2506.

Bogardus C, Tataranni PA. Reduced early insulin secretion in the etiology of type 2 diabetes mellitus in Pima Indians. *Diabetes* 2002;51(suppl 1):S262–S264.

Khoury MJ, McCabe LL, McCabe ER. Population screening in the age of genomic medicine. *N Engl J Med* 2003;348:50–58.

McKusick VA. *Mendelian Inheritance in Man: A Catalogue of Human Genes and Genetic Disorders.* 12th ed. Baltimore: Johns Hopkins Press; 1998.

National Center for Biotechnology Information. Available at www.ncbi.nlm.nih.gov

Vincent GM. The long-QT syndrome: Bedside to bench to bedside. *N Engl J Med* 2003;348:1837–1838.

Watson JD, Crick FH. Molecular structure of nucleic acids: A structure for deoxyribose nucleic acid. *Nature* 1953;171: 737–738.

Watson JD, Steitz J. *Molecular Biology of the Gene.* 4th ed. Menlo Park, CA: Benjamin/Cummings; 1987.

Chapter 63

Effects of Exercise on Cardiovascular Health

Chin K. Kim, Srikanth Ramachandruni, Eileen M. Handberg, Richard S. Schofield, Edith E. Bragdon, and David S. Sheps

With approximately 1.5 million new cases each year, coronary heart disease (CHD) is the leading cause of mortality and morbidity in the United States. Epidemiologic studies show that low levels of habitual physical activity and physical fitness are associated with markedly increased all-cause mortality rates. Sedentary lifestyle has a relative risk of 1.9 for CHD, compared with active occupations. As many as 250,000 deaths per year in the United States, approximately 12% of the total, may be attributable to a lack of regular physical activity. Despite being considered a modifiable risk factor for CHD, the number of Americans with a sedentary lifestyle continues to increase. However, it is never too late to change behavior and achieve health benefits. Even a midlife increase in physical activity is associated with a decreased risk of death and disability. Epidemiologic research has shown that physical activity has protective effects of varying strength against several chronic diseases, including CHD, hypertension, non–insulin-dependent diabetes mellitus, anxiety, and depression. Guidelines from the Centers for Disease Control and Prevention and the American College of Sports Medicine (ACSM), as well as the Surgeon General's Report on Physical Activity and Health, strongly recommend at least 30 minutes of moderate-intensity physical activity on most, preferably all, days of the week. More recent recommendations suggest additional benefit from an hour of daily exercise. In addition to the recommendations to increase activity related to aerobic capacity, the guidelines encourage participation in activities that promote flexibility and strength.

If adopted, these guidelines would result in substantial improvements in physiologic and psychological health. The psychological benefits of exercise include positive changes in mood; relief from tension, depression, and anxiety; and increased ability to cope with daily activities. These benefits bring about positive changes in self-perception, well-being, self-confidence, and awareness and may result in more health-promoting behaviors.

Increasing physical activity is extremely important, but achieving a higher level of fitness is even more important, especially for individuals who are at high risk for CHD or have experienced a cardiac event and require rehabilitation. The physical activity guidelines targeted to increase physical activity promote health but do not necessarily result in physical fitness. Some substantial improvements in cardiovascular risk factors (resting BP, lipid levels, body composition, insulin sensitivity) have been demonstrated in studies that prescribed more rigid exercise training programs. The AHA and ACSM position statements

on exercise training cite extensive data regarding improvements in exercise capacity and other measures in patients with or without CHD after regular exercise training to moderate or high levels of exertion. This chapter addresses more specific issues related to exercise, primary and secondary prevention, and the rationale for exercise prescription to patients with heart failure.

PRIMARY PREVENTION

There is a strong inverse relation between physical activity and the risk of coronary disease and death. Similar cardiovascular benefit from fitness also exists in both sexes and across different races and ethnic groups (Fig. 63-1).

Several studies in men support a role for physical activity in reducing the risk of mortality. In nonsmoking, retired men aged 61 to 81 years who had other risk factors controlled, the distance walked daily at baseline inversely predicted the risk for all-cause mortality during a 12-year follow-up. Of 10,269 Harvard alumni born

Figure 63-1

Effects of Exercise on Cardiovascular Health
Primary Prevention

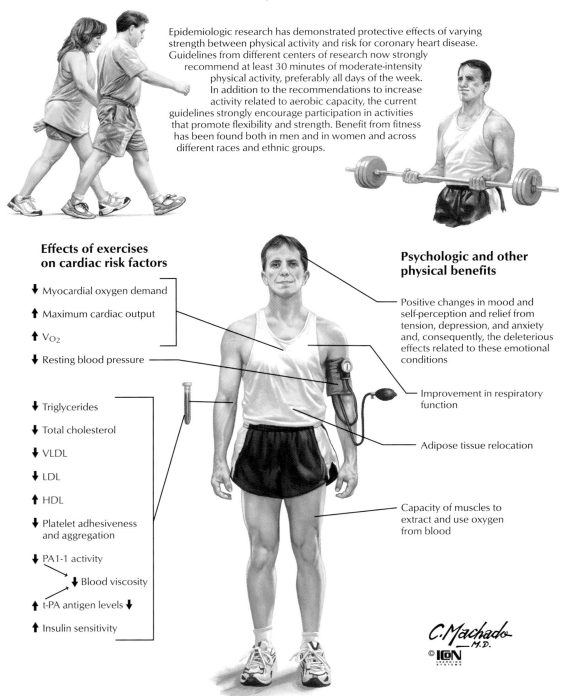

Epidemiologic research has demonstrated protective effects of varying strength between physical activity and risk for coronary heart disease. Guidelines from different centers of research now strongly recommend at least 30 minutes of moderate-intensity physical activity, preferably all days of the week. In addition to the recommendations to increase activity related to aerobic capacity, the current guidelines strongly encourage participation in activities that promote flexibility and strength. Benefit from fitness has been found both in men and in women and across different races and ethnic groups.

Effects of exercises on cardiac risk factors

↓ Myocardial oxygen demand

↑ Maximum cardiac output

↑ V_{O_2}

↓ Resting blood pressure

↓ Triglycerides

↓ Total cholesterol

↓ VLDL

↓ LDL

↑ HDL

↓ Platelet adhesiveness and aggregation

↓ PA1-1 activity

　　↓ Blood viscosity

↑ t-PA antigen levels ↓

↑ Insulin sensitivity

Psychologic and other physical benefits

Positive changes in mood and self-perception and relief from tension, depression, and anxiety and, consequently, the deleterious effects related to these emotional conditions

Improvement in respiratory function

Adipose tissue relocation

Capacity of muscles to extract and use oxygen from blood

C. Machado
M.D.
© ICON
LEARNING
SYSTEMS

The physical activity guidelines are targeted to increase physical activity to promote health, but will not necessarily result in physical fitness, and should not diminish the importance of achieving physical fitness.

between 1893 and 1932, those individuals who began moderately vigorous sports between 1960 and 1977 had a reduced risk of all-cause and CHD-related death over an average of 9 years of observation compared with those who did not increase sports participation. This finding was independent of the effects of lower BP or lifestyle behaviors related to low cardiac risk, such as cessation of smoking and maintenance of lean body mass. Data on the leisure-time physical activity levels of men participating in the Multiple Risk Factor Intervention Trial (MRFIT) support a reduction of risk for all-cause and CHD-related fatalities associated with moderate or high (as compared to low) levels of leisure time spent in physical exercise. The effect was retained when confounding factors, including baseline risk factors and MRFIT intervention group assignments, were controlled. Mortality rates for the high and moderate physical activity groups were similar. The Lipid Research Clinics Mortality Follow-Up Study found that men with a lower level of physical fitness, as indicated by HR during phase 2 (submaximal exercise) of the treadmill test, are at significantly higher risk than physically fit men are for death as a result of cardiovascular causes within 8.5 years.

In women as well, higher physical activity level is related to improved health outcome. The Iowa Women's Health Study observed 40,417 postmenopausal women for 7 years; moderate and vigorous exercise was associated with a reduced risk of death. This reduction of risk exists for all-cause mortality and specifically for deaths as a result of cardiovascular and respiratory causes. Women who increase their frequency of activity from rarely or never to four or more times per week have a reduced risk of death. The Women's Health Initiative (73,743 postmenopausal women) and the Nurses' Health Study (72,488 women aged 40–65 years) assigned subjects into quintiles based on energy expenditure. Age-adjusted risk decreased incrementally from the lowest to the highest energy expenditure group, was statistically significant when other cardiovascular risk factors were controlled, and was similar in white and black women. In addition, energy expenditure from vigorous exercise or walking and time spent walking (but not pace) were all linked to a

lowered risk for the development of CHD. The inverse relation between CHD risk and activity level has also been observed in groups of patients with other high-risk factors, including smokers and women with high cholesterol levels, although not for hypertensive women.

In one study of postmenopausal women, the odds ratios for nonfatal myocardial infarction (MI), adjusted for confounding factors, decreased across the second, third, and fourth quartiles of energy expenditure compared with the lowest quartile. Exercise equivalent to 30 to 45 minutes of walking 3 days per week decreased the risk for MI by 50%.

Studies show that in black and white men and women, lack of exercise is associated with a higher risk of 5-year all-cause mortality, independent of age, male sex, low income, BP, or a number of cardiovascular measures (e.g., left ventricular [LV] ejection fraction, abnormal ECG) or other physiologic measures (e.g., glucose level, creatinine level). A community-based study of elderly (aged 65 years or older) adults with no history of heart disease showed that walking at least 4 hours weekly significantly reduced the risk of hospitalization due to cardiovascular disease events during the subsequent 4 to 5 years.

SECONDARY PREVENTION

Research findings suggest that exercise and fitness are beneficial in patients with established diagnoses of CHD (Fig. 63-2). In a large study of men with established heart disease, regular light to moderate activity (such as 4 hours per weekend of moderate to heavy gardening or 40 minutes per day of walking) was associated with a reduced risk of all-cause and cardiovascular mortality compared with a sedentary lifestyle. Another large study assessed men's health status and physical fitness during two medical examinations scheduled approximately 5 years apart; subjects were followed up for adverse outcomes for an additional 5 years. Men who were unfit at both examinations had the highest subsequent 5-year death rate (122/10,000 man-years); the death rate was substantially lower in initially unfit men who improved their fitness (68/10,000 man-years) and lowest in the group who maintained their fitness from the first to the second examination (40/10,000 man-years). For

Figure 63-2

Secondary Prevention

It has been found that exercise of light to vigorous intensity (moderate to heavy gardening, jogging, cycling, swimming, etc.) and fitness are beneficial in patients with established diagnoses of coronary heart disease, including those who experienced myocardial infarction, lowering mortality from acute myocardial infarction and frequency of angina pectoris, increasing functional capacity and reduction of myocardial work.

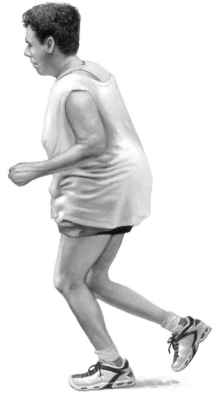

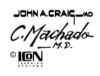

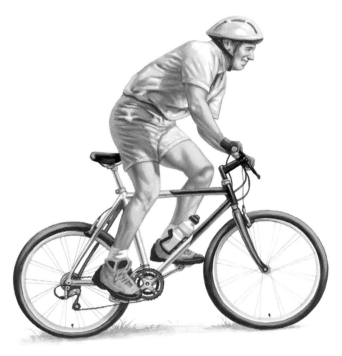

Studies have also shown that intensive exercise on a regular basis associated with a low-fat, low-cholesterol diet may be associated with regression in atherosclerotic coronary lesions, an increase in myocardial oxygen consumption, and a decrease in stress-induced myocardial ischemia.

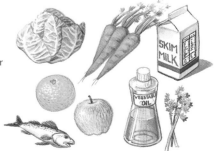

each minute that the maximal treadmill exercise time at the second examination exceeded the initial treadmill time, the mortality risk decreased almost 8%. These results were retained when subjects were stratified by health status, demonstrating that unhealthy as well as initially healthy individuals benefited from exercise fitness.

Exercise intervention experiments have documented better health and survival even in patients who have experienced an MI. In one randomized study, patients were enrolled in a rehabilitation program of three 30-minute periods of exercise weekly, while other patients—matched by age, sex, coronary risk factors, site and level of cardiac damage, and acute-phase complications—served as controls. At 9 years after the initial MI, the rate of death caused by acute MI and the frequency of angina pectoris were lower in the treatment group. In the National Exercise and Heart Disease Project, male post-MI patients were randomly assigned to a 3-year program of supervised regular vigorous exercise (jogging, cycling, or swimming) or to regular care not involving an exercise program; follow-up at 3, 5, 10, 15, and 19 years determined total and cardiovascular-related mortality. A moderate advantage of the treatment versus control condition in reducing the risk of all-cause and cardiovascular death was seen at the first follow-up time point but diminished and eventually reversed as the time since baseline increased, perhaps indicating that the benefits of an intensive exercise program are time limited. Nevertheless, each metabolic equivalent unit by which the participants' work capacity increased from the outset to the completion of the 3-year program yielded an incremental reduction in total and cardiovascular-related mortality; this finding suggests increasing exercise fitness did promote survival and that failure to observe a long-term benefit in the treatment group versus the control group may have resulted from crossover between the two groups during the protracted follow-up period.

Results of a large meta-analysis of 10 randomized clinical trials of post-MI patients showed that cardiac rehabilitation with exercise reduced all-cause mortality by 24% and cardiovascular death by 25% versus control subjects. However, the risk of nonfatal recurrent MI did not differ between groups.

Exercise training plays an important role in post-MI rehabilitation. Significant increases in functional capacity (10–60%) and reductions of myocardial work at standardized exercise workloads (10–25%) have been observed after 12 weeks of post-MI cardiac rehabilitation. That exercise training after an MI may also improve ventricular remodeling and LV function was demonstrated in the Exercise in Left Ventricular Dysfunction trial. The AHA guidelines on physical activity in secondary prevention after MI, bypass surgery, and clinical ischemia recommend attendance at supervised facilities where symptoms, HR, and BP can be monitored. A symptom-limited exercise test is essential for all patients before starting an exercise program.

Limiting Coronary Atherosclerotic Progression

A few prospective, randomized intervention studies have evaluated the influence of exercise training on the progression of coronary atherosclerosis. In one study, patients with a history of stable angina were randomized to receive a behavioral intervention (2 or more hours per week of intensive exercise group training sessions, at least 20 minutes per day of exercise, and a low-fat, low-cholesterol diet) or usual care. After 1 year, 32% of the treatment group versus 9% of the control group had regression in atherosclerotic coronary lesions, and, conversely, 48% of the control group versus 23% of the treatment group had progression of lesions; all of these differences were statistically significant. Other changes in the treatment group included reductions in weight, total cholesterol level, and triglyceride level and increases in HDL level, work capacity, and myocardial oxygen consumption. Stress-induced myocardial ischemia also decreased from the intervention, which was presumably attributable to enhanced myocardial perfusion. At 6-years' follow-up, the progression of CAD was still significantly retarded in the treatment group. Retrospective analysis of exercise intensity and angiographic data revealed that eliciting a regression of coronary stenosis necessitates expenditure of at least 2200 kcal/week (equivalent to 5–6 hours of exercise).

In the Stanford Coronary Risk Intervention Project, patients received a behavioral risk reduction intervention or usual care. Intervention programs were similar to those in the aforementioned studies, but smoking cessation and pharmacologic treatment of lipid profiles (according to established treatment guidelines) were added. Evaluations at 4 years after baseline revealed that the risk reduction intervention significantly improved levels of LDL, apolipoprotein B, HDL, and triglycerides and body weight, exercise capacity, and intake of dietary fat and cholesterol. Changes in the control group were much more modest. The rate of coronary stenosis progression and the number of hospitalizations were also lower for the intervention group, although each group experienced the same number of deaths.

The Lifestyle Heart Trial used an intervention program designed by Ornish et al. Measures were undertaken to transform lifestyle behaviors, including a low-fat vegetarian diet, aerobic exercise, stress management training, smoking cessation, and group psychosocial support. Follow-up angiograms at 1 and 5 years after baseline showed average relative decreases in stenosis of 4.5 and 7.9%; conversely, individuals in the control group showed 5.4 and 27.8% average relative *worsening* of stenoses. The 5-year risk of adverse cardiac events was also significantly greater in the control group.

These investigations show that programs introducing intensive measures to alter coronary risk–promoting behaviors, especially via exercise training and cholesterol reduction, can limit or even reverse the progression of coronary stenoses. Although the associated changes in coronary diameter were relatively small and therefore unlikely by themselves to explain the accompanying improvements in myocardial perfusion, improvements in vascular tone and reduction in the risk of plaque rupture (see chapter 2) may well have contributed to the observed outcomes.

PHYSIOLOGY OF EXERCISE EFFECTS ON CARDIOVASCULAR HEALTH
Oxygen Supply and Demand

Ventilatory oxygen uptake is increased by exercise training via enhanced maximum cardiac output (blood volume ejected by the heart per minute, which determines the amount of blood delivered to exercising muscles) and muscles' capacity to extract and use oxygen from blood. Increased exercise capacity in turn favorably affects hemodynamic, hormonal, metabolic, neurologic, and respiratory function. Exercise training reduces the myocardial oxygen demand associated with a given level of work, as represented by a decrease in the product of HR times systolic arterial BP, and allows persons with coronary artery disease to attain a higher level of physical work before reaching the threshold at which an inadequate oxygen level results in myocardial ischemia (Table 63-1).

Lipids

A recommended exercise-training regimen constructively alters lipid and carbohydrate metabolism. The positive effect of a low–saturated fat, low-cholesterol diet on blood lipoprotein levels is enhanced by a strict regular exercise regimen in overweight adults. Training also influences adipose tissue relocation, which is thought to be important in lowering cardiovascular risk. Intense endurance training also enhances insulin sensitivity and has a highly salutary effect on fibrinogen levels in healthy older men.

The beneficial effects of exercise on lipids are implicated in the primary and secondary preven-

Table 63-1
Benefits of Exercise Training

- Reduces all-cause mortality risk
- Reduces cardiovascular mortality risk
- May limit atherosclerotic progression
- Enhances oxygen uptake
- Reduces myocardial work
- Constructively alters lipid and carbohydrate metabolism
- Influences adipose relocation
- Enhances insulin sensitivity
- Reduces the conversion of HDL cholesterol into LDL and VLDL
- May suppress platelet adhesiveness and aggregation
- Increases activity of mitochondrial enzymes
- Lowers blood pressure
- Improves functional capacity and peak oxygen consumption in congestive heart failure

tion of heart disease. Kraus et al. examined the effects of graded exercise on serum cholesterol in sedentary and overweight adults with hyperlipidemia who completed a 6-month protocol. Comparing the three treatment exercise programs—high-amount, high-intensity exercise; low-amount, high-intensity exercise; or low-amount, moderate-intensity exercise—with controls, all exercising groups showed improvements in plasma lipoprotein levels, including a decrease in VLDL triglycerides and an increase in the size of LDL particles. Increased HDL cholesterol level and particle size occurred only in the high-amount, high-intensity group; the largest improvements in LDL measures were also seen only in this group. These effects were independent of weight loss, and higher amounts of exercise were associated with greater benefits in lipoproteins.

Mechanisms that link exercise with an improved lipoprotein profile may include increased lipoprotein lipase activity and reduced hepatic lipase activity, leading to HDL increases and decreased conversion of cardio-protective HDL2 into smaller HDL3 particles. Exercise reduces the conversion of HDL cholesterol into LDL and VLDL by decreasing serum concentrations of cholesterol ester transfer protein. It increases the conversion of HDL3 to HDL2 by increasing levels of serum lecithin cholesterol acyltransferase.

Hemostatic Factors

Platelets, plasma fibrinogen, plasminogen activator inhibitor type 1 (PAI-1) activity, tissue-type plasminogen activator (t-PA) antigen, and increased plasma viscosity affect the pathogenesis and progression of cardiovascular disease. Although exercise acutely increases platelet adhesiveness and aggregability, exercise training blunts this postexercise effect. After 8 weeks of exercise, resting, and postexercise, platelet adhesiveness and aggregability in one study were lower in the training group but undiminished in the control group. Therefore, endurance exercise training seems to suppress platelet adhesiveness and aggregation. Deconditioning may reverse the effects of platelet adhesiveness and aggregability to the pretraining state. Decreased PAI-1 activity, t-PA antigen levels, and blood viscosity occur with moderate-intensity exercise.

Diabetes

Exercise increases the activity of mitochondrial enzymes, which improves muscle energetics. Large studies have shown that even modest levels of exercise also increase insulin sensitivity. Women with diabetes who exercise moderately or vigorously for at least 4 hours per week have a 40% lower risk of the development of coronary disease than those with lower exercise levels. Low physical activity in men with diabetes predicts coronary disease independently of the effects of age.

Blood Pressure

Maintaining a habitual exercise routine can lower BP by as much as 5 to 15 mm Hg in patients with critical hypertension; mean reductions of 4 to 5 mm Hg systolic pressure and 3 to 5 mm Hg diastolic pressure are widely reported. Just as perseverance with an exercise program elicits a hypotensive response, detraining is associated with an increase in BP toward the pre-exercise level. Reductions in circulating norepinephrine level, plasma volume, and cardiac index parallel the reduction in BP and are likely involved in the antihypertensive consequences of exercise. Reduced systemic vascular resistance resulting from decreased sympathetic activity probably also affects BP.

RECOMMENDED EXERCISE LEVELS

A lifelong appropriate regimen should include 30 to 60 minutes of physical activity at least 5 days per week. Exertion to the point of fatigue, breathlessness, and sweating is recommended, although achieving the target HR may not be necessary. Bicycling, jogging, and brisk walking may be performed for short periods several times a day or for a single, longer period. For secondary prevention, low-risk CHD patients with no ischemia or arrhythmia should exercise under supervision to achieve an HR reserve (maximal minus resting HR) above the resting HR. Eventually, as tolerance develops, resistance exercises can be included. High-risk patients with ischemia or arrhythmia require close supervision to achieve an HR of at least 10 beats/min below the rate associated with the abnormality.

ROLE OF EXERCISE TRAINING IN CONGESTIVE HEART FAILURE

Congestive heart failure (CHF) is a growing problem in the industrialized world and has reached epidemic proportions in the United States. Although the central effects of CHF are pulmonary and peripheral vascular congestion, many patients believe that exercise limitation is the most troubling feature. Traditional therapies, such as angiotensin-converting enzyme inhibitors, β-blockers, and spironolactone, show impressive reductions in mortality with somewhat less significant improvement in functional capacity. Therapies targeted at functional capacity improvement are also needed. Once prohibited in heart failure out of concern for patient safety, exercise training is now recognized as a therapeutic option for improving functional capacity in patients with heart failure (Fig. 63-3).

These benefits of exercise in heart failure bring to mind the lack of correlation between cardiac mechanical function and functional capacity in patients with heart failure. LV ejection fraction is a poor index of exercise capacity in patients with chronic CHF; therefore, other factors must contribute to exercise intolerance in CHF. The physiologic mechanisms for exercise intolerance in heart failure, albeit incompletely understood, help to explain the potential benefits of exercise training.

Among the factors contributing to exercise limitation are impaired LV systolic and diastolic function, baroreflex desensitization, sympathetic nervous system activation, impaired vasodilator capacity, skeletal muscle abnormalities, and abnormalities of pulmonary function. Skeletal muscle abnormalities in patients with CHF include atrophy of highly oxidative, fatigue-resistant (type I) muscle fibers; increased glycolytic, less fatigue-resistant (type II) muscle fibers; decreased mitochondrial oxidative enzyme concentration and activity; reduced mitochondrial volume and density; and reduced muscle bulk and strength. As heart failure progresses, patients become more physically limited as a result of pulmonary congestion and therefore reduce physical activity, causing a downward spiral in which cardiac limitation aggravates skeletal muscle deconditioning. The increases in circulating cytokines, known to be part of the heart failure syndrome, further worsen muscle atrophy.

Reduced peak skeletal muscle blood flow with exercise limitation also reduces shear stress and thereby depletes tissue vasodilator reserve.

Pulmonary abnormalities are also common in CHF, including reduced lung volumes and respiratory muscle strength and endurance; increased airway resistance with reduced flow rates; reduced diffusion capacity as a result of alveolar edema; and increased ventilatory drive, minute ventilation, respiratory rate, and dead space/tidal volume ratio. The effects of training on these ventilatory abnormalities in patients with CHF include reduction in minute ventilation, reduced perceived sense of dyspnea, and improved respiratory muscle function.

The well-documented, abnormal activation of neurohormones in chronic heart failure is associated with a poor prognosis. An exercise training program can correct the increased plasma levels of angiotensin II, aldosterone, arginine vasopressin, and atrial natriuretic peptide in chronic heart failure to near control values. Decreased HR variability (HRV), which is markedly abnormal in patients with CHF, is a further marker of sympathetic activation. A physical conditioning program can improve HRV and endothelial dysfunction in patients with chronic heart failure.

Clinical trials of exercise training in CHF show improvements in exercise time, functional capacity, and peak oxygen consumption. Exercise training seems to be safe and generally well tolerated in patients with CHF. One randomized trial found a reduction in cardiac events, an improvement in Minnesota Living With Heart Failure scores, and, most importantly, an improved survival rate in patients with CHF who were randomized to exercise training. These important findings have increased interest in the development of a multicenter, randomized trial of exercise training in heart failure. The planned Heart Failure—A Controlled Trial Investigating Outcomes of Exercise Training (HF-ACTION) trial, sponsored by the National Institutes of Health, is powered to show mortality differences between exercise training and standard care groups.

Exercise training in patients with heart failure is best initiated within a traditional phase II (outpatient) cardiac rehabilitation program. Patients should be prescreened by a cardiologist to assess the clinical risk for training initiation. Most

Figure 63-3   ## Exercise Training in Congestive Heart Failure

Once prohibited in heart failure, exercise training has only recently been recognized as a viable therapeutic option for improvement of functional capacity. Most of the abnormalities seen in CHF can be improved or even reversed by exercise training.

Some of the Abnormalities Seen in CHF That Can Be Improved or Even Reversed by Exercise Training

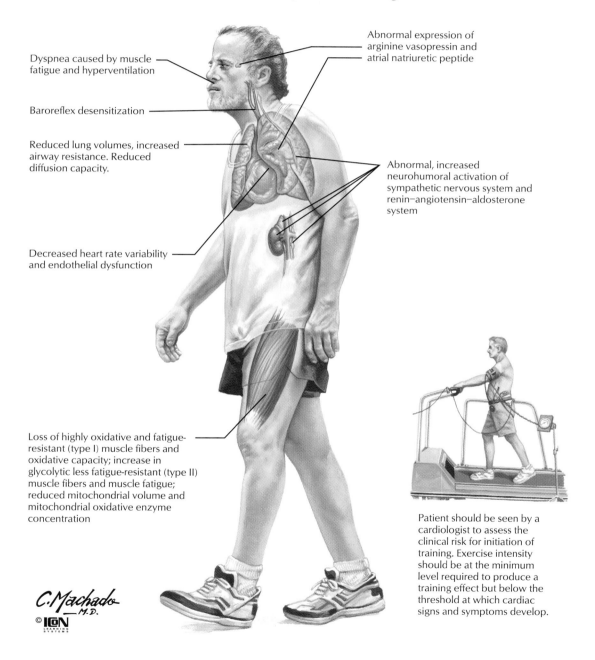

Dyspnea caused by muscle fatigue and hyperventilation

Baroreflex desensitization

Reduced lung volumes, increased airway resistance. Reduced diffusion capacity.

Decreased heart rate variability and endothelial dysfunction

Abnormal expression of arginine vasopressin and atrial natriuretic peptide

Abnormal, increased neurohumoral activation of sympathetic nervous system and renin–angiotensin–aldosterone system

Loss of highly oxidative and fatigue-resistant (type I) muscle fibers and oxidative capacity; increase in glycolytic less fatigue-resistant (type II) muscle fibers and muscle fatigue; reduced mitochondrial volume and mitochondrial oxidative enzyme concentration

Patient should be seen by a cardiologist to assess the clinical risk for initiation of training. Exercise intensity should be at the minimum level required to produce a training effect but below the threshold at which cardiac signs and symptoms develop.

C. Machado
—M.D.
© ICN
LEARNING
SYSTEMS

patients with New York Heart Association (NYHA) class I to III symptoms can exercise safely; however, patients with NYHA class IV symptoms, recent MI, unstable angina, severe aortic stenosis, uncontrolled arrhythmias, significant hypotension (SBP <85 mm Hg), or acute myocarditis should be excluded. Chronotropic response may be blunted in patients with CHF, so the level of perceived exertion and dyspnea should be used as a termination point and should be no higher than 11 to 14 on the Borg scale (light to somewhat difficult exertion). Patients with heart failure require prolonged warm-up and cool-down periods compared to healthy individuals and should avoid resistance training initially. Patients also should be counseled to avoid exercise after meals. Usual recommended activities include walking and cycling, although arm ergometry (e.g., using arm motion, instead of leg motion, to peddle an upright stationary bicycle) and rowing are well suited for individuals whose walking or cycling is limited by arthritis or conditions other than cardiovascular fatigue.

Exercise intensity should be at the minimum level needed to produce a training effect but below the threshold at which cardiac signs and symptoms develop. A baseline maximal oxygen consumption (MVo_2) study can be helpful in designing the exercise prescription but is not mandatory. Target intensity should begin at 40% of the MVo_2 and progress to 75% of the MVo_2 (roughly 70–85% of peak HR) over 4 to 6 weeks. Initially, the frequency of exercise generally should be three times per week. Maximal oxygen consumption plateaus when the frequency of exercise exceeds 3 to 5 sessions per week, and the injury rate increases exponentially. In frail or high-risk individuals, two sessions per week may also be effective for initial conditioning. The frequency of exercise should eventually increase to five sessions per week.

Exercise sessions should begin with a 10- to 15-minute warm-up and end with a 10- to 15-minute cool down. The initial duration of exercise should be 10 to 20 minutes. Interval training may be required in markedly deconditioned patients, with 2 to 6 minutes of exercise alternating with 1 to 2 minutes of rest. Duration should increase gradually to 20 to 40 minutes per session. After 12 weeks, patients can pro-

ceed to unsupervised exercise and can consider light to moderate resistance training.

FUTURE DIRECTIONS

During the next decade, important questions related to the effects of exercise on CHF may be answered. The HF-ACTION trial seeks to determine whether exercise training prolongs life in patients with CHF. If the results favor exercise training, there should be greater willingness on the part of insurers to cover costs of cardiac rehabilitation in CHF patients and thereby greater access to this therapy. Renewed interest in diastolic as opposed to systolic heart failure offers an opportunity to study the pathophysiology of exercise intolerance in CHF. Patients with diastolic heart failure are frequently just as symptomatic as patients with systolic heart failure; therefore, investigation into the mechanisms of exercise intolerance in diastolic dysfunction could help to define more precisely the causes of exercise intolerance in systolic heart failure as well.

REFERENCES

Dorn J, Naughton J, Imamura D, et al. Results of a multicenter randomized clinical trial of exercise and long-term survival in myocardial infarction patients: The National Exercise and Heart Disease Project (NEHDP). *Circulation* 1999;100:1764–1769.

Ekelund LG, Haskell WL, Johnson JL, et al. Physical fitness as a predictor of cardiovascular mortality in asymptomatic North American men: The Lipid Research Clinics Mortality Follow-Up Study. *N Engl J Med* 1988;319:1379–1384.

Fried LP, Kronmal RA, Newman AB, et al. Risk factors for 5-year mortality in older adults. *JAMA* 1998;279:585–592.

Giannuzzi P, Temporelli L, Corra U, et al. Attenuation of unfavorable remodeling by exercise training in postinfarction patients with left ventricular dysfunction: Results of the Exercise in Left Ventricular Dysfunction (ELVD) trial. *Circulation* 1997;96:1790–1797.

Kraus, WE, Houmard, JA, Duscha, BD, et al. Effects of the amount and intensity of exercise on plasma lipoproteins. *N Engl J Med* 2002;347:1483–1492.

McKelvie RS, Teo KK, McCartney N, et al. Effects of exercise training in patients with congestive heart failure: A critical review. *J Am Coll Cardiol* 1995;25:789–796.

Ornish D, Scherwitz LW, Billings JH, et al. Intensive lifestyle changes for reversal of coronary heart disease. *JAMA* 1998;280:2001–2007.

Pate RR, Pratt M, Blair SN, et al. Physical activity and public health: A recommendation from the Centers for Disease Control and Prevention and the American College of Sports Medicine. *JAMA* 1995;273:402–407.

Pina IL, Apstein CS, Balady GJ, et al. Exercise and heart failure: A statement from the American Heart Association Committee on Exercise, Rehabilitation, and Prevention. *Circulation* 2003;107:1210–1225.

Chapter 64

Lipid Abnormalities and Risk Factor Reduction

Ross J. Simpson, Jr and Sidney C. Smith, Jr

For most individuals at risk of coronary heart disease, elevated serum lipid levels are the dominant modifiable risk factor. Lipid levels can be modified by several types of interventions—appropriate dietary, exercise, and drug programs to lower key components of serum lipid levels—which together represent the most important strategies for reducing an individual's risk for CHD. This chapter reviews mechanisms by which key blood lipid components and the other CHD risk modifiers can be altered favorably.

Low-density lipoprotein cholesterol (LDL-C) levels are strongly associated with atherosclerosis and CHD events. The lowering of LDL-C levels with drug and diet therapies is consistently related to a reduction in CHD events. The Heart Protection Study demonstrated that, regardless of the initial cholesterol value, the lowering of LDL-C with the HMG CoA inhibitor simvastatin substantially lowered the risk for subsequent CHD events. The Heart Protection Study reaffirmed the primary importance of reducing LDL-C levels in individuals at high risk for CHD events and provided strong evidence that LDL-C reduction should remain the focus of preventive efforts.

High-density lipoprotein cholesterol (HDL-C) levels are influenced by diet, exercise, alcohol, exogenous estrogens, obesity, smoking, diabetes, and certain drugs (e.g., diuretics and anabolic steroids). Of these factors, exercise, estrogens, and alcohol are known to increase HDL-C. However, it should be emphasized that treatment with estrogens is not recommended as a primary or secondary prevention measure for atherosclerotic cardiovascular disease and that the cardiovascular benefits of alcohol have been demonstrated in surveys of individuals and only among those whose alcohol consumption is in the range of 1 to 3 oz per day. Initiation of alcohol consumption to reduce cardiovascular risk is not recommended because of the potential for alcohol abuse. A strong inverse relationship exists between HDL-C levels and CHD risk. However, clinical evidence is not adequate to support the primary use of therapies to increase HDL-C to reduce CHD events independent of lowering LDL-C or triglyceride levels. Moreover, the results of therapy with drugs that raise HDL-C levels often are not as consistent as are the results of drug therapies used to lower LDL-C levels. In the absence of compelling data from large populations of both genders, the National Cholesterol Education Program recommends that increased HDL-C not be the primary therapeutic goal and recommends instead that the initial focus be on reducing LDL-C. Increased HDL-C remains a secondary goal. Although recent studies were done on small numbers of individuals using various strategies to increase HDL-C, large randomized clinical trials will be needed to ascertain whether therapies that raise HDL-C levels are useful as a primary strategy for CHD prevention.

Triglycerides are important plasma lipids found in varying concentrations in all plasma lipoproteins. The relationship between plasma triglycerides and CHD is debated. Moderately elevated triglycerides are often found in the nephrotic syndrome, the metabolic syndrome, diabetes, and hypothyroidism. Although triglyceride levels appear to be associated with CHD, there is only limited evidence that lowering triglyceride levels has a protective effect in terms of CHD events. Therapies to lower triglyceride levels are well established and include treatment of the underlying diseases, such as diabetes, reduction of the dietary intake of simple carbohydrates, weight loss, alcohol avoidance, and increased exercise. In patients with diabetes, control of diabetes with a HbA1C goal of less than 7% should be the first therapeutic strategy. Very high levels of triglycerides (>500 mg/dL) are associated with the development of pancreatitis and should be treated aggressively with therapy targeted to lower triglycerides.

DIAGNOSTIC APPROACH

Lipids are commonly measured by β-quantification: total cholesterol, triglycerides, and HDL-C levels are measured directly; LDL-C levels are estimated by the Friedewald equation (LDL-C = total cholesterol − HDL-C − [triglycerides/5]). The LDL-C measurement is useful for monitoring lipid therapy and for assessing a patient's risk for a CHD event. In general, as with the other lipid profile components, measurement of LDL-C on a single occasion is not a basis for therapeutic intervention. For patients for whom long-term therapy is indicated, two fasting measurements of the lipoprotein profile, taken at least 1 week apart, should be obtained.

Direct measurement of LDL-C levels, particle size, and particle density can be accomplished by ultracentrifugation, gradient gel electrophoresis, and magnetic resonance imaging methods. Measurement of Lp(a) and other lipid fractions may provide additional information on the lipid lipoprotein characteristics of the serum. However, detailed clinical studies that indicate the utility of drugs that target these individual lipid components have yet to be reported. In many patients, it is useful to measure these components to further assess risk and, occasionally, to guide therapy. However, the primary focus is still on lowering LDL-C through drug therapy, diet, and exercise.

Lipid management requires the assessment of the patient's short-term risk for CHD events. The therapy and specific goals are then based on the patient's absolute risk for a CHD event. The National Cholesterol Education Program, Adult Treatment Panel III recommends that patients with established coronary disease, diabetes, carotid artery disease, or lower extremity arterial disease be considered to be in the highest risk group (10-year risk >20%). Increasingly, the metabolic syndrome and diabetes are becoming dominant cardiovascular risk factors, as the incidence of obesity in the United States and industrialized countries continues to increase (Fig. 64-1; see also chapter 54). In the absence of such disease, patients' global risk should be determined by the Framingham risk equation. Global risk is considered high if the 10-year risk is greater than 20%. The global risk of patients in the intermediate-risk (10-year risk of 10–20%) and low-risk (10-year risk <10%) groups should be considered in light of the presence or absence of major CHD risk factors. The critical CHD risk factors are age (≥45 years for men, ≥55 years for women), a history of premature CHD in a first-degree relative, current cigarette smoking, the presence of hypertension, and HDL-C below 40 mg/dL. Patients with two or more major risk factors in addition to high LDL-C are considered to be at intermediate risk; patients with one major risk factor in addition to high LDL-C are considered to be at low risk. Then, using the Framingham risk equation, the 20-year probability of the development of a CHD event can be estimated for the patients with two or more risk factors. When the number of risk factors is 0 to 1, the Framingham scoring is not needed.

MANAGEMENT AND THERAPY

Therapy is based on the probability of a CHD event and the estimated risk. In patients with CHD or a CHD risk equivalent (e.g., cerebrovascular disease, lower extremity arterial disease, or diabetes), therapy to lower LDL-C levels should be aggressive. These patients require drug therapy to achieve the recommended LDL-C goals of less than 100 mg/dL. The Heart Protection Study strongly suggested that even high-risk patients whose LDL-C level is below 100 mg/dL benefit from further lowering LDL-C by the addition of statin therapy to their regimen.

The goal for patients in the intermediate-risk group (a 10-year 10–20% risk of a CHD event) is an LDL-C level below 130 mg/dL. For patients in the low-risk group (10-year risk <10%) the goal is an LDL-C level below 160 mg/dL. The majority of patients in this lower-risk group will not require drugs to achieve their LDL-C goal. Lower LDL-C goals may be appropriate for patients with familial hyperlipidemia or for patients with a strong positive family history of CHD.

Figure 64-1

Metabolic Syndrome

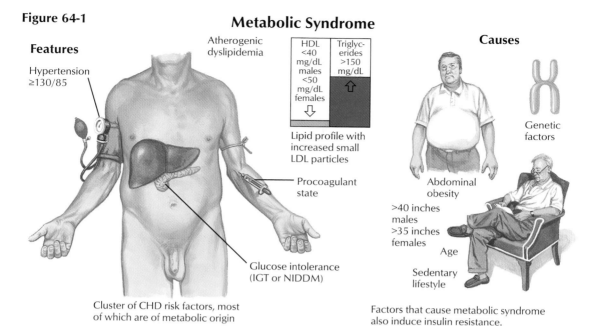

Features

Atherogenic
dyslipidemia

HDL <40 mg/dL males <50 mg/dL females ⇩	Triglyc- erides >150 mg/dL ⇧

Lipid profile with
increased small
LDL particles

Hypertension
≥130/85

Procoagulant
state

Glucose intolerance
(IGT or NIDDM)

Cluster of CHD risk factors, most
of which are of metabolic origin

Causes

Genetic
factors

Abdominal
obesity

>40 inches
males
>35 inches
females

Age

Sedentary
lifestyle

Factors that cause metabolic syndrome
also induce insulin resistance.

Insulin resistance (biochemical basis of metabolic syndrome)

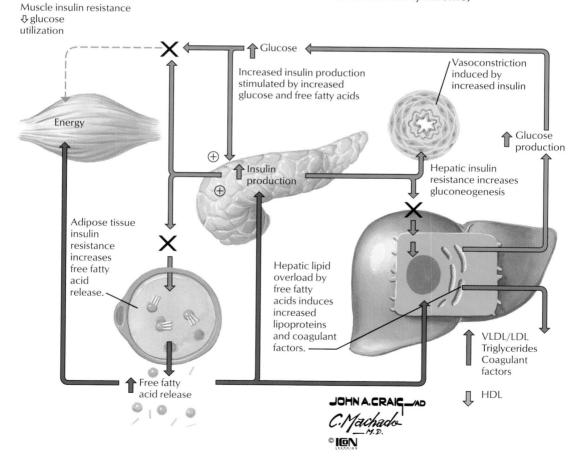

Muscle insulin resistance
⇩ glucose
utilization

Glucose

Increased insulin production
stimulated by increased
glucose and free fatty acids

Vasoconstriction
induced by
increased insulin

Energy

Glucose
production

Insulin
production

Hepatic insulin
resistance increases
gluconeogenesis

Adipose tissue
insulin
resistance
increases
free fatty
acid
release.

Hepatic lipid
overload by
free fatty
acids induces
increased
lipoproteins
and coagulant
factors.

Free fatty
acid release

VLDL/LDL
Triglycerides
Coagulant
factors

HDL

JOHN A. CRAIG—MD

C. Machado
M.D.

© ICON

The Adult Treatment Panel III recommends that the primary therapeutic target be LDL-C and not HDL-C, triglycerides, or other lipid fractions. This recommendation is based on clinical trial results and epidemiologic evidence showing that lowering LDL-C levels substantially reduces the risk of future CHD events. Other lipid fractions, particularly HDL-C and triglyceride levels, should be secondary therapeutic targets until the LDL-C level is within the goal range.

A low HDL-C level is a strong predictor of future CHD events. However, because of the lack of large randomized trials showing that raising HDL-C levels with drugs is effective and safe in reducing CHD events, therapy should be aimed at lowering LDL-C levels. Similarly, elevated triglyceride levels may pose an additive risk for patients with high LDL-C levels, multiple risk factors, diabetes, or established CHD. Reduced triglyceride levels should be a secondary goal provided these levels are below 500 mg/dL. When triglycerides are elevated but below this value, hypothyroidism, the nephrotic syndrome, the metabolic syndrome, and obesity are the likely causes of the elevation. Thus, therapy should focus on these conditions and lipid-lowering treatment should be directed at the LDL-C level. When triglyceride levels exceed 500 mg/dL, primary therapy should be directed at lowering triglycerides, through the use of a fibrate or nicotinic acid, with an important goal being the prevention of pancreatitis.

Specific Management

Appropriate diet therapy and exercise are highly effective in helping patients manage their cholesterol levels and CHD risk (Fig. 64-2). Clinical trials showing the efficacy of statin drugs and other drug therapies are built on effective diet counseling and therapy. Patients should receive dietary counseling by a trained physician, nurse, or nutritionist. The Adult Treatment Panel III recommends that daily saturated fat intake be limited to less than 7% of calories and daily cholesterol intake be limited to less than 200 mg. Plant stanols and sterols, such as those found primarily in certain margarines are recommended in quantities up to 2 g/d. Trans fatty acids and hydrogenated fats found in margarines and other foods should be avoided.

Monosaturated fatty acids and fish oils are also encouraged through increased intake of fish and other foods found in traditional Mediterranean diets. Calorie restriction is recommended for patients who are overweight. In addition, a fish oil mixture containing 2 to 5 g of alpha omega-3 fatty acids is a promising dietary supplement to reduce triglycerides.

Exercise is another important component of the management of dyslipidemia (see also chapter 63). Exercise counseling make take the form of a referral to a formal rehabilitation or wellness program, a formal physical fitness assessment, an exercise prescription, or an increase in the patient's daily living activities. One helpful home measurement device is a "step counter." A step counter records the number of steps a patient takes in a normal day. The patient is then able to increase the step counts toward a specific count goal depending on the patient's baseline activity level. Another strategy is to ask what type of physical activities the patient enjoys and negotiate with the patient to achieve a higher level and a greater frequency of these or similar activities. All patients undergoing cholesterol treatment with drugs should receive periodic diet, exercise, and reinforcement counseling sessions from their primary care physician or other specialist.

Drug Therapy

Drug therapy (Fig. 64-3) is now predominantly based on the use of HMG CoA reductase inhibitors (statins). Statins are effective at lowering LDL-C and have an excellent safety profile. They inhibit cholesterol synthesis, thereby increasing LDL-C receptors on the liver cell membrane and potentiating LDL-C clearance from the blood. On average, statin therapy can reduce LDL-C levels by up to 50%, in a dose-dependent manner, and may lower triglycerides by 30% while simultaneously raising HDL-C by up to 15%.

The recommended starting dose of each statin varies on the ability of the drug to lower LDL-C. Statins generally have a predictable dose-response relationship with regard to LDL-C. For each doubling of the statin dose, there is an approximate 6% further lowering of the LDL-C level. Statin drugs may be combined with cho-

Figure 64-2

Non-Drug Therapy

Targets of therapy

Smoking

Obesity and
decreased exercise
⬆LDL
⬇HDL
⬆Triglycerides
⬆blood pressure

High saturated fat diet
⬆LDL

High salt diet
⬆blood pressure

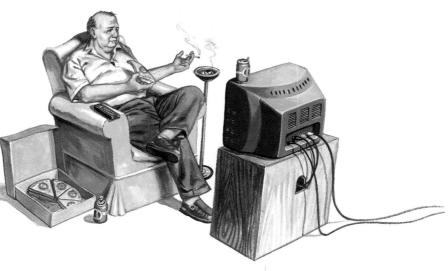

Nutrition and life habit modification

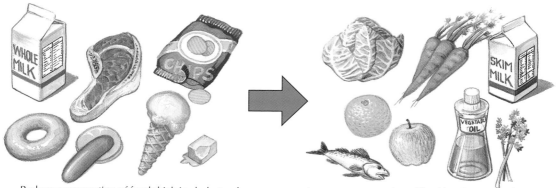

Reduce consumption of foods high in cholesterol,
saturated and *trans* fatty acids, and salt. Decrease
total caloric intake.

Increase consumption of food low in saturated
fat and high in fiber.

Control weight.

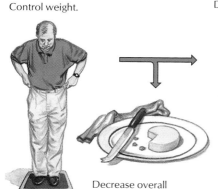

Decrease overall
caloric intake.

Daily physical activity

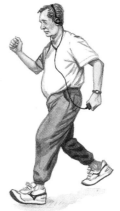

Stop smoking.

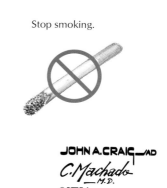

JOHN A. CRAIG—AD
C. Machado—
M.D.
©ICON

Figure 64-3

Mechanism of Action of Lipid-Lowering Drugs

Ezetimibe.
Localizes at intestinal brush border of small intestine Blocks absorption of intestinal cholesterol

Statins (HMG-CoA reductase inhibitors).
Reduce cholesterol synthesis, lowering intracellular cholesterol, which stimulates LDL receptor synthesis

Bile acid sequestrants.
Bind bile acids in gut, decreasing intracellular cholesterol content, which stimulates LDL receptor synthesis

Nicotinic acid.
Decreases hepatic production of VLDL

Fibric acids.
Stimulate PPAR α nuclear receptor, increasing LPL synthesis and decreasing Apo C-III synthesis

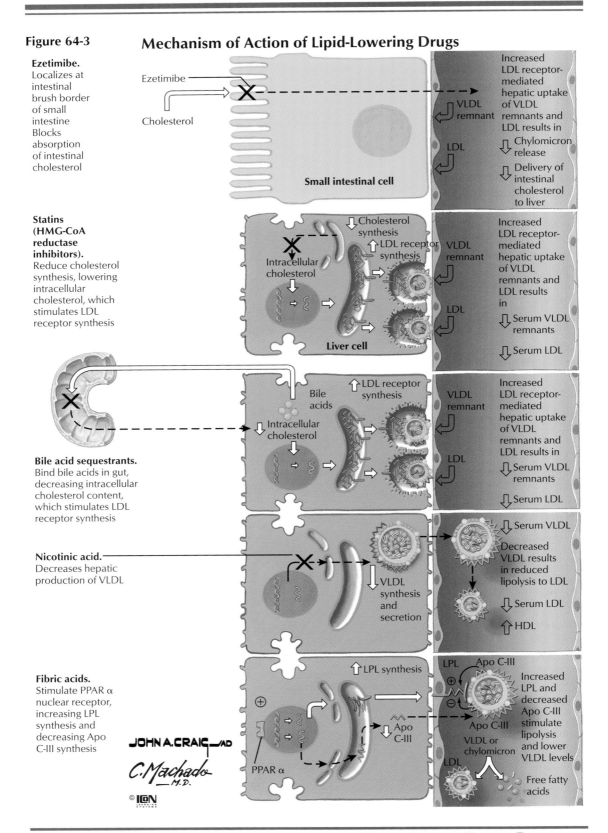

JOHN A. CRAIG—MD
C. Machado—M.D.
© ICON

lesterol-binding resins to provide an additive effect on the lowering of LDL-C.

Although these drugs are well tolerated, there is a small risk of myopathy, particularly at higher doses or when the statins are combined with fibrates or niacin. Interactions with antibiotics and drugs used to treat HIV or to prevent organ rejection may also lead to rhabdomyolysis. Patients who develop muscle aches or pains should consult their physician about discontinuing their statin drug and should have their serum creatinine phosphokinase level measured.

Liver toxicity can also occur with statins and is manifested as increased liver enzymes to more than three times the upper limit of normal. This may occur at higher doses and can be avoided by monitoring the transaminase enzymes and, if necessary, discontinuing the medication.

Second-line medications include bile acid sequestrants such as cholestyramine (4–6 g/day), colestipol (5–20 g/day), or colesevelam (2.6–2.8 g/day). These drugs prevent bile acid reabsorption and potentiate LDL-C uptake by liver LDL-C receptors. At maximum doses, they can reduce LDL-C by up to 30% in a dose-dependent manner. However, bile acid sequestrants should be avoided in patients with elevated triglyceride levels because they may further increase triglyceride values. These drugs are not systemically absorbed and their side effects are generally limited to their potential to interfere with the absorption of vitamins and other drugs and to complaints of constipation and bloating. These drugs are usually taken in combination with a statin.

Another second-line medication is nicotinic acid, which acts to reduce tissue lipase activity and very-low-density lipoprotein synthesis. Moderate to high doses of nicotinic acid may lower LDL-C levels by as much as 25%, decrease triglyceride levels by as much as 50%, and raise HDL-C levels by as much as 35%. The side effects of the drug include flushing, elevated blood sugar, hyperuricemia, abdominal pain, and, in rare cases, hepatotoxicity. Nicotinic acid is available in intermediate-release (1–5 g/day), extended-release (1–2 g/day), and long-acting (1–2 g/day) forms. It is highly effective and has a demonstrated safety record. Compliance is dependent on the form of medication used and the availability of experienced counseling. Compliance can be improved through the use of the extended-release form, starting the patient at 500 mg/day to be taken in the late evening with a snack, an aspirin 30 minutes before taking the niacin, and gradually increasing the dose.

Niacin can be also combined with a statin drug to treat patients with extremely high levels of cholesterol. This must be done with care and, as with the statins, it is important to monitor liver enzymes and watch for symptoms of muscle pains. When niacin is combined with a statin, lower doses of the statin, as recommended in the package insert, should be used.

Fibrates (gemfibrozil 600 mg twice a day; fenofibrate 160 mg once a day) are particularly effective at lowering triglycerides and, to a lesser extent, LDL-C. Fibrates have an effect on lipoprotein lipase activity and can be expected to lower LDL-C by as much as 20% (particularly fenofibrate), to raise HDL by up to 20%, and to lower triglycerides by up to 50%. The side effects of fibrates are dyspepsia, the possible development of gallstones, and myopathy, particularly when combined with statins. Fibrates are contraindicated in patients with renal or hepatic diseases.

Plasmapheresis

Patients with familial hypercholesterolemia (in which LDL-C values exceed 300 mg/dL) are at high risk for CHD. These patients usually cannot reach their target LDL-C levels and may require plasmapheresis. Plasmapheresis appears to be effective and safe at lowering LDL-C. Regional centers throughout the United States offer plasmapheresis on a biweekly basis.

FUTURE DIRECTIONS

Additional diagnostic tests to more precisely define patients' risk of developing CHD events and to better characterize their lipid profile are being developed. These include blood tests to assess new risk factors and quantitative measurements to assess early atherosclerotic disease. Diagnostic tests include the high-sensitivity C-reactive protein assay to measure chronic inflammation; assessment of lipid particle size and density; electron beam tomography to assess calcium scores in the coronary arteries; carotid Doppler ultrasound to test intima–media thickness ratios; and the ankle–brachial index for peripheral vascular disease.

New drugs that raise HDL-C levels, selectively inhibit the absorption of cholesterol and highly effective HMG CoA blockers, are under development or are newly available. Ezetimibe is a highly specific inhibitor of cholesterol absorption in the intestine and reduces the LDL-C by approximately 17%. This drug may be combined with a statin to provide a potent effect on LDL-C lowering.

The combination of new diagnostic tests to better identify individuals at risk for CHD events and expanded therapies to treat dyslipidemia should result in major advances in the prevention of the epidemic of CHD.

REFERENCES

Gotto AM Jr. *Contemporary Diagnosis and Management of Lipid Disorder*. 2nd ed. Newtown, PA: Handbooks in Health Care; 2001.

Greenland P, Smith SC Jr, Grundy SM. Improving coronary heart disease risk assessment in asymptomatic people: Role of traditional risk factors and noninvasive cardiovascular tests. *Circulation* 2001;104:1863–1867.

MRC/BHF Heart Protection Study collaborative group. MRC/BHF Heart Protection Study of cholesterol lowering therapy with simvastatin in 20,536 high-risk individuals: A randomized placebo-controlled trial. *Lancet* 2002;360:7–22.

Pearson TA, Mensah GA, Alexander RW, et al. AHA/CDC Scientific Statement: Markers of Inflammation and Cardiovascular Disease, Application to Clinical and Public Health Forum. A statement for healthcare professionals from the Centers for Disease Control and Prevention and the American Heart Association. *Circulation* 2003;107:499–511.

Third Report of the National Cholesterol Education Program Expert Panel on the Detection, Evaluation, and Treatment of High Blood Cholesterol in Adults (Adult Panel III). Grundy S, Chair. Bethesda, MD: National Heart, Lung, and Blood Institute, 2001. See also *JAMA* 2001;285:2486–2497.

Working Group on Lipoprotein Measurement. Recommendations on Lipoprotein Measurement. Bethesda, MD: National Institutes of Health and National Heart, Lung, and Blood Institute. NIH Publication No. 95-3044, September 1995.

Chapter 65

Cardiovascular Effects of Air Pollutants

Wayne E. Cascio, Milan J. Hazucha, Philip A. Bromberg, and Robert B. Devlin

The established risk factors for the development of coronary artery disease include age, hypertension, lipid abnormalities, diabetes, and tobacco use. These factors are targets for modification in prevention programs (see chapters 54, 60, and 64); yet they account for only about 50 to 75% of cases of coronary artery disease and cardiac events. Other factors, including factors related to the environment, must contribute independently or must modify the established factors to produce cardiovascular disease and trigger cardiac events. The best-studied environmental factor that may influence cardiovascular morbidity and mortality rates is air pollution. Of the various air pollutants, the evidence for a causative role in cardiovascular diseases is strongest for fine particles derived primarily from combustion. However, the effects of air pollutants on the cardiovascular system are not well studied and are generally not appreciated by health care providers. The major air pollutants include particulate matter (PM), carbon monoxide (CO), ozone, nitrogen oxides, and sulfur dioxide (SO_2). This chapter reviews the possible links between air PM and cardiovascular disease and discusses the plausible physiologic mechanisms for these associations.

PARTICULATE MATTER

Particulate matter is not a single compound but a mixture of materials, all of which have a carbonaceous core, and associated materials such as organic compounds, acids, metals, crustal material, and biological material, including pollen, spores, and endotoxin. Combustion processes, such as those in automobiles and power plants, account for most PM, but particles generated by mechanical processes and windblown dust contribute to the mass of PM. The particles are classified as "ultrafine," "fine," and "coarse" on the basis of their size. Ultrafine $PM_{2.5}$ and PM_{10} have an equivalent aerodynamic diameter of less than 0.1 μm, 2.5 μm, and 10 μm, respectively. Particles larger than 10 μm in diameter are usually not respirable. Particles of crustal origin are more likely to be in the coarse fraction, whereas particles produced by combustion are more likely to be in the fine fraction. Cooking, smoking, dusting, and vacuuming generate indoor PM. Outdoor PM penetrates easily into homes and buildings and increases indoor levels of PM.

The US Environmental Protection Agency has statutory responsibility (Clean Air Acts) to regulate ambient air pollutants, including but not limited to PM, CO, nitrogen dioxide (NO_2), ozone, and SO_2. The levels of permissible air pollutants are established by the doses at which a measurable health risk is anticipated. This risk assessment is based on scientific data that are updated periodically and published as the US National Ambient Air Quality Standards Criteria document. The national air quality standards for the allowable levels of $PM_{2.5}$ and PM_{10} averaged over 24 hours are 65 μg/m^3 and 150 μg/m^3, respectively.

Epidemiologic studies show associations between PM and mortality rates, but the biological mechanisms are unknown. In part, the controversy over the cardiovascular effects of some pollutants is due to the limited number of controlled human exposure studies and the reliance on epidemiologic studies showing associations between fluctuating levels of air pollution and cardiovascular health. Also, the strong correlation among the various outdoor air pollutants to increase cardiovascular risk makes it difficult to attribute observed cardiovascular effects to specific components of air pollution. Nevertheless, time-series and cross-sectional epidemiologic studies show an association between exposure to airborne PM and cardiovascular morbidity and mortality rates. The association appears to be strongest with fine particles. The deeper penetration of fine particles into the lung before deposition may contribute to the apparent biological activity of these particles. These findings implicate the aerodynamic diameter, the source, and the composition of PM as factors that affect health.

The causal connection between inhaled particles depositing on respiratory surfaces and cardiovascular health effects remains problematic. Because the association of PM air pollution with the cardiovascular mortality rate is acute, the mechanism(s) may involve myocardial infarction and arrhythmic sudden cardiac death. The intermediate effects of exposure to ambient air PM include changes in blood proteins (affecting viscosity and coagulation), endothelial function, and neural modulation of the heart. Because such changes might increase the risk of cardiovascular events such as thrombosis and arrhythmia, the study of the mechanisms responsible for these endpoints represents a common thread linking recent observational epidemiologic and controlled experimental human exposure studies.

Possible cardiovascular effects associated with PM exposure can be categorized as acute or chronic (Fig. 65-1). Acute exposure to PM increases heart rate and blood pressure and decreases oxygen saturation. Exposure to PM affects pulmonary oxygen transport and neural modulation of the sinus node and the vascular system, although the magnitude of these changes is small. An increase in heart rate might be caused by an increase in the sympathetic input to the heart or a decrease in the parasympathetic input. Exposure to PM decreases cardiac vagal input, as suggested by a decrease in heart rate variability (HRV). Yet the association between changes in HRV and ambient PM concentrations is inconsistent. Whether the differences relate to the chemical composition of PM, associated co-pollutants, the age and the gender of the exposed individual, or the influence of concurrent cardiac disease, medications, or the HRV methodology is not known. Nor is it known whether change in HRV associated with PM exposure represents an independent measure of risk.

There are at least three possible mechanisms by which PM may induce changes in cardiac physiology: a neural reflex from afferents in the lung that interact with PM directly or indirectly through associated pulmonary inflammation; secondary effects of inflammatory cytokines, acute-phase reactants produced in the lung, or both; and direct effects of adsorbed constituents of PM on cardiac membrane currents responsible for impulse formation and propagation. The observations that inhalation of fine-particulate air pollution and ozone causes arterial vasoconstriction and that sympathetic activation reduces endothelium-dependent flow-mediated vasodilation might provide a mechanistic link between the changes in HRV and the changes in vascular reactivity, a known risk for cardiac events. Because sudden shifts in neural input to the heart may be arrhythmogenic, changes in HRV imply that arrhythmia formation is a potential mechanism.

The effects of chronic exposure to fine-particulate air pollution have been inferred from the linking of cardiovascular risk factors and estimated air pollution exposure to the cause of death for approximately 500,000 individuals over a period of 16 years. These observational studies have shown that fine-particulate air pollution increased the rate of all-cause mortality from cardiopulmonary causes and lung cancer. The risk of cardiopulmonary mortality was most strongly associated with fine particles (as compared with larger particles) and was greatest in nonsmokers (possibly because the relative increase in fine-particle exposure was less in smokers). Although the mechanisms are unknown, possible explanations of the risk include acceleration of the progression of atherosclerosis secondary to increased oxidative stress or systemic inflammation, and modulation of factors that enhance coronary plaque instability or electrical instability. No data show that PM causes or accelerates atherosclerosis in humans, although it is quite plausible that PM accentuates chronic inflammation, and chronic inflammation is causally linked to the development of atherosclerosis. For instance, high-sensitivity C-reactive protein correlates with cardiac events. C-reactive protein is produced in the liver in response to the cytokines IL-1, IL-6, and

Cardiovascular Effects of Air Pollutants

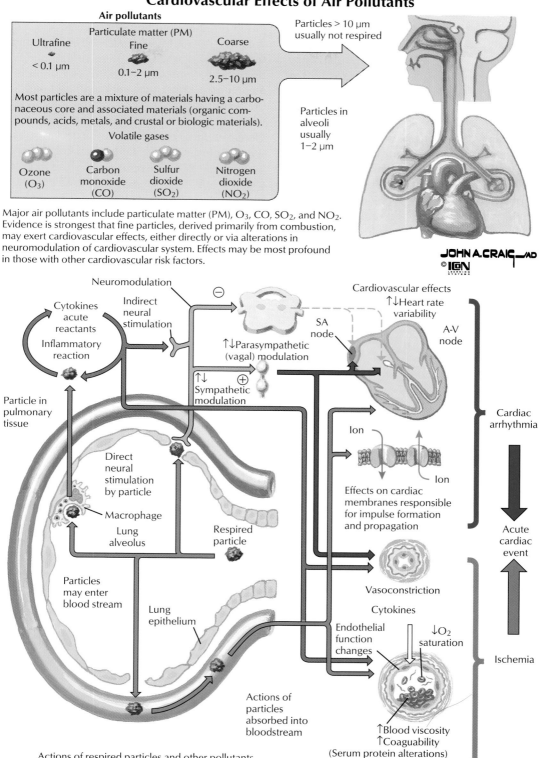

Air pollutants

Particulate matter (PM)

Ultrafine
< 0.1 μm

Fine
0.1–2 μm

Coarse
2.5–10 μm

Particles > 10 μm usually not respired

Most particles are a mixture of materials having a carbonaceous core and associated materials (organic compounds, acids, metals, and crustal or biologic materials).

Volatile gases

Ozone (O₃)

Carbon monoxide (CO)

Sulfur dioxide (SO₂)

Nitrogen dioxide (NO₂)

Particles in alveoli usually 1–2 μm

Major air pollutants include particulate matter (PM), O₃, CO, SO₂, and NO₂. Evidence is strongest that fine particles, derived primarily from combustion, may exert cardiovascular effects, either directly or via alterations in neuromodulation of cardiovascular system. Effects may be most profound in those with other cardiovascular risk factors.

JOHN A. CRAIG—MD
©ICON LEARNING SYSTEMS

Neuromodulation

Cytokines acute reactants
Inflammatory reaction

Indirect neural stimulation

↑↓Parasympathetic (vagal) modulation

↑↓ Sympathetic modulation

Cardiovascular effects
↑↓Heart rate variability

SA node

A-V node

Particle in pulmonary tissue

Direct neural stimulation by particle

Macrophage

Lung alveolus

Respired particle

Ion

Ion

Effects on cardiac membranes responsible for impulse formation and propagation

Cardiac arrhythmia

Acute cardiac event

Particles may enter blood stream

Lung epithelium

Vasoconstriction

Cytokines

Endothelial function changes

↓O₂ saturation

Ischemia

Actions of particles absorbed into bloodstream

↑Blood viscosity
↑Coaguability
(Serum protein alterations)

Actions of respired particles and other pollutants

tumor necrosis factor α. Measurement of cytokines, and even high-sensitivity C-reactive protein, may provide a mechanism to assess cardiovascular risk in response to PM exposure. Because of the complexity of the mechanisms that regulate the initiation and progression of atherosclerosis, and the complex constituents of PM, absolute proof of a causal effect of PM on the development of atherosclerosis is unlikely.

It is possible that PM has a direct effect on cardiac autonomic function or on cardiac repolarization and that PM increases the individual's susceptibility to myocardial ischemia and ventricular fibrillation during regional myocardial ischemia. Chronic exposure to airborne PM might initiate cellular signaling that affects the expression of cellular proteins important to electrical impulse formation and conduction in the heart. These proteins might include structural proteins, as well as voltage- and ligand-gated channels and ion exchangers. Thus, cardiac deaths associated with exposure to PM are likely to result from the interaction of the direct effects of PM on vascular function, cardiac electrophysiology, autonomic regulation, and/or coronary thrombosis in individuals at high risk for sudden cardiac death.

Exposure to second-hand tobacco smoke is a reasonable model for understanding how exposure to PM mediates changes in the cardiovascular system and contributes to cardiac events. Acute exposure activates platelets and decreases endothelial function in humans, whereas chronic exposure accelerates the formation of atherosclerosis.

CARBON MONOXIDE

Carbon monoxide (CO) is produced by combustion and binds avidly to hemoglobin, thereby reducing the capacity of blood to deliver oxygen to the tissues. Within the tissue, CO may bind to cytochrome P-450, cytochrome oxidase, and myoglobin, affecting intracellular function. The individuals most susceptible to these effects are those with flow-limiting coronary disease.

A study of the chronic health effects of CO exposure in a comparison of bridge and tunnel workers showed that the relative risk of coronary artery disease was greater in tunnel workers. Prolonged exposure to CO and attendant

carboxyhemoglobin (COHb) concentration in excess of 10% increased heart rate, systolic blood pressure, red blood cell mass, and blood volume. CO has been implicated in atherogenesis and in increased risk of myocardial infarction. In general, controlled exposure to CO reduces the time to onset of electrocardiographic evidence of exercise-induced ischemia and angina in individuals with ischemic heart disease and increases the frequency of ventricular arrhythmias during exercise. These effects occur at COHb levels as low as 2.9%. The baseline COHb in healthy nonsmokers is 0.5 to 1.0%. Prolonged exposure to 9 ppm CO would produce a blood COHb level of approximately 2%. Thus, the national air quality standards for CO (35 ppm averaged over 1 hour and 9 ppm averaged over 8 hours) should provide protection even for a sensitive population with ischemic heart disease.

SULFUR DIOXIDE

Sulfur dioxide is a gas produced by coal-burning power plants, smelters, refineries, pulp mills, and food processing plants. Typical ambient air reactions include formation of sulfuric acid (acid rain) and sulfates. A positive correlation exists between SO_2 and hospital admissions, the mortality rate in elderly individuals, and the documented presence of cardiovascular disease. It is often difficult to separate the contributions of individual components of air pollution and attribute them to health effects. For example, the total mortality rate was estimated to increase by 5% for each 38 parts per billion (ppb) increase in SO_2; yet the effects were no longer significant when respirable particles were included in the statistical model. Thus, SO_2 is likely to be a surrogate marker of PM because of the common sources of SO_2 and PM.

NITROGEN DIOXIDE

Nitrogen dioxide and nitric oxide (NO) are highly reactive gases produced by gasoline and diesel fuel combustion, electric power generation, and solid waste disposal. NO_2 is also a major indoor air pollutant produced by gas stoves and gas heaters. Both gases (NO_x) are critical components of the photo-oxidation cycle and ozone formation. NO is also produced endogenously and can reach concentrations in excess of 1 ppm. The ultimate fate of NO_2 and NO in ambient air and biological fluids is the formation of nitrite and nitrate.

Nitric oxide has strong antioxidant properties that could benefit the cardiovascular system. Experimental data suggest that NO is an important mediator controlling coronary perfusion and cardiac muscle metabolism. NO_2, a strong airway irritant, is primarily associated with chronic respiratory effects. Children and adults with existing respiratory disease are at increased respiratory risk from NO_2 inhalation. Increased levels of NO_2 and black carbon are positively associated with delayed cardiac arrhythmias. A positive association also exists between NO_2 and elevated, but statistically not significant, risk of myocardial infarction.

OZONE

Ozone is a secondary air pollutant formed in the atmosphere by photochemical reactions involving primary pollutants, volatile organic compounds, and NO_x. Exposure to ozone irritates mucous membranes, decreases lung function, increases the reactivity of airways, and causes airway inflammation. Consequently, ozone exposure can cause symptoms of nonischemic chest pain and decreased exercise capacity. Whether ozone exposure contributes to more serious cardiovascular disease or events remains uncertain. Increases in ozone concentration may be associated with an increased cardiovascular mortality rate. In one study, an increase in ozone of 21.3 ppb increased the cardiovascular disease mortality rate by 2.5% and the respiratory disease mortality rate by 6.6%; the effect of ozone was independent of the effects of other pollutants.

FUTURE DIRECTIONS

More information is needed to establish the cardiovascular health effects of specific pollutants. The dose dependence of these effects is important for determining air quality standards. Environmental concentrations of air pollutants vary substantially, as do the sources of these pol-

lutants. Source apportionment is important for identifying the origin of the various constituents with health effects. Because significant differences exist at home, outdoors, at work, and at school, the degree of exposure is expected to depend on the time spent in these different environments. Of particular importance is the potential effect of air pollutants on children, because children spend a greater proportion of their time outdoors.

Many questions about the cardiovascular effects of air pollutants remain. Does the interaction of air pollutants lead to additive, synergistic, or reduced health effects? What are the chronic effects of exposure, and do these effects differ from those of transient exposure? Do individuals become tolerant to chronic exposure? Why do individuals with existing cardiovascular and pulmonary disease appear to have a greater susceptibility to the effects of air pollution? What is the role of PM-induced systemic inflammation in the development and progression of atherosclerotic vascular disease? Further investigation, particularly controlled human and animal exposure studies, is needed to answer these questions.

REFERENCES

Air pollution and health effects. Health Effects Institute. Boston. Available at: http://www.healtheffects.org.

Air pollution and health effects and regulations. Environmental Protection Agency of the U.S. Government. Available at: http://www.epa.gov.

Gold D, Litonjua A, Schwartz J, et al. Ambient pollution and heart rate variability. *Circulation* 2000;101:1267–1273.

Goldberg MS, Burnett RT, Brook J, Bailar JC III, Valois M-F, Vincent R. Associations between daily cause-specific mortality and concentrations of ground-level ozone in Montreal, Quebec. *Am J Epidemiol* 2001;154:817–826.

Otsuka R, Watanabe H, Hirata K, et al. Acute effects of passive smoking on the coronary circulation in healthy young adults. *JAMA* 2001;286:436–441.

Peters A, Dockery D, Muller J, Mittleman M. Increased particulate air pollution and the triggering of myocardial infarction. *Circulation* 2001;103:2810–2815.

Pope CA III, Burnett RT, Thun MJ, et al. Lung cancer, cardiopulmonary mortality, and long-term exposure to fine particulate air pollution. *JAMA* 2002;287:1132–1141.

Samet J, Dominici F, Curriero F, Coursac I, Zeger S. Fine particulate air pollution and mortality in 20 U.S. cities, 1987-1994. *N Engl J Med* 2000;343:1742–1749.

Note: Page numbers followed by *t* and *f* indicate tables and figures, respectively.